D1797403

# GASTROINTESTINAL ENDOSONOGRAPHY

Jacques Van Dam, M.D., Ph.D.
Director, Endoscopic Gastrointestinal Oncology
Associate Director, Gastrointestinal Endoscopy
Brigham and Women's Hospital

Assistant Professor of Medicine
Harvard Medical School
Boston, Massachusetts

Michael V. Sivak, Jr., M.D.
Chief, Division of Gastroenterology
University Hospitals of Cleveland

Professor of Medicine
Case Western Reserve University School of Medicine
Cleveland, Ohio

**W.B. SAUNDERS COMPANY**
*A Division of Harcourt Brace & Company*
Philadelphia • London • Toronto • Montreal • Sydney • Tokyo

W.B. Saunders Company
*A Division of Harcourt Brace & Company*

The Curtis Center
Independence Square West
Philadelphia, Pennsylvania 19106

**Library of Congress Cataloging-in-Publication Data**

Gastrointestinal endosonography / [edited by] Jacques Van Dam, Michael V. Sivak, Jr. — 1st ed.
p. cm.
ISBN 0–7216–7989–7
1. Endoscopic ultrasonography. 2. Gastrointestinal system—Ultrasonic imaging. I. Van Dam, Jacques. II. Sivak, Michael V.
[DNLM: 1. Gastrointestinal System—ultrasonography. 2. Endosonography—methods. 3. Gastrointestinal Diseases—ultrasonography. WI 141 G25785 1999]
RC804.E59G37 1999
616.3'307543—dc21
DNLM/DLC 98–20110

GASTROINTESTINAL ENDOSONOGRAPHY ISBN 0–7216–7989–7



Printed in the United States of America

Last digit is the print number: 9 8 7 6 5 4 3 2 1

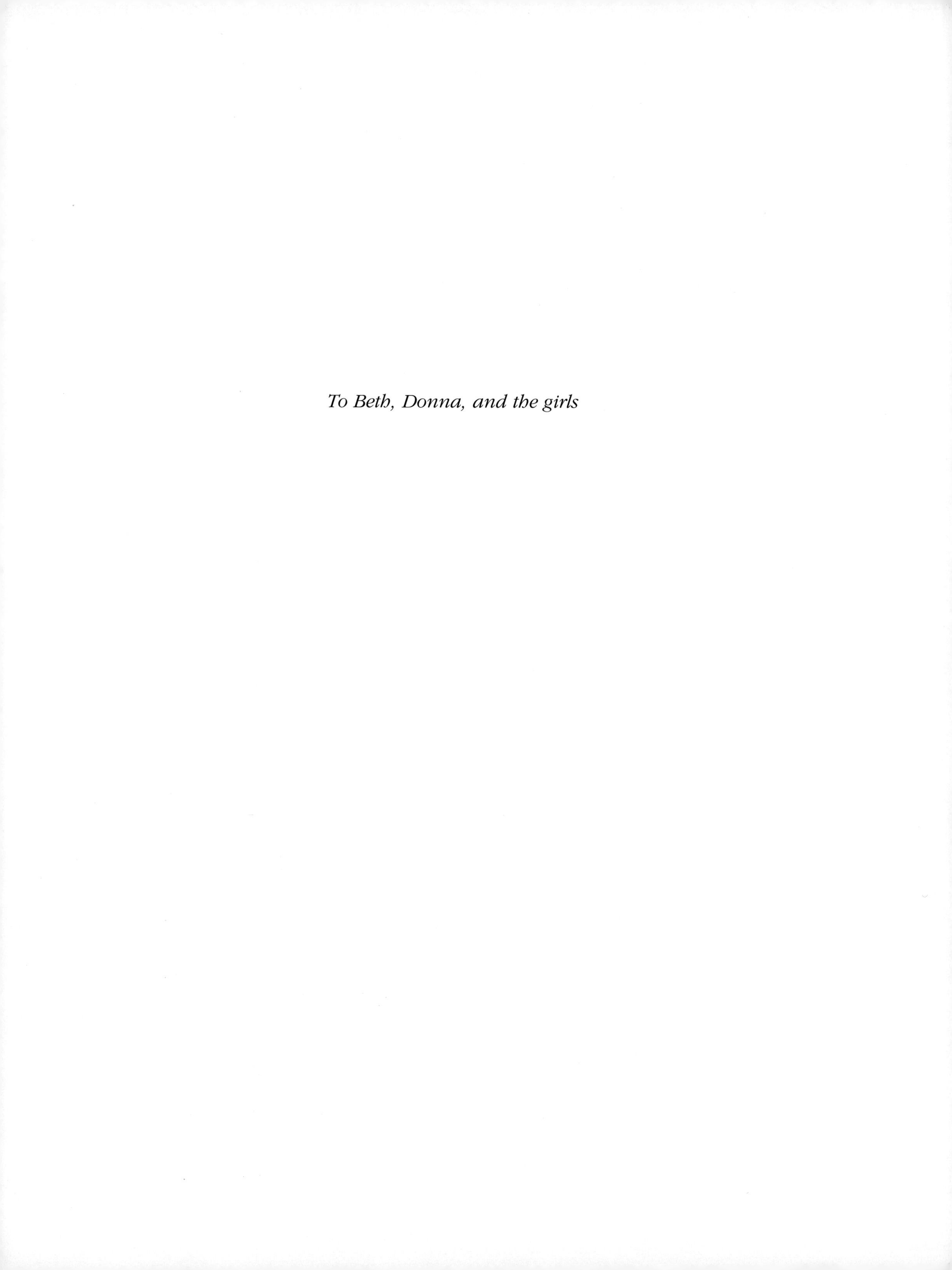

*To Beth, Donna, and the girls*

# ABOUT THE ARTIST

Joseph Pangrace graduated from the Cleveland Institute of Art with a Bachelor of Fine Arts degree in Medical Illustration. In his 15 years at the Cleveland Clinic Foundation, Joe has concentrated his talents in creating illustrations pertaining to cardiothoracic surgery, colorectal surgery, and gastroenterology. Working at a major medical institution such as the Cleveland Clinic has enabled Joe to create a large volume of illustrations for medical journals, surgical atlases, textbooks, and slide and video presentations. Joe is an active member of the Association of Medical Illustrators.

# CONTRIBUTORS

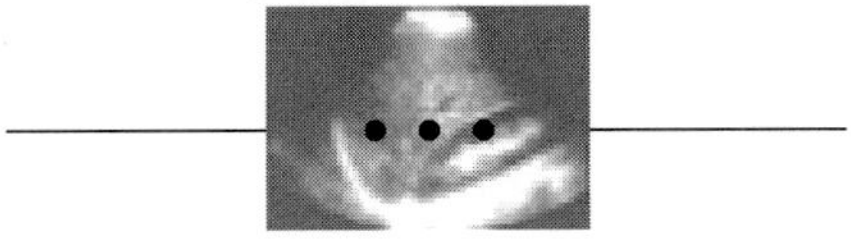

**Luigi Barbara, M.D.**
Professor of Internal Medicine, University of Bologna; Head, Department of Medicine and Gastroenterology, Policlinico S. Orsola, Bologna, Italy
*Chapter 20, Endosonographic Evaluation of the Patient with Portal Hypertension: The Bologna Experience*

**Kenneth F. Binmoeller, M.D.**
Associate Professor of Medicine, University of California at San Diego School of Medicine; Director, Gastrointestinal Endoscopy, University of California at San Diego Medical Center, San Diego, California
*Chapter 25, Endosonography in Pancreatic Disease: Interventional Endosonography*

**Paolo Bocus, M.D.**
Post-Graduate Fellow, University of Bologna; Department of Medicine and Gastroenterology, Policlinico S. Orsola, Bologna, Italy
*Chapter 8, The Gut Wall*
*Chapter 16, Needle Biopsy of Subepithelial Lesions*
*Chapter 17, Gastric Lymphoma, Infiltrative Disorders, and Large Gastric Folds*
*Chapter 20, Endosonographic Evaluation of the Patient with Portal Hypertension: The Bologna Experience*

**Giancarlo Caletti, M.D.**
Associate Professor of Gastroenterology, University of Bologna; Chief of Endoscopy, Department of Medicine and Gastroenterology, Policlinico S. Orsola, Bologna, Italy
*Chapter 8, The Gut Wall*
*Chapter 16, Needle Biopsy of Subepithelial Lesions*
*Chapter 17, Gastric Lymphoma, Infiltrative Disorders, and Large Gastric Folds*
*Chapter 20, Endosonographic Evaluation of the Patient with Portal Hypertension: The Bologna Experience*

**Marcia Irene F. Canto, M.D.**
Assistant Professor of Medicine, Johns Hopkins University School of Medicine; Director of Therapeutic Endoscopy and Endoscopic Ultrasonography, Johns Hopkins University Hospital, Baltimore, Maryland
*Chapter 4, Practical Guide to Using the Linear Array Echoendoscope*

**Marc F. Catalano, M.D.**
Associate Clinical Professor of Medicine, Medical College of Wisconsin; Staff Gastroenterologist, St. Luke's Medical Center, Pancreatic Biliary Center, Milwaukee, Wisconsin
*Chapter 21, Endosonographic Evaluation of the Patient with Portal Hypertension: The Cleveland Experience*

**Amitabh Chak, M.D.**
Assistant Professor of Medicine, Case Western Reserve University; Head, Section of Gastrointestinal Endoscopy, Division of Gastroenterology, University Hospitals of Cleveland, Cleveland, Ohio
*Chapter 2, The Radial Scanning Echoendoscope*

**Kenneth J. Chang, M.D.**
Assistant Professor of Medicine, University of California at Irvine; Head, Gastrointestinal Oncology, UCI Medical Center; Director, Interventional Endoscopy Center, Chas Family Comprehensive Cancer Center, Orange, California
*Chapter 4, Practical Guide to Using the Linear Array Echoendoscope*

**Meinhard Classen, M.D.**
Professor of Internal Medicine, Technical University of Munich; Director of II Department of Medicine, Medizinische Klinik und Poliklinik der Technischen, Universität München, Munich, Germany
*Chapter 11, Pitfalls in Endosonographic Imaging*
*Chapter 13, Staging Esophageal Cancer: The Munich Experience*
*Chapter 19, Staging Gastric Cancer: The Munich Experience*
*Chapter 22, Endosonography of the Retroperitoneum: Normal Anatomy Using the Radial Scanning Echoendoscope*
*Chapter 24, Endosonographic Staging of Pancreatic Cancer*
*Chapter 27, Endosonography of the Colon and Rectum: Normal Anatomy Using the Radial Scanning Echoendoscope*

**Alberto Ferrari, M.D.**
Academic Department of Medicine and Gastroenterology, University of Bologna, Bologna, Italy
*Chapter 20, Endosonographic Evaluation of the Patient with Portal Hypertension: The Bologna Experience*

**Robert H. Hawes, M.D.**
Professor of Medicine, Medical University of South Carolina; Director of Endoscopy, Medical University of South Carolina Medical Center, Charleston, South Carolina
*Chapter 28, Endoscopic Ultrasound Staging of Rectal Cancer*

**Thomas E. Herbener, M.D.**
Assistant Professor of Radiology, Case Western Reserve University; Director of Ultrasound, Vice-Chairman of Clinical Affairs, Department of Radiology, University Hospitals of Cleveland, Cleveland, Ohio
*Chapter 1, Fundamentals of Ultrasonography*

**Michael B. Kimmey, M.D.**
Professor of Medicine, University of Washington; Director of Endoscopy, University of Washington Medical Center, Seattle, Washington
*Chapter 5, High-Resolution Endoluminal Sonography of the Upper Gastrointestinal Tract: The Linear Scanning Ultrasound Probe*

**Charles J. Lightdale, M.D.**
Professor of Clinical Medicine, Columbia University; Director, Clinical Gastroenterology, Columbia-Presbyterian Medical Center, New York, New York
*Chapter 9, Normal EUS Anatomy: The Esophagus and Stomach*
*Chapter 14, Postoperative Recurrence of Esophageal Cancer*
*Chapter 18, Staging Gastric Cancer: The New York Experience*
*Chapter 26, Neuroendocrine Tumors*

**Ji-Bin Liu, M.D.**
Research Assistant Professor of Radiology, Thomas Jefferson University School of Medicine; Department of Radiology, Thomas Jefferson University Hospital, Philadelphia, Pennsylvania
*Chapter 6, High-Resolution Endoluminal Sonography of the Upper Gastrointestinal Tract: The Radial Scanning Ultrasound Probe: Part I*

**Lawrence S. Miller, M.D.**
Associate Professor of Medicine, Temple University; Director of Endoscopic Research, Temple University Hospital, Philadelphia, Pennsylvania
*Chapter 6, High-Resolution Endoluminal Sonography of the Upper Gastrointestinal Tract: The Radial Scanning Ultrasound Probe: Part I*

**Svein Ødegaard, M.D., Ph.D.**
Professor of Medicine, University of Bergen, Haukeland University Hospital, Bergen, Norway
*Chapter 5, High-Resolution Endoluminal Sonography of the Upper Gastrointestinal Tract: The Linear Scanning Ultrasound Probe*

**Thomas W. Rice, M.D.**
Head, Section of General Thoracic Surgery, The Cleveland Clinic Foundation, Cleveland, Ohio
*Chapter 12, Staging Esophageal Cancer: The Cleveland Experience*

**Enrico Roda, M.D.**
Professor of Gastroenterology, University of Bologna; Chairman and Director, Department of Medicine and Gastroenterology, Policlinico S. Orsola, Bologna, Italy
*Chapter 8, The Gut Wall*
*Chapter 16, Needle Biopsy of Subepithelial Lesions*
*Chapter 17, Gastric Lymphoma, Infiltrative Disorders, and Large Gastric Folds*

**Thomas Rösch, M.D.**
Assistant Professor of Internal Medicine, Technical University of Munich; Director of Endoscopy, II Department of Medicine, Medizinische Klinik und Poliklinik der Technischen, Universität München, Munich, Germany
*Chapter 11, Pitfalls in Endosonographic Imaging*
*Chapter 13, Staging Esophageal Cancer: The Munich Experience*
*Chapter 19, Staging Gastric Cancer: The Munich Experience*
*Chapter 22, Endosonography of the Retroperitoneum: Normal Anatomy Using the Radial Scanning Echoendoscope*
*Chapter 24, Endosonographic Staging of Pancreatic Cancer*
*Chapter 27, Endosonography of the Colon and Rectum: Normal Anatomy Using the Radial Scanning Echoendoscope*

**Thomas J. Savides, M.D.**
Associate Professor of Clinical Medicine, University of California at San Diego School of Medicine; Division of Gastroenterology, University of California at San Diego Medical Center, San Diego, California
*Chapter 28, Endoscopic Ultrasound Staging of Rectal Cancer*

**Hans Seifert, M.D.**
Professor of Medicine, Johann-Wolfgang-Goethe-Universität; Chief of Endoscopy Unit, Medizinische Klinik II, Klinikum der Johann-Wolfgang-Goethe-Universität, Frankfurt, Germany
*Chapter 25, Endosonography in Pancreatic Disease: Interventional Endosonography*

**Nib Soehendra, M.D.**
Professor of Surgery, Director, Department of Surgical Endoscopy, University Hospital Eppendorf, Hamburg, Germany
*Chapter 25, Endosonography in Pancreatic Disease: Interventional Endosonography*

**Mark J. Sterling, M.D.**
Assistant Professor of Clinical Medicine, University of Medicine and Dentistry of New Jersey; Chief of Gastrointestinal Endoscopy, UMDNJ University Hospital, Newark, New Jersey
*Chapter 23, Endosonography in Pancreatic Disease: Differential Diagnosis*

**Thomas Togliani, M.D.**
Department of Medicine and Gastroenterology, Policlinico S. Orsola, Bologna, Italy
*Chapter 8, The Gut Wall*
*Chapter 16, Needle Biopsy of Subepithelial Lesions*
*Chapter 17, Gastric Lymphoma, Infiltrative Disorders, and Large Gastric Folds*

**Jacques Van Dam, M.D., Ph.D.**
Assistant Professor of Medicine, Harvard Medical School; Director, Endoscopic Gastrointestinal Oncology, Associate Director, Gastrointestinal Endoscopy, Brigham and Women's Hospital, Boston, Massachusetts
*Chapter 10, The TNM Classification for Staging Gastrointestinal Malignancies*

**Frank Van de Mierop, M.D.**
Consultant, University Hospital Gasthuisberg, Catholic University of Leven; Director of Endoscopy, Saint Augustinus Hospital, Belgium
*Chapter 9, Normal EUS Anatomy: The Esophagus and Stomach*
*Chapter 14, Postoperative Recurrence of Esophageal Cancer*
*Chapter 18, Staging Gastric Cancer: The New York Experience*
*Chapter 26, Neuroendocrine Tumors*

**Rosalind U. van Stolk, M.D.**
Assistant Professor of Medicine, Ohio State University; Director, Center for Colon Polyps and Cancer, The Cleveland Clinic Foundation, Cleveland, Ohio
*Chapter 15, Subepithelial Lesions*

**Maurits J. Wiersema, M.D.**
Clinical Assistant Professor of Medicine, Indiana University School of Medicine, Indianapolis, Indiana
*Chapter 3, The Linear Array Echoendoscope*

**Kenjiro Yasuda, M.D.**
Vice Director, Department of Gastroenterology, Kyoto 2nd Red Cross Hospital, Kyoto, Japan
*Chapter 7, High-Resolution Endoluminal Sonography of the Upper Gastrointestinal Tract: The Radial Scanning Ultrasound Probe: Part II*

**Gregory Zuccaro, Jr., M.D.**
Head, Section of Gastrointestinal Endoscopy, The Cleveland Clinic Foundation, Cleveland, Ohio
*Chapter 12, Staging Esophageal Cancer: The Cleveland Experience*
*Chapter 23, Endosonography in Pancreatic Disease: Differential Diagnosis*

# FOREWORD

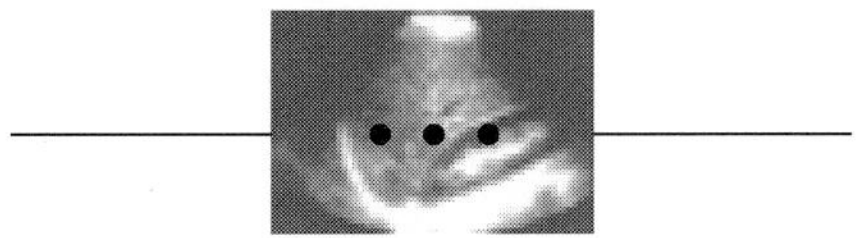

The coupling of endoscopy, both diagnostic and therapeutic, with ultrasound (EUS) constitutes the most difficult and time consuming endoscopic procedure performed today. Although ERCP also is a technically difficult procedure, the production of its radiographic images is relatively easy and accurate once ductal cannulation is achieved. Not so with EUS, which requires basic knowledge of ultrasound, cross sectional anatomy of thorax, abdomen, and pelvis, almost constant multidirectional manipulation of the transducer in the tip of the instrument, plus use of controls on the electronic processor keyboard to obtain and record diagnostic images.

EUS provides detailed intramural and adjacent extramural images not obtainable by any other method. It is an exciting experience to be able to "electronically dissect" the entire wall and adjacent viscera. Only histologic examination of a surgically resected lesion can provide more pertinent clinical information. EUS is the method *par excellence* for T-staging enteric malignancies, evaluating submucosal tumors, localizing neuroendocrine tumors of the pancreas, and taking biopsies from para-enteric lymph nodes and masses. TNM stage-based treatment protocols will require EUS staging as an essential part of pre- and post-therapy evaluation. Numerous other applications discussed in this text are under investigation to establish additional valid indications.

The greatest current challenge is to develop effective methods, both cognitive and hands-on technical, to teach EUS. The learning curve is gradual and prolonged. Remuneration is not one of the driving forces to enhance interest and clinical use of EUS. The problems in learning EUS and the lack of fiscal incentive have made rapid expansion and wide availability more difficult than for endoscopic procedures.

Previous textbooks have been of good quality and very helpful, but served primarily as atlases, correlating endoscopy, ultrasound images, and histopathology. The information provided by the editors and multiple other expert endosonographers in this book is comprehensive, current, and clear even for those who have no prior experience with EUS. The narrative style is uniform and reflects expert editorial blending of expression that provides a unique consistency in form, grammar, and clarity. The abundant, high quality image reproductions with many line drawings provide the advantages of an atlas with far more explanatory narrative than previously available on this subject. Distinctive features of this text are the thorough objective reviews of the physical characteristics, technical operation, risks, and proper procedure performance for all current instruments and accessories for ultrasound-guided diagnosis and therapy.

*Gastrointestinal Endosonography* is a timely publication at this stage in the evolution of endosonography and will be the definitive text on EUS as it enters its third decade of clinical application. Many advances in instrumentation, new clinical indications, and therapeutic applications lie ahead, but for now and into the new millennium, this text will be the ultimate resource to guide the quest of clinicians toward mastery of gastrointestinal endosonography.

H. Worth Boyce, Jr., M.D.
University of South Florida
College of Medicine
Tampa, Florida

# PREFACE

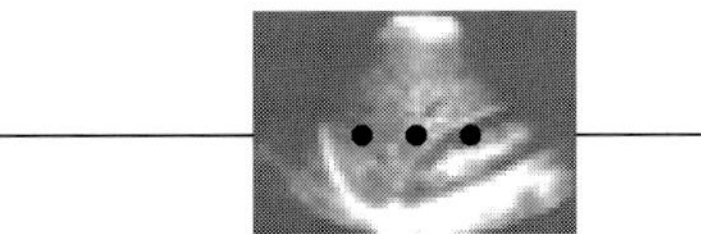

A little more than two centuries have elapsed since the first attempts to see into the human body. For decades, the unaccommodating twists and turns of the gut and the lack of adequate illumination remained problematic. To a great extent, technology has surmounted these impediments. Despite these splendid achievements, however, the fundamental objective of seeing the inner aspect of the gut has not changed. In this context, endoscopic ultrasonography (EUS)—and the ability to see into and beyond the wall of the gastrointestinal tract—represents the only significant advance in endoscopic thinking and technology that has occurred for many decades.

The idea for this book came from the several international symposia on EUS that we have organized. It was readily apparent from these meetings that knowledge of this novel and unique field of gastrointestinal endoscopy was markedly limited and that true expertise in EUS resided in a small cadre of pioneering endoscopists who were almost exclusively responsible for its development. Thus, the major intent of this book is the wider dissemination of their knowledge and experience. It also became evident that the complex, highly technical essence of EUS meant that the price for initiation into the "club" of experts—great expenditures of time and effort—will always be high. As a result, the significant contributions of EUS to patient care are largely underappreciated by the vast majority of physicians who are not directly involved with this type of procedure, even many gastroenterologists and gastrointestinal surgeons. Much of the content of the book is therefore suitable for the nonendosonographer who requires a better understanding of EUS in the interest of improved patient care.

There are two attributes of proficiency in EUS: technique and interpretation. Whereas novice endosonographers often have the prerequisite endoscopic skills, they invariable possess not the slightest familiarity with the use of ultrasound to create images, let alone endosonographic interpretation. In addition to contributions from many of the pioneering experts, a major element in our plan for this book, meant to enhance interpretive skill and make EUS more familiar for the nonendosonographer, has been the use of drawings. For the purpose of illustrating the salient points of EUS imaging, we were fortunate to engage a talented medical artist, Joe Pangrace, whose fine work broadens the educational dimension of the book.

To the many expert endosonographers who have been more than generous in their contributions of time and knowledge to this book, we extend our thanks and appreciation.

Jacques Van Dam, M.D., Ph.D.
Michael V. Sivak, Jr., M.D.

# NOTICE

# CONTENTS

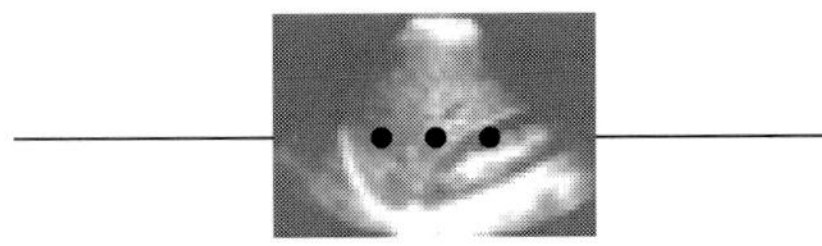

## SECTION I

Introduction to Endosonography: Technical Considerations ................................1

CHAPTER 1
Fundamentals of Ultrasonography 3
Thomas E. Herbener, M.D.

CHAPTER 2
The Radial Scanning Echoendoscope 19
Amitabh Chak, M.D.

CHAPTER 3
The Linear Array Echoendoscope 29
Maurits J. Wiersema, M.D.

CHAPTER 4
Practical Guide to Using the Linear Array Echoendoscope 45
Marcia Irene F. Canto, M.D., and Kenneth J. Chang, M.D.

CHAPTER 5
High-Resolution Endoluminal Sonography of the Upper Gastrointestinal Tract: The Linear Scanning Ultrasound Probe 67
Michael B. Kimmey, M.D., and Svein Ødegaard, M.D., Ph.D.

CHAPTER 6
High-Resolution Endoluminal Sonography of the Upper Gastrointestinal Tract: The Radial Scanning Ultrasound Probe: Part I 81
Lawrence S. Miller, M.D., and Ji-Bin Liu, M.D.

CHAPTER 7
High-Resolution Endoluminal Sonography of the Upper Gastrointestinal Tract: The Radial Scanning Ultrasound Probe: Part II 95
Kenjiro Yasuda, M.D.

SECTION II

Introduction to Endosonography: Getting Started ....................................101

CHAPTER 8

The Gut Wall 103

Giancarlo Caletti, M.D., Paolo Bocus, M.D., Thomas Togliani, M.D., and Enrico Roda, M.D.

CHAPTER 9

Normal EUS Anatomy: The Esophagus and Stomach 109

Charles J. Lightdale, M.D., and Frank Van de Mierop, M.D.

CHAPTER 10

The TNM Classification for Staging Gastrointestinal Malignancies 115

Jacques Van Dam, M.D., Ph.D.

CHAPTER 11

Pitfalls in Endosonographic Imaging 123

Thomas Rösch, M.D., and Meinhard Classen, M.D.

SECTION III

Endosonography of the Esophagus...........129

CHAPTER 12

Staging Esophageal Cancer: The Cleveland Experience 131

Thomas W. Rice, M.D., and Gregory Zuccaro, Jr., M.D.

CHAPTER 13

Staging Esophageal Cancer: The Munich Experience 139

Thomas Rösch, M.D., and Meinhard Classen, M.D.

CHAPTER 14

Postoperative Recurrence of Esophageal Cancer 147

Charles J. Lightdale, M.D., and Frank Van de Mierop, M.D.

SECTION IV

Gastric Endosonography .......................151

CHAPTER 15

Subepithelial Lesions 153

Rosalind U. van Stolk, M.D.

CHAPTER 16

Needle Biopsy of Subepithelial Lesions 167

Giancarlo Caletti, M.D., Paolo Bocus, M.D., Thomas Togliani, M.D., and Enrico Roda, M.D.

CHAPTER 17
Gastric Lymphoma, Infiltrative Disorders, and Large Gastric Folds 175
Giancarlo Caletti, M.D., Paolo Bocus, M.D., Thomas Togliani, M.D., and Enrico Roda, M.D.

CHAPTER 18
Staging Gastric Cancer: The New York Experience 185
Charles J. Lightdale, M.D., and Frank Van de Mierop, M.D.

CHAPTER 19
Staging Gastric Cancer: The Munich Experience 195
Thomas Rösch, M.D., and Meinhard Classen, M.D.

SECTION V

Portal Hypertension ............................201

CHAPTER 20
Endosonographic Evaluation of the Patient with Portal Hypertension: The Bologna Experience 203
Giancarlo Caletti, M.D., Paolo Bocus, M.D., Thomas Togliani, M.D., Enrico Roda, M.D., Alberto Ferrari, M.D., and Luigi Barbara, M.D.

CHAPTER 21
Endosonographic Evaluation of the Patient with Portal Hypertension: The Cleveland Experience 213
Marc F. Catalano, M.D.

SECTION VI

Retroperitoneal Endosonography .............227

CHAPTER 22
Endosonography of the Retroperitoneum: Normal Anatomy Using the Radial Scanning Echoendoscope 229
Thomas Rösch, M.D., and Meinhard Classen, M.D.

CHAPTER 23
Endosonography in Pancreatic Disease: Differential Diagnosis 235
Gregory Zuccaro, Jr., M.D., and Mark J. Sterling, M.D.

CHAPTER 24
Endosonographic Staging of Pancreatic Cancer 245
Thomas Rösch, M.D., and Meinhard Classen, M.D.

CHAPTER 25
Endosonography in Pancreatic Disease: Interventional Endosonography 251
Kenneth F. Binmoeller, M.D., Hans Seifert, M.D., and Nib Soehendra, M.D.

CHAPTER 26
Neuroendocrine Tumors 263
Charles J. Lightdale, M.D., and Frank Van de Mierop, M.D.

SECTION VII
Endosonography of the Colon and Rectum ........................................ 269

CHAPTER 27
Endosonography of the Colon and Rectum: Normal Anatomy Using the Radial Scanning Echoendoscope 271
Thomas Rösch, M.D., and Meinhard Classen, M.D.

CHAPTER 28
Endoscopic Ultrasound Staging of Rectal Cancer 279
Thomas J. Savides, M.D., and Robert H. Hawes, M.D.

Index 291

Color Plates follow.

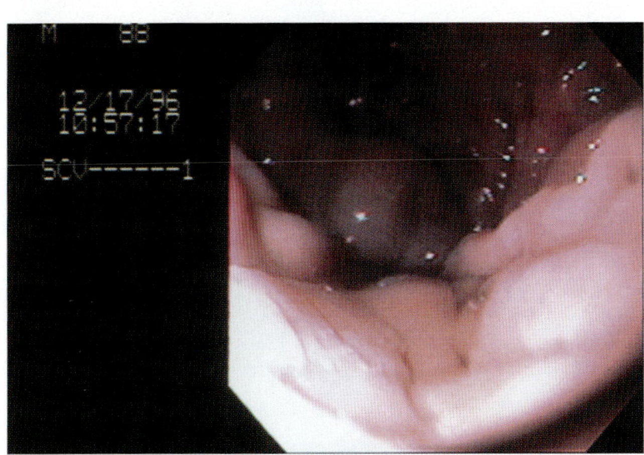


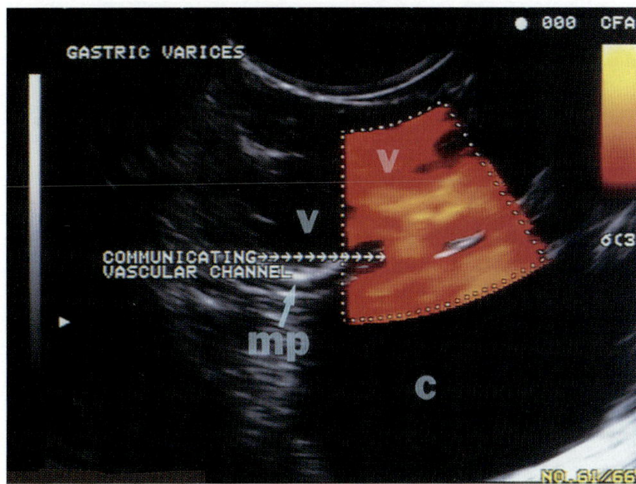


A B

**FIGURE 3-2**

An 88-year-old male presented with dysphagia secondary to a Schatzki's ring and was found to have (**A**) a submucosal mass in the cardia suspicious for gastric varices (retroflex view of cardia). EUS with Ultrasound Angio™ color Doppler.(**B**) demonstrates the gastric varices (v) with communicating vessels traversing the muscularis propria (mp) and entering a large perigastric collateral (c). The patient was found to have splenic vein thrombosis.

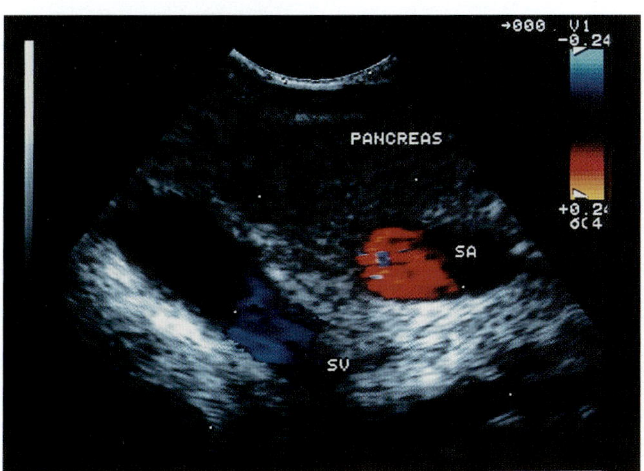


**FIGURE 3-3**

Transgastric imaging from the mid body demonstrates the pancreas, with the adjacent splenic artery (SA) highlighted in red by color Doppler and the splenic vein (SV) highlighted in blue. These vessels can be followed into the hilum of the spleen by withdrawing the instrument. By advancing and rotating the probe, the splenic vein may be seen to course into the portal vein and the splenic artery can be followed down to the level of the celiac trunk.

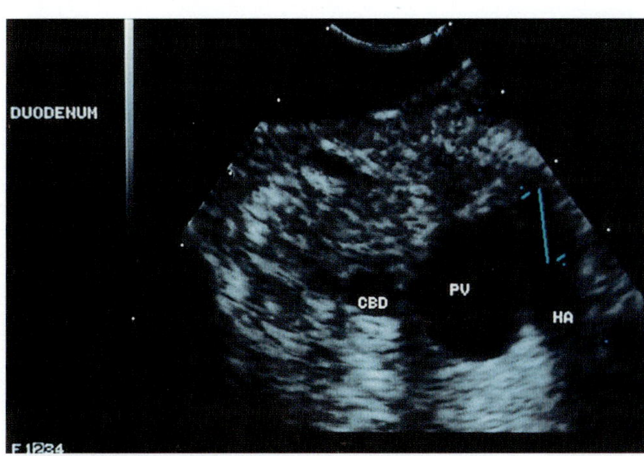


**FIGURE 3-4A**

The portal triad comprising the common bile duct (CBD), portal vein (PV), and hepatic artery (HA) visualized from the second segment of the duodenum.

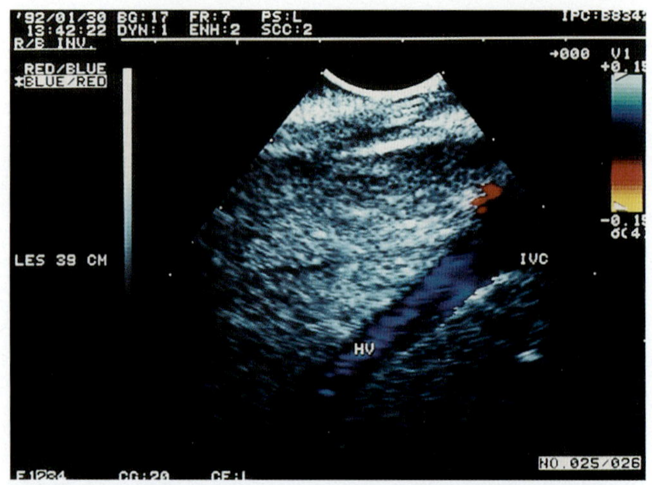


FIGURE 3–5

Imaging at the level of the lower esophageal sphincter (LES) demonstrates one of the hepatic veins (HV) entering into the inferior vena cava (IVC) as highlighted with the blue color Doppler signal. By rotating the transducer, hepatic veins from the right and left lobe can be seen converging toward the inferior vena cava.

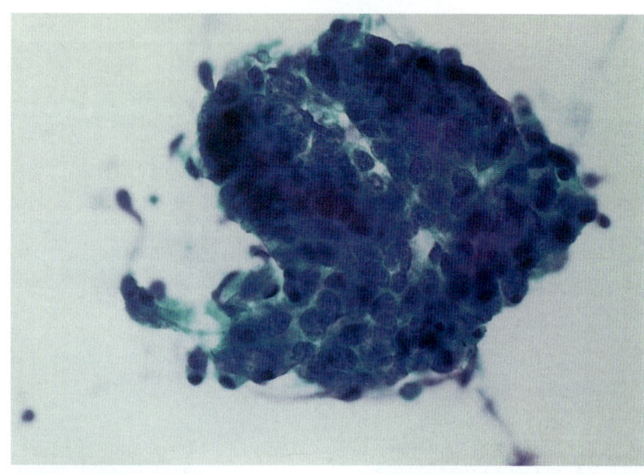

FIGURE 3–8C

Cytology demonstrated an adenocarcinoma.

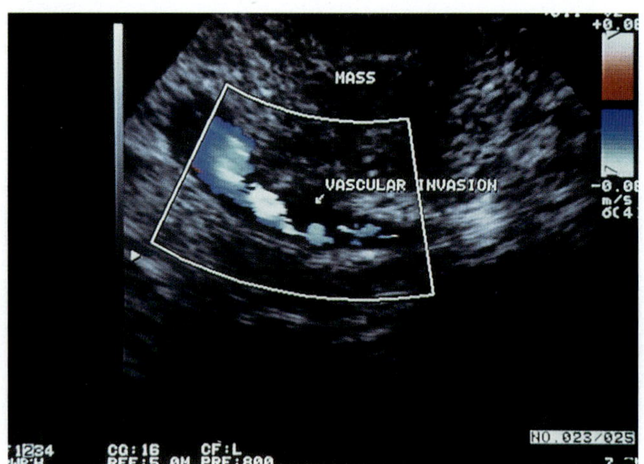


FIGURE 3–8A

Transduodenal sagittal imaging with the Pentax FG-32UA at 7.5 MHz demonstrates a pancreatic head mass. Invasion of the superior mesenteric vein is highlighted with color Doppler by the velocity increase (white area) seen at the level of the stenosis.

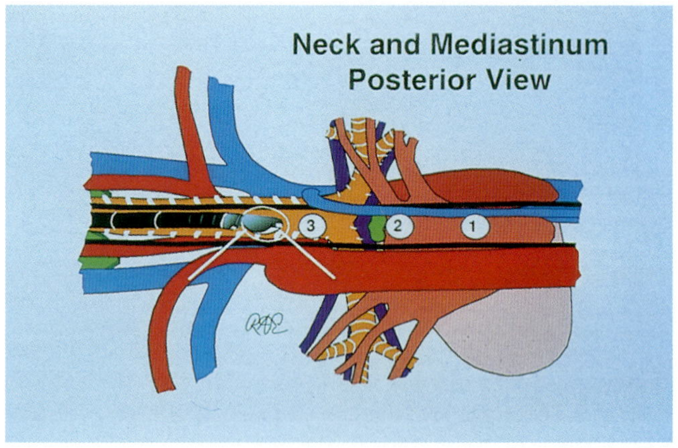


FIGURE 4–4

Diagram of echoendoscope imaging positions (stations 1–3) in the esophagus and anatomic relations of the esophagus with mediastinal structures.

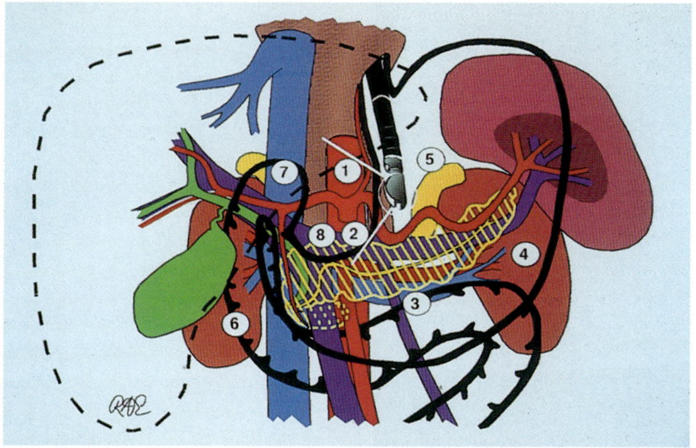


**FIGURE 4–10**

Diagram of linear array echoendoscope positions for imaging abdominal structures. (Reprinted with permission from Chang K. Gastroenterologic Endoscopy.)

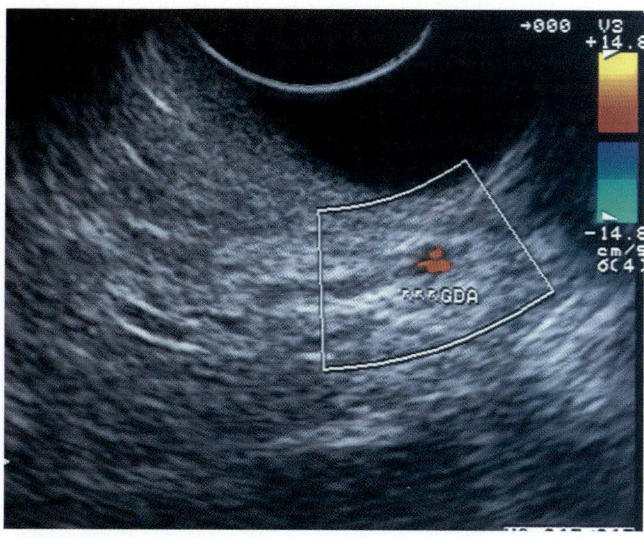


**FIGURE 4–23**

Color flow image of the gastroduodenal artery (GDA) just outside the duodenal wall.

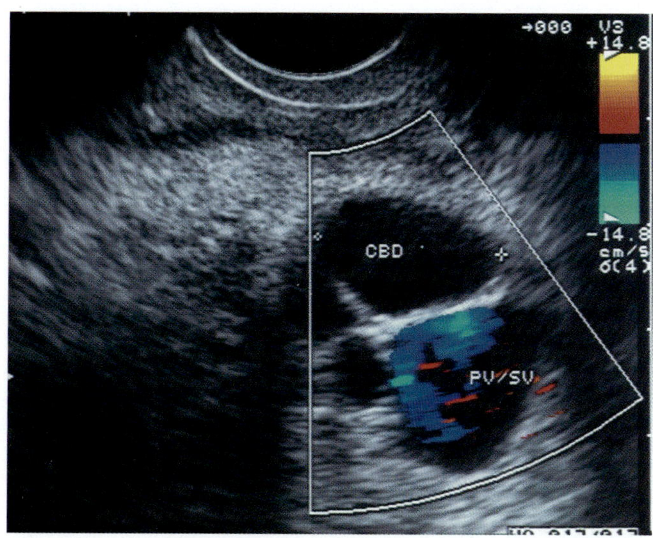


A

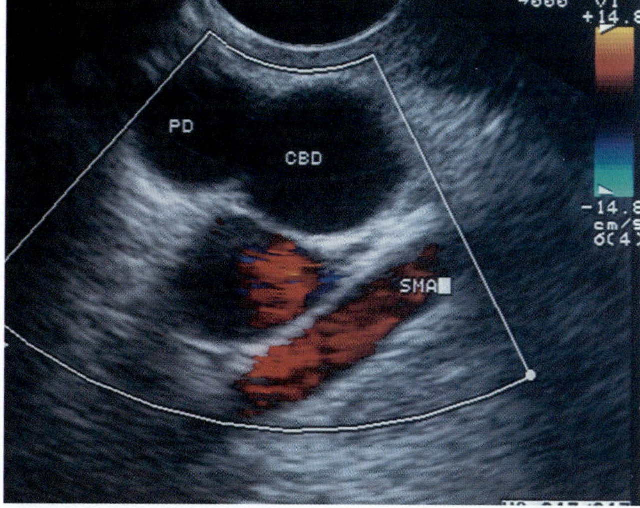


B

**FIGURE 4–25A, B**

Color flow images from the duodenum. (**A**) A dilated common bile duct (CBD) and portal vein (PV) deep to it. The portal vein has color, which is absent in the CBD. (**B**) A dilated pancreatic duct (PD) and common bile duct (CBD) without color flow, unlike the superior mesenteric artery (SMA) and portal vein.

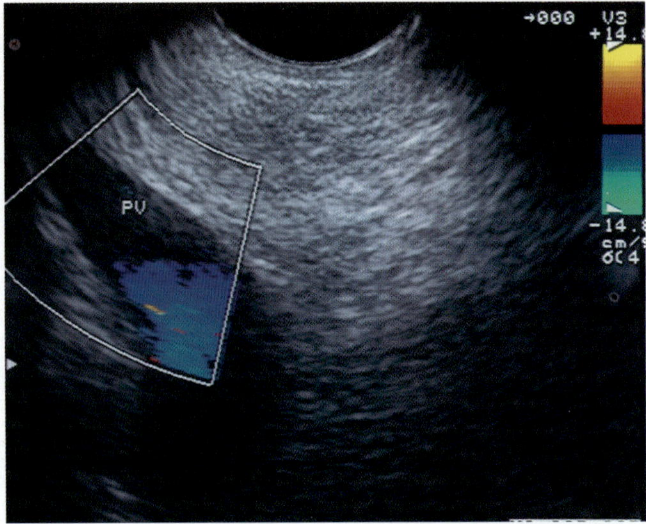


**FIGURE 4-26A**

Color flow image waveform of the portal vein from the duodenum. The superior mesenteric vein (SMV) has a similar color flow and Doppler waveform (continuous venous hum).

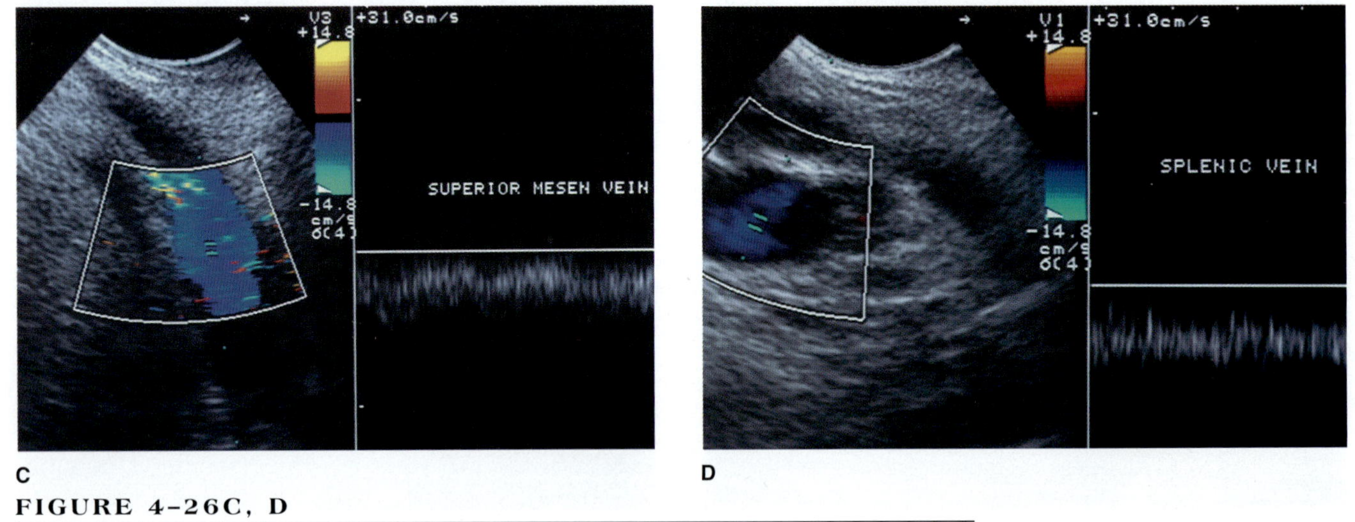


**FIGURE 4-26C, D**

(**C**) Color flow and Doppler waveform of the splenic vein imaging from the stomach at the level of the pancreatic body (**D**).

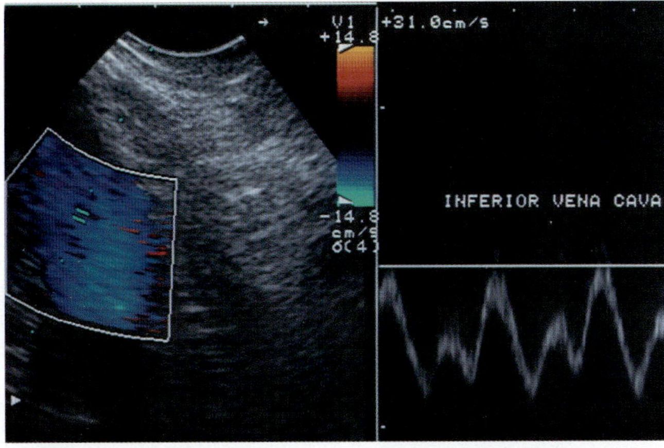


**FIGURE 4-27**

Color flow image and typical sawtooth Doppler waveform of inferior vena cava (IVC) with the transducer in the distal descending duodenum.

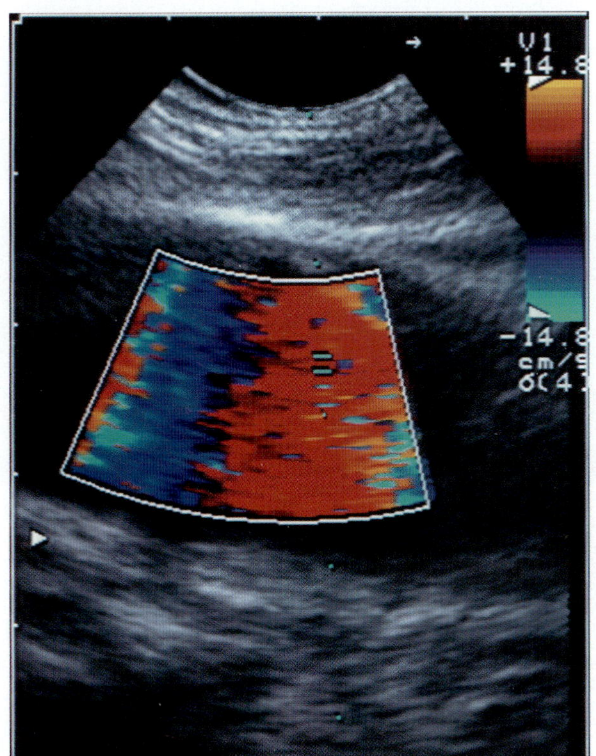


**FIGURE 4-28A**

Color flow of the aorta, showing characteristic arterial pattern—sharp upstroke, slower downstroke, and substantial diastolic flow.

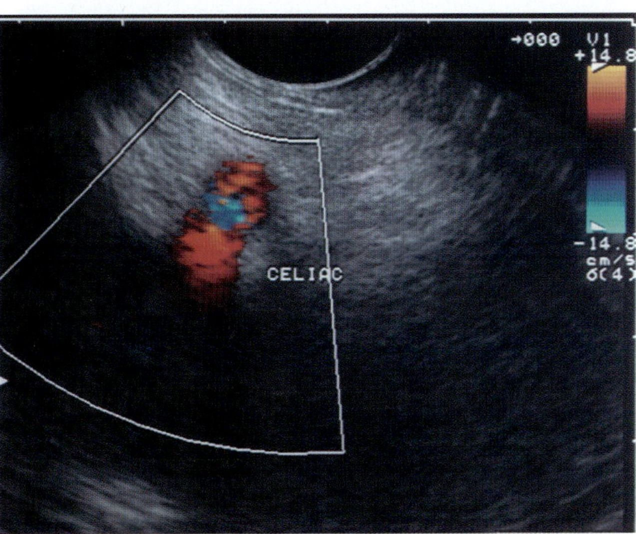


**FIGURE 4-29**

Color flow of the celiac artery; scanning from the stomach.

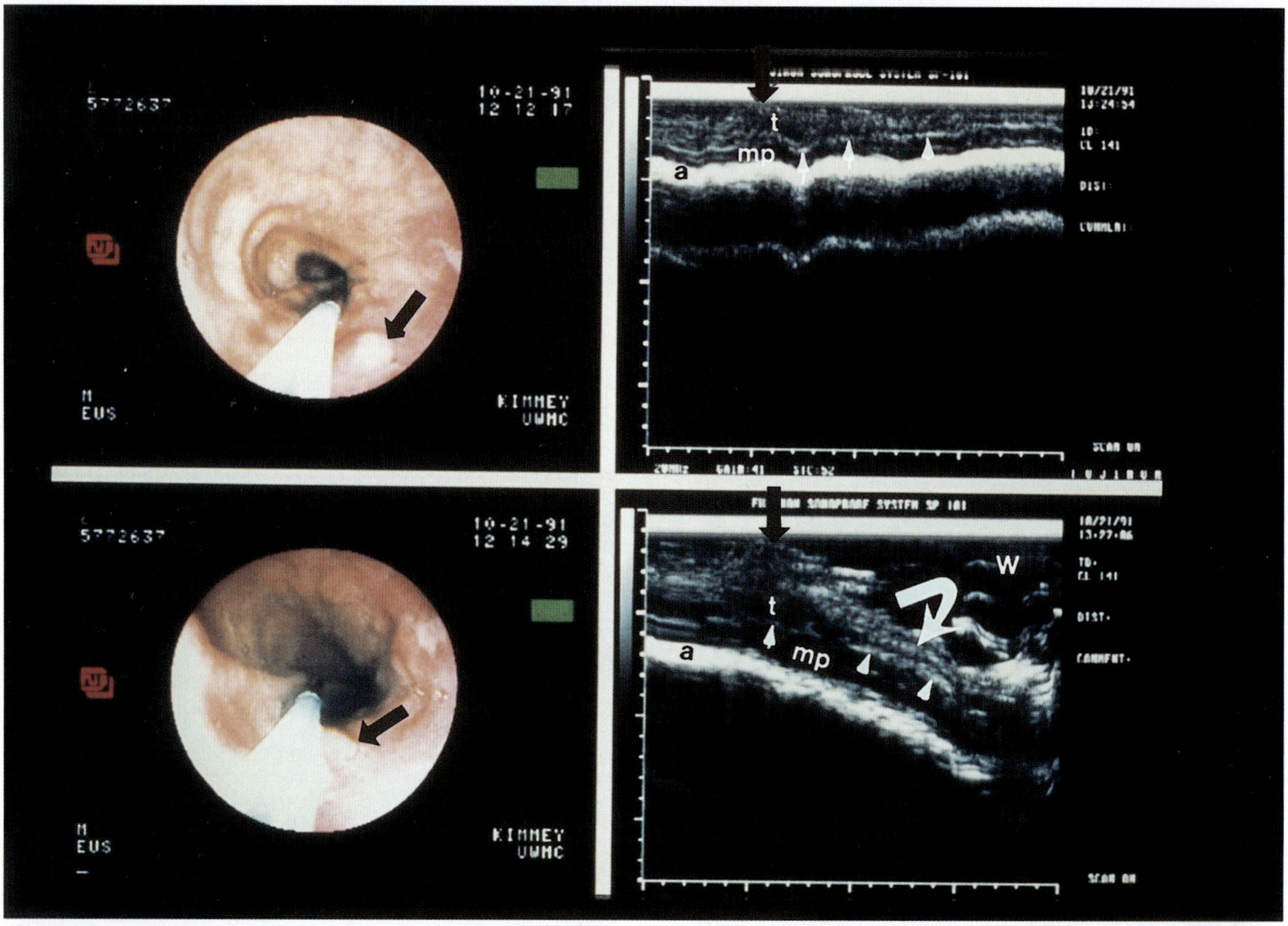

FIGURE 5-4

A nodule in Barrett's esophagus (large straight black arrow) is seen on both endoscopic and ultrasound images. The ultrasound image corresponds to the endoscopic image on the left in this four-on-one format. The hypoechoic expansion of the second ultrasound layer is due to an area of intramucosal carcinoma (t). Layers corresponding to the interface between the lamina propria and muscularis mucosae (large curved white arrow), submucosa (small white arrowheads), muscularis propria (mp), and adventitia (a) are also shown in these images made by scanning through water (W).

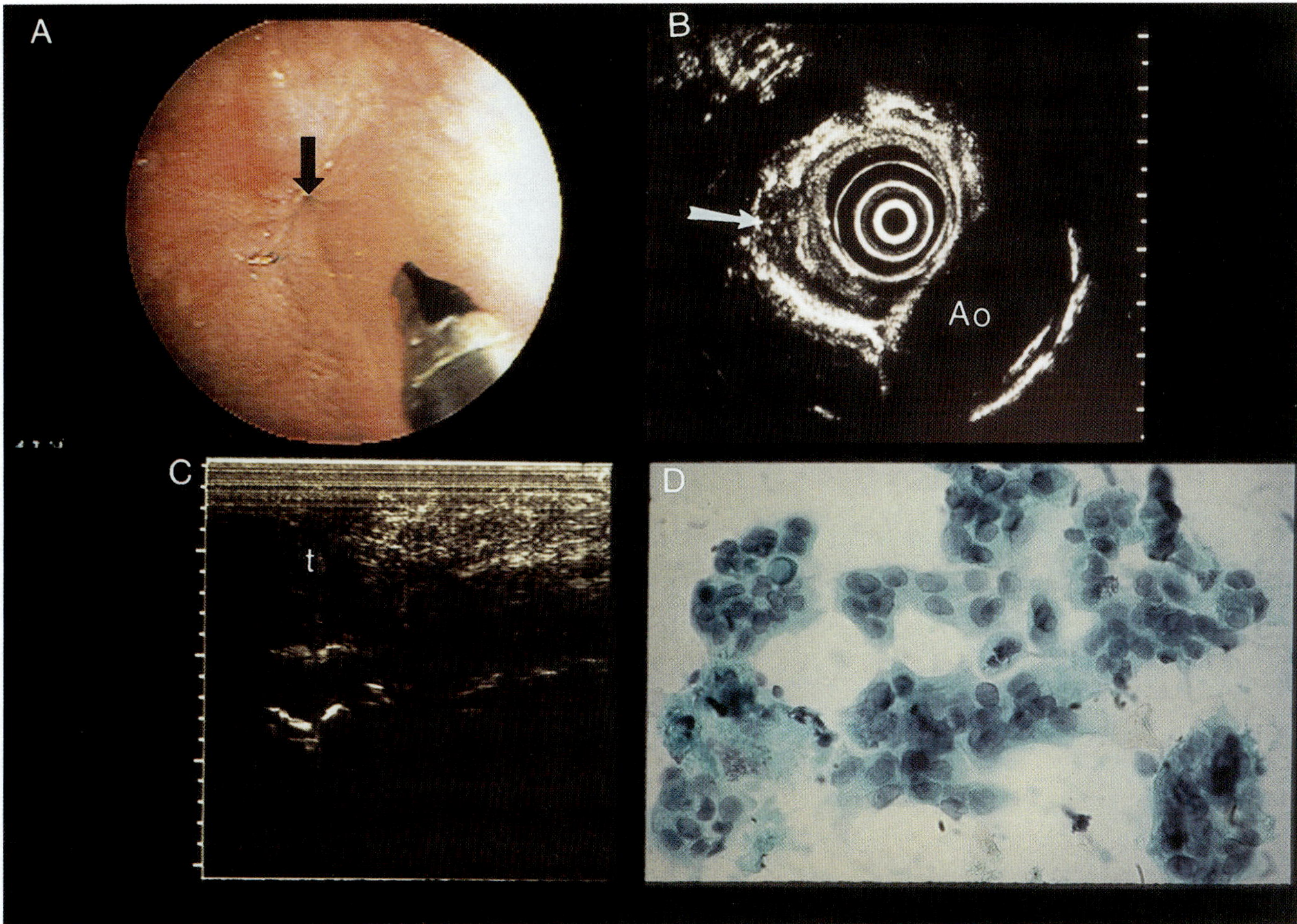


**FIGURE 5-5**

(**A**) Extrinsic invasion of the esophagus produced a tight, impassable stricture (arrow) as shown on the endoscopic image. (**B**) Conventional endosonography from above the stricture also showed a mass (arrow) invading the esophageal wall opposite from the descending aorta (Ao). (**C**) Imaging down into the stricture with a linear probe showed the quadrant containing the tumor mass (t). (**D**) Immediately following probe imaging an aspirating needle was directed into the area of thickened esophagus, revealing these malignant cells.

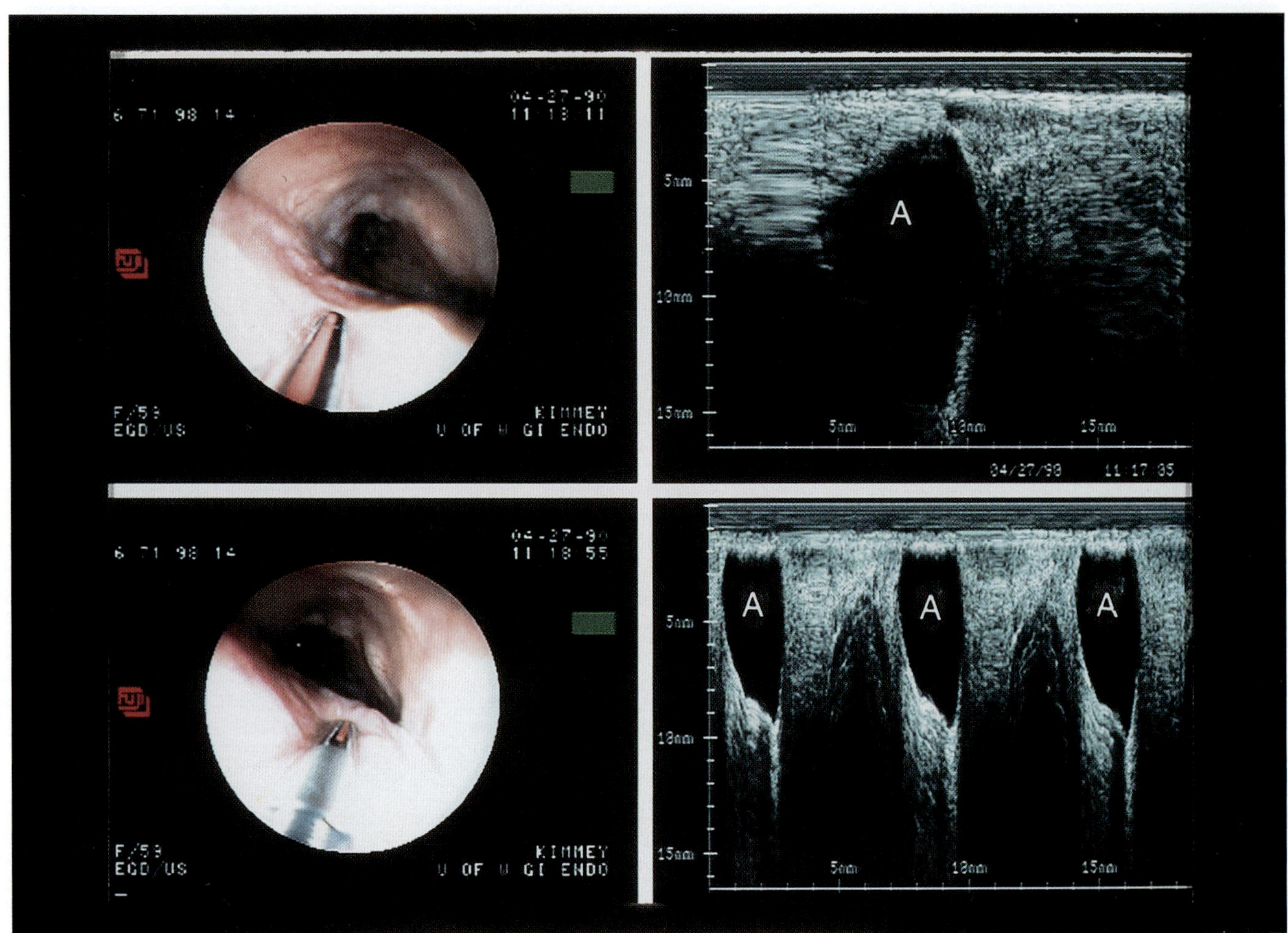


**FIGURE 5–6**

A large anechoic vessel (A) is imaged adjacent to the esoph-ageal wall on B mode scanning (upper two pictures). The horizontal axis represents mechanical movement of the probe over the esophageal wall. When the probe is held in one position over the vessel and the horizontal axis is changed to time, an M mode image is produced (bottom right image) and the vessel (A) can be seen to have arterial pulsation.

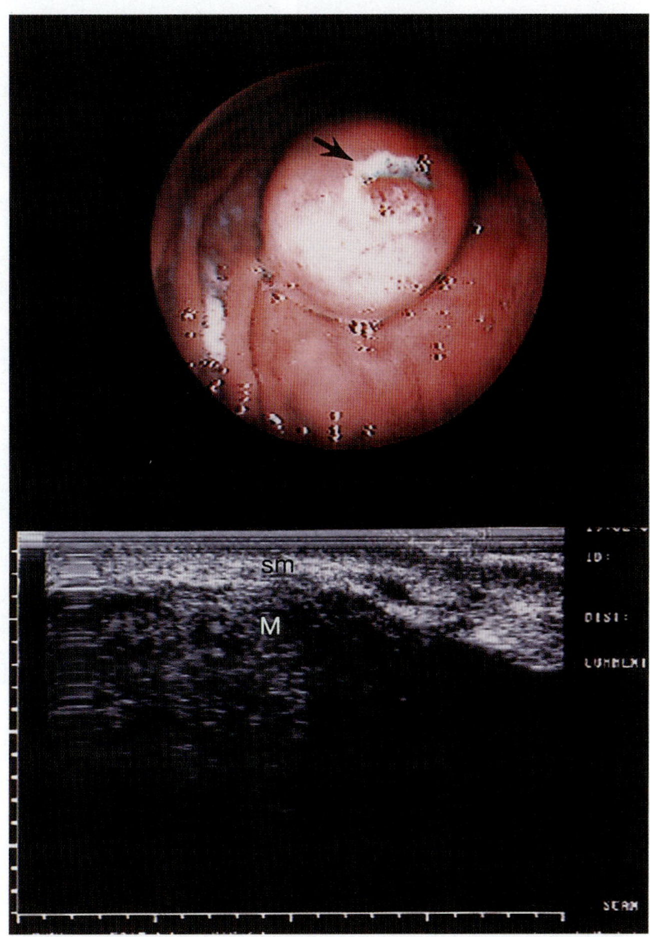


**FIGURE 5–12**

This ulcerated (arrow on top photo), polyploid subepithelial mass in the stomach was found at surgery to be a leiomyosarcoma. The linear probe image (bottom) shows a hypoechoic mass (M) below the submucosa (sm), but incomplete tissue penetration does not allow full evaluation of the size, extent, and presence of lobulation of the mass, which might suggest the presence of a malignant neoplasm.

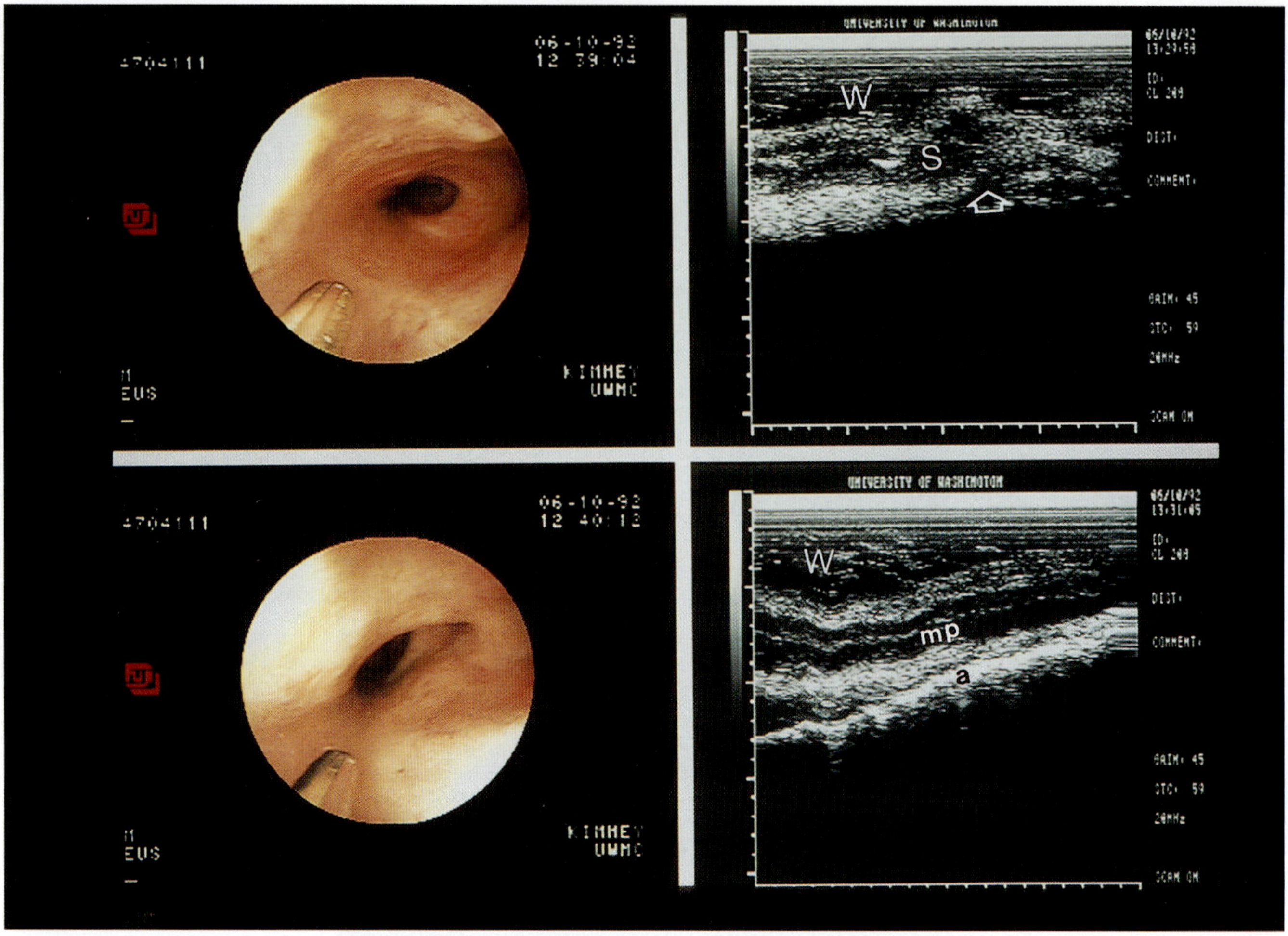

**FIGURE 5-16**

A slightly depressed area of the esophagus (upper left) where a T3 squamous cell carcinoma had been treated with chemo-therapy and radiation therapy without resection two years previously. The image reveals persistent disruption of the normal wall layers (upper right image). Wall detail is shown by imaging through a small amount of water (W) in the lumen.
A hypoechoic area extends through into the adventitia (open arrow) and is caused by scar (S) at the location of the previous tumor. Normal wall layers are shown from imaging an area of esophagus distal to the scar (bottom left and right).

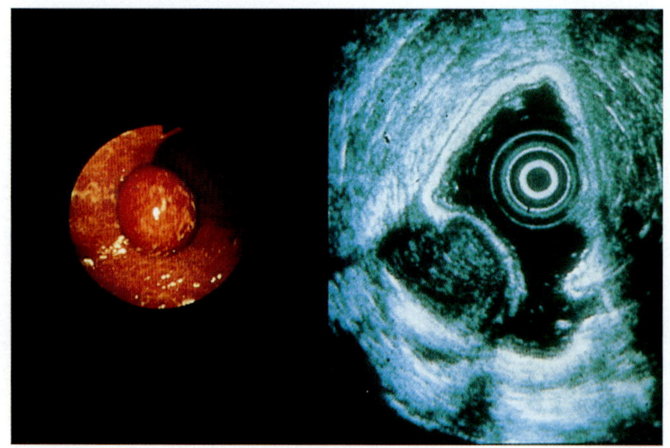


**FIGURE 15-3A, B**

(**A**) Endoscopic photograph of a gastric leiomyoma. The lesion is covered by endoscopically and histologically normal gastric mucosa. The mass lesion projects into the lumen of the stomach and may produce symptoms of bleeding if ulcerated.
(**B**) Endoscopic ultrasound of the leiomyoma pictured in (A). The endosonograph shows the typical appearance of a hypoechoic lesion contiguous with the muscularis propria layer (fourth, hypoechoic layer) of the gastrointestinal tract wall.

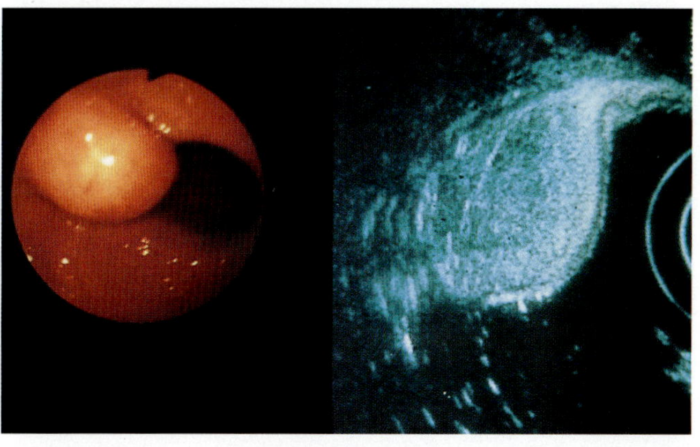

A B

FIGURE 15-5A,B

(**A**) Endoscopic photograph of a gastric lipoma. The lesion is covered by endoscopically and histologically normal gastric mucosa. The mass lesion projects into the lumen of the stomach and may produce symptoms of bleeding if ulcerated. (**B**) Endoscopic ultrasound of the lesion pictured in (A). The endosonograph shows the typical appearance of a hyperechoic lesion contiguous with the submucosal layer (third, hyperechoic layer) of the gastrointestinal tract wall.

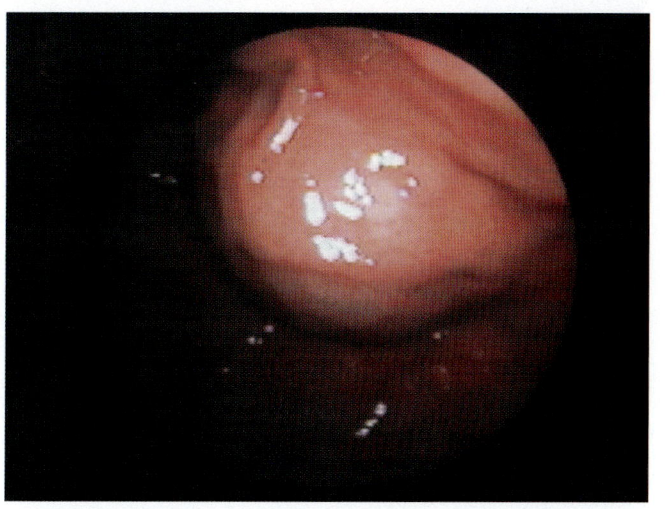

A

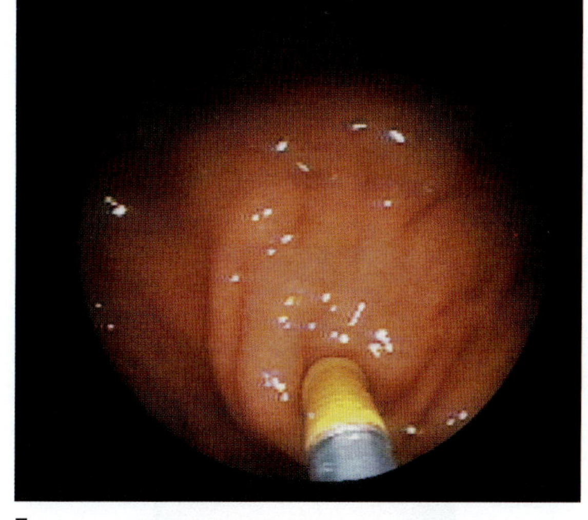

E

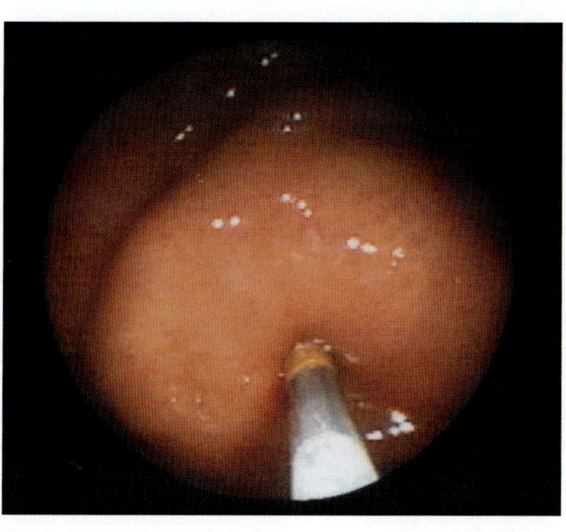

D

FIGURE 15-9A, D, E

(**A**) A gastric subepithelial lesion detected by endoscopy. (**D**) A sclerotherapy needle is inserted into the cyst endoscopically. (**E**) The cyst is drained. (Reprinted with permission from Ferrari AP, Van Dam J, Carr-Locke DL. Endoscopy 27:270, 1995.)

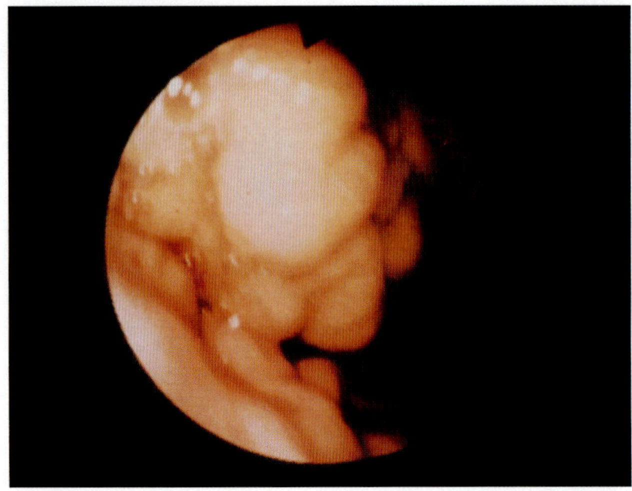

**FIGURE 15-7A**

Endoscopic photograph of gastric varices. The lesion is covered by endoscopically and histologically normal gastric mucosa. The serpentine lesion projects into the lumen of the stomach and may produce symptoms of profound bleeding similar to that of esophageal varices.

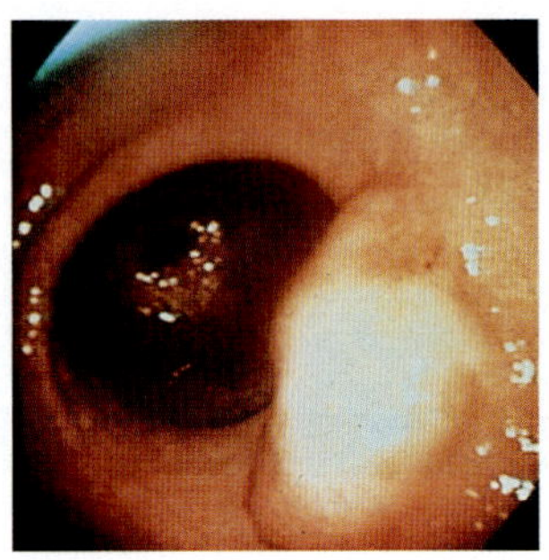

**FIGURE 15-8A**

Gastric cyst. The endoscopic photograph shows a gastric subepithelial lesion at the junction of the gastric antrum and body. The lesion is covered by endoscopically and histologically normal gastric mucosa.

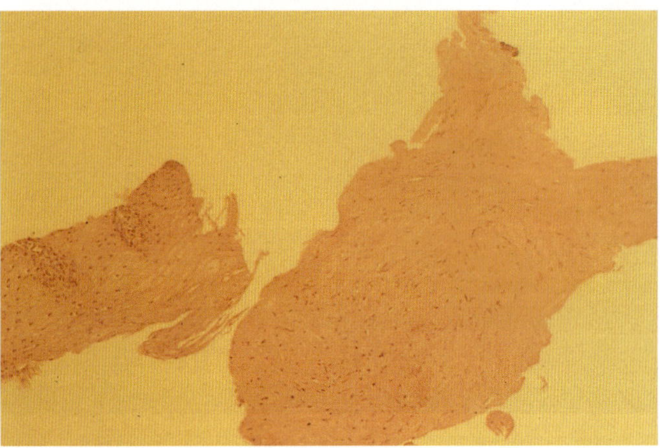

**FIGURE 16-4**

Guillotine needle sample of an esophageal leiomyoma. (hematoxylin–eosin, ×100)

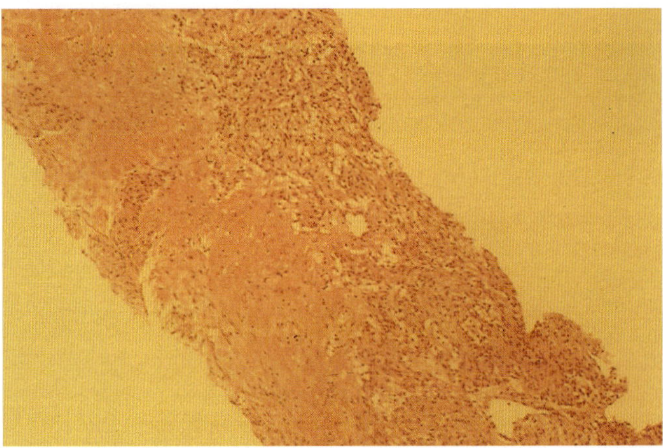

**FIGURE 16-8**

Guillotine needle sample of a duodenal leiomyoblastoma. (hematoxylin–eosin, ×100)

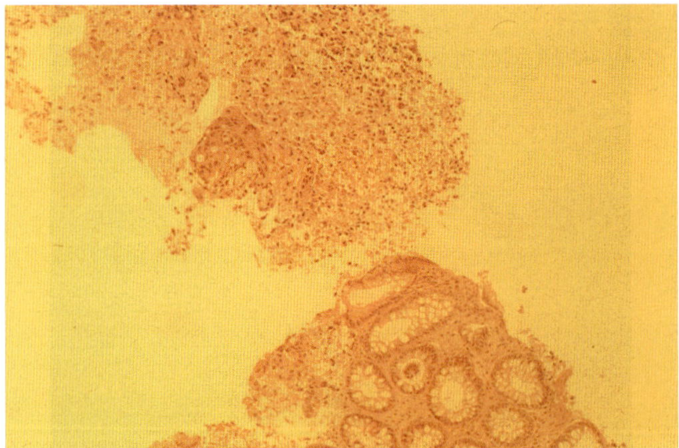

**FIGURE 16-9**

Guillotine needle sample of a submucosal cancer recurrence of the rectum. (hematoxylin–eosin, ×100)

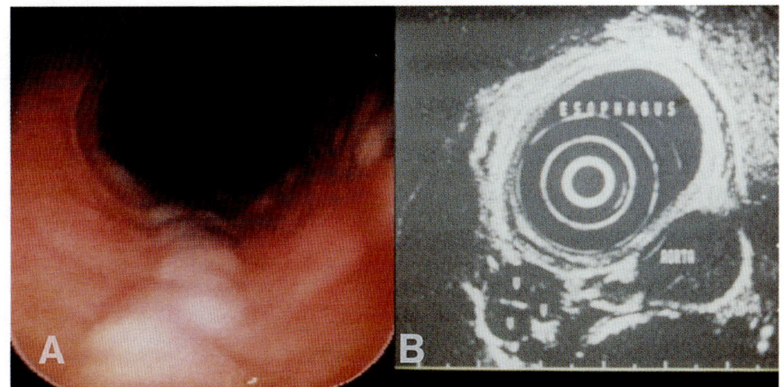


**FIGURE 21-8A, B**

(**A**) Endoscopic image of the esophagus showing Grade I esophageal varices. (**B**) EUS image of the esophagus demonstrating Grade I esophageal varices.

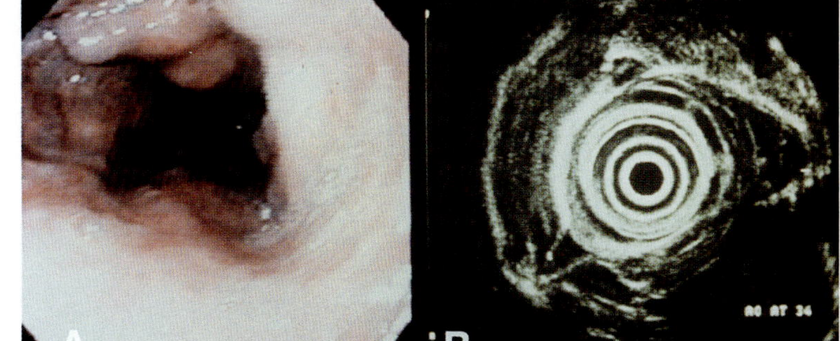


**FIGURE 21-9A, B**

(**A**) Endoscopic image of the esophagus showing Grade II esophageal varices. (**B**) EUS image of the esophagus demonstrating Grade II esophageal varices.

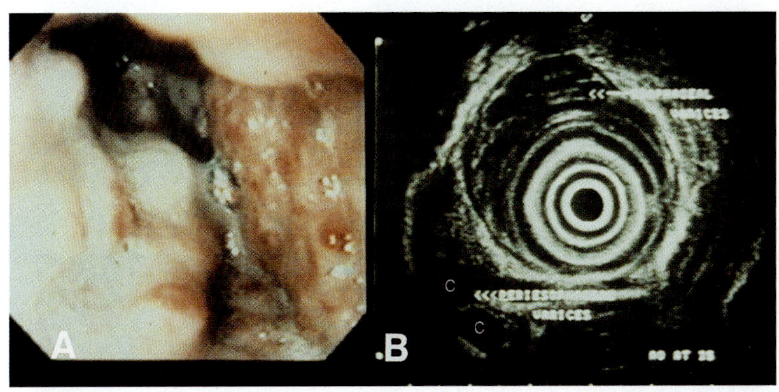


**FIGURE 21-10A, B**

(**A**) Endoscopic image of the esophagus showing Grade III esophageal varices. (**B**) EUS image of the esophagus demonstrating Grade III esophageal varices. Also shown are periesophageal collateral veins (c).

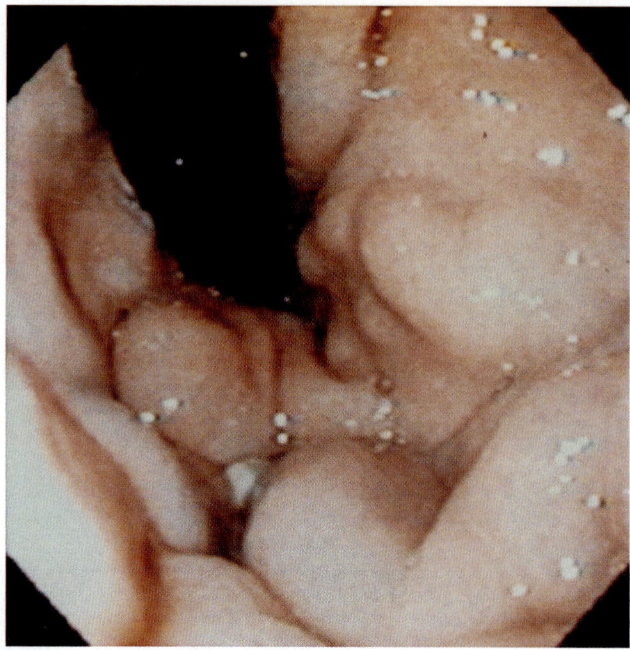

**FIGURE 21-11**

Endoscopic photographs demonstrating typical nodular varices within the gastric fundus and cardia.

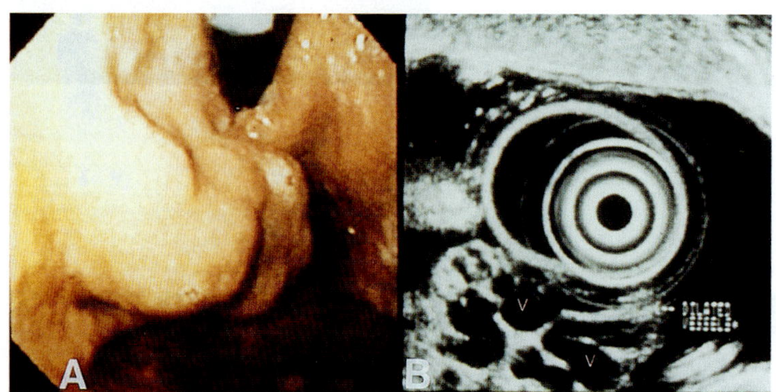


**FIGURE 21-12A, B**

(**A**) Endoscopic image showing lobulated gastric varices in the fundus of the stomach. (**B**) EUS image of the same patient, demonstrating rounded echo-free structures beneath the mucosal and submucosal layers consistent with gastric varices (v).

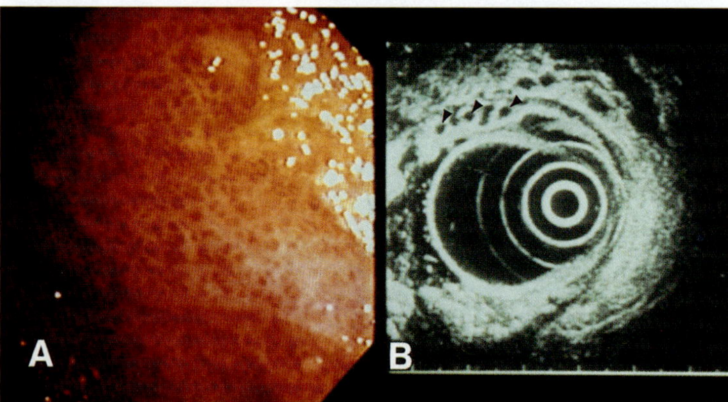


**FIGURE 21-13A, B**

(**A**) Endoscopic image showing diffuse subepithelial hemorrhages in a patient with portal hypertension consistent with Grade V PHG. (**B**) EUS image of the same patient, demonstrating small (2–3 mm), round, echo-free structures consistent with PHG.

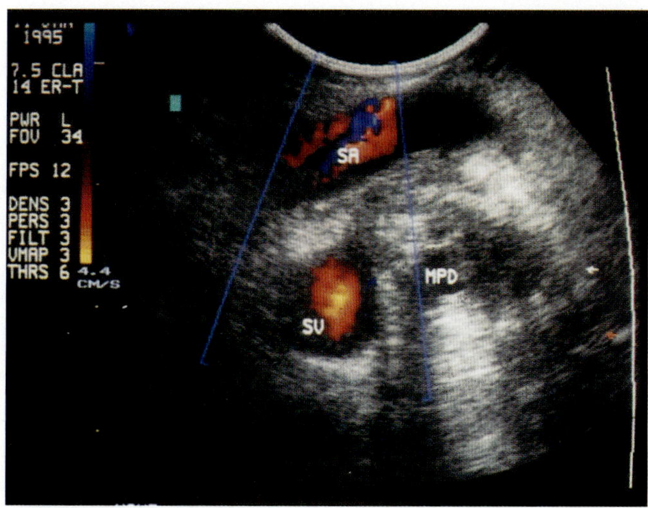


**FIGURE 25-4**

Endosonographic image demonstrating the use of color Doppler to identify vascular structures. SA = splenic artery, SV = splenic vein, MPD = main pancreatic duct (dilated).

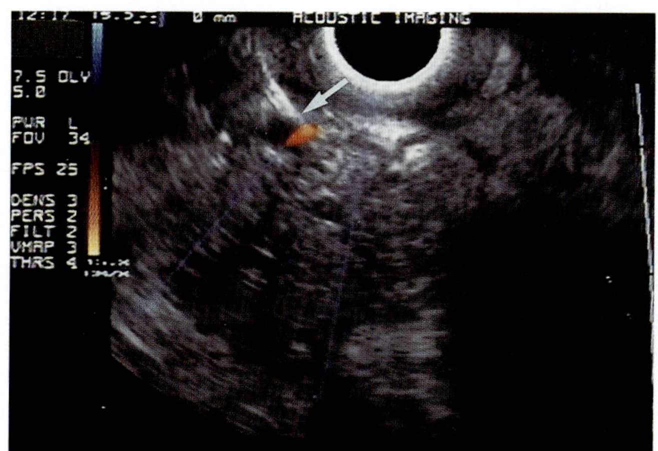


**FIGURE 25-6**

Doppler imaging showing a small vessel interposed between the needle (arrow) and target lesion (pancreatic head tumor), illustrating the importance of Doppler scanning prior to FNA.

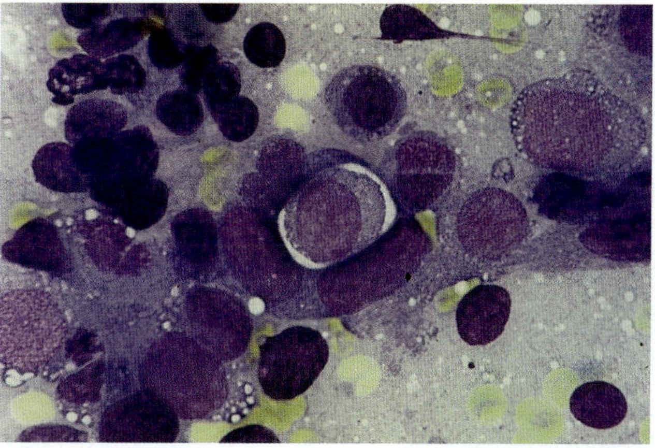

**FIGURE 25-11**

Cytologic smear of a pancreatic fine-needle aspirate showing enlarged, polymorphic nuclei diagnostic of a pancreatic malignancy (adenocarcinoma). (Hematoxylin–esosin, ×400)

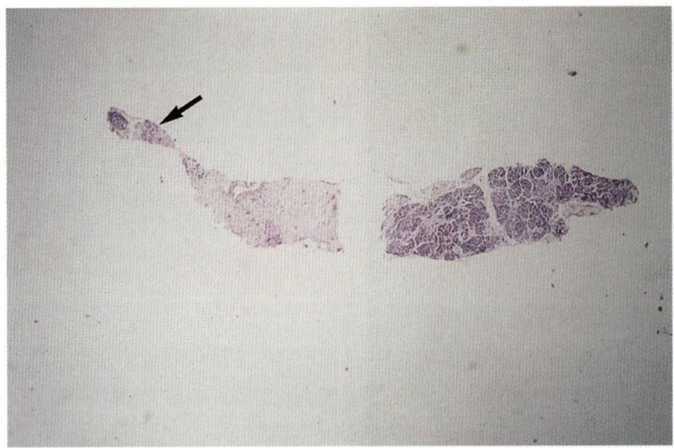

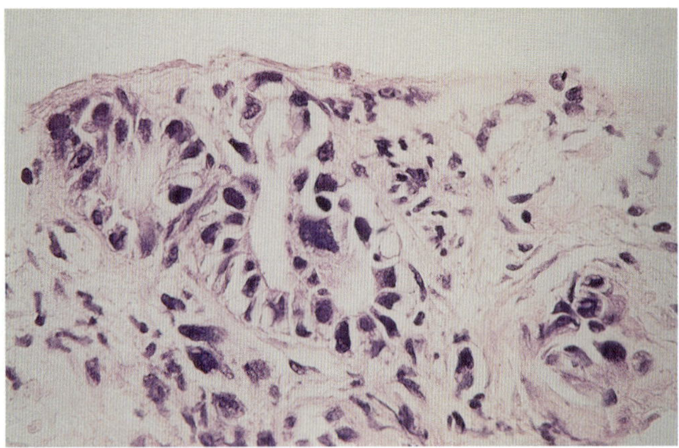

**A** **B**

**FIGURE 25-12A, B**

Histologic sections of a pancreatic fine-needle biopsy. (**A**) 3-cm core specimen, fragmented in the middle. Histology shows adenocarcinoma (left fragment, arrow) accompanied by changes of chronic pancreatitis (right fragment). (Hematoxylin–eosin ×50) (**B**) Magnified view of area below arrow shows highly atypical epithelial cells forming primitive glandular structures diagnostic of adenocarcinoma. (Hematoxylin–eosin, ×400)

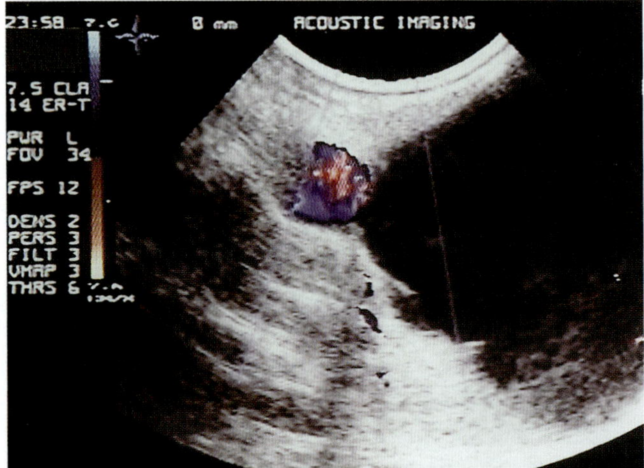


**FIGURE 25-14**

Endosonographic image with Doppler showing a large vessel adjacent to a pseudocyst.

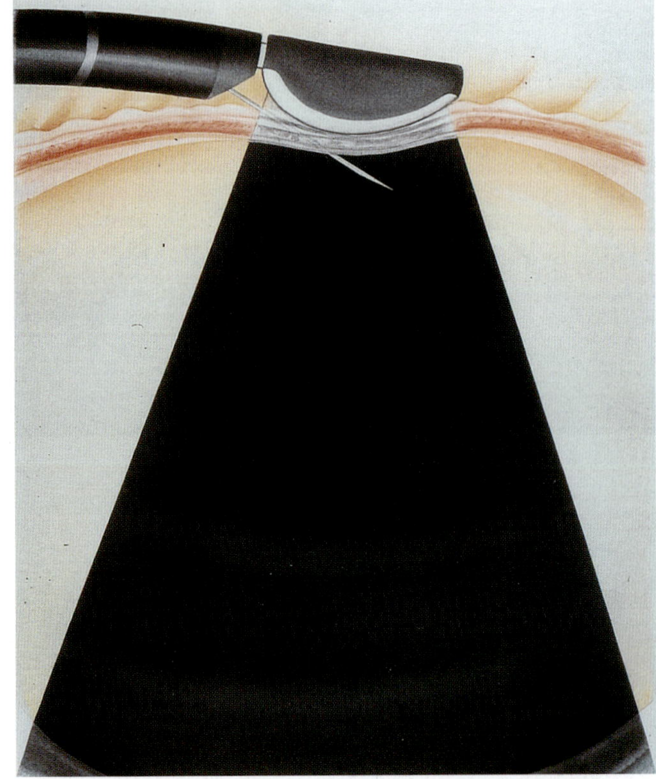

**FIGURE 25-16B**

Endosonography guided pseudocyst puncture and drainage. Schematic diagram of pseudocyst puncture.

# SECTION

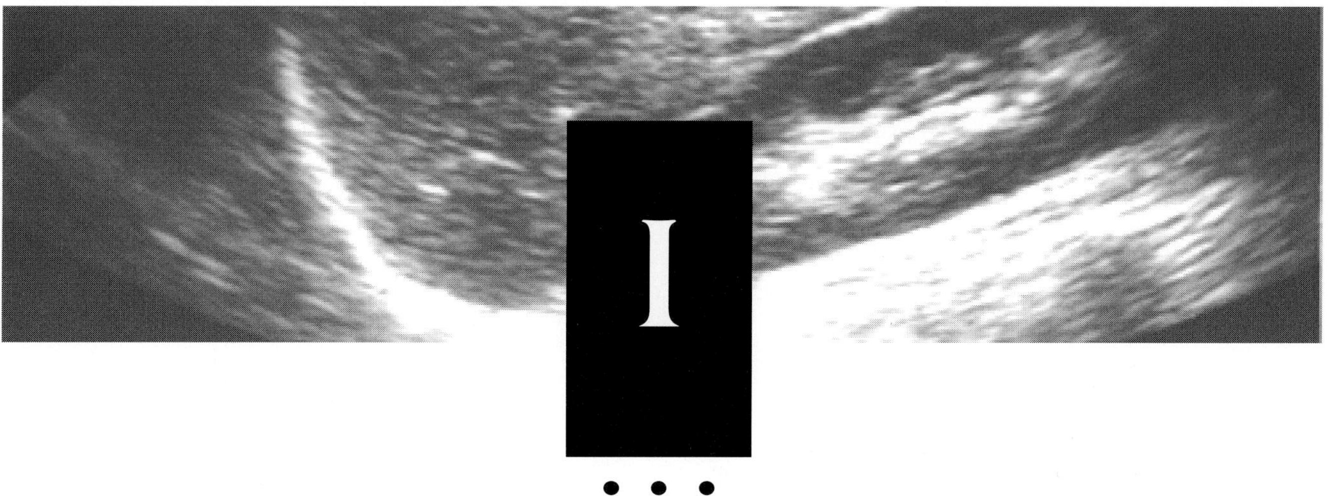

# I

# Introduction to Endosonography: Technical Considerations

CHAPTER

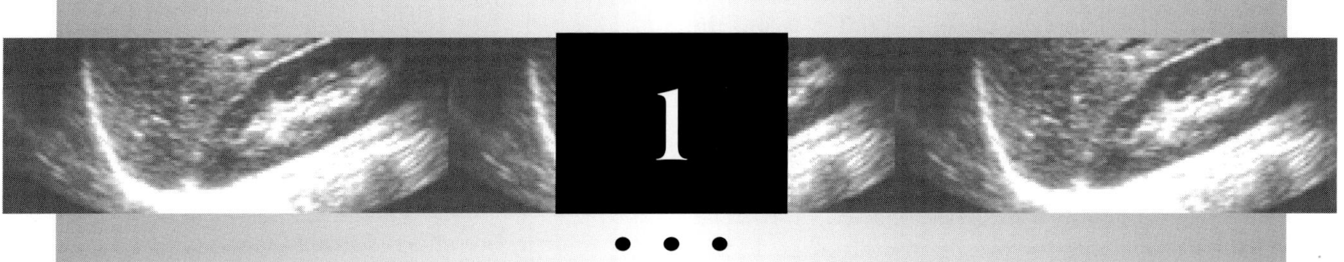


# Fundamentals of Ultrasonography

Thomas E. Herbener

## Ultrasound Physics

Sound is a form of energy that propagates through a medium in the form of repetitive longitudinal or compression waves (Fig. 1–1). Several characteristics of sound are important to understanding how sound, and hence ultrasound, behaves and interacts with matter. First, sound is a form of **energy**. We can therefore discuss such aspects of sound as the amount—or *intensity*—of sound energy in a particular sound wave. We can also discuss the dissipation—or *attenuation*—of sound energy as it travels through a medium. Second, sound, like light, travels in the form of a **wave**, which can be described in terms of its *frequency* and *wavelength*. Thus the manner in which sound interacts with matter can be explained based on such wave properties as *reflection* and *refraction*. Finally, sound requires a **medium** through which it must travel. Sound cannot travel through a vacuum, but it can travel through media such as human tissue.

### Sound as a Wave

Sound as a wave is characterized by its frequency, velocity, and wavelength. The frequency of sound is the number of cycles per second expressed in terms of hertz (Hz), where (1 Hz = 1 cycle per second). Audible sound, for example, ranges from 15 Hz to 20 kHz (1 kHz = 1000 cycles per second). But ultrasound (US) used for diagnostic purposes is in the megahertz (1 MHz = 1,000,000 cycles per second) range of 1–30 MHz. (Experimentally US frequencies of 60 MHz have been explored.) For diagnostic ultrasound, transducers used in standard abdominal or pelvic ultrasound generally utilize frequencies in the range of 2.5–7.0 MHz. Most probes for endoscopic ultrasound (EUS) range from 5 to 25 MHz. The particular frequency of the ultrasound utilized is important for image quality and depth of penetration of the ultrasound beam.

Velocity is, of course speed. And the velocity of sound in human tissue tends to be fairly constant. The standard average velocity of sound through water—and through most human soft tissue—is 1540 meters per second (m/sec), though it may vary slightly in different soft tissues (1–4). In fat, for example, sound velocity is approximately 1450 m/sec. In some human tissue the velocity is very different. In bone, for instance, sound velocity is 4100 m/sec (3). The velocity of sound in a particular tissue depends on that tissue's density and elastic properties. Thus the type of tissue affects the time it takes for sound to be emitted from the transducer face and travel through the tissue, be reflected, and travel back to the transducer for reception and image formation. But for all practical purposes, velocity may be considered constant in human tissue.

The wavelength of sound is the distance between each longitudinal wave or compression wave traveling through a medium (Fig. 1–2). The wavelength of ultrasound is usually quite small (1 mm or less) and varies according to the formula

$$\lambda = C/F$$

where $\lambda$ is wavelength, $C$ is the (constant) velocity and $F$ is the frequency (1–4). Since the velocity of sound in human tissue is fairly constant, its wavelength varies with frequency.

The wavelength of the sound being utilized influences how well certain objects can be imaged: it affects both the clarity of the image and the accuracy with which the image depicts the true object.

All of these characteristics—frequency, wavelength, and velocity—affect the manner in which any given transducer with a specific frequency, and hence a specific wavelength, of ultrasound can produce an image of high quality.

An ultrasound image is produced when an ultrasound transmitter (the *probe* or *transducer*) emits US waves. These waves travel into tissue, then are reflected back to the transducer as *echoes*. Thus the transducer acts as a receiver to detect the echoes. These echoes are processed to form an image of the object being examined. Since the velocity of ultrasound in tissue is constant, the time it takes for sound to travel from the transducer, be reflected from a target, and echo back to the transducer is directly related to the distance of the target from the transducer. That is, the time it takes echoes from various targets to return to the transducer determines the distances at which these echoes are placed in the image. The image produced comes from a multitude of echoes from a subject; these echoes are collected, placed at various depths, and formulated into a readable image.

Reflection is the property of sound that allows us to produce images with ultrasound. Without reflection, none of the beam emitted from a transducer would return for image production. Reflection occurs because of a property of tissue known as *acoustic impedance* ($Z$), which is a measure of how well matter transmits or propagates sound waves. Because acoustic impedance is related to the velocity of sound traveling through the tissue and the density of the tissue, it varies with the type of tissue. When sound strikes an interface between two tissues, say fat and liver tissue, some of the beam is transmitted through this interface and some of the beam is reflected back from this interface. How much of the sound is transmitted through or reflected back depends on the difference in acoustic impedance between the two tissues (Fig. 1–3). If there is little difference in acoustic impedance between two tissues, reflection at the interface is low, permitting a high degree of transmittance of the sound forward. This is usually the case

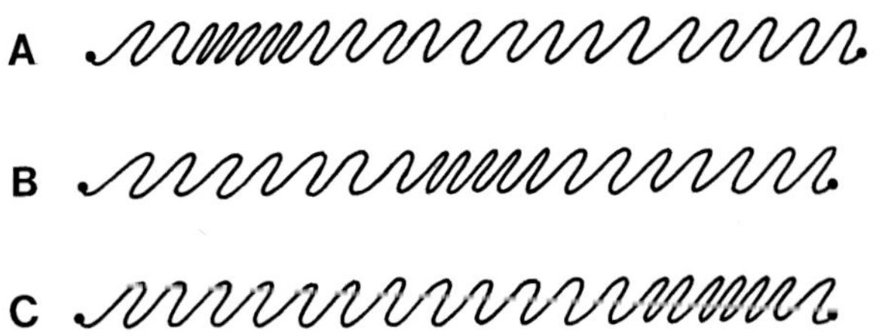

A
B
C

**FIGURE 1–1**

Sound travels through a medium the same way a compression wave travels through a coiled spring.

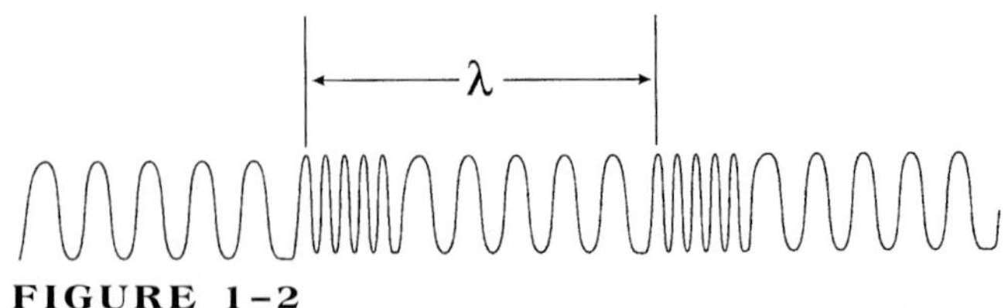


**FIGURE 1–2**

The wavelength ($\lambda$) of a sound wave is the distance from the beginning of one wave to the beginning of the next.

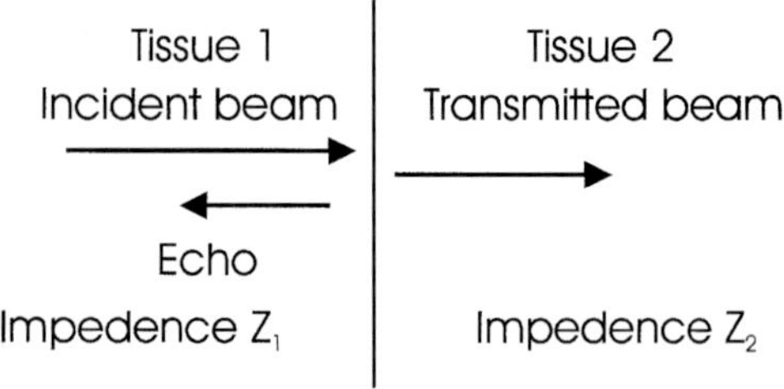


**FIGURE 1–3**

An interface between two tissues of differing acoustic impedance ($Z$). If the difference between $Z_1$ and $Z_2$ is great, a large amount of the incident beam is reflected as an echo. If the difference between $Z_1$ and $Z_2$ is small, a large amount of the incident beam is transmitted.

as acoustic impedance varies only slightly among most human tissues.

But if there is a large difference in acoustic impedance between two tissues, reflection at the interface is high while transmittance is low. The capacity of tissues and interfaces between tissues to reflect sound determines how well ultrasound can form an image. If two tissues have a large discrepancy in acoustic impedance, sound will be so reflected at the interface that no image can form beyond the interface; that is, no sound can penetrate beyond this interface (Fig. 1–4). For example, an interface between air and soft tissue results in such a large discrepancy in acoustic impedance that all of the sound is reflected at this interface; that is, ultrasound cannot image deep to such an interface. Thus ultrasound cannot image normal lung parenchyma because the interface between the soft chest wall and the air-filled lung is so highly reflective.

*Acoustic coupling agents* can be used to improve transmittance of sound across interfaces between substances widely divergent in acoustic impedance. Ultrasound gel, which is used in abdominal and pelvic ultrasound, is such an agent. Without it, the vast difference in acoustic impedance between the transducer face, the adjacent air, and the patient's skin would cause all the sound emitted from the transducer to be reflected at the skin surface. No sound could penetrate into the patient to produce an image. The acoustic gel serves to narrow the discrepancy gap. With the gel between the face of the probe and the skin surface, the discrepancy in impedance is lowered, so the ultrasound emitted from the transducer can more easily be transmitted through the skin surface. In EUS, a water-filled balloon serves the same purpose. The water acts as an acoustic coupling agent to allow transmittance of sound from the endoscopic ultrasound probe through the mucosa of the esophagus, stomach, and so on. Without this water coupling agent, the differences in acoustic impedance between the probe and the adjacent mucosa would be so great that most of the ultrasound would be reflected at this interface and little ultrasound would be transmitted into the adjacent tissues for imaging.

As with light waves, the angle of reflection (*r*) of ultrasound from an interface is equal to the angle of incidence (*i*) of the ultrasound beam on the interface (Fig. 1–5). This is important in ultrasound image production, which depends on the quantity of echoes reflected back to the transducer to produce an image. Sound that strikes an interface orthogonally (at a 90° angle) is reflected back to the transducer at nearly a 90° angle. If an incident beam of ultrasound strikes a surface at a nonperpendicular angle, the echoes are reflected at an angle equal to the angle of incidence. But these echoes are not directed back toward the transducer; rather, they are reflected into surrounding tissues. When ultrasound is reflected nonorthogonally (or at an angle different from that directed back to the transducer), the echoes are *scattered* into surrounding tissues. Scattering means that the reflected ultrasound beam is dissipated and diffused through the tissue (Fig. 1–6). Most human tissues present an incident ultrasound beam with many irregular interfaces that cause a great degree of scattering of the reflected echoes. These echoes are repeatedly reflected and further scattered until, eventually, they are reflected back to the trans-

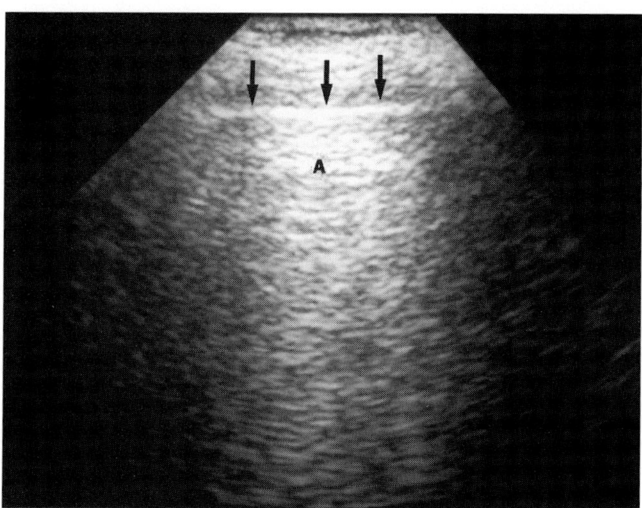


**FIGURE 1–4**

An ultrasound image of the chest shows chest wall–lung interface (arrows). Because of the great reflection of sound at this interface, no image deep to the interface can be made and only artifact (A) is seen deeper.

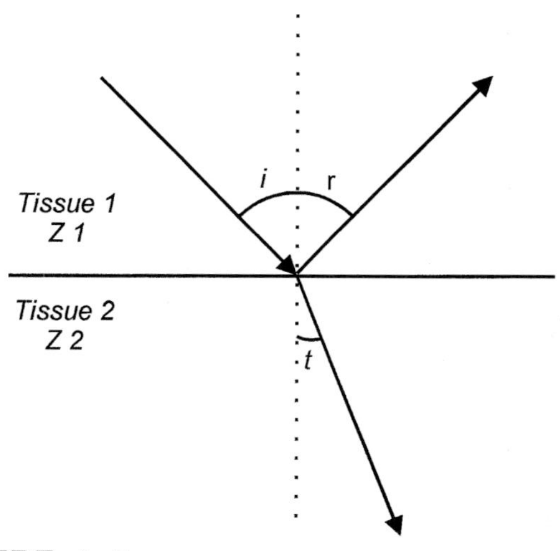


**FIGURE 1–5**

An ultrasound beam striking an interface between tissue 1 and 2. $Z_1$ = acoustic impedance of tissue 1; $Z_2$ = acoustic impedance of tissue 2; *i* = angle of incidence (perpendicular to the interface); *r* = angle of reflection; *t* = angle of transmittance. ***Note:*** $i = r$. Angle $t < i$, showing that the ultrasound beam is refracted, or bent, toward the midline.

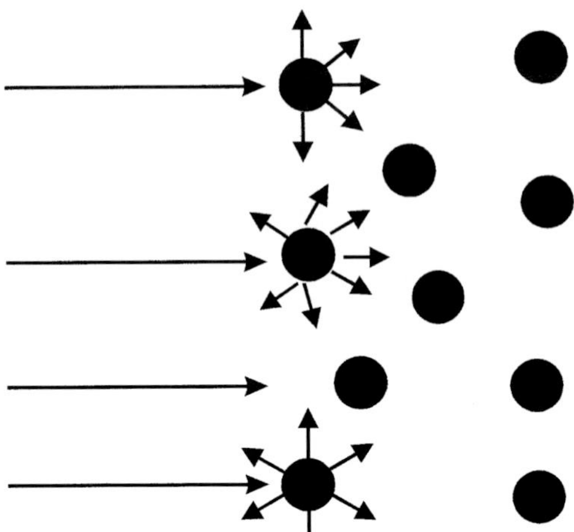

**FIGURE 1–6**

Ultrasound waves strike reflectors in a tissue. Since the reflectors present interfaces with varying angles to the incident beam, echoes are reflected at various angles and are scattered throughout the tissue.

ducer for image formation. This diffuse scattering of the incident ultrasound beam in tissue results in a variegated image. Human liver, for example, yields a diffuse back-scatter, resulting in the overall appearance, or "texture" of the liver (Fig. 1–7).

Smooth surfaces tend to reflect ultrasound in a single given direction, which is related to the angle of incidence. Smooth surfaces, then, are referred to as *specular reflectors.* In the human body specular reflectors include the diaphragm, the curved capsule of the liver, the curved surface of the gallbladder, and the capsule of the kidney. Irregular surfaces that reflect ultrasound in multiple directions are known as *diffuse reflectors.* Such diffuse reflectors scatter the reflected ultrasound beam in a manner that gives these tissues characteristic ultrasonic texture, such as the homogeneous texture of the liver or the bright sonographic texture of fat.

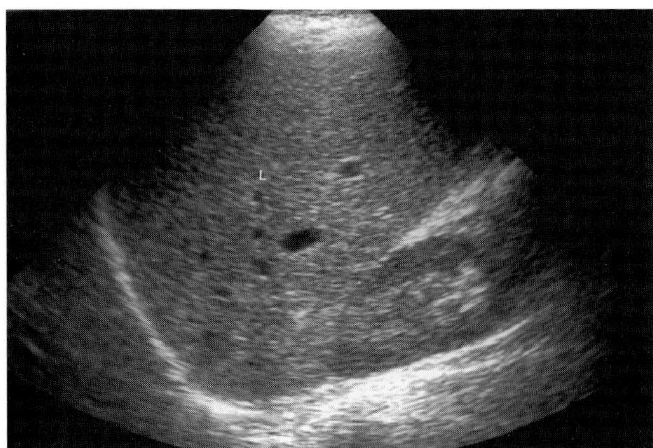


**FIGURE 1–7**

Multiple interfaces in tissue, such as the liver (L), cause reflection and scattering of the sound beam. As the sound is reflected and scattered, echoes eventually return to the ultrasound probe, creating an image of the liver with an ultrasound texture.

Like light, ultrasound can also be *refracted.* That is, sound waves may be "bent," or refracted, in a different direction (see Fig. 1–5). This bending can occur with slight irregularities in the velocity of ultrasound. Although the velocity of ultrasound in human tissue is usually fairly constant at 1540 m/sec, that velocity can change with the density and elastic properties of tissue. When sound travels through two tissues of very different densities, the velocity varies and the beam bends. Refraction can cause artifacts in diagnostic ultrasound.

## Sound as Energy

Sound can also be described in terms of energy. The amount of energy within a sound wave, described in terms of its intensity or *amplitude,* is related to the loudness of the sound. Similarly, the intensity or amplitude of ultrasound waves refers to the amount of energy in those waves. Like that of sound, the intensity of ultrasound is usually expressed in decibels (dB), which is a relative ratio between two different sound or ultrasound waves. (Audiophiles will recognize the term *decibel* as a measure of the loudness of audible sound.) A decibel is, in fact, a logarithmic ratio, so that increasing the intensity from 1 to 2 dB increases intensity not twice but by a factor of 10 (1–4). The decibel level is thus the energy level or "loudness" of both sound and ultrasound waves.

As ultrasound travels through tissue, it loses energy. That is, it attenuates as it passes through a medium. Reflection and scattering cause attenuation—and so does absorption. *Absorption* arises because a small amount of the sound energy is converted to friction-induced heat. The amount of absorption depends on inherent properties of the medium and on the frequency of the sound. For example, viscosity of the medium affects absorption. Less viscous materials like fluids absorb less sound energy than do more viscous materials like soft tissue or bone.

Because fluids do not absorb sound energy significantly, the sonographer can use them in strategic ways. The water that fills the balloon around the EUS probe is a good acoustic coupling agent because it does not absorb or attenuate the ultrasound beam to any significant degree. Similarly, transabdominal sonographers may fill the stomach or urinary bladder with water. In this way the ultrasound beam is less attenuated and better visualization of the pancreas or deep pelvic organs becomes possible.

Bone absorbs sound, greatly attenuating it. For example, the spine and ribs absorb so well that ultrasound does not penetrate through them. Fat also absorbs and attenuates sound. If the fat content of liver is increased, as with fatty infiltration, the sonographer can note that the ultrasound beam directed at the liver is greatly attenuated—a finding that can aid in the diagnosis of a fatty liver. Likewise, gallstones or renal calculi also absorb and attenuate ultrasound. Little ultrasound is transmitted through such stones, giving a characteristic—often diagnostic—shadowing (Fig. 1–8).

The frequency of the sound wave also greatly affects the amount of absorption or attenuation. In soft tissue, the relationship between frequency and absorption is linear: As the frequency of the sound wave increases, the absorption of sound increases. Therefore an ultrasound probe whose frequency is 20 MHz has a higher degree of sound absorption or attenuation as it travels through tissue than does a 5-MHz probe. This will greatly affect imaging since higher frequency transducers cannot penetrate as deeply as lower frequency transducers. In EUS, for example, a 5-MHz transducer penetrates to approximately 8 cm but a 10-MHz transducer can only penetrate to about 4 cm.

The ability to penetrate to deeper tissues depends on how quickly the incident sound beam is attenuated. Moreover, the reflected sound beam, or collection of echoes, is attenuated in the same fashion as the incident beam. That is, just as the incident beam is reflected, scattered, and absorbed by tissue, so also is the reflected sound beam. When the reflected sound waves or echoes finally reach the transducer, their intensity is so diminished with respect to the original incident waves that no image can be produced unless their energy is amplified. Consequently, all ultrasound units have mechanisms to amplify these echoes for image production.

## Ultrasound Image Production

The basic physics of sound determines how an ultrasound image is actually formed by an ultrasound unit. An ultrasound unit produces an ultrasound beam with a transducer, then utilizes that same transducer to receive the returning echoes. Transducers, therefore, are both transmitters and receivers. Typically, transducers transmit sound in pulses, then listen for returning echoes between those transmitted pulses.

The transducer consists of small crystals housed in plastic. The crystals are *piezoelectric crystals,* meaning that when stimulated by an electric pulse, they vibrate or "ring." And when the crystal rings, it produces sound waves. Multiple piezoelectric crystals are usually aligned in a transducer head and produce sound waves in response to computer-controlled electric pulsing (Fig. 1–9). As reflected echoes return to the transducer, the sound wave induces the piezoelectric crystal to ring, whereupon the crystal generates an electric pulse. It is this series of electric pulses produced by the transducer crystals during receiver mode that is processed to form an ultrasound image.

Each piezoelectric crystal resonates over a band of frequencies. But it resonates best at a specific frequency known as its *resonant frequency.* This is the frequency at which the transducer will produce ultrasound—e.g., 5 or 10 MHz. Newer transducers employ crystals with wider bands of frequencies, so these transducers can provide multiple frequencies of ultrasound. That is, these new transducers can function at several different frequencies. For example, such a transducer may be

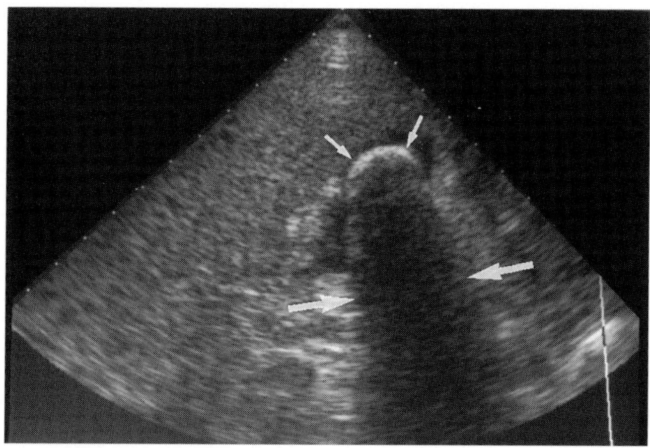

A

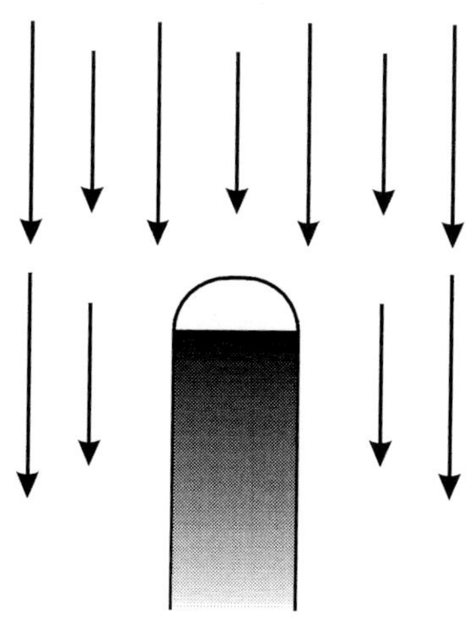

B

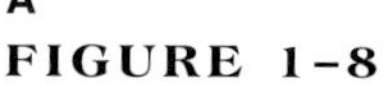

**FIGURE 1–8**

(**A**) A gallstone (small arrows) in the gallbladder is causing posterior acoustic shadowing (large arrows). (**B**) Diagram of acoustic shadowing shows an incident ultrasound beam (arrows) striking a stone (curved surface). The dark area deep to the stone is devoid of echoes, representing shadowing.

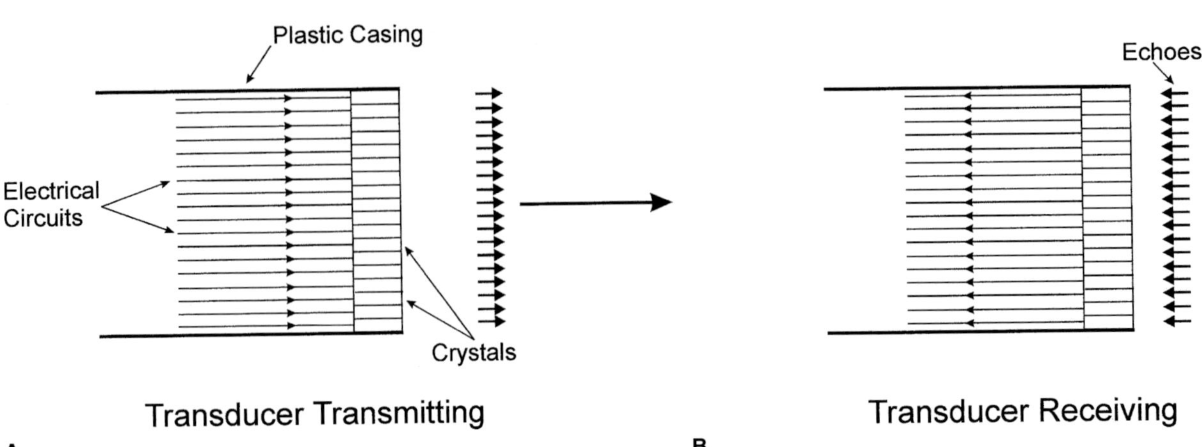


**FIGURE 1–9**

(**A**) *Transmitting*: Ultrasound transducer with piezoelectric crystals stimulated by electric impulses to transmit sound waves. (**B**) *Receiving*: Ultrasound transducer receiving returning echoes that stimulate crystals to produce electric impulses along the electric circuits.

able to produce 2.5-, 3-, and 4-MHz frequencies of ultrasound from the same series of crystals.

Ultrasound from a transducer is produced when electric pulses stimulate vibration in the crystals within the transducer head, setting up a series of ultrasound waves from each crystal. Most transducer heads contain multiple crystals that send out multiple small ultrasound waves to form a unified ultrasound beam. This is the beam that is transmitted into the tissue being interrogated. As this beam advances into the tissue, it is reflected and refracted, scattered and absorbed. Eventually, however, echoes return to the transducer front. These echoes cause the transducer crystals to vibrate, thereby generating electric pulses. All this takes time—a time interval that is measured by the ultrasound unit. The time it takes an echo to return to the transducer is related to the velocity of sound in tissue and thus to the distance between the reflecting interface and the transducer. And since the velocity of sound in tissue is relatively fixed at 1540 m/sec, the determining factor in the time interval is, in fact, the distance between the target and the transducer. As many echoes return to the transducer at many different times, different depths of echoes are created (Fig. 1–10); and as a series of echoes accumulates, an image begins to take form.

The strength or amplitude of returning echoes depends on the attenuation of the sound emitted from and returning to the transducer through a given tissue as well as on the strength of the interaction of the sound at various interfaces. The greater the distance that sound travels, the greater the degree of attenuation of the transmitted sound reaching this distance, and the greater the attenuation of the returning echo. Most returning echoes in diagnostic ultrasound are extremely attenuated. Therefore, to create a visible image, the returning echoes must be amplified. Since the amplification is performed in response to attenuation losses, it must be directly proportional to this attenuation. This is done electronically by *time gain compensation (TGC)*. The time gain compensation mechanism increases the amplitude of returning echoes directly proportionately to the amount of time it takes for these echoes to return. Echoes that arise deep in tissue—and hence take longer to return to the transducer—are also the most attenuated and weakest signals returning. Therefore, these weak echoes are more highly amplified by the time gain compensation mechanism of the ultrasound machine. The time gain compensation, also known as the TGC mechanism, is usually expressed on the equipment as a curve, which can be controlled by adjusting either the TGC knob or a series of TGC slide bars.

As echoes return to the transducer, they cause the piezoelectric crystals in the transducer to vibrate and produce electric pulses. These electric signals are ana-

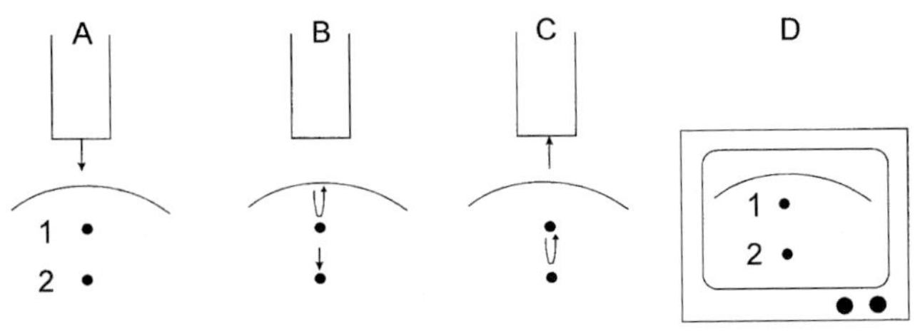


**FIGURE 1–10**

(**A**) Transducer emits an ultrasound wave (arrow) toward targets 1 and 2 at different depths. (**B**) Target 1 reflects an echo (curved arrow) while the sound wave (straight arrow) continues down to target 2. (**C**) Echo (straight arrow) from target 1 reaches the transducer while the deeper target 2 is reflecting an echo (curved arrow). (**D**) Ultrasound image of targets 1 and 2 placed at appropriate correlating depths.

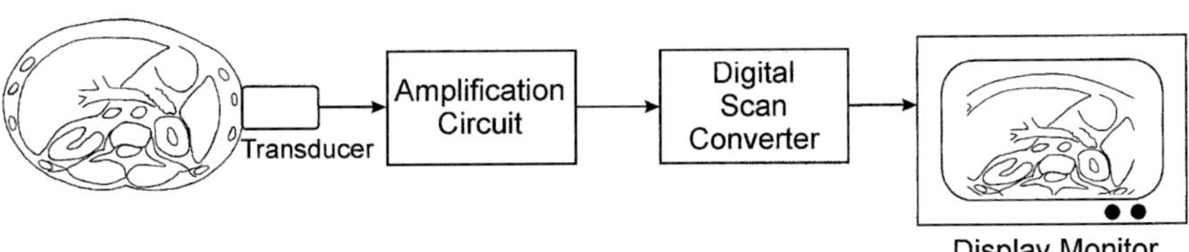


**FIGURE 1-11**

Simplified diagram of ultrasound unit processing information returning from a transducer to create an image on a display monitor.

lyzed and processed through complex circuitry to produce an image on a video screen. Basically, the electrical signals coming from the transducer are digitized in a unit known as a digital scan converter (Fig. 1–11). This digitized information undergoes processing and amplification, resulting in a collage of points that form an image on a video screen. The whiteness or blackness of each point (or pixel) depends on the amplitude of the echo that pixel represents. Echoes with high amplitude or energy produce a pixel that is fairly bright on the video screen, while echoes of low amplitude produce darker pixels on the video screen. Various shades of black, white, and gray comprise the ultrasound image, and these shades directly correspond to the amplitudes of the multitude of echoes creating the image.

One final note on how the video image is formed may be helpful. Most modern ultrasound provides "real-time" imaging, meaning that the image being observed corresponds exactly to the subject being examined; thus it moves or changes over "real" time. One "sees," for example, the liver or kidney moving with respiration or the heart beat. To achieve this real-time effect, multiple images or frames must be produced rapidly enough so that the eye perceives smooth motion on the video screen. The human eye detects flickering if the frame rate drops below 16 frames or refreshed images per second (2). Each video image is constructed with a series of vertical lines consisting of pixels of shades of gray (Fig. 1–12). The more vertical lines there are per image, the better the clarity of image. There is, however, a trade-off: The more lines per image, the longer each image takes to form, and therefore the lower the frame rate. In addition, the depth of tissue examined will affect the frame rate. Echoes from deeper tissue take longer to return to the transducer for processing. Therefore, examination of deeper tissues takes longer to form an image, thus decreasing the frame rate. When one examines deep tissues, the image often begins to flicker because the time required to refresh each image is so long that 16 frames cannot be created in 1 second. Many ultrasound units allow for adjustment of frame rate to keep the real-time imaging fairly smooth, making the image as clear as possible.

## Transducers

Two types of transducers are utilized in ultrasound units: mechanical and electronic array (Fig. 1–13). Mechanical

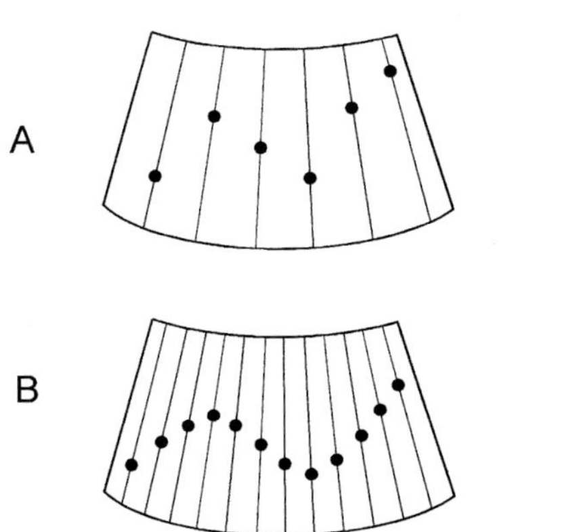


**FIGURE 1-12**

Real-time US images are created one frame, or one complete image, at a time. Each frame or image is created by a series of vertical scan lines. Fewer scan lines per frame, as in (**A**), allows quicker formation of the frame and more frames per second. More scan lines, as in (**B**), allows for a clearer, more representative image of the subject but take longer to create, resulting in fewer frames per second.

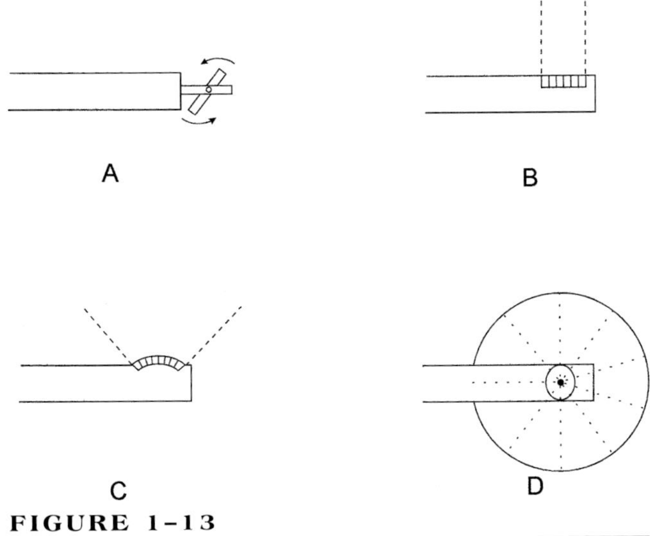


**FIGURE 1-13**

Transducers: (**A**) Mechanical transducer with rotating crystals. (**B**) Electronic array with crystals arranged in a straight line, giving a linear beam profile (dotted lines). (**C**) Curved electronic array with crystals arranged in curved fashion, giving a sector-type beam profile (dotted lines). (**D**) Radial beam profile (dotted lines) created by crystals typically rotating at the end of the probe.

transducers employ crystals mounted in a casing; these crystals are either oscillated back and forth or rotated through a given distance. The image formed is either a sector format encompassing a 45–90° arc or a radial image encompassing 360°. Electronic arrays are made up of multiple small crystals arranged either in a straight line (linear array) or over a curved surface (curved array). These crystals do not move as in the mechanical transducers; rather, the crystals are independently stimulated by electronic means. By adjusting the manner in which the crystals are stimulated, a linear image format or a sector image format can be created. In addition, such transducers can be electronically steered and focused.

## Knobology

Most ultrasound units have various controls whose function and effect on image quality the sonographer must understand. But since the types and labels of these controls vary depending on the unit's manufacturer, the discussion here is limited to general terms.

GAIN is the term used to describe the increase in amplitude necessary to register echoes returning to the US transducer. Most units have an overall gain control that adjusts the amplitude of all echoes returning to the transducer (Fig. 1–14). Most units have a TGC control which adjusts the amplitude of specific echoes at specific depths. Typically, the TGC is set so that the echoes are amplified proportionately to the depth from which they arise (Fig. 1–15). Overall gain is usually set at a level so that background noise just disappears. If the overall gain is set inappropriately, the image may be so bright or so dark that information such as subtle contrast between structures is lost.

The POWER setting available on US units allows control of the power output of the transducer. These output settings must meet FDA requirements for power deposition in human tissue. To date no biological hazards for diagnostic ultrasound have been demonstrated; however, the physician utilizing ultrasound should adhere to the ALARA principle—as low as reasonably achievable (5–8). This approach means that the power setting should be just high enough to achieve diagnostic objectives, and no higher.

DEPTH controls regulate how deep into tissue the imaging will extend. Depth of imaging can be adjusted

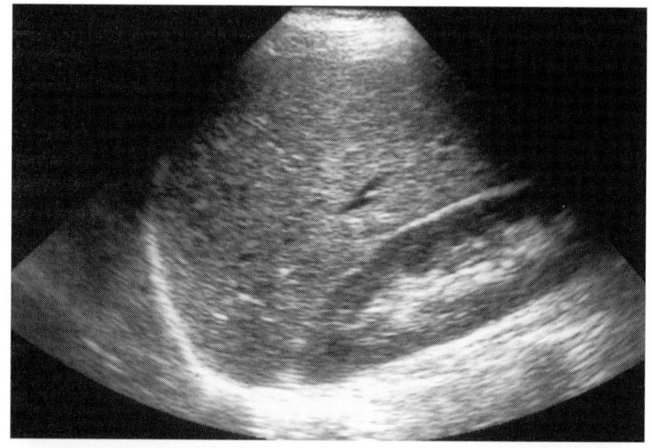

A

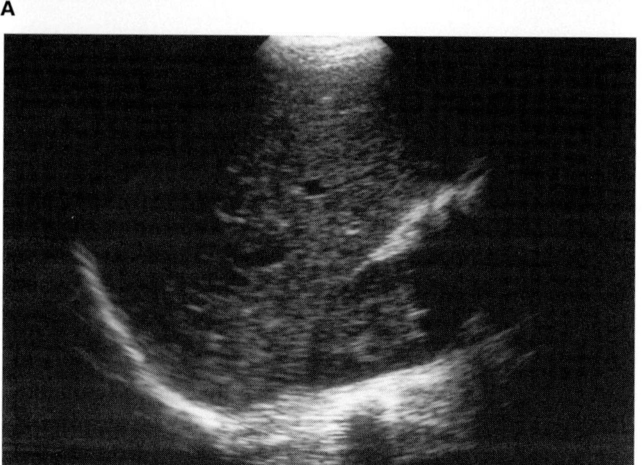

B

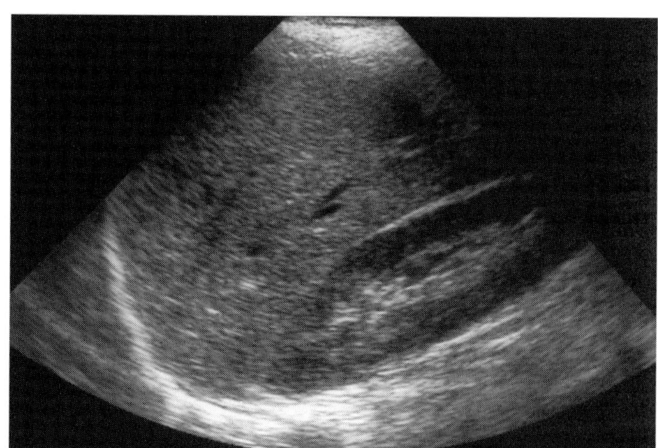

C

**FIGURE 1–14**

Gain control: (**A**) Gain settings too high, information lost. (**B**) Gain settings too low, information lost. (**C**) Appropriate gain settings, providing even level echoes.

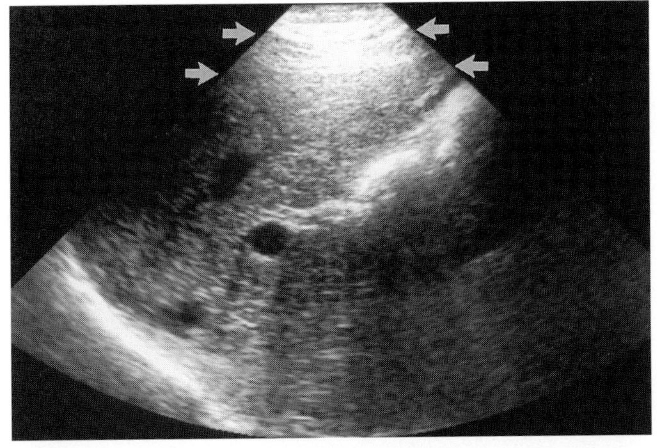

A

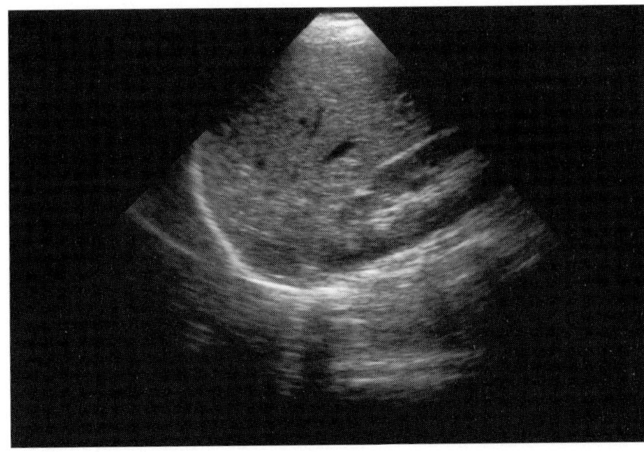

C

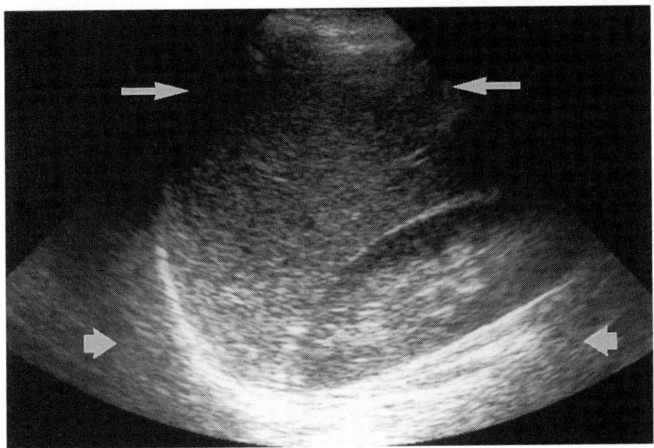

B

**FIGURE 1–15**

TGC settings: (**A**) Near-field (arrows) gain set too high. (**B**) Near-field (long arrows) gain set too low and far-field (arrowheads) gain set too high. (**C**) TGC set for even level gain at all depths.

to image only superficially or at greater depths. The major limiting factor is the depth to which the ultrasound beam can penetrate. Another limit is the fact that the deeper one images, the slower the frame rate for real-time imaging.

The FOCAL DEPTH or FOCAL ZONE is the level at which the ultrasound beam is best focused or its narrowest profile (see Fig 1–18). The optimum lateral resolution will occur at this level. Most ultrasound units allow for adjustment of the focal depth or zone.

Finally, several controls may be available to control image quality. By adjusting image contrast or log compression one can adjust the range of shades between the blackest black and whitest white in the image (Fig. 1–16). If the range is too narrow, the image will be high in contrast—having mostly black and white pixels—so subtle shades of gray (and hence helpful information) may be lost. Conversely, if the contrast range is too wide, the image may be too gray, and again, information is lost. Appropriate contrast setting varies depending on the subject being examined. Many units also provide PREPROCESSING and POSTPROCESSING adjustment to control other aspects of the image, including sharpness, edge-enhancement, graininess, smoothness of motion, and so on.

## Image Quality

The two main characteristics that describe ultrasound image quality are contrast sensitivity and spatial resolution. The *contrast sensitivity* of a system is its ability to detect differences in echo amplitudes (1–3). The varying amplitudes of echoes returning to the transducer yield varying shades of brightness on the image screen. High-amplitude echoes returning to the transducer are projected as very bright pixels on the image screen while low-amplitude echoes are projected as darker pixels on the image. High contrast sensitivity permits very subtle differences in echo amplitude to be detected while low contrast sensitivity does not. In practical terms, if the contrast sensitivity is high, lesions in the liver or pancreas with subtle differences in echogenicity can be distinguished from the adjacent normal tissue. Low contrast sensitivity would not allow such lesion detection. Contrast in an image can be adjusted by the

A

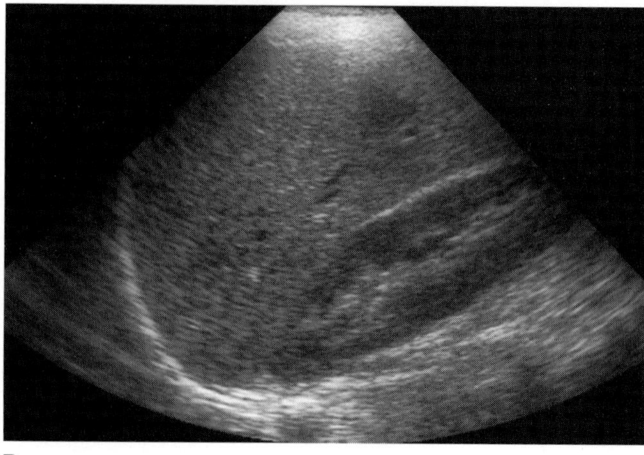

B

**FIGURE 1–16**

Image contrast: (**A**) Image contrast high, resulting in few shades of gray. The echoes are either very black or very white. (**B**) Image contrast low, so the image is very gray with little difference between the blackest black and whitest white.

overall gain, TGC, log compression (contrast), and postprocessing.

The second characteristic of ultrasound image quality is *spatial resolution*. This is the capacity of a system to demonstrate two points clearly as two distinct points. High spatial resolution demonstrates two separate points clearly even when the points lie a minute distance apart. Low spatial resolution would show two points as a single, blurred point. In EUS, spatial resolution translates into the ability of the system to clearly define the closely spaced layers of the esophageal or stomach wall as distinctly separate layers.

There are two components to spatial resolution in ultrasound (1–4, 6, 9–13). The first is *lateral resolution,* which concerns distinguishing separate points lying in a plane horizontal to the ultrasound beam. The shape of the ultrasound beam—the beam profile—determines the lateral resolution of a particular system. The ultrasound beam has three dimensions: length, width, and thickness. The thinner the beam, the better the lateral resolution (Fig. 1–17). The size of the transducer, the frequency of the transducer, and the focusing of the beam all affect the shape and hence thickness of the beam Smaller transducers allow for thinner ultrasound beams. The higher the frequency of the ultrasound utilized, the less the divergence of the ultrasound beam, the thinner the beam, and the better the lateral resolution. Focusing is also important for optimum lateral resolution (Fig. 1–18). With focusing, the beam can be prevented from diverging and forced to converge to a narrow three-dimensional beam to allow for high lateral resolution. Focusing can be done either with a lens attached to the transducer or by electronic means. With electronic focusing, the focal zone can be adjusted to varying depths. Modern array systems have focusing that can occur electronically at all levels to provide a sharp image at all depths.

*Axial resolution,* the second componet of resolution, refers to the ability of a system to depict two points in a plane parallel to the ultrasound beam. Axial resolution is determined by the pulse length that the transducer emits. Sound is emitted from the transducer in pulses—little packets of sound—at ~1000 pulses per second (3). This allows the transducer to act as a receiver between each discrete transmitted pulse. The length of the transmitted pulse determines the axial resolution (Fig. 1–19). The shorter the duration of each pulse, the better the axial resolution. The duration of each pulse (spatial pulse length) is determined by the type of crystals used in the transducer and the frequency of the sound emitted. The higher the frequency,

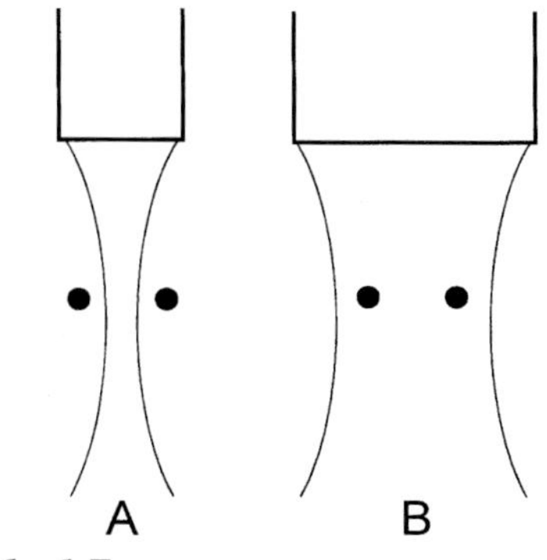


**FIGURE 1–17**

Lateral resolution depends on the US beam thickness. In (**A**) the beam is thin and can resolve the two distinct points. In (**B**) the beam is thick and cannot resolve the points.

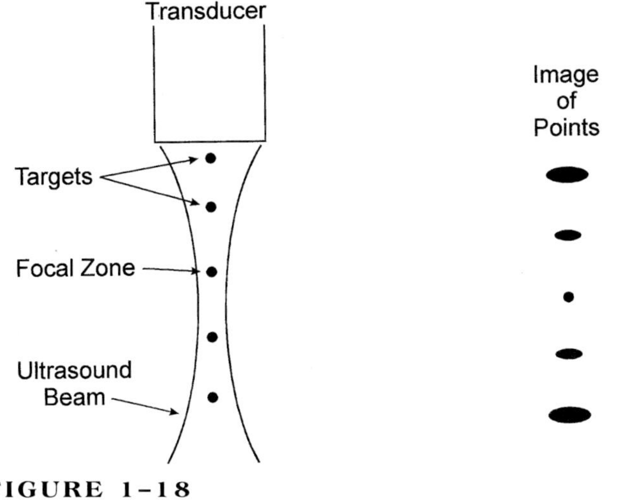


**FIGURE 1–18**

Focusing of an US beam causes the beam to narrow, allowing for improved lateral resolution. Point targets are shown. At the focal zone, the point targets are imaged clearly as points. Away from the focal zone, the beam widens and the points are distorted and blurred.

the shorter the pulse length. Therefore, the higher the frequency, the better the axial resolution.

In conclusion, the best resolution—including both lateral and axial resolution—can be achieved with higher frequency ultrasound. The compromise is that higher frequency ultrasound is also attenuated to a greater degree, so that deeper tissues are not well "imaged." To optimize resolution, one should use the highest frequency transducer that allows adequate penetration to the area of interest.

## Artifacts

With ultrasound imaging, multiple artifacts can cause confusion, and even misdiagnosis, if the sonographer is not familiar with them. This section addresses some of the artifacts routinely seen with ultrasound imaging.

### Reverberation

Reverberation artifact occurs when there is a reflected echo. In this case, on its journey back to the transducer, the returning echo hits an interface that is itself a strongly reflecting surface. The returning echo is again reflected back away from the transducer, and this type of back-and-forth reflection may happen several times before the echoes eventually return to the transducer (1,2,10,12,14). The depth at which an echo is placed in an image is directly proportional to the time it takes the echo to return to the transducer; thus, echoes first reflecting back and forth (reverberating) in a structure and only then returning to the transducer will generate a series of artifactual echoes that lie deep to the more superficial interface (Fig. 1–20). Classic areas for reverberation artifacts are those in which echogenic interfaces are next to fluid-filled structures, such as the near field of the urinary bladder or the near field of the gallbladder. On endoscopic ultrasound,

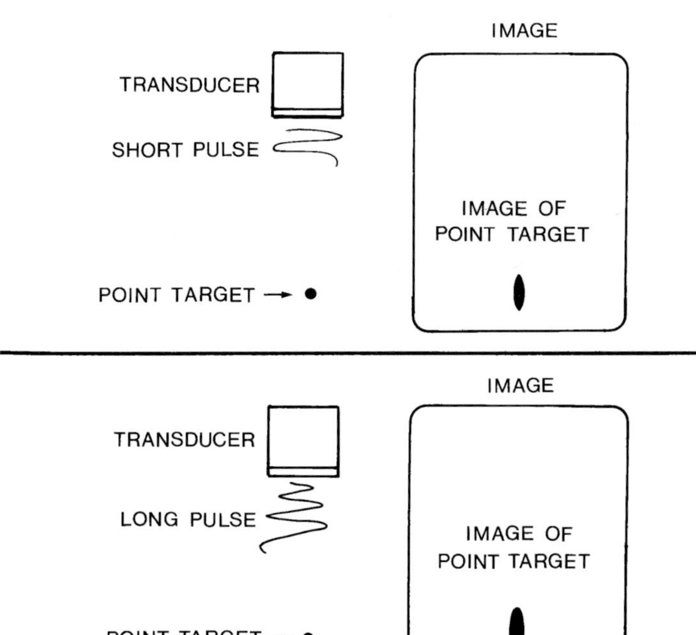


**FIGURE 1–19**

Axial resolution is determined by the duration of the pulse of US waves emitted by the transducer. If the pulse is short, a point target is more clearly imaged as a point, with better axial resolution. If the pulse is long, a point target is distorted or blurred, with poorer axial resolution.

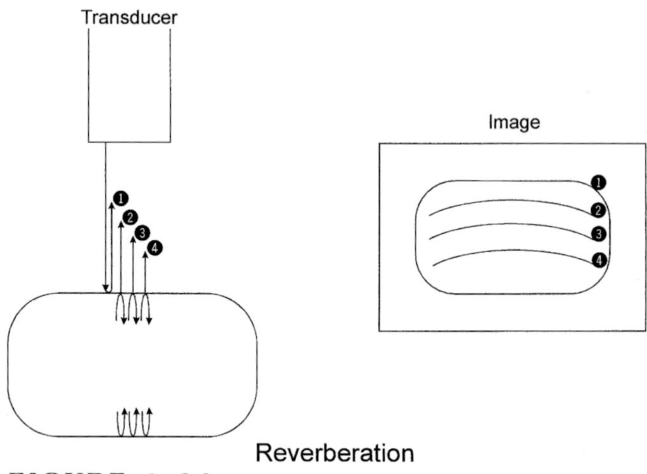


FIGURE 1-20

Reverberation artifact occurs when echoes bounce back and forth within a structure, then slowly return to the transducer (1, 2, 3, 4). Since the depth at which the echo is placed in the image depends on the time to return to the transducer, echoes 1, 2, 3, and 4 are placed at successively deeper levels. Echo 1 represents the echo from the true interface. Echoes 2, 3, and 4 are reverberation artifacts.

reverberation artifact is often seen within the water-filled balloon or water-filled stomach adjacent to the transducer (Fig. 1–21). The difficulty in interpretation lies in the fact that the reverberation artifact often obscures the near field. In addition, it causes artifactual echoes that can mimic debris, such as sludge in the gallbladder or the urinary bladder. This artifact can be diminished by adjusting the near-field gain (i.e., via the TGC curve).

## Ring-Down Artifact

Ring-down artifact, which is similar to reverberation artifact, can be seen when ultrasound strikes a structure that begins to resonate or ring, in much the same way that a tuning fork or fine crystal rings when struck. The structure is induced to vibrate for a long period of time, sending echoes back to the transducer as long as it continues to vibrate (10). Since the ultrasound machine places these echoes at a depth that correlates with time, one can see that if echoes are returning over a long period of time, they are slowly placed at deeper and deeper depths. The resulting trail of echoes extends deep to the ringing structure (Fig. 1–22). The deeper this trail goes, the less intense the echoes will be, hence the name "ring-down" artifact. Common structures that generate ring-down artifact are metal clips, metallic fragments (such as bullet fragments), and gas. For example, gas within bowel is highly reflective, demonstrating ring-down artifact deep to its highly reflective surface. This appearance can be diagnostic of gas within the bowel, the biliary tree, or even an abscess cavity.

## Shadowing

Shadowing occurs when US waves strike a structure that both reflects and absorbs a large amount of the ultrasound. Since the beam is either strongly reflected or absorbed by the structure, an area devoid of echoes is seen deep to the structure (see Fig. 1–8). This echo-poor area is known as a shadow. Classically, structures that produce shadowing are bony structures like the spine and ribs, stones such as gallstones or renal calculi,

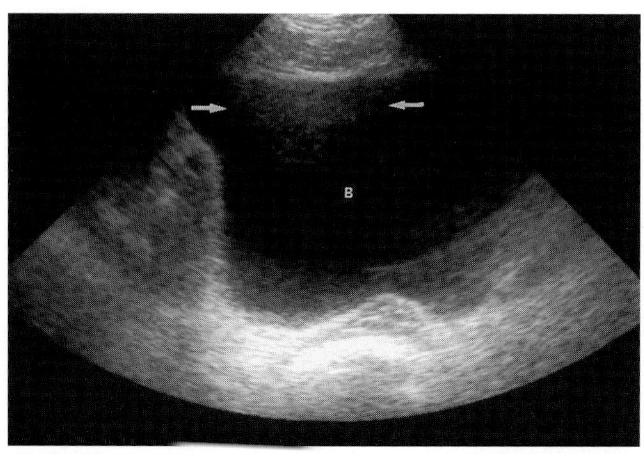


A

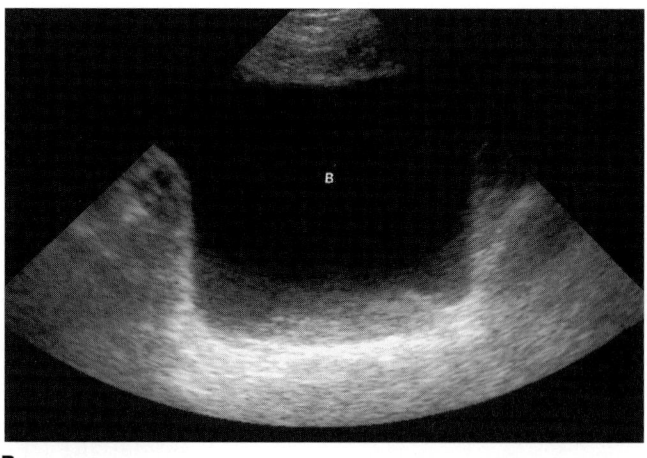


B

FIGURE 1-21

(**A**) Reverberation artifact (arrows) in the anterior urinary bladder (B). (**B**) Reverberation artifact improved by lowering the near-field gain via the TGC control.

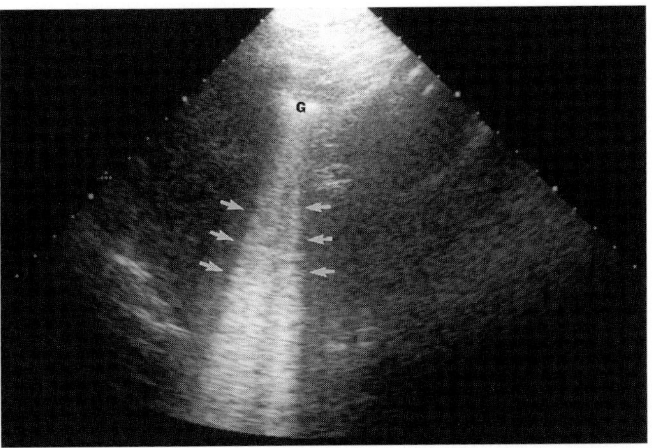


A

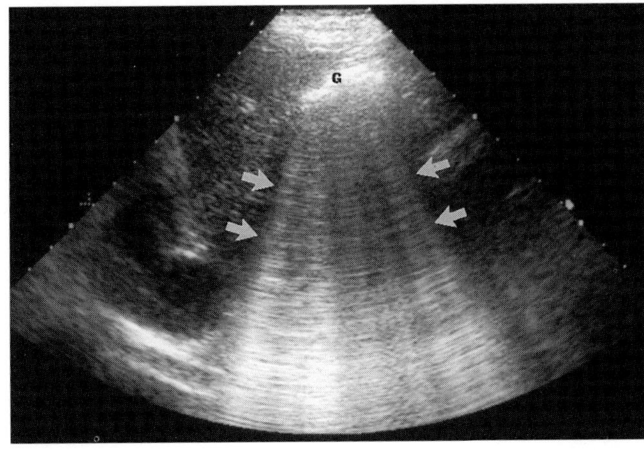


B

**FIGURE 1–22**

(**A**) Ring-down artifact (arrows) from gas (G) in the biliary tree. (**B**) Ring-down artifact (arrows) from gas (G) in the bowel.

and calcified granulomata or lymph nodes (Fig. 1–23). Whether a structure will shadow or not depends on the composition of the structure and how the US beam interacts with it (1,9,10,11,14,15). For example, the best way to produce shadowing from a gallstone is to use a high-frequency transducer and place the focal zone at the same depth as the stone so that the US beam is thinnest at the level of the stone. The higher frequency ultrasound will be absorbed to a greater degree, causing more shadowing from the stone.

Shadowing can be used to aid in diagnosis. For example, echogenic mobile structures that shadow in the gallbladder are nearly always gallstones. Lack of shadowing in this case may simply imply sludge balls or even blood clot. In addition, reference is sometimes made to "dirty" versus "clean" shadowing. Clean shadowing is the dark, echo-poor shadow seen deep to a stone or bony structure. Dirty shadowing is actually ring-down artifact typically produced deep to gas-containing structures. Being able to make the distinction will aid in correct sonographic diagnosis.

## Enhancement

Enhancement occurs deep to a structure that does not attenuate much sound but does allow a large amount of sound to be transmitted through it (Fig. 1–24). Such structures typically contain either fluid or tissue that does not attenuate the ultrasound. Therefore, the intensity of sound reaching tissues deep to such structures is high, and the reflected echoes from these deeper tissues is higher. This results in brighter echoes behind

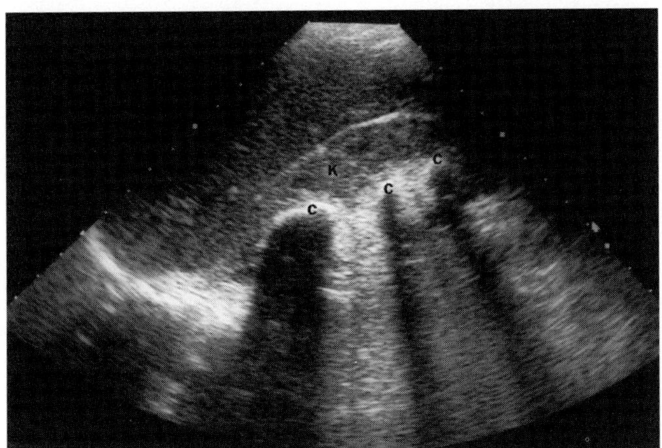


**FIGURE 1–23**

Shadowing (arrows) from renal calculi (C) in the kidney (K).

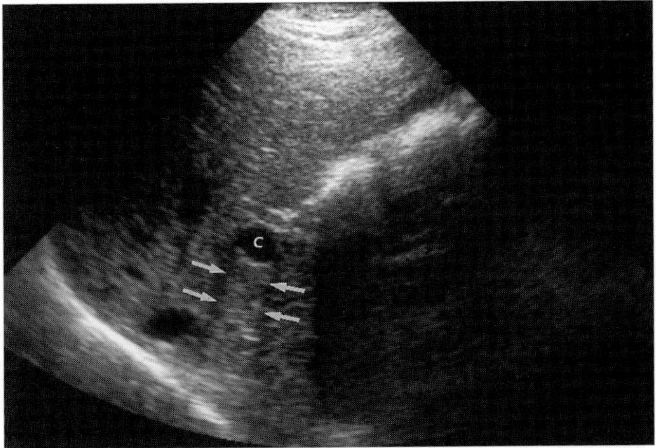


**FIGURE 1–24**

Enhancement is the brighter echoes (arrows) seen deep to a hepatic cyst (c).

these less attenuating structures (1,10,11,14,15). Classic structures that allow enhancement of sound behind them are fluid-filled structures such as the gallbladder, vascular structures such as the portal vein or hepatic veins, cysts such as hepatic cysts, the urinary bladder, and various fluid collections such as pseudocysts, abscesses, and hematomas. In addition, certain solid lesions such as hemangiomas of the liver and lymphomatous nodules may not attenuate sound and hence permit enhancement.

## Off-Axis Artifacts and Section-Thickness Artifacts

Because the US beam has a three-dimensional profile, the beam may be thicker than the structure being examined (Fig. 1–25) (1,2,9–12,14). If that is the case, echoes may be spuriously placed into this structure on the image display. A classic example is the artifactual appearance of echoes in a fluid-filled structure such as a cyst or the gallbladder. These artifactual echoes may mimic sludge or debris. The echoes arise from tissue lying adjacent to the cyst or gallbladder, and are produced by the wider portion of the US beam. Such artifacts can be minimized by placing the focal zone—the narrowest portion of the ultrasound beam—at the same depth as the cyst or gallbladder.

## Refraction Artifact

Because sound has wave characteristics, it can be refracted when it undergoes a change in velocity traveling from one tissue to another (see Fig. 1–5). Such refraction can lead to refraction artifacts. In this case, certain structures may appear to be lying in slightly different positions in the image than they actually do in the body (14). Refraction of the sound beam may also occur at the curved surfaces of rounded structures, such as blood vessels, the gallbladder, or the urinary bladder. In these cases, the ultrasound is refracted away from the rounded structure, leading to shadowing that extends deep to the edges of the structures (Fig. 1–26).

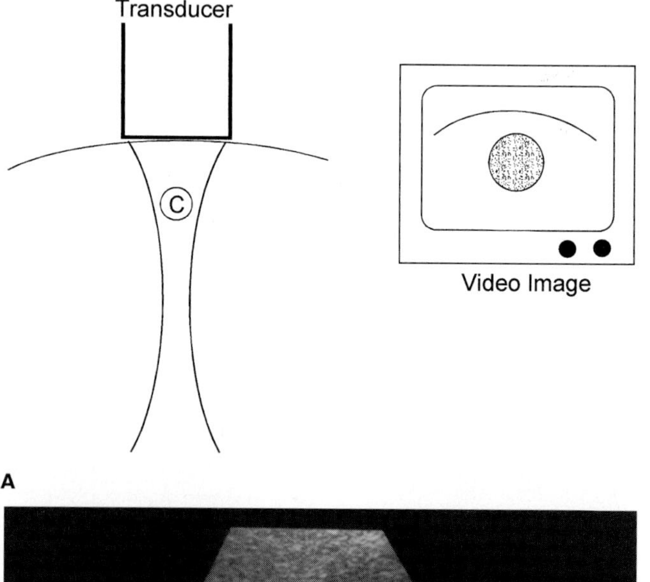


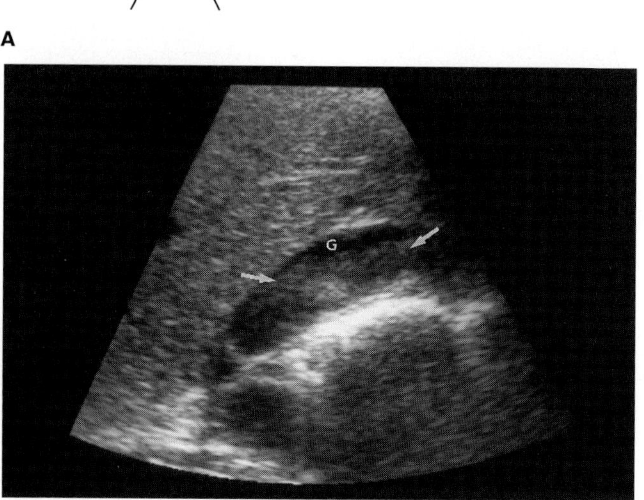


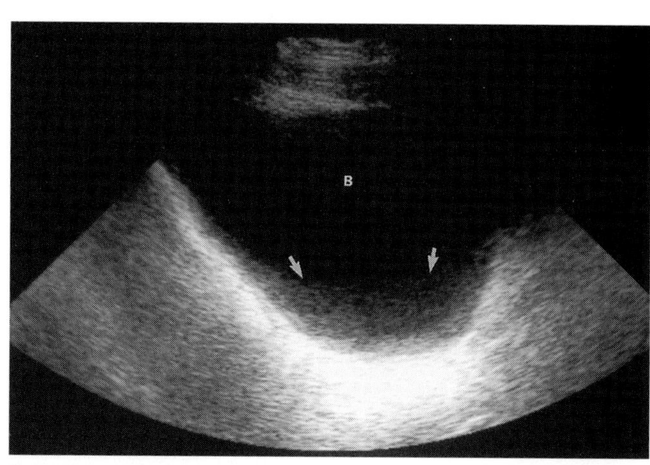


**FIGURE 1–25**

(**A**) Ultrasound beam whose width is greater than the diameter of a cyst (C). The video image on the right therefore shows a cyst with artifactual echoes in it rather than an anechoic cyst. (**B**) Artifactual echoes (arrows) placed within the gallbladder (G) owing to off-axis artifacts that mimic sludge. (**C**) Off-axis artifactual echoes (arrows) in the urinary bladder (B).

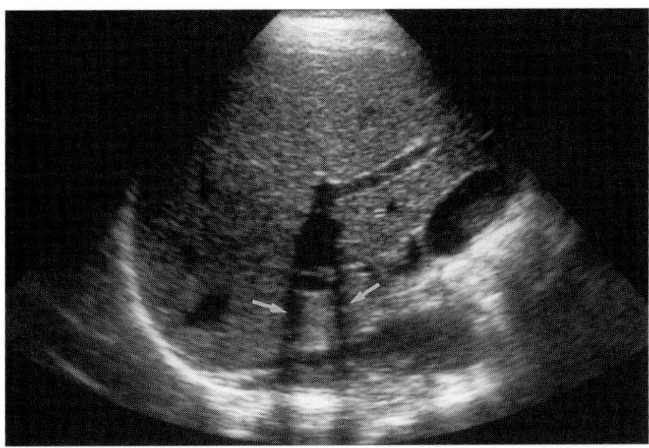

**FIGURE 1–26**

Refraction artifact caused by refraction of the US beam as it strikes the rounded edge of the portal vein, causing shadowing (arrows) deep to the vein edges.

## Mirror-Image Artifact

Mirror-image artifact occurs when there is a highly reflective surface such as the hemidiaphragm or rectal gas that functions as an acoustic mirror. Sound bounces off the acoustic mirror, is reflected off an adjacent interface back to the acoustic mirror, and then is reflected back to the transducer (Fig. 1–27). The ultrasound machine cannot determine how the returning echoes were created; it places the echoes at a depth corresponding to the time it took for them to return to the transducer and orients them in the direction in which the transducer is pointing (10). Classic examples of mirror- imaging artifact occur at the right hemidiaphragm where lesions in the liver appear above the diaphragm. Another classic location is in the pelvis where the highly reflective gas in the rectum acts as an acoustic mirror and artifactually creates a fluid collection deep to the bladder (14).

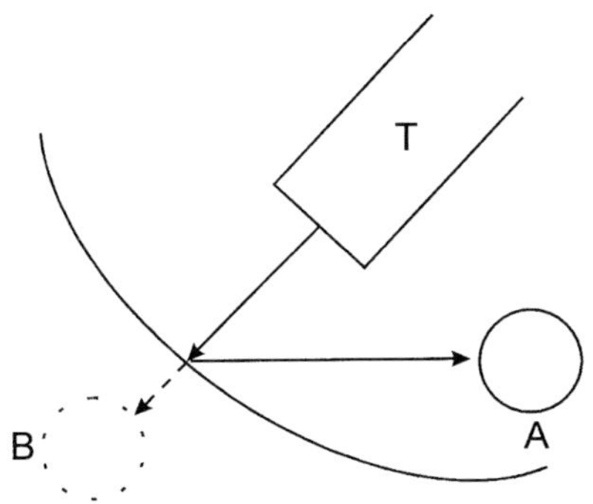


A

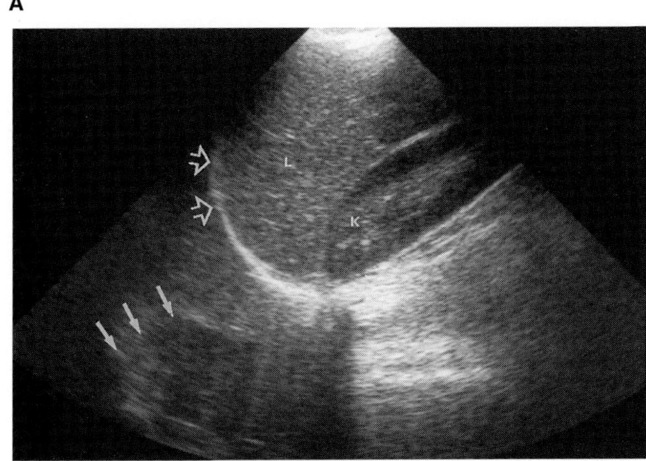


B

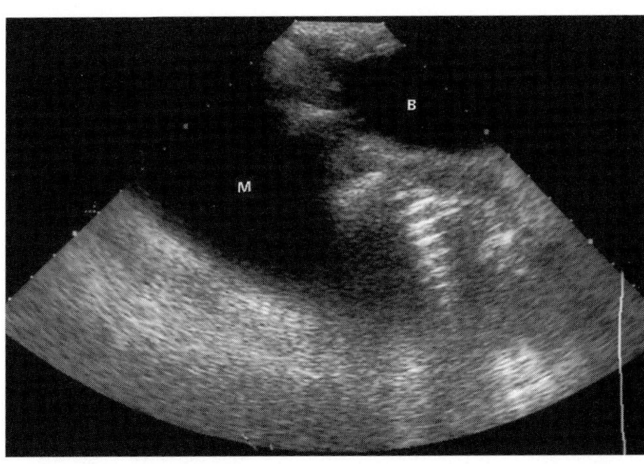


C

**FIGURE 1–27**

(**A**) Diagrams of mirror-image artifact occurring at the hemidiaphragm causing the subject at A to artifactually appear above the diaphragm at B. (**B**) Mirror image of right kidney (long arrows) above the right hemidiaphragm (arrowheads). True right kidney (K), liver (L). (**C**) Mirror image of the urinary bladder (M) seen deep to true urinary bladder (B).

## References


1. Burns PN. Ultrasound imaging and Doppler: Principles and instrumentation. In: Ultrasonography of the Urinary Tract, 3d ed. Baltimore: Williams & Wilkins, 1991, pp 1–33.
2. Curry RTS, Dowdey JE, Murry RC. Ultrasound. In: Christensen's Physics of Diagnostic Radiology, 4th ed. Philadelphia: Lea and Febiger, pp 323–371.
3. Sprawls P. Ultrasound imaging. In: Physical Principles of Medical Imaging. Aspen Publishers, Inc., 1989, pp 389–406.
4. Zagzebski JA. Physics and instrumentation in Doppler and B mode ultrasonography. In: Introduction to Vascular Ultrasonography, 3d ed. Philadelphia: W. B. Saunders, 1992, pp 19–44.
5. Frizzell LA. Conclusions regarding biological effects of ultrasound for diagnostically relevant exposures. J Ultrasound Med 13:69–72, 1994.
6. Halpern EJ. Effect of focal zone on a curved array transducer. Invest Rad 28:7–10, 1993.
7. Merritt CRB. Safety issues in diagnostic ultrasound. Syllabus Special Course: Ultrasound 1991. Radiologic Society of North America, Inc., 1991, pp 73–80.
8. Wu J, Cubberley F, Gormley G, Szako TL. Temperature rise generated by diagnostic ultrasound in a transcranial phantom. Ultrasound Med Biol 21:561–568, 1995.
9. Burns PN. Principles of ultrasound. Syllabus Special Course: Ultrasound 1991. Radiologic Society of North America, 1991, pp 33–55.
10. Cooperberg PL. Artifacts in ultrasound. Syllabus Special Course: Ultrasound 1991. Radiologic Society of North America, 1991, pp 57–72.
11. Kremkau FW, Taylor KJ. Artifacts in ultrasound imaging. J Ultrasound Med 5:227–237, 1986.
12. Laing FC. Commonly encountered artifacts in clinical ultrasound. Semin Ultrasound CT, MR 4:27, 1983.
13. McDicken WN. Diagnostic Ultrasonic Principles in Use of Instruments. New York: John Wiley and Sons, 1981.
14. Sanders RC. Atlas of Ultrasonographic Artifacts and Variants. Chicago: Medical Publishers, Inc., 1986.
15. Sprawls P. Ultrasound productions and interactions. In: Physical Principles of Medical Imaging. Aspen Publishers, Inc., 1989, pp 371–388.

CHAPTER

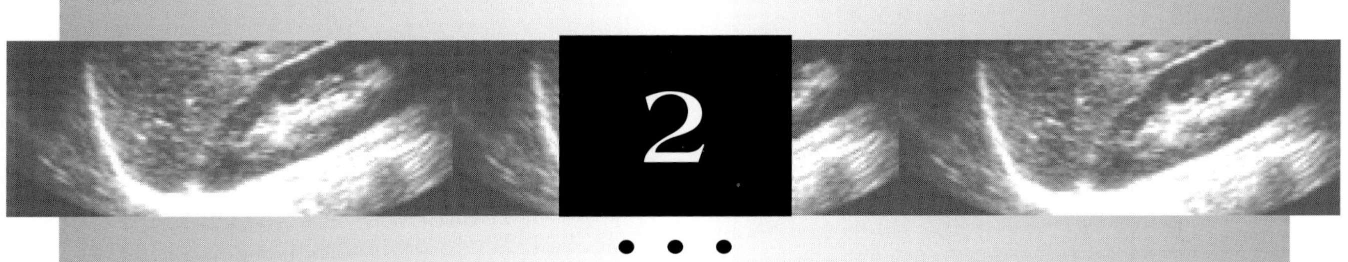

# The Radial Scanning Echoendoscope

Amitabh Chak

Endoscopic ultrasonography has emerged as a significant advance in diagnostic gastrointestinal endoscopy. A high-frequency transducer placed at the tip of an endoscope enables endoscopists to obtain high-resolution transmural sonographic images of the intestinal wall and surrounding structures. Intraluminal sonographic imaging is a marked improvement over transabdominal sonographic imaging, largely because of the endoscopist's ability to place the transducer in close proximity to lesions, avoiding intervening air, fat, and bone.

Two types of endosonographic instruments have been developed (1–4): sector (or radial) scanning instruments with a scanning plane perpendicular to the axis of the endoscope, and linear or convex array instruments that scan in a plane parallel to the axis of the endoscope (see Fig. 2–1). Each method has its inherent advantages and disadvantages. Sector scanning instruments have had wider appeal because these instruments produce a radial 360° image, which is easier to orient. The endosonographic images in the transverse plane produced with this type of instrument are similar to computed tomographic (CT) images, and are more familiar to gastroenterologists.

The EU-M20 system for endoscopic ultrasound, commercially available from Olympus America, Inc. (Lake Success, New York), is the latest in a series of radial scanning instruments with mechanically rotated transducers. This chapter explains the features of this sector scanning system and details its operation. The next chapter deals with the Pentax/Hitachi system for endoscopic ultrasound, which is designed for convex scanning with a sonographic image plane parallel to the endoscope.

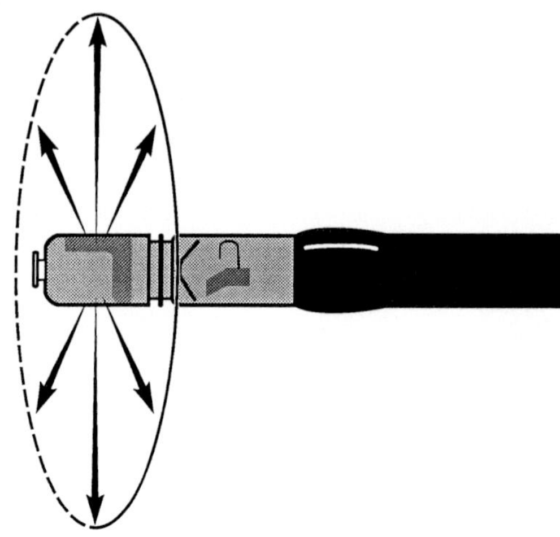

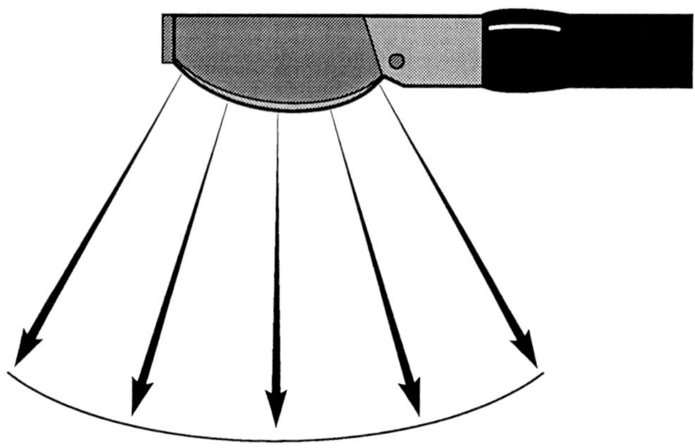

**FIGURE 2–1**

The plane of sonographic imaging with radial scanning ultrasound endoscopes (top) and convex array ultrasound endoscopes (bottom).

## Features and Components of the EU-M20

The EU-M20 is a portable ultrasound unit that produces a pulsed B-mode radial image. It is designed for use with the mechanically rotating transducers of Olympus ultrasound endoscopes and endoscopic probes. The switchable frequencies of 7.5 and 12 MHz available with these endoscopes are ideal for high-resolution intraluminal real-time sonography. Compared to the previous generations of Olympus ultrasound units, viz. EU-M2 and EU-M3, the EU-M20 offers several major improvements including more compact, lighter weight endoscopes with improved maneuverability; a more durable motor drive; submersible endoscopes for disinfection; and several pre- and postprocessing features for image analysis and documentation. The basic system consists of an image processing unit with attachable keyboard, a pulse unit, a display monitor, a Polaroid camera, a remote control as well as a foot switch, and a water pump—all of which can be mounted on a trolley designed for the system (see Fig. 2–2). The image processing unit can be connected to video recorders as well as hard-copy devices. A trackball, which greatly eases movement of electronic cursors on the displayed image, is also available. The system is designed for use with the ultrasound gastroscope, duodenoscope, and colonoscope (GF-UM20, JF-UM20, and CF-UM20, respectively) of the UM20 series, but can also be used with the ultrasound endoscopes of the UM3 series. A 7.5-MHz ultrasound probe, the Olympus UM-1W, which can be passed through the biopsy channel of an endoscope, is also available for use in countries other than the United States.

### Control Panel, Remote Control and Foot Control

The EU-M20 unit is equipped with a membrane keyboard (Fig. 2–3). Because it is flat, it can easily be cleaned by wiping with alcohol. The disadvantage of this design is that the keys respond only when a fair amount of pressure is applied. Typing labels on images can be somewhat frustrating when using this keyboard. LEDs mounted on the upper right corner of function switches are off when the function is nonoperational (e.g., during freeze), turn green when the function can

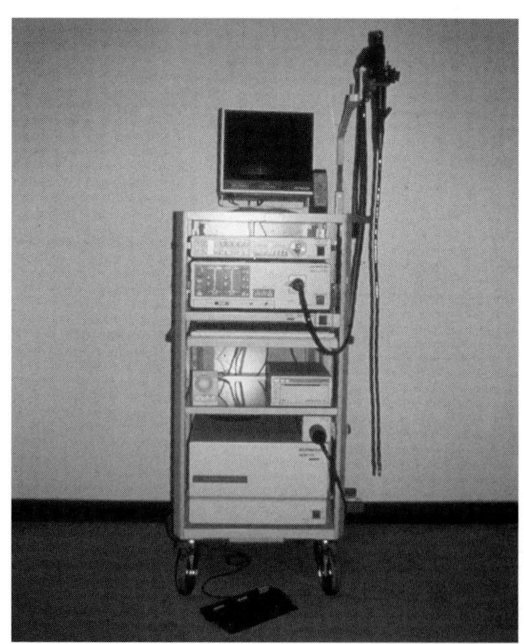

**FIGURE 2–2**

Trolley-based EU-M20 system: The endoscope is hanging on the right; the display monitor is on the top of the trolley; and the EU-M20 processor is on the bottom shelf. Foot controls can be seen on the floor in front of the trolley. The trackball is seen to the left on the shelf just above the EU-M20 processor.

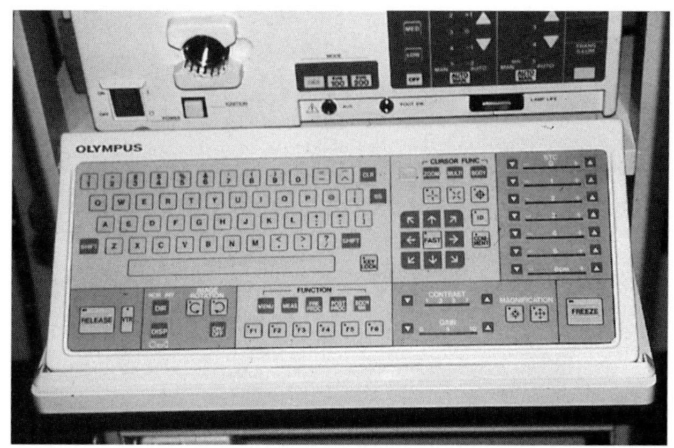

**FIGURE 2–3**

Keyboard control panel of the EU-M20.

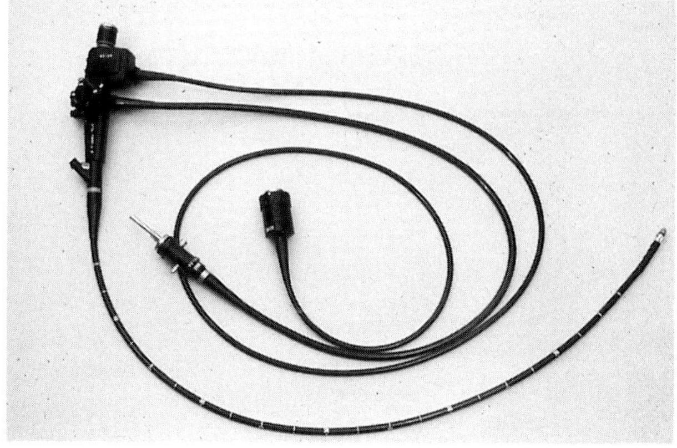

**FIGURE 2–4**

The Olympus GF-UM20 ultrasonic gastrofiberscope.

be selected, and turn orange when the function is usable. A standard alphanumeric and character keyboard for labeling is located on the upper left corner of the panel. Buttons that control recording devices, direction of scanning, choice of sector displayed, rotation of the image, processing functions, gain, contrast, magnification, and image freeze are positioned from left to right at the bottom of the panel. The sensitivity time control (STC) for each of the seven dynamic ranges is at the right of the panel. Controls for movement of the cursor are situated in between the STC and the alphanumeric keyboard. Cursor movement using directional arrows can be painfully slow when labeling or measuring lesions during an examination. A trackball, which allows faster and easier cursor movement, is available as a separate attachment; it is highly recommended.

An infrared transmitter which allows remote control of all the functions located at the bottom of the control panel is also available with the system. This feature has limited use because the endoscopist is positioned next to the standard control panel, and hence has no need for remote controls. On the other hand, the foot control (shown on the floor in Fig. 2–2) that allows activation of the image recording unit, pauses the VCR, and controls image freeze is extremely useful: it allows the endoscopist to control recording while keeping both hands on the endoscope.

## Endoscopes

The Olympus GF-UM20 (Fig. 2–4), JF-UM20-7.5/12 (Fig. 2–5), and CF-UM20-7.5/12 (Fig. 2–6) are respectively the ultrasonic gastrofiberscope, duodenofiberscope, and colonofiberscope available for use with the EU-M20 system. Detailed specifications of these instruments are given in Table 2–1. The 20 series designation signifies that the instruments are completely waterproof, and can be submerged for thorough cleaning and disinfection. The objective eyepiece, tip deflection controls, biopsy channels (see Fig. 2–7), elevator (JF-UM20 only), and shaft of these instruments are largely the same as standard Olympus fiberscopes. These scopes contain a dc motor with a flexible shaft that rotates the transducer at the tip of the endoscope. This motor is mounted in a housing between the eyepiece and tip deflection controls, as shown in (Figure 2–7). These endoscopes are easier to maneuver than their predecessors because the drive motor is lighter and more compact. Balloons can be mounted into grooves around the transducer housing and need not be tied down to maintain a seal (Fig. 2–8). The GF-UM20 has forward oblique optics, the JF-UM20 has side viewing optics, and the CF-UM20 has forward optics. The GF-UM20 and the JF-UM20 have a rounder, slimmer tip than their predecessors, which facilitates

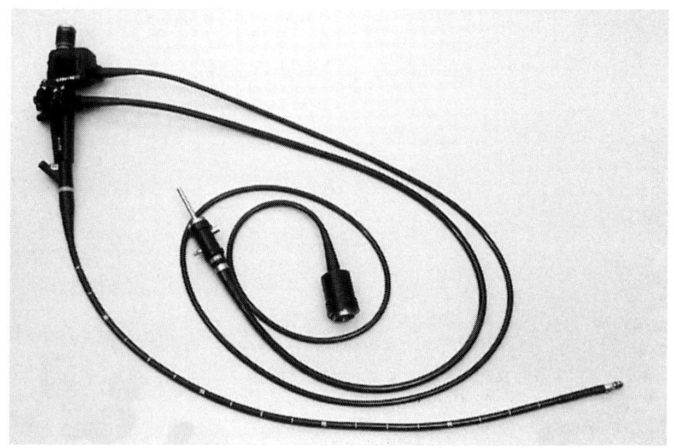

**FIGURE 2–5**

The Olympus JF-UM20 ultrasonic duodenofiberscope.

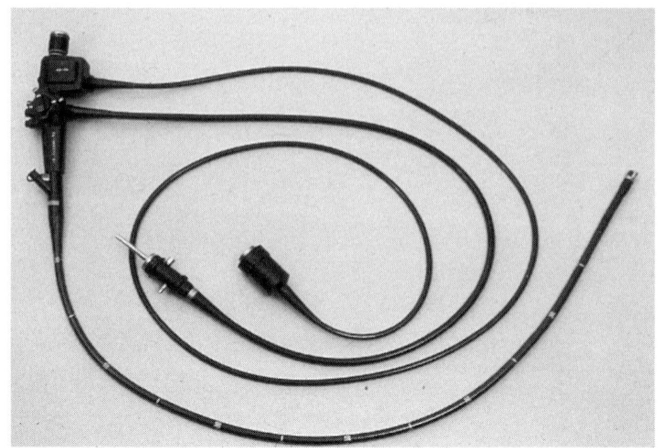

**FIGURE 2–6**

The Olympus CF-UM20 ultrasonic colonofiberscope.

esophageal intubation, insertion through the pylorus, and traversal through mild to moderate strictures.

## Valve Features

Suction valves and air/water valves on these ultrasound endoscopes have a two-step button. The normal endoscopic functions of lens cleaning with water or suctioning via the biopsy channel can be performed by pressing the appropriate valve to the first step. In addition, water can be introduced into the balloon around the transducer by pushing the air/water valve fully to the second step. This water can be aspirated out of the balloon by pushing the suction valve fully to the second step. These two-step valves allow the endoscopist to control balloon distension without relinquishing the endoscope shaft or deflection controls.

**TABLE 2–1**

**Specifications of UM20 Ultrasound Endoscopes**

| | GF-UM20 | JF-UM20 | CF-UM20 |
|---|---|---|---|
| Shaft diameter | 11.7 mm | 11.2 mm | 13.7 mm |
| Tip diameter | 13.2 mm | 12.5 mm | 17.4 mm |
| Shaft length | 105.5 cm | 125 cm | 132.5 cm |
| Channel diameter | 2 mm | 2.2 mm | 2.8 mm |
| Angulation: | | | |
| Up/Down | 130° | 120°/90° | 180° |
| Left/Right | 90° | 90°/110° | 160° |
| Optical direction | 45° Forward oblique | Side | Forward |
| Angle of view | 80° | 80° | 120° |
| Ultrasound frequency | Switchable 7.5/12 MHz | 7.5 or 12 MHz | 7.5 or 12 MHz |
| Focal distance | 30 mm (7.5 MHz) 25 mm (12 MHz) | 30 mm (7.5 MHz) 25 mm (12 MHz) | 30 mm (7.5 MHz) 25 mm (12 MHz) |

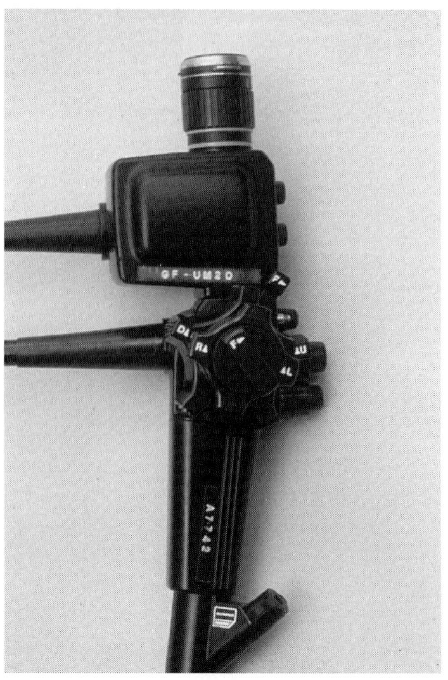


**FIGURE 2–7**

The head of the GF-UM20 ultrasound endoscope showing eyepiece, drive motor in housing, tip deflection controls, and biopsy port. The frequency switch button, release button, freeze button, and two-step suction and air/water valves (in order, from top to bottom) can be seen in profile on the right.

## Electronic Controls on Endoscopes

A freeze button mounted above the suction valve allows the endoscopist to rapidly capture images (seen in profile in Fig. 2–7). A release button mounted on the drive

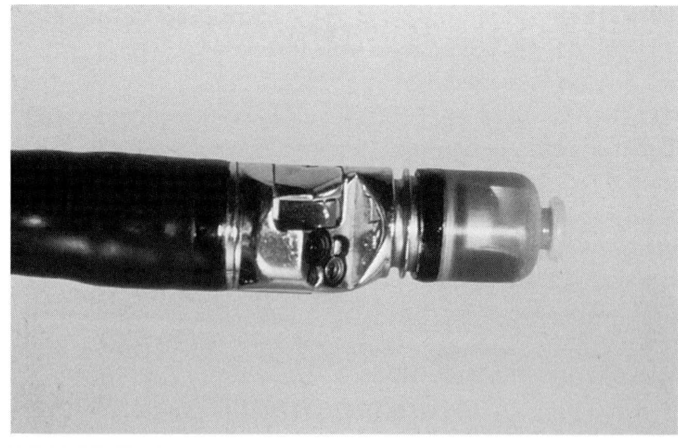

**FIGURE 2–8**

Tip of the GF-UM20. The plastic-encased transducer can be seen at the tip, with a black sealing ring at the bottom of the transducer casing. The metal groove below the transducer casing is for balloon attachment. The oblique optics and biopsy channel are seen in the metallic portion just below the groove.

motor above the freeze control operates the photo documentation unit connected to the EU-M20 (seen in profile in Fig. 2–7). The GF-UM20 is the only instrument in this series that has both a 7.5-MHz and a 12-MHz transducer contained in the casing at the tip of the scope. Thus, this particular endoscope can be operated at either frequency. A frequency switch that allows selection of frequencies is mounted on the GF-UM20 just above the release switch (seen in profile in Fig. 2–7).

### Uses

The combination of a limited angle of view and a long rigid tip makes these instruments more difficult to maneuver than standard endoscopes. Endoscopic examination with these instruments cannot substitute for routine endoscopy. Biopsy forceps or cytology needles introduced through the biopsy channels of these endoscopes are not imaged in the perpendicular sonographic plane. No technique for obtaining tissue samples under sonographic guidance using these instruments has yet been developed. Thus, most endoscopists prefer standard endoscopy for obtaining biopsies or needle aspiration cytology.

Established indications for endosonography generally involve the upper tract and surrounding structures. Therefore, the gastrofiberscope (GF-UM20) is the ultrasound endoscope used most often by endosonographers. The JF-UM20 optics and elevator are designed to allow placement of catheters into the pancreaticobiliary system. With this endoscope, however, one cannot perform most of the complex maneuvers necessary for ERCP. Thus, this instrument is rarely, if ever, used. The forward optics of the CF-UM20 are necessary for colonoscopy. The radial ultrasound image produced by this instrument contains a 60° wedge defect because the optics of the CF-UM20 are mounted adjacent to the transducer. Aside from the staging of rectal cancers, no indications have yet been established for the ultrasound examination of the lower tract. Many ultrasound endoscopists prefer to use the GF-UM20 for examination of the rectum because the image does not contain a wedge defect. Thus, the use of the CF-UM20 is generally limited to investigational protocols and select cases.

## Catheter Probes

Catheter probes for use with the EU-M20 have been under development. The UM-1W, which has a 3.4-mm diameter, a rotating 7.5-MHz transducer, a 15-mm rigid tip, and a 15-mm focal distance, was the first commercially available probe. Because this probe had limited penetration depth and poor lateral resolution (3,4), no significant clinical applications were developed for it.

The next-generation commercially available probes from Olympus, the UM-2R and UM-3R, offer scanning frequencies of 12 and 20 MHz, respectively. They have a diameter of 2.4 mm, allowing passage of most endoscopes through the accessory channel. Imaging with these probes appears to be much better than that obtainable with their predecessor. Clinical applications are still under development (5,6). It appears that these probes may be useful for staging early superficial gastric or esophageal cancers. They may also find limited applicability in the imaging of stenotic lesions and small submucosal tumors, as well as in intraductal imaging of pancreatic or biliary strictures.

## Esophagoprobe

A specialized blind ultrasonic probe designed for the staging of stenotic esophageal cancers has also been developed for the Olympus EU-M20 system. Termed the esophagoprobe, this probe has a design similar to that of the standard echoendoscope. However, in order to make it slimmer, the fiberoptics and accessory channel have been eliminated. This probe has a 7.9-mm diameter and a bougie-shaped tip with a channel for over-the-guide wire insertion. This scanning frequency is fixed at 7.5 MHz. Binmoeller et al. (7) have demonstrated the utility of this probe in staging highly stenosing esophageal cancers that cannot be traversed with conventional echoendoscopes.

## Preliminary Procedures

### Initial Setup for Imaging

Initial adjustments need to be made to the EU-M20 after it has been installed. The name of the hospital can be entered by activating the menu. Once entered, the name is stored in memory and subsequently appears on top of all images. After the resistance switch in the back of the monitor has been turned on, brightness and contrast on the monitor should be adjusted using the sliding switches mounted in the front on the display panel. The display monitor has a gray scale on the left. Brightness should be at a level such that the low end of the scale is black. Contrast should be adjusted such that characters can be read clearly from a distance. The gain button on the control panel changes the intensity of the ultrasound. Too high a gain gives a whited-out image, whereas too low a gain gives a dark image with limited penetration. Generally, the gain should be set at the lower end of the scale. It may need to be increased by one or two steps when performing examinations on overweight patients. The sensitivity time controls (STC) on the right side of the control panel allow adjustment of the echo intensity from various depths. The STC is used to compensate for the loss of intensity in echoes at increasing depths due to attenuation. Usually, the STC is set at the lowest level at depths close to the transducer and increases gradually at farther distances. The STC of the EU-M20 needs to be set for each frequency. But each setting is stored in memory, so that the STC seldom needs resetting. Contrast in the image can be further adjusted by using the contrast button on the control panel.

Preprocessing adjustments may include the automatic gain control (AGC) and edge enhancement. AGC allows discrimination of weaker signals which can be obscured by powerful echoes near the transducer. This feature is seldom needed for gastrointestinal applications, and is usually turned off. Edge enhancement can help sharpen differences between tissues with different densities. Layers on an endosonographic image of the normal gastrointestinal wall are generally easily distinguishable, even without the use of edge enhancement. The postprocessing feature on the EU-M20 allows adjustment of the brightness of the displayed image according to the intensity of the echo. Examinations are generally performed in a linear postprocessing mode, where the brightness is directly proportional to the intensity of the echo signal. It is a good idea for beginners to become familiar with the various preprocessing and postprocessing features of the EU-M20 by imaging various objects in a container of water.

## Pre-examination Preparation

Patient preparation for endoscopic ultrasonography is the same as that for other endoscopic examinations. Preprocedural therapy with oral simethicone (8) or mucolytic-antifoam solution (9) has been reported to improve imaging of the upper gastrointestinal tract. This therapy should be seriously considered in patients who, having undergone gastric resection, often have a lot of bile in their gastric remnants. For rectal examinations, it is a good idea to clean out the colon with a standard preparation for colonoscopy because small amounts of stool can interfere with imaging.

### *Endoscope Attachment*

Like other endoscopes, the ultrasound endoscope is readied by attachment of the umbilical cord to the light source, suction tubing, and water bottle. The ultrasound connecting cord must be connected to the pulse unit on the EU-M20 prior to turning on the EU-M20 system. If it is attached after the unit has been turned on, the processor does not recognize the endoscope, and the display remains blank.

### *Balloons*

The balloon applicator that accompanies the instrument can be used to slide the balloon over the transducer casing at the tip of the ultrasound endoscope. Alternatively, the balloon can be grasped at the lower edge with two hands, stretched, and then pulled over the transducer casing. The lower edge of the balloon must be completely in the groove below the transducer (see Fig. 2–8). The upper edge of the balloon must be seated around the protrusion at the tip of the transducer casing. It is not necessary to tie the balloon into the groove with a thread (this technique is useful with older instruments). Balloon inflation with water can be tested by turning on the light source. Initially, the balloon will inflate with air, which can be removed by suction. Small holes in the balloon will be revealed when water is infused into the balloon. The balloon should not be inflated beyond a diameter of 5 cm. Balloons should be handled carefully with the tips of fingers, avoiding contact with fingernails or sharp objects. Balloons should not be reused. Because latex can degrade with time, balloons should be inspected for color changes if they have been stored for a long period.

### *Water Pump*

The water pump available with the system is convenient to use because it can be activated with a foot pedal. Water may also be infused through the biopsy port with a syringe, but this method is inconvenient and often leads to air-bubble formation. The water pump that accompanies the system should be filled with water and readied prior to any examination. Experienced endosonographers have individual preferences for the source of the water they use with the water infusion pump. Degassed water, spring water, or sterile water are used at different institutions because they contain fewer air bubbles than tap water. A metal one-way valve, the Olympus MD-744, which can be inserted into the biopsy port is commercially available for use with this water pump. Unfortunately, one must exert continuous pressure on this valve with one hand for water to flow, which is usually not practical during examinations. A blunt needle attached to the end of the water pump tubing is a more practical method for infusing water through the biopsy port. A disposable three-way plastic Luer lock connector can be positioned before the blunt needle. This allows the endoscopist to shut off water infusion as needed.

Once the endoscope is readied and the EU-M20 system has been turned on, the patient's name and identification number can be entered by pressing the ID button on the right-hand side of the control panel. Immediately before the introduction of the ultrasound endoscope into a patient, it is a good idea to test the endoscope. Function of the transducer can be tested by pressing the freeze button. Transducer rings should appear on the display monitor, and the gentle whir of the drive motor should be heard. Dipping the transducer in a cup of water should eliminate the air artifact. A piece of gauze in the water cup functions as a good test object. If a wedge defect is seen in the image or a "flare" is present, then the transducer has a leak and air or dust has entered the casing (3). Servicing of the endoscope is necessary if this defect is significant. The appearance of "snow" on the display screen is indicative of electric interference (3). This may be related either to other equipment in the room or to the electric outlet itself. Monitoring devices, such as pulse oximeters, should be turned off. If the snow persists, the outlet needs to be changed or an electric filter needs to be placed in the line. After the transducer has been checked, water should be infused into the balloon to check for leaks, and then the water should be aspirated out. Gentle fingertip pressure on the balloon while holding the transducer tip pointed down serves to suction out small air bubbles trapped in the balloon. This maneuver is especially important if the endoscope has been hanging for some time, as air bubbles tend to build up in the line. The video recorder and any hardcopy devices that are to be used should be activated. The foot control can then be used to record real-time ultrasonography during the examination. Video recording of the entire examination is recommended for beginners. With experience, ultrasound endoscopists learn to record select parts of the examination.

## The Examination

Endoscopic examination with the upper ultrasound endoscopes resembles endoscopy performed with a duodenoscope. Esophageal intubation, which is partially blind, is made somewhat more difficult because of the length of the rigid tip. The tip of the endoscope should be maneuvered with gentle pressure across the back of the tongue, as the long tip could easily perforate the posterior pharynx. The upper ultrasound endoscope, the GF-UM20, can also be used for examination of the rectum and distal sigmoid colon. Intubation of the remainder of the colon requires the forward-viewing colonic instrument, the CF-UM20. The rigid, long tip of this instrument makes colonoscopy technically more difficult. As mentioned previously, endoscopic view with these ultrasound endoscopes is very limited, and does not substitute for routine endoscopy. The endoscopic capability of these instruments should be viewed as a means to position the transducer adjacent to a lesion, which can then be examined by ultrasonography. (Organ-specific endoscopic ultrasonography is discussed in subsequent chapters of this textbook and need not be detailed here.)

Once the transducer has been positioned endoscopically, ultrasonographic real-time scanning is begun by pressing the freeze button located on the control panel, the endoscope, the foot control, or the remote. Endoscopic ultrasonography is generally performed by one of two methods: (1) the balloon contact method; (2) the water instillation method.

In the first method, the balloon around the transducer is inflated with water by pressing the air/water valve all the way down. This allows the transducer to move away from the wall of the gastrointestinal tract, bringing the wall and the area of interest closer to the focal plane of the instrument. The balloon also helps displace luminal air which interferes with imaging. Pressing the suction valve to the first step helps to remove the remainder of the luminal air, collapsing the bowel wall around the balloon. Frequent, sometimes constant, suctioning is required to prevent air from interfering with the image. Intermittent infusion of small amounts of water with the water pump can also be helpful in displacing trapped air when examining structures with the balloon contact method. At this point, the endoscopic view is lost, and the ultrasound picture guides further maneuvering of the transducer. This balloon contact method can be used to view the duodenal and esophageal wall, and for viewing the retroperitoneum.

The second method, the water instillation method, is used when viewing the wall of the stomach or rectum. In this method, it is essential to infuse several hundred milliliters of water through the biopsy port with the aid of the water pump. This helps distend the gastrointestinal wall and also replaces the intraluminal air with water. The balloon around the transducer is inflated with water in order to move the transducer away from the wall, bringing the wall into focus. Generally, tip deflection and torque on the endoscope can move the transducer in such a way that it focuses in on different sectors of the distended gastric or rectal wall.

The ultrasound examination is usually begun only after the balloon has been inflated and the air has been satisfactorily removed, either by suctioning (balloon contact method) or by water infusion. Scanning should be initiated only after the radial image is nearly free of air artifact. Scanning is performed by using tip deflection, torque on the shaft, and movement of the endoscope forward or backward. Small, controlled movements are required during scanning, as the angle of the transducer, which determines the imaging plane, can change quite rapidly.

Scanning should usually be started at a frequency of 7.5 MHz, a range of 9 or 12 cm, and a 360° display.

The video recorder can be turned on (using the foot control or the keyboard) when a satisfactory image is obtained. Once the area of interest has been identified, the image can be magnified by pressing the appropriate button on the lower right-hand corner of the control panel. The range setting—the farthest distance displayed on the image—appears on the right side of the monitor (lower ranges correspond to higher magnification). Pressing the display button (labeled DISP) at this point allows the selection of a suitable 180° sector of the imaging plane, further focusing in on the lesion of interest. Changing the displayed sector also allows further increase in magnification (decrease in range). If the lesion is not completely imaged in a 180° sector, the image rotation buttons on the control panel can be used to rotate the image in a clockwise or counterclockwise direction as needed. By convention, the scanning direction (labeled DIR) is always set such that the ultrasound image corresponds to the orientation of a standard CT scan of the chest when the esophagus is examined. The multiple image control (MULTI) allows the endoscopist to display a number of images on the display, with one image being the live display. This feature has limited practical use.

The frequency for scanning can be changed from 7.5 to 12 MHz on the GF-UM20 by pressing the frequency button on the endoscope. Increasing the frequency from 7.5 to 12 MHz improves the resolution of the image, but limits the depth of penetration. The 12-MHz image may be useful for examining small areas of a lesion at high magnification. Generally, most questions can be adequately answered with the 7.5-MHz image, and expert endosonographers do not need the higher resolution image.

## Freeze and Labeling

While scanning, when a lesion is seen in sharp focus and the image contains features of interest, the image should be captured by quickly pressing the freeze button located on the endoscope or the foot control. An assistant can also operate the freeze button on the keyboard or on the remote for this purpose. Identified structures on a frozen image can be labeled by pressing the comment button. A cursor appears on the screen. This cursor can be positioned with the arrow controls, or can be rapidly moved around with the trackball. The alphanumeric keyboard is used for labeling. Images can also be labeled subsequently during review of videotapes. When recording an examination, the endoscopist can easily indicate which organ is being imaged by pressing the body mark control. By pressing the mark reference switch, an arrow on top of the anatomic drawing can be activated. This arrow can be moved with the arrow controls or the trackball to indicate the anatomic location being scanned. This feature is useful when the videotape is subsequently reviewed.

## Measurements

Sizes of various structures can be measured by pressing the "+" or "×" cursors located above the arrow controls on the control panel or on the trackball. Distance (in millimeters) is measured by positioning a cursor at one edge of the lesion, pressing the mark reference button (⊕), then moving the cursor to the other edge of the lesion. Measurements appear on the right lower corner of the display. By activating the measurement menu, the EU-M20 also allows the measurement of circumference and area of an adjustable ellipse or a traced boundary, in a manner similar to distance measurement. Again, the + or × cursors are positioned at one edge, set in place by pressing the mark reference button (⊕), then moved to an appropriate measuring location by the arrow controls or trackball. A histogram function is also available within the measurement function. This function computes a gray-scale distribution of a desired area on the sonographic image, which can be demarcated either with a box (HIST_B) or traced (HIST_T) with the help of cursor controls. Theoretically, such a measurement could help quantify abstract qualities of an ultrasound image, such as inhomogeneity and echogenicity. However, given that each ultrasound unit has its own standard settings, patients are examined at different settings of gain and contrast, and echo characteristics of normal tissues vary from patient to patient, the histogram function has found little use.

## Image Recording and Review

Pertinent parts of the ultrasound examination should generally be recorded, either by videotape or hard-copy device. Beginners should consider taping the entire examination for subsequent review. A ¾-inch video recorder or a super VHS recorder provides the highest quality reproduction of images. Other video formats, such as VHS and Beta, can also be used but suffer from a loss in image quality. During video recording, it is a good idea to freeze interesting images for 5–10 seconds. Image labeling and measurement of structures can be performed either during the examination or subsequently while reviewing the videotape. The videotape can be reviewed by pressing the VTR option in the menu. During VTR playback, measurements of imaged structures can be made by pressing the measurement function switch, selecting the EU-M20 option, then calibrating to the appropriate magnification range by pressing the magnification switches. After calibration, it is necessary to exit back to the main menu. At this point, the cursors will become activated (as shown by a lit LED), and measurements can be made.

The EU-M20 comes with a Polaroid camera unit, the MD-901. This unit contains an internal video monitor. Brightness and contrast on the video image projected to the camera can be adjusted by opening the side door on the unit. The eight-exposure black-and-white Polaroid 667 pack that is available for this unit provides adequate hard copies. A Polaroid photograph of a frozen ultrasound image can be made during the examination by pressing the release button (if the camera has previously been programmed in the EU-M20 menu as the selected hard-copy unit), or a photograph can be obtained later by activating the shutter on the Polaroid unit during playback. Many endosonographers find it inconvenient to take photographs during examinations because of the time taken to develop the Polaroids. Thermoprinters with pushbutton activation are a convenient alternative to the Polaroid images. Other hard-copy devices can be coupled with the EU-M20 to get a more durable, higher quality image. By selecting the gamma option in the EU-M20 menu, adjustments can be made on the EU-M20 signal, optimizing the signal for the selected photographic equipment.

## Care and Cleaning

The transducer, in its casing at the tip of the ultrasound endoscope, is the part of the instrument that is most susceptible to damage, and should always be handled gently. Care should be taken that the transducer not strike anything while the endoscope is being hung. A piece of foam with a small cylindrical hole in the center can be placed around the transducer for protection. Care should also be exercised while removing the balloon. Balloons can be grasped with a piece of gauze and peeled off the transducer. This should be done gently, as excessive pulling force has been known to jar the transducer seal off. Since the UM20 endoscopes are completely immersible, they can be cleaned and disinfected in a manner similar to other Olympus OES-20 endoscopes. Because of the high pressures generated in some of the newer endoscope washers, it is advisable to clean these instruments by hand, avoiding the use of these washers. The control panel on the EU-M20 can be cleaned by wiping with alcohol or other disinfectant.

## References


1. Caletti G, Bolondi L, Barbara L. Instrumentation and scanning techniques. In Kawai K (ed): Endoscopic Ultrasonography in Gastroenterology. New York: Igaku-Shoin, 1988, pp 1–17.
2. Sasai T. Development of ultrasonic endoscope. In Kawai K (ed): Endoscopic Ultrasonography in Gastroenterology. New York: Igaku-Shoin, 1988, pp 18–34.
3. Rösch T, Classen M. Instruments, preparation, and general aspects of the endosongraphic examination. In: Gastroenterologic Endosonography: Textbook and Atlas: New York: Thieme Medical Publishers, 1992, pp 1–13.
4. Boyce HW, Boyce GA. Endoscopic Ultrasonography: Instruments and Techniques, Vol 2. Gastrointestinal Endoscopy Clinics of North America, 1992, pp 575–599.
5. Yasuda K. Development and clinical use of ultrasonic probes. Endoscopy 26:816–817, 1994.
6. Chak A, Canto M, Stevens PD, Lightdale CJ, Van de Mierop F, Cooper G, Pollack BJ, Sivak MV. Clinical applications of a new through-the-scope ultrasound probe: Prospective comparison with an ultrasound endoscope. Gastrointest Endosc 1997 (in press).
7. Binmoeller KF, Seifert H, Seitz U, Izbicki JR, Kida M, Soehendra N. Ultrasonic esophagoprobe for TNM staging of highly stenosing esophageal carcinoma. Gastrointest Endosc 41:547–552, 1995.
8. Beroni G, Gumina C, Conigliaro R, et al. Randomized placebo-controlled trial of oral liquid simethicone prior to upper gastrointestinal endoscopy. Endoscopy 24:268–270, 1992.
9. Yiengpruksawan A, Lightdale CJ, Gerdes H, Botet JF. Mucolytic-antifoam solution for reduction of artifacts during endoscopic ultrasonography: A randomized controlled trial. Gastrointest Endosc 37:543–546, 1991.

CHAPTER

3

# The Linear Array Echoendoscope

Maurits J. Wiersema

The accuracy of endosonography in staging gastrointestinal malignancies has been established (1–5). Most studies have been performed using radial mechanical scanning instruments. The centripetal pattern of neoplasm growth together with the luminal nature of gastrointestinal tumors has supported the radial orientation for imaging. Unfortunately, to achieve this goal, manufacturers have been forced to rely on mechanical systems, with their inherent problems of reliability. This has occurred at a time when electronic and crystal technology has advanced to a sufficient degree to permit real-time duplex and color Doppler imaging with transcutaneous probes. The necessity for transoral passage of the endoscopic probes has placed physical restrictions on the equipment—a limitation that is partially responsible for the continued acceptance of mechanical units among gastroenterologists. This contrasts with the radiology community where electronic array probes, with their Doppler capabilities, are the standard.

The Pentax and Hitachi Corporations (Pentax Precision Instrument Corporation, Orangeburg, New York; and Mitsubishi Corporation, Conshohocken, Pennsylvania) have collaborated to develop an endoscopic convex linear array probe. Unlike in radial scanning instruments, the scan plane is parallel to the long axis of the endoscope, offering a different image orientation. Certain advantages and disadvantages arise with this configuration. As the number of studies describing the performance of this equipment is limited, comparison is difficult (6,7). However, several new applications including endosonography-guided fine needle aspiration biopsy (EUS FNA), duplex endosonography, endosonography-guided cholangiopancreatography (EGCP), and endosonography-guided celiac plexus neurolysis (EUS CPN) have been described (8–17). This chapter outlines the capabilities of this equipment and the unique features that may augment the clinical utility of gastrointestinal endosonography.

## Equipment

The Pentax ultrasound probe (Fig. 3–1) is a completely immersible fiberoptic oblique forward viewing instrument with a 100° linear convex array ultrasound transducer mounted on the end of the endoscope. The scan plane of the ultrasound transducer is oriented parallel to the long axis of the instrument. A 2-mm biopsy channel permits the passage of accessories into the scan plane of the instrument. A balloon is placed over the ultrasound housing to allow for acoustic coupling and may be filled via a syringe and valve on the endoscope body. Additionally, water may be placed into the gastrointestinal lumen through the biopsy channel to assist in acoustic coupling. The equipment operates at 5 and 7.5 MHz with variable focal depths which are adjusted electronically. In addition, a probe with a larger biopsy channel (2.4-mm diameter) equipped with an elevator has been introduced (FG-36UX). This probe has the advantage of permitting stent placement, it also facilitates EUS FNA because resistance is reduced when passing the biopsy needle (18). Additionally, filling (and emptying) of the balloon has been incorporated into the endoscope valve housing. When either instrument is used with the Hitachi 515C or the newer 525 ultrasound console, both duplex and color Doppler imaging are possible. The probes may also be used with less costly and more portable consoles lacking Doppler capabilities. A unique feature available with the Hitachi

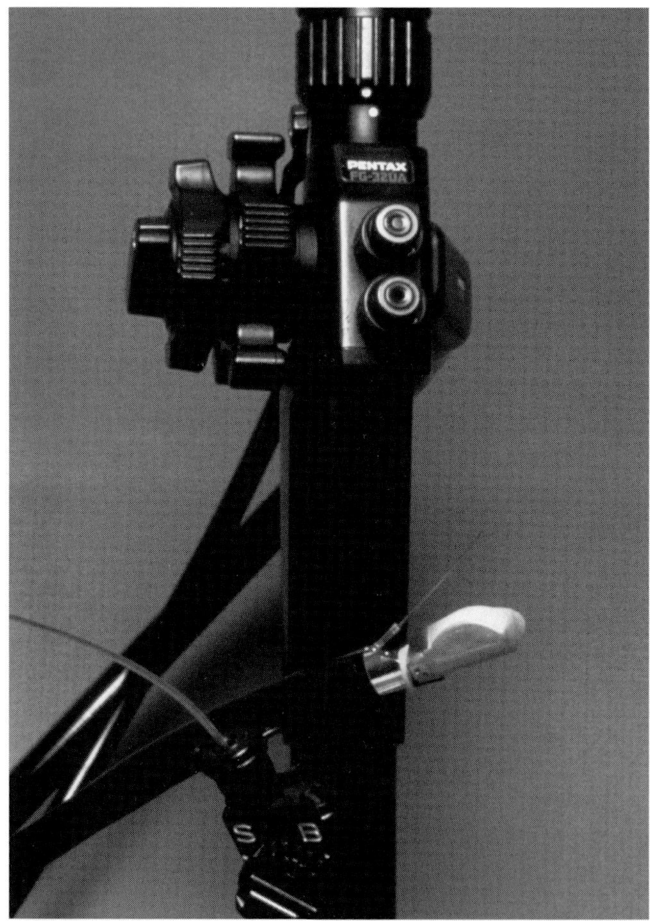


A

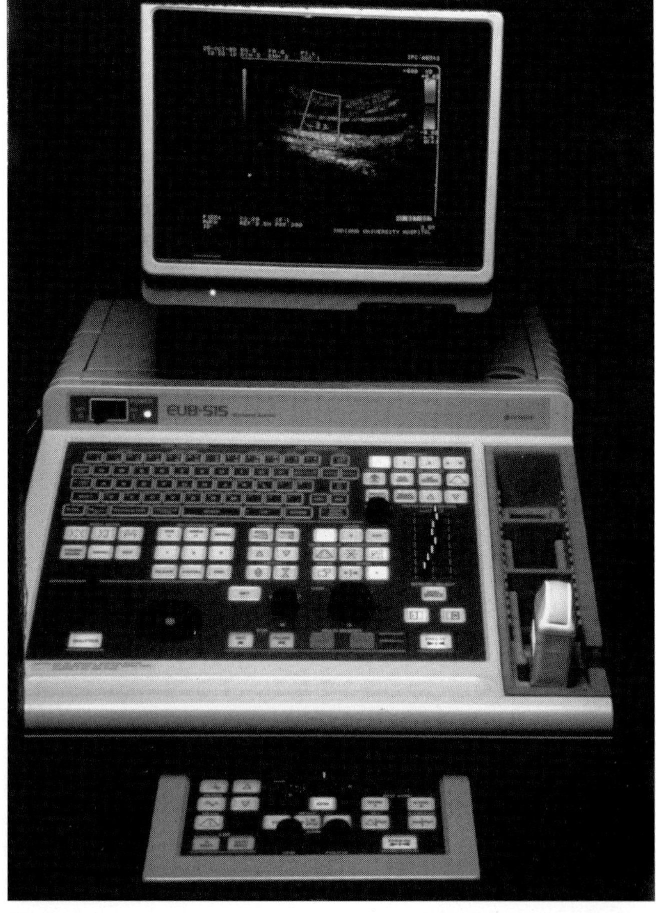


B

**FIGURE 3–1**

(**A**) Pentax FG-32UA ultrasound endoscope with prototype Wilson–Cook catheter exiting from the biopsy channel. The needle is extended from the sheath and lies in the imaging plane of the transducer. (**B**) The Hitachi 515C console allows pulsed and color Doppler imaging. The console may be used with other probes including those for transabdominal imaging.

console is the option of image storage. Specifically, after freezing the image, the last several seconds of ultrasound scanning are stored in memory and may be scrolled through to allow selection of the best image. This is especially useful for endosonography since respiratory and/or cardiac movement may blur the image precisely at the time that it is frozen. This option also works with duplex and color Doppler.

The Doppler capability with the Pentax unit is unique among endosonography probes. Multiple imaging modes are possible, including pulsed Doppler (with greater sensitivity owing to higher sampling rates) and duplex imaging, which allows continuous display of the B-mode image and Doppler waveform simultaneously. Color Doppler imaging superimposes flow velocities from a region of interest on the real-time B-mode image. The color is determined by the direction of flow relative to the transducer. The Hitachi 525 console has incorporated the technology of Ultrasound Angio™ (Diasonics Ultrasound, Santa Clara, California). This technique produces a display of blood that has visual properties similar to standard angiography (Fig. 3–2). The amplitude of the returning signal (color intensity) is dependent on the density of red blood cells and the size of the vessel within the sampling region. A major advantage of Ultrasound Angio is its ability to detect flow at right angles to the ultrasound beam. This new feature facilitates identification of blood vessels and will conceivably enhance the efficiency of performing EUS exams.

## Normal Anatomy

The linear scan plane of the Pentax instrument provides an orientation to the gastrointestinal tract and adjacent organs different from that of the radial scanning probes. The five-layer pattern of the gastrointestinal wall is best visualized when imaging at 7.5 MHz. Within the esophagus, a parasagittal scan plane allows a linear view of the thoracic aorta. Tumor staging, however, requires a 360° rotation of the probe to allow a complete survey. Similar principles apply to the stomach and duodenum, but complete rotation while maintaining acoustic coupling with the gastrointestinal wall is fairly difficult. The head of the pancreas is most easily visualized with the probe placed against the major papilla. At this level, such vascular structures as the gastroduodenal artery may be distinguished from the common bile duct and main pancreatic duct using Ultrasound Angio. The remainder of the pancreas is best visualized from the stomach, where the body and tail may be followed in close proximity to the splenic artery and vein (Fig. 3–3).

The portal vein is typically imaged from the duodenum (bulb and second portion) or stomach at the level of the confluence with the splenic vein (Fig. 3–4). The proper hepatic artery is seen from the duodenum adjacent to the portal vein, and the common hepatic artery is seen from the stomach as a branch from the celiac trunk. The splenic artery and vein are visualized adjacent to the pancreas along the posterior wall of the

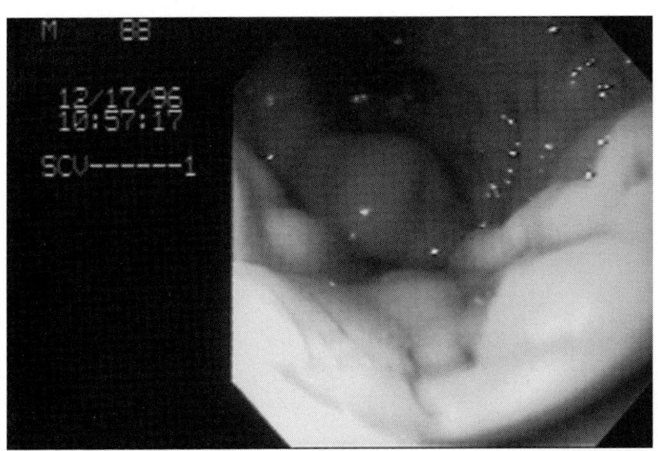


A

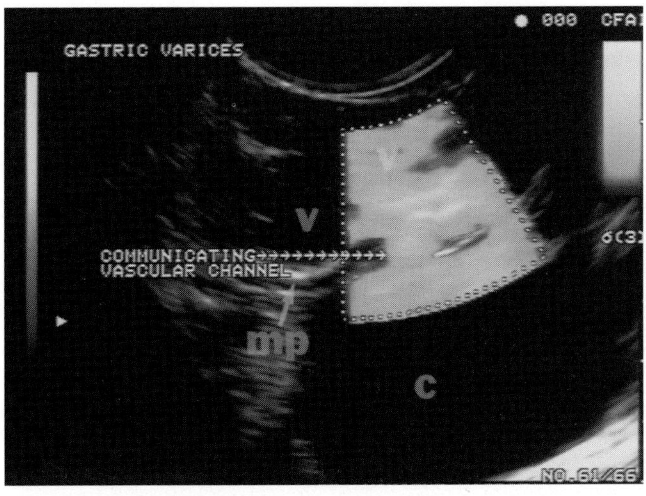


B

**FIGURE 3–2**

An 88-year-old male presented with dysphagia secondary to a Schatzki's ring and was found to have (**A**) a submucosal mass in the cardia suspicious for gastric varices (retroflex view of cardia). EUS with Ultrasound Angio™ color Doppler. (**B**) demonstrates the gastric varices (v) with communicating vessels traversing the muscularis propria (mp) and entering a large perigastric collateral (c). The patient was found to have splenic vein thrombosis. (*See color insert for color plate.*)

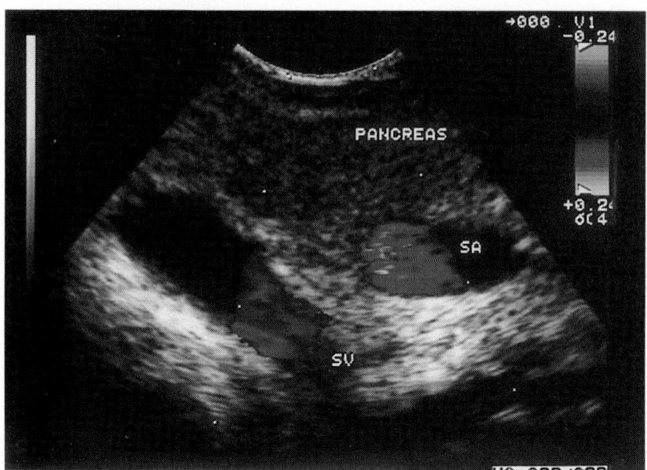


**FIGURE 3-3**

Transgastric imaging from the mid body demonstrates the pancreas, with the adjacent splenic artery (SA) highlighted in red by color Doppler and the splenic vein (SV) highlighted in blue. These vessels can be followed into the hilum of the spleen by withdrawing the instrument. By advancing and rotating the probe, the splenic vein may be seen to course into the portal vein and the splenic artery can be followed down to the level of the celiac trunk. (*See color insert for color plate.*)

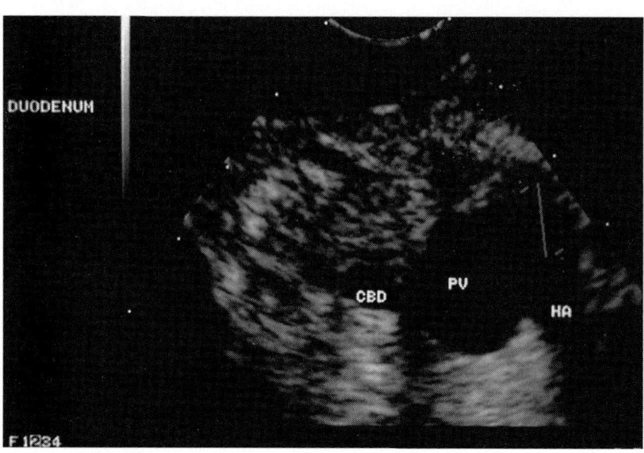


A

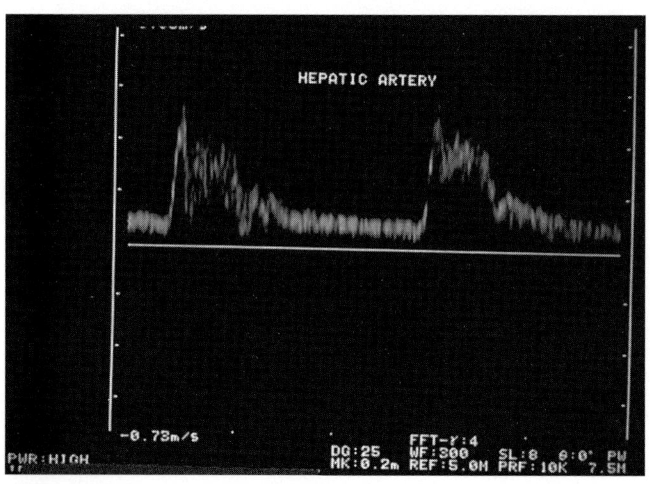


B

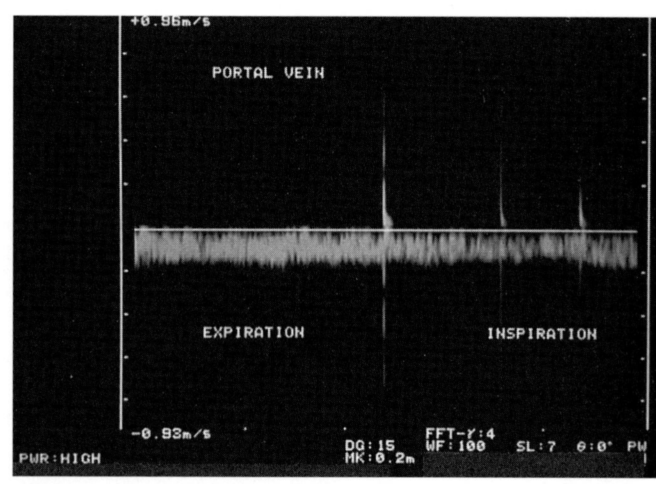


C

**FIGURE 3-4**

(**A**) The portal triad comprising the common bile duct (CBD), portal vein (PV), and hepatic artery (HA) visualized from the second segment of the duodenum. (*See color insert for color plate.*) (**B**) The Doppler gate has been placed at the location of the hepatic artery and the flow profile is seen. The systolic peak is rounded and there is flow through diastole. (**C**) The pulsed Doppler signal of the portal vein is a broad-spectrum waveform with minimal cardiac variation; its velocity increases during expiration and decreases on inspiration.

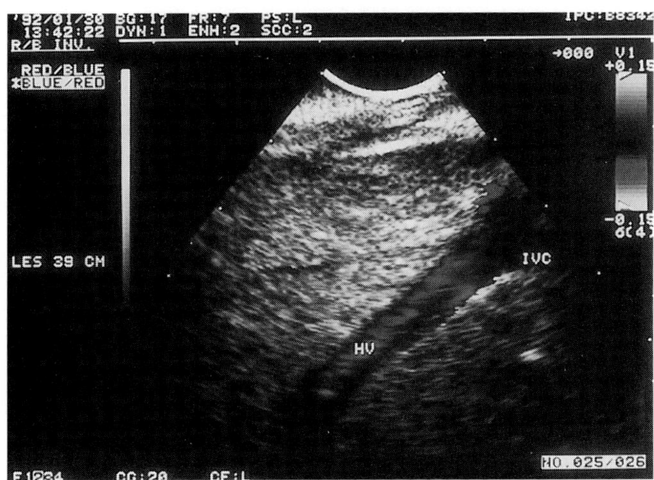


**FIGURE 3-5**

Imaging at the level of the lower esophageal sphincter (LES) demonstrates one of the hepatic veins (HV) entering into the inferior vena cava (IVC) as highlighted with the blue color Doppler signal. By rotating the transducer, hepatic veins from the right and left lobe can be seen converging toward the inferior vena cava. (*See color insert for color plate.*)

stomach. The hepatic veins course at an acute angle into the inferior vena cava and can be best visualized from the cardia (Fig. 3–5).

## Tumor Staging

Virtually all of the reported tumor-staging work done with endosonography has employed the Olympus radial scanning equipment. Whether the linear orientation and Doppler capabilities of the Pentax probe offer any advantage requires additional study. We prospectively evaluated 45 patients with malignancies (esophageal 8, mediastinal 5, gastric 3, duodenal/ampullary 3, pancreas 16, biliary 5, and rectal 5) and 8 patients with submucosal masses using the Pentax (FG-32UA) and Olympus (EUM3, EUM20) probes (Figs. 3–6, 3–7) (6). Patients underwent an exam with each probe, then the videotapes and films were reviewed in a blind fashion. The TNM system was employed for tumor staging.

Twelve of the patients with malignancies had surgical pathology correlation to allow assessment of tumor-

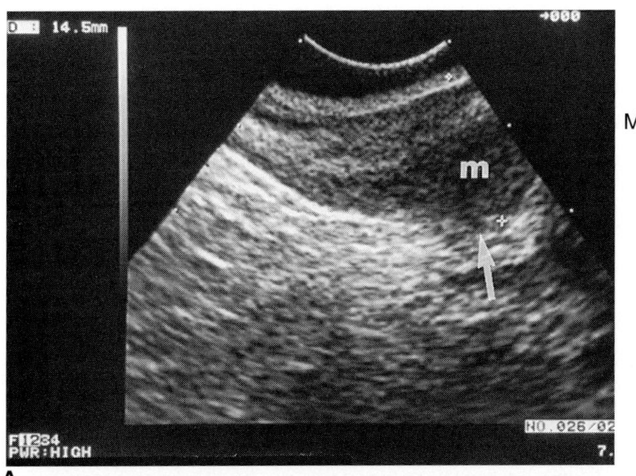


A

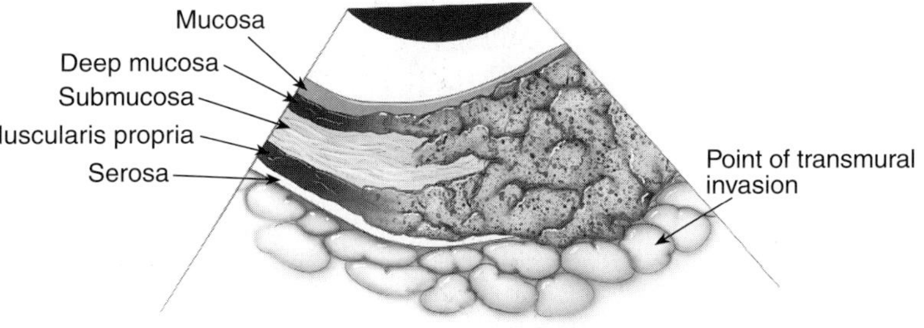


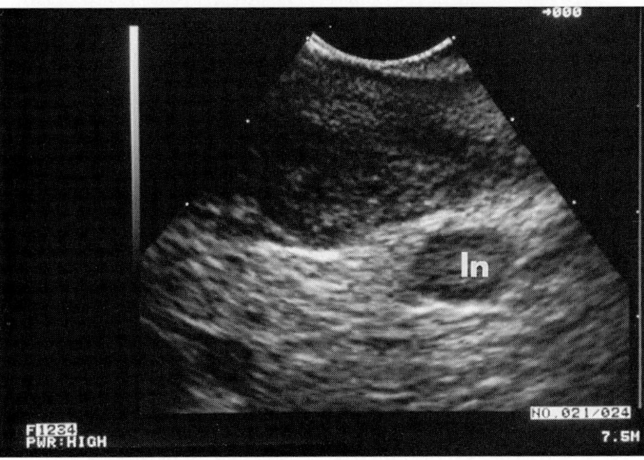


B

**FIGURE 3-6**

A 53-year-old woman presented with abdominal pain and was subsequently found to have a linitus plastica appearance of the stomach on endoscopy. Pinch forceps biopsies were nondiagnostic. (**A**) Endosonography demonstrates the transition zone from a five-layered gastric wall to complete destruction and thickening of the wall (m). Transmural invasion is seen (arrow). (**B**) At a different level a regional hypoechoic lymph node is identified (ln). Endosonography-guided fine-needle aspiration biopsy was performed and the patient was found to have a non–Hodgkin large cell lymphoma.

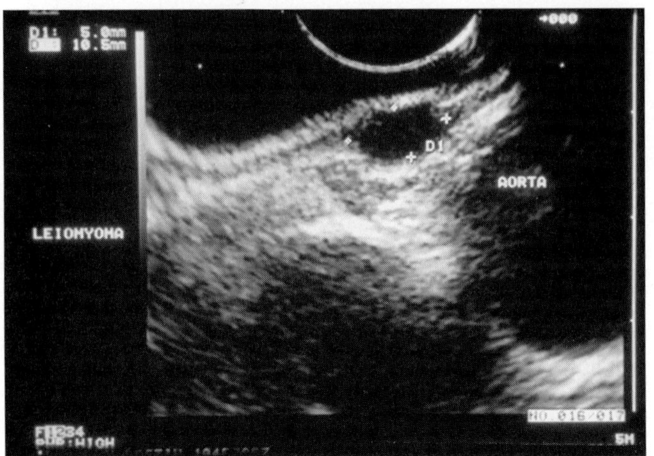


**FIGURE 3–7**

Transesophageal imaging demonstrates a hypoechoic mass arising from the muscularis propria. Fine-needle aspiration biopsy revealed spindle cells consistent with a leiomyoma.

staging accuracy. For these patients, the T-staging accuracy was the same for both the Pentax and Olympus systems (75%, 9/12). The Pentax system failed to identify splenic vein invasion in one patient. The Olympus system was unable to identify a T1 ampullary mass (9 × 13 mm) visualized with the Pentax system. Both instruments overstaged a T2 gastric adenocarcinoma as T3 and a large T1 ampullary lesion (30 mm) as a suspected pancreatic invasion. One patient with pancreatic carcinoma was found to have vascular invasion at surgery; therefore, a palliative procedure was done and lymph node staging was not available. The N-staging accuracy was 64% (7/11) for the Pentax system and 73% (8/11) for the Olympus system.

For all patients with gastrointestinal malignancies, review of the Pentax and Olympus exams resulted in the same T stage in 80% of patients (32/40) and the same N stage in 93% of patients (37/40). With pancreatic carcinoma, in three cases the Olympus system found splenic vein ($n$ = 2) or portal vein invasion ($n$ = 1) that the Pentax system did not detect (splenic vein invasion confirmed in one patient at surgery). Metastatic staging agreement was seen in all cases, except for two patients with esophageal carcinoma. Each system failed to detect celiac lymph nodes seen by the other instrument.

Five patients with mediastinal tumors were examined. In the single patient with surgical correlation, the Pentax system correctly predicted an absence of esophageal invasion whereas the Olympus system reported invasion. In all other cases both systems provided equivalent information. Two patients had malignant mediastinal lymphadenopathy confirmed by EUS FNA.

With submucosal tumors, equivalent findings were found in seven of eight cases (88%). Four of these patients had histologic ($n$ = 1) or cytologic ($n$ = 3) confirmation, and in these individuals 100% agreement was found between the Olympus and Pentax systems.

Mortensen et al. (7) found that, when using the Pentax probe, a correct preoperative assessment of resectability could be made in 38 of 42 patients (91%). When subdivided by tumor location, the resulting accuracy of operability assessment remained consistent: esophageal carcinoma 91%, gastric carcinoma 94%, and pancreatic carcinoma 87%. Although specific TNM staging results were not provided, they found that the clinically important question of surgical resectability could be reliably addressed using the Pentax probe.

## Endosonography-Guided Fine-Needle Aspiration Biopsy

Endoscopic ultrasound permits detailed imaging of gastrointestinal tumors and has been demonstrated to be a sensitive method for detecting mediastinal lymphadenopathy in non–small cell lung cancer (1–5,19–22). Endosonography is not equivalent to histology; although certain features may suggest a malignant origin, tissue sampling is still required to confirm the diagnosis (23, 24). Several recent reports have described using the Pentax probe in conjunction with a flexible small-gauge biopsy needle to sample luminal lesions and masses extrinsic to the gastrointestinal tract (8–14). After localizing the region of interest with the Pentax system, the fine-needle aspiration catheter is advanced into the mass while visualizing the process with endosonography. The maximum depth of penetration that can reliably be achieved depends on the needle length, but has been reported to be up to 35 mm. When the needle tip is seen to lie within the lesion as visualized with endosonography, suction is applied to the proximal end of the catheter assembly using a 10-mL syringe. Simultaneously, small to-and-fro movements are made with the needle while observing the process on the ultrasound screen. The aspirated material may then be smeared onto glass slides and processed.

In a multicenter study EUS FNA was performed in 457 patients with 554 lesions (25). Clinical ($n$ = 218) or histopathologic ($n$ = 256) confirmation of the final diagnosis was available in 192 lymph nodes, 145 extraluminal mass lesions (e.g., pancreas, liver), 115 gastrointestinal wall lesions (e.g., gastric ulcer, submucosal mass), and 22 cystic lesions (Figs. 3–8 to 3–10). Table 3–1 lists the operating characteristics among these types of lesions. Both the sensitivity and accuracy of EUS FNA for lymph nodes and extraluminal masses were superior to those for gastrointestinal wall lesions ($p \leq .02$). The accuracy of EUS FNA in patients with previously failed biopsy procedures was 81% (73/90,

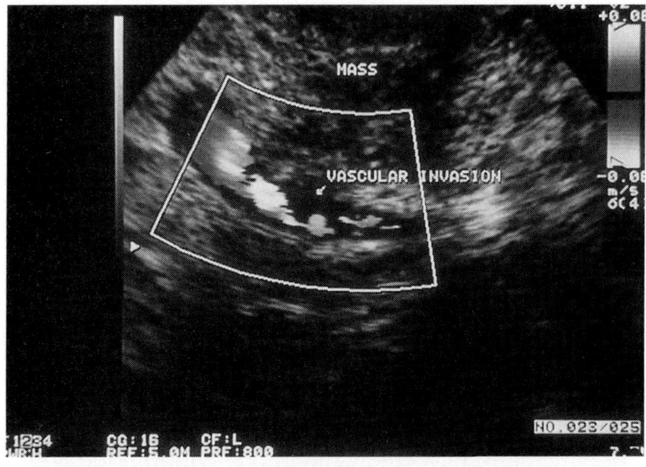


A

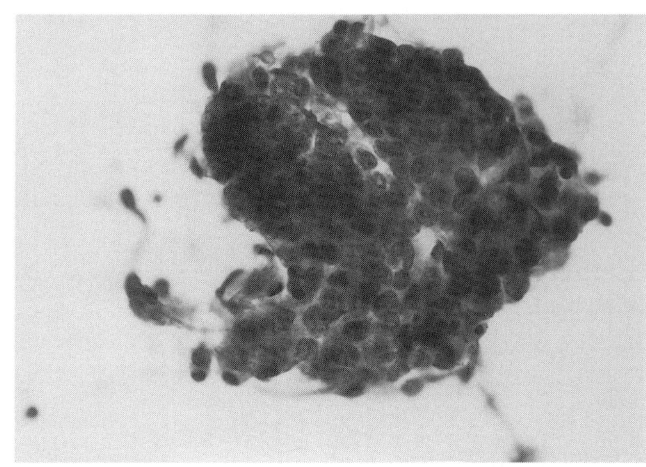

C

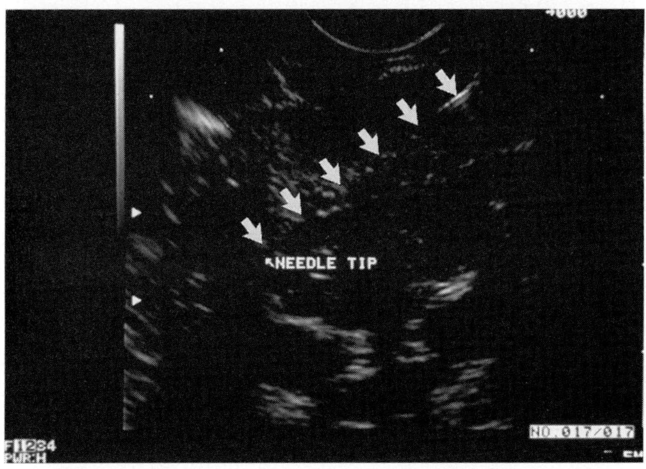


B

**FIGURE 3–8**

(**A**). Transduodenal sagittal imaging with the Pentax FG-32UA at 7.5 MHz demonstrates a pancreatic head mass. Invasion of the superior mesenteric vein is highlighted with color Doppler by the velocity increase (white area) seen at the level of the stenosis. (**B**) Because previous CT-guided fine-needle aspiration biopsy failed to provide a diagnosis, fine-needle aspiration biopsies were performed under endoscopic ultrasound guidance (arrows outline the course of the needle). (**C**) Cytology demonstrated an adenocarcinoma. (*See color insert for color plates of **A** and **C***).

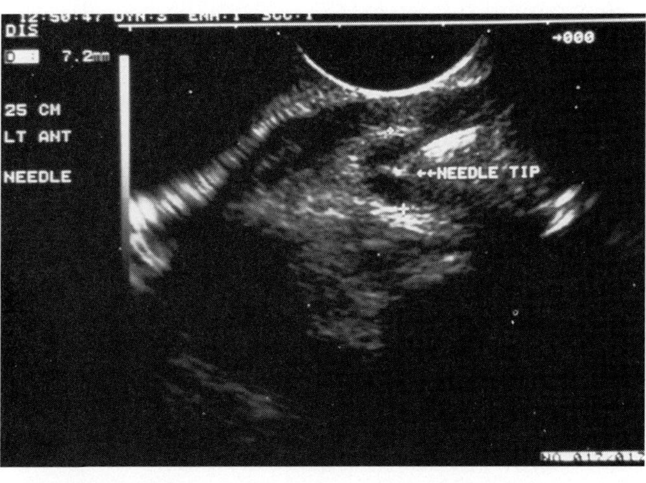


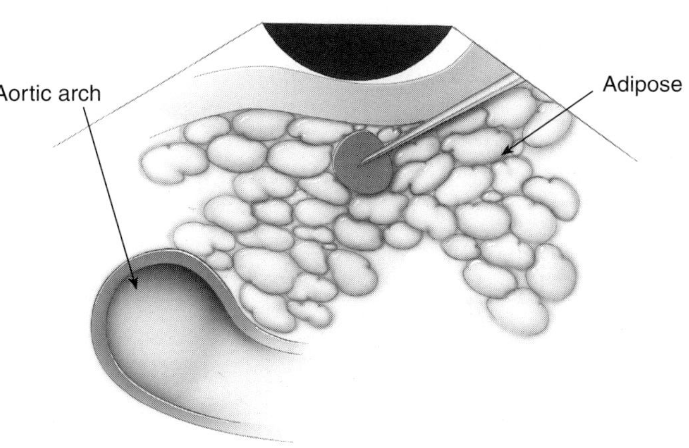


**FIGURE 3–9**

Transesophageal sagittal imaging reveals a 7-mm periesophageal lymph node with the aspiration needle coursing into it. The patient presented with dysphagia and a remote history of breast cancer. Cytology demonstrated adenocarcinoma consistent with a recurrence of her breast cancer. Cranial direction is to the right.

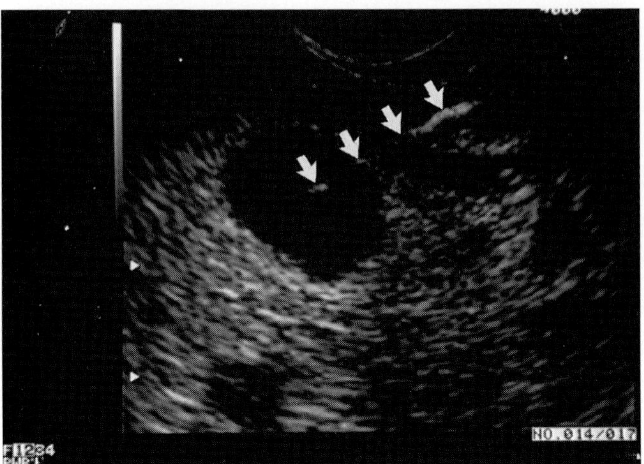

**FIGURE 3–10**

Transgastric imaging demonstrates a 16-mm liver metastasis with the aspiration needle entering the lesion (arrows). The patient presented with abdominal pain and was found to have a pancreatic head mass on CT without evidence of liver metastasis. Cytology demonstrated a non–Hodgkin large cell lymphoma.

$p < .001$). Attendant cytopathology assistance during sampling offered improved negative predictive value in extraluminal masses. Five nonfatal complications occurred, for a rate of .5% (95% CI: .1–.8%) in solid lesions versus 14% (95% CI: 6–21%) in cystic lesions ($p < .001$).

Subjective assessments of lymph node echotexture and border pattern were not available for analysis. EUS size criteria were used to predict if a lymph node was benign or malignant. At a cutoff of 10 mm in long axis dimension (i.e., all lymph nodes less than or equal to this size are considered benign; those larger than this size, malignant), the operating characteristics of EUS FNA versus EUS alone were as follows: sensitivity 92% versus 86% (n.s.), specificity 93% versus 24% ($p < .001$), accuracy 92% versus 69% ($p < .001$). A receiver operating-characteristic curve was generated by varying the long axis size threshold required for a lymph node to be considered malignant. The highest accuracy (75%) occurred with the EUS size criterion of 5 mm, providing a sensitivity of 99% and specificity of 2%.

In a more recent analysis comparing EUS FNA with EUS alone in lymph node evaluation, 148 patients underwent EUS FNA of 211 lymph nodes for staging and/or primary diagnostic purposes (26). No complications occurred. The median number of needle passes was 2, ranging from 1 to 10. In 128 patients CT was performed prior to the EUS exam. Adequate followup occurred in 143 patients (mean age 61 years, range 16–93 years) with 204 lymph nodes. In this group, 86 lymph nodes were ultimately found to be benign and 118 malignant. EUS criteria including lymph node width, length, echotexture, border, and shape were recorded at the time of the exam; and the lymph node was classified as benign or malignant based on these features. These results were then correlated with EUS FNA cytology and the final diagnosis. The final diagnosis for a lymph node was based on clinical followup, including repeat radiographic imaging and/or nonsurgical biopsies ($n$ = 103, median duration for benign lymph nodes 358 days, range 90–1239 days; and median duration for malignant lymph nodes 259 days, range 7–866 days) or surgery within 30 days of the EUS FNA ($n$ = 40). All patients with malignant lymph nodes were followed at least to their death or 90 days. The mean width and length of malignant lymph nodes were greater than those of benign lymph nodes (width = 16 versus 9 mm, length = 23 versus 14 mm; $p = .0001$ for both). The operating characteristics of EUS FNA versus EUS alone were as follows: sensitivity for malignant lymph nodes 85% versus 83% (n.s.), specificity for benign lymph nodes 93% versus 44% ($p < .0001$), accuracy 88% versus 67% ($p < .001$), positive predictive value 99% versus 67% ($p < .001$), negative predictive value 89% versus 67% ($p < .002$). Separate analysis for lymph node staging in 77 patients with gastrointestinal malignancies was done, as shown in Table 3–2. For all patients, CT performed prior to the

**TABLE 3–1**

EUS FNA Operating Characteristics

| | | | Predictive Value | | |
|---|---|---|---|---|---|
| Lesion | *Sensitivity* (%) | *Specificity* (%) | *Positive* (%) | *Negative* (%) | *Accuracy* (%) |
| Lymph node ($n$ = 192) | 92 | 93 | 100 | 86 | 92 |
| Extra-intestinal mass ($n$ = 145) | 88 | 95 | 100 | 88 | 90 |
| Gastrointestinal wall ($n$ = 103) (excluding stromal tumors) | 61 | 79 | 100 | 76 | 67 |
| Cystic lesions ($n$ = 22) | 22 | 89 | 100 | 100 | 77 |

Sensitivity is proportion of correctly diagnosed malignant lesions. Specificity is proportion of correctly diagnosed benign lesions.

Reprinted with permission from Wiersema MJ, Villman P, Giovannini M, Chang KJ, Wiersema LM. Endosonography guided fine needle aspiration biopsy: Diagnostic accuracy and complication assessment. Gastroenterology 112:1087–1095, 1997.

**TABLE 3-2**

Operating Characteristics of EUS FNA versus EUS Alone in the Staging of Lymph Nodes in 77 Patients with Gastrointestinal Malignancies

| | EUS FNA (%) | EUS alone (%) | *p* |
|---|---|---|---|
| Sensitivity | 80 | 77 | n.s. |
| Specificity | 94 | 53 | <.001 |
| Accuracy | 87 | 66 | <.001 |
| PPV | 98 | 64 | <.001 |
| NPV | 91 | 68 | .01 |

Sensitivity is for malignant lymphadenopathy ($n$ = 59) and specificity is for benign lymphadenopathy ($n$ = 53). PPV = positive predictive value, NPV = negative predictive value.

Reprinted with permission from Harada N, Wiersema M, Wiersema L. Endosonography guided fine needle aspiration biopsy (EUS FNA) in the evaluation of lymphadenopathy: Staging accuracy of EUS FNA versus EUS alone. Gastrointest Endosc (abstract 1997).

**TABLE 3-3**

Operating Characteristics of EUS FNA versus EUS Alone in the Evaluation of Mediastinal Lymphadenopathy

| | EUS FNA (%) | EUS alone (%) | *p* |
|---|---|---|---|
| Sensitivity | 88 | 83 | n.s. |
| Specificity | 92 | 46 | <.001 |
| Accuracy | 90 | 69 | .006 |
| PPV | 100 | 71 | .001 |
| NPV | 83 | 63 | n.s. |

Sensitivity is the proportion of correctly diagnosed malignant lymph nodes ($n$ = 42). Specificity is the proportion of correctly diagnosed benign lymph nodes ($n$ = 26). PPV = positive predictive value, NPV = negative predictive value.

Reprinted with permission from Wiersema M, Harada N, Daiehagh P, Beltz HF, Pfeiffer M, Allen K, Griffith G, Wiersema LM. Evaluation of mediastinal lymphadenopathy with transesophageal endosonography guided fine needle aspiration biopsy. Acta Endoscopia 28(1):7–19, 1998.

EUS exam failed to visualize the biopsied lymph node in 57% of cases ($p < .001$). In 40% of all cases, EUS FNA confirmed distant metastastic lymphadenopathy that was detected by CT in just 50% of these patients ($p < .001$). This study suggests that, without sacrificing sensitivity, improvements in EUS lymph node staging accuracy can be accomplished with EUS FNA through enhanced specificity.

The esophagus affords an excellent acoustic window to the mediastinum, thereby extending the utility of EUS in evaluating the mediastinum for evidence of lymph node metastases in patients with lung cancer (19–22). We have described our initial experience employing transesophageal real-time ultrasound-guided FNA to sample deep mediastinal lymph nodes not endoscopically identifiable by luminal compression (8,9). This experience has been extended to 48 patients who underwent EUS FNA of 71 lymph nodes (mean width 19 mm, range 4–70 mm; mean length 28 mm, range 9–80 mm) without complications (27). Comparing the performance of EUS FNA to EUS alone using criteria similar to those described above, we found that EUS FNA had superior specificity and similar sensitivity, resulting in improved accuracy (Table 3–3). In 9 patients who had 12 lymph nodes ≤10 mm in width and ≤15 mm in length, EUS FNA provided the correct diagnosis in all cases. Size and echo features were not found to be reliable means for differentiating benign from malignant lymph nodes ($p < .005$). In 17 of 18 patients (94%) with non–small cell lung cancer, EUS FNA cytology confirmed the N0–N3 stage.

The ability to sample mediastinal lymph nodes has important implications in the treatment of non–small cell carcinoma of the lung. In patients with lung carcinoma and mediastinal lymphadenopathy, EUS FNA may be considered a method for providing histologic confirmation of inoperability. Certainly, those patients found to have ipsilateral mediastinal lymph nodes could be directed to neoadjuvant treatment in hopes of improving their chances of a surgical cure. The potential cost saving as a result of this technique may be substantial in that patients would be redirected to nonsurgical treatments when inoperable disease is defined. Pulmonologists and thoracic surgeons now have an additional technique to assist them in the preoperative staging of patients with non–small cell lung cancer.

## Endosonography-Guided Cholangiopancreatography

The proximity of the distal bile duct to the duodenum permits detailed imaging with endosonography. Complete assessment of the entire extent of the biliary tree is not possible with endosonography, however. We have examined the feasibility of performing endosonography-guided cholangiopancreatography (EGCP) in those patients who have had failed attempts at ERCP (16). The technique employs passage of a small-gauge needle through the duodenal wall into the bile duct under endosonography visualization. Doppler capabilities assist in allowing positive identification of the bile duct via absence of any flow. In 8 of 10 patients who underwent this procedure, cholangiography was successful (Fig. 3–11). No complications occurred in this limited group. In five patients, abnormalities were identified, resulting in a subsequent repeat ERCP with pre-cut sphincterotomy to allow biliary access. Because EGC has the benefit of avoiding manipulation of the major papilla and hence the pancreatic duct, its use should minimize the potential for pancreatitis. Additional studies are needed to determine the clinical applicability and complications of this technique.

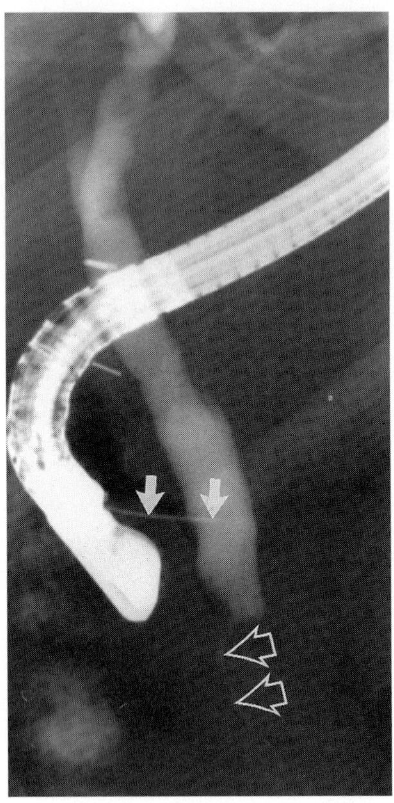

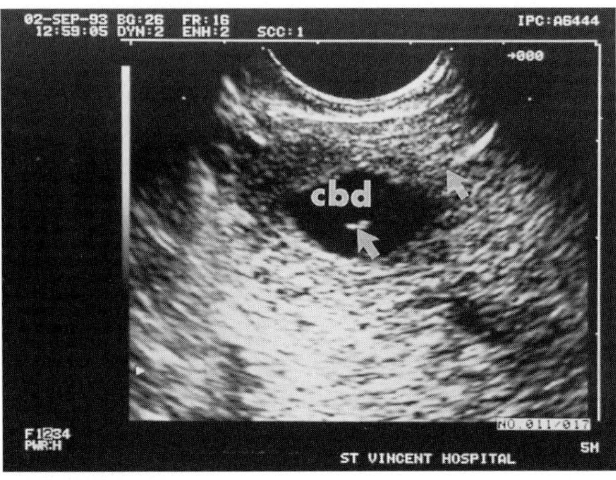


A B

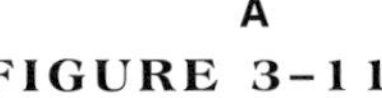

**FIGURE 3–11**

A 59-year-old female presented with painless jaundice and biliary dilation without evidence of a mass on CT scan. At ERCP, cholangiography and pancreatography were unsuccessful. Endosonography-guided cholangiography was performed and the needle (closed arrows) can be seen within the distal common bile duct (CBD) on both ductography (**A**) and endosonography (**B**). A distal common bile duct stricture (open arrows, **A**) is identified which was found to be secondary to chronic pancreatitis at surgery.

## Duplex Endosonography

Transcutaneous ultrasonography (TUS) with Doppler has become increasingly useful in the evaluation of disorders of the abdominal vasculature (28–38). Specific indications include investigating thrombosis of the portal, splenic, or hepatic veins; evaluating the patency of surgical shunts; and, in some patient populations, screening for renovascular hypertension. TUS has multiple advantages, including its noninvasive nature with minimal patient risk and short exam time. However, both duplex and color Doppler scanning of intra-abdominal vessels can be limited by intervening adipose tissue, bowel gas, ascites, or bone. When ultrasonography fails, angiography is often necessary to make a diagnosis; however, the invasive nature of the test, exposure to radiation, and the need for contrast agents makes it a less attractive alternative. Endosonography avoids some of the difficulties encountered with TUS because the transducer can be positioned within the lumen of the gastrointestinal tract. The proximity of the stomach and duodenum to the mesenteric vasculature permits detailed imaging of these structures with endosonography. With the recent addition of Doppler capabilities, functional characterization can also be made. We have examined the feasibility of performing Doppler ultrasonographic examinations of the abdominal vessels using endosonography.

We prospectively evaluated twenty asymptomatic subjects and reliably identified the portal vein, splenic vein, splenic artery, and hepatic artery in all subjects (15). Subsequently, owing to clinical suspicion of compromise of an intra-abdominal vessel, 11 patients underwent duplex TUS and endosonography. Patency of the portal or splenic vein was defined when a continuous low-velocity pulsed and color Doppler signal were seen within the vessel. Venous thrombosis was demonstrated by the absence of flow within the vessel with or without the finding of stationary echoes (solid thrombosis) within the lumen (28–33). Transcutaneous US with Doppler failed to visualize the vessel in question well enough to allow assessing patency/stenosis in 11 of the patients. However, EUS with Doppler visualized the appropriate vessel(s) in 10 out of 11 patients and provided information regarding the characteristics of the flow (TUS accuracy 0% versus EUS 91%, $p < .001$). This included six patients with splenoportal thrombosis, three patients with splenoportal patency, and two patients with splenorenal shunts (Figs. 3–12, 3–13). In three patients with thrombosis of the splenic and/or portal veins, the vessels had an internal hypoechoic appearance, but flow was not present. That is, B-mode imaging alone would have suggested patency.

These results suggest that duplex endosonography may be considered when transcutaneous Doppler ultrasound is unsuccessful. The recent addition of Ultrasound Angio should expand the applications by improving sensitivity. This technique provides the clinician an alternative to angiography. Moreover, it allows for a concordant endoscopic evaluation which may be necessary for therapeutic purposes.

## Endosonography-Guided Celiac Plexus Neurolysis

EUS CPN is a new technique in which the linear echoprobe is used to inject material into the region of the celiac ganglia (17). The celiac ganglia are located anterolateral to the aorta at the level of the L1 vertebral body, but may also be found between T12 and L2. The most consistent relationship appears to be with the origin of the celiac artery. Transgastric endosonography with the linear electronic array probe permits sagittal imaging of the aorta. The celiac artery can typically be identified from the proximal stomach (15). The celiac ganglion is not visualized as a discrete structure on

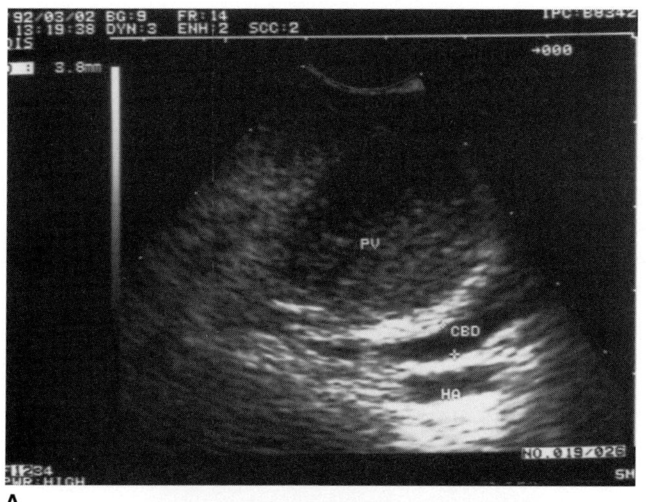

A

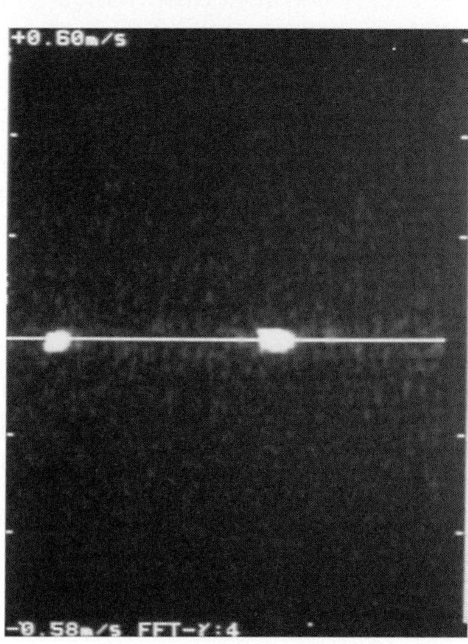

B

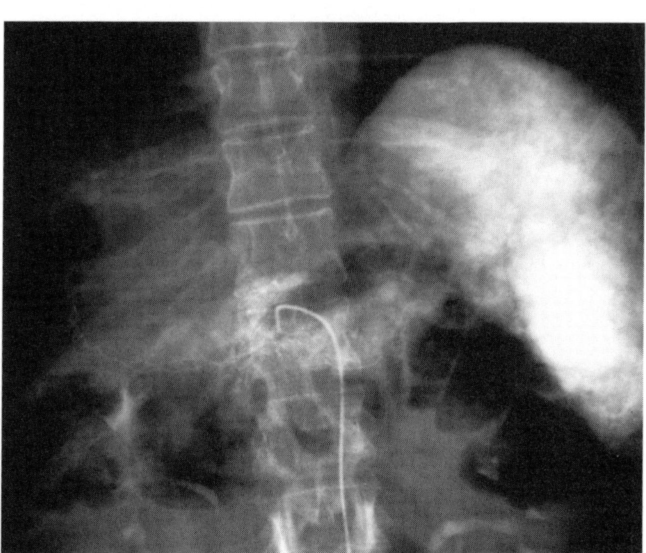
C

**FIGURE 3–12**

Transduodenal imaging from the bulb in a 44-year-old patient with a history of cryptogenic cirrhosis and gastrointestinal bleeding demonstrates (**A**) the portal vein (PV) with echogenic material within it as well as the adjacent common bile duct (CBD) and hepatic artery (HA). (**B**) Pulsed Doppler interrogation of the portal vein did not demonstrate any evidence of flow. Transcutaneous ultrasound could not confirm the presence or absence of flow. (**C**) On the venous phase of the arteriogram, flow was seen within the splenic vein; however, there is no evidence of any portal vein flow. The spleen is highlighted with contrast.

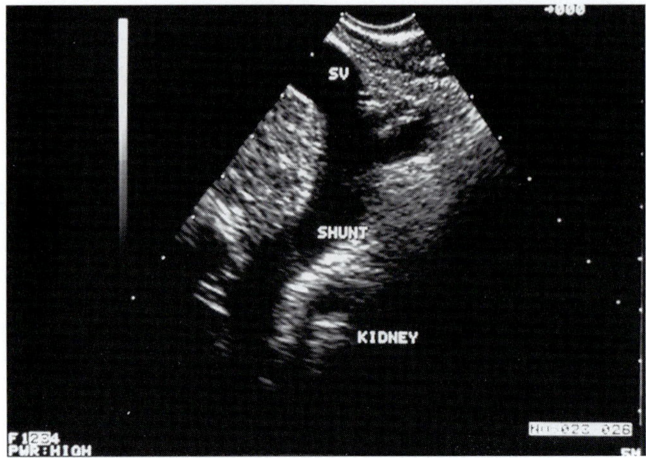


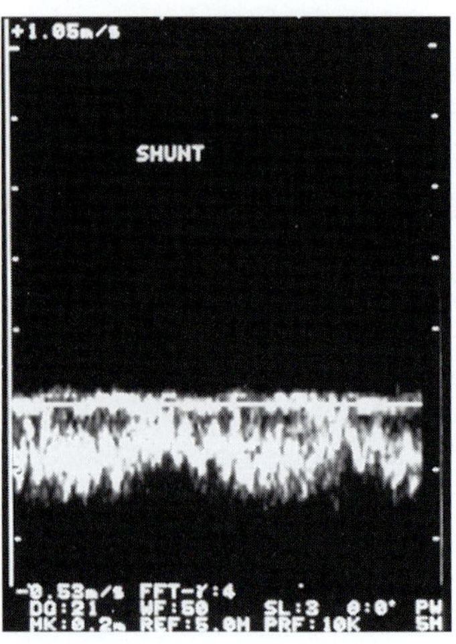


A

B

**FIGURE 3–13**

A 23-year-old patient with a prior splenorenal shunt for decompression of varices presented with recurrent gastrointestinal bleeding and esophageal varices. (**A**) Endosonography from the mid body of the stomach demonstrates the splenic vein (SV)/shunt anastomosis seen adjacent to the left kidney. (**B**) Doppler interrogation of the shunt demonstrates flow toward the left kidney, as expected. Transcutaneous ultrasound was unable to confirm the presence or absence of flow.

endosonography. Instead, at the level of the celiac artery, the probe may be rotated (either direction) until the celiac artery origin is no longer visualized but the aorta can still be seen. Using these landmarks, material may be injected bilaterally. Prior to the procedure the absence of a coagulopathy or thrombocytopenia should be confirmed. A 23-gauge 4-cm ultrasound aspiration needle (Wilson-Cook, Winston-Salem, North Carolina) is prepared by flushing the device with .9% saline. A syringe with 5 mL of saline is attached to the hub of the needle. The needle assembly is placed through the biopsy channel. When the aspiration catheter is identified as protruding from the biopsy channel, the needle is advanced into the patient. The needle is placed immediately adjacent and anterior to the lateral aspect of the aorta under direct EUS visualization. An aspiration test is then performed. If no blood is obtained, 3 mL of .25% preservative-free bupivacaine (Winthrop-Breon, New York) is injected. This is followed by 10 mL of dehydrated 98% absolute alcohol (American Regent Laboratories, Luitpold Pharmaceuticals, Shirley, New York). Some centers have employed steroid solutions, but we prefer the bactericidal ethanol because an endoscopic approach lacks sterility. In all patients, with the injection of alcohol an echogenic cloud can be identified on EUS (Fig. 3–14). The needle is then withdrawn from the patient and flushed with .9% saline; then the same process is performed on the opposite side of the aorta.

The potential risks of the procedure (in addition to the risk related to the endoscopy) include hypotension, diarrhea, and neuropathic pain. Rarely, paraplegia may occur, but has been described only with the posterior approach (39–41). During the examination, normal saline should be administered to counteract any potential hypotension arising from the neurolysis. The average time required to perform the CPN component of the exam is 15 minutes. Post-procedure patients are checked for orthostasis and other complications prior to discharge (recovery period approximately 2 hours). We have not found hospitalization to be necessary post procedure.

We prospectively evaluated patients with intractable abdominal pain secondary to chronic pancreatitis (9 patients, mean age 43 years, range 32–54) or intra-abdominal malignancy (58 patients, mean age 66 years, range 40–86) who underwent EUS CPN using 98% ethanol (42). Pre/post-procedure pain medication usage and pain scores measured with a visual analog scale (range 0–10) were recorded. The median followup for chronic pancreatitis was 273 days (range 14–365 days) and malignant disease was 114 days (range 12–593 days). Initial pain scores between the two patients groups were similar (Fig. 3–15). At each followup interval, the mean pain score for patients with malignancy was less than baseline ($p < .001$) and less than in patients with chronic pancreatitis ($p < .05$). In patients with chronic pancreatitis, the pain score improvement post-EUS CPN was not significant. Pain medication usage decreased or was stable in 78–100% of patients with chronic pancreatitis and 72–81% of patients with malignancy during the followup intervals. The Kaplan–Meier estimate for median duration of pain control was 2 weeks for patients with chronic pancreatitis and 20 weeks for patients with malignant disease

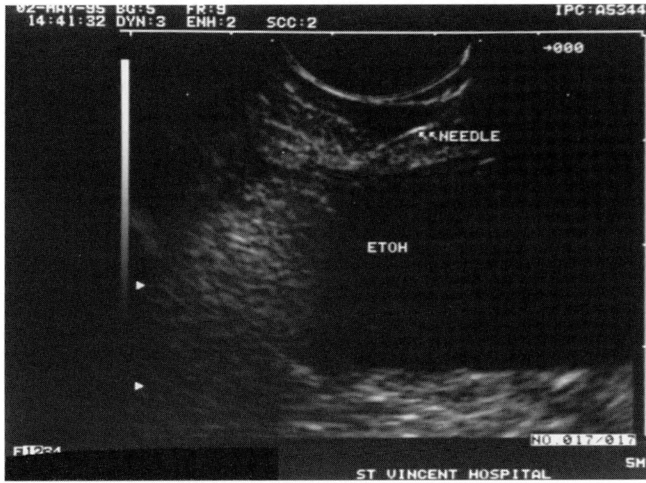


A

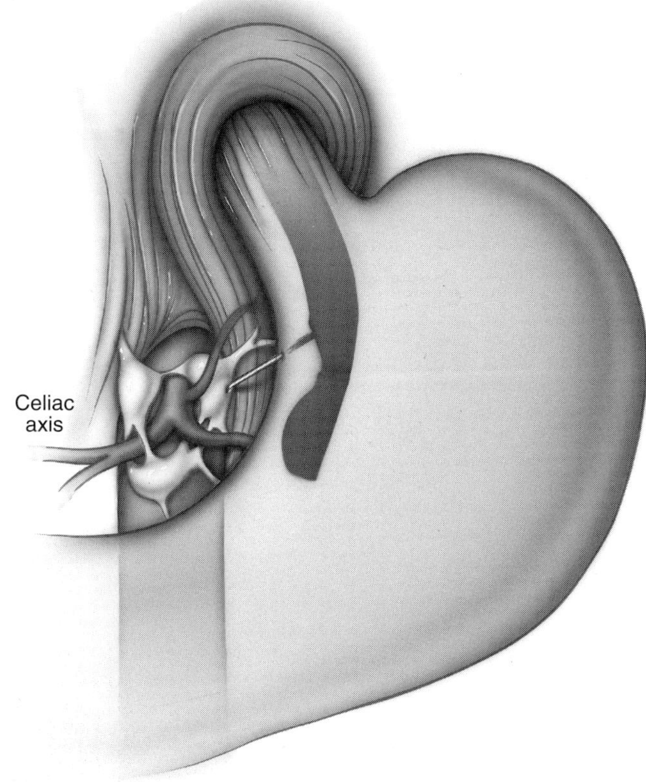


B

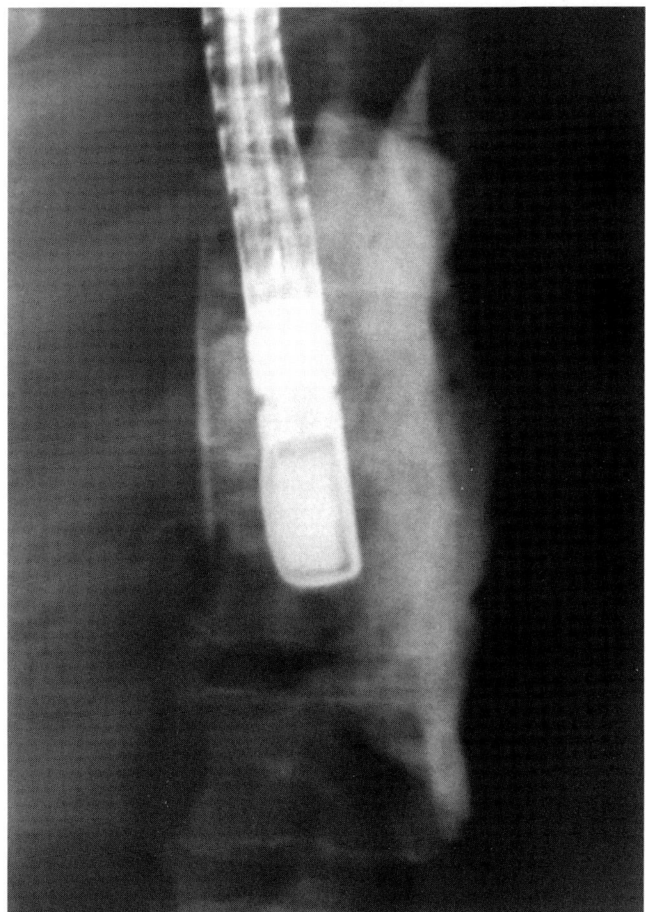

C

**FIGURE 3-14**

Parasagittal transgastric US scan obtained with the linear echoprobe demonstrates a longitudinal view of the aorta. The probe is rotated toward the patient's left (cranial direction is to the right). The needle is advanced along the lateral aspect of the aorta. Anesthetic material can then be injected after an aspiration test has been performed. (**A**) Alcohol injection results in an echogenic cloud adjacent to the aorta. The illustration demonstrates the echoprobe position within the stomach when performing the EUS CPN. (**B**) Fluoroscopic monitoring demonstrates left periaortic distribution of contrast (**C,** supine). The procedure is then repeated on the patient's right side. (Reprinted with permission from Wiersema MJ, Wiersema LM. Endosonography-guided celiac plexus neurolysis. Gastrointestinal Endoscopy 44(6):656–662, 1996.)

($p$ = .008). For those patients with malignancy, 38–52% had pain scores of 0 during each followup interval and 32% had pain scores of ≤50% of baseline at the time of their death. Complication frequency was similar in the chronic pancreatitis (33%) versus malignant group (21%) and was minor in nature (transient diarrhea or transient increase in pain). None of the patients was specifically hospitalized for the EUS CPN. These results suggest that EUS CPN is a safe pain control method that should be limited to patients with malignancy.

## Summary

The linear echoprobe allows EUS FNA, EGCP, Doppler imaging, and shows promise in EUS CPN. All of these

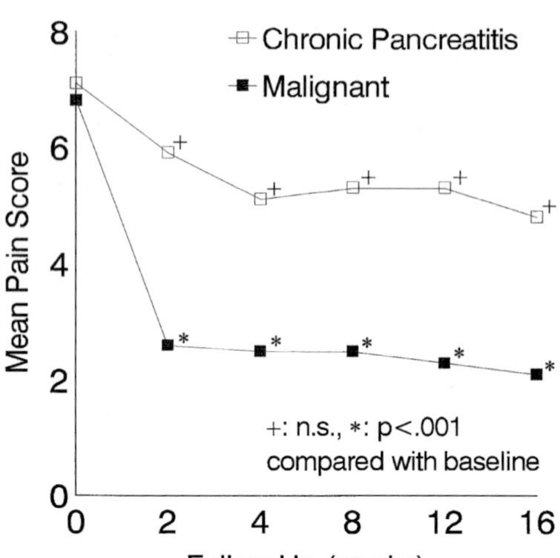


**FIGURE 3-15**

Comparison of baseline and followup mean pain scores for patients with chronic pancreatitis and intra-abdominal malignancy treated with EUS CPN. Initial mean pain scores were similar between the two groups. In the patients with chronic pancreatitis followup mean pain scores were not significantly different from baseline. In patients with malignancy, post-procedure mean pain scores were less than baseline ($p < .001$) and also less than those in patients with chronic pancreatitis ($p < .05$) at each followup interval through 16 weeks. (Reprinted with permission by Wiersema M, Harada N, Wiersema L. Endosonography guided celiac plexus neurolysis (EUS CPN) for abdominal pain: Efficacy in chronic pancreatitis and malignant disease. Acta Endoscopia 28(1):67–79, 1998.)

imaging/therapeutic capabilities are unique to this probe owing to its electronic design and transducer orientation. Preliminary studies support the ability to obtain accurate staging information with the device; however, the limitations have not been as vigorously addressed as with the radial scanning probes. The addition of biopsy capabilities appears to improve lymph node staging accuracy through an improvement in specificity when compared with EUS alone. Further studies are needed to examine the tumor staging capabilities of the Pentax probe as well as the role EUS FNA may play in patient management.

## References

1. Botet JF, Lightdale CJ, Zauber AG, Gerdes H, et al. Preoperative staging of esophageal cancer: Comparison of endoscopic US and dynamic CT. Radiology 181(2):419–425, 1991.
2. Botet JF, Lightdale CJ, Zauber AG, Gerdes H, et al. Preoperative staging of gastric cancer: Comparison of endoscopic US and dynamic CT. Radiology 181(2):426–432, 1991.
3. Tio TL, Lohen P, Coene P, Udding J, et al. Endosonography and computed tomography of esophageal carcinoma. Gastroenterol 96:1478–1486, 1989.
4. Rosch T, Braig C, Gain T, Geuerbach S, et al. Staging of pancreatic and ampullary carcinoma by endoscopic ultrasonography. Comparison with conventional sonography, computed tomography, and angiography. Gastroenterol 102(1):188–199, 1992.
5. Tio TL, Cheng J, Wijers OB, Sars PR, Tytgat GN. Endosonographic TNM staging of extrahepatic bile duct cancer: Comparison with pathological staging. Gastroenterol 100:1351–1361, 1991.
6. Wiersema MJ, Chak A. Prospective comparative evaluation of a linear electronic array ultrasound endoscope and a radial mechanical ultrasound endoscope. Gastrointest Endosc 39(2):51a, 1993.
7. Mortensen MB, Hovendal C. Curved array endosonography in the preoperative assessment of resectability of upper GI cancer. Gastroenterol 104(4):431a, 1993.
8. Wiersema MJ, Kochman ML, Chak A, Cramer HM, Kesler KA. Real-time endoscopic ultrasound-guided fine-needle aspiration of a mediastinal lymph node. Gastrointest Endosc 39(3):429–431, 1993.
9. Wiersema MJ, Kochman ML, Cramer HM, Wiersema LM. Preoperative staging of non–small cell lung cancer: Transesophageal US-guided fine-needle aspiration biopsy of mediastinal lymph nodes. Radiology 190:1–4, 1994.
10. Vilmann P, Jacobsen GK, Henriksen FW, Hancke S. Endoscopic ultrasonography with guided fine needle aspiration biopsy in pancreatic disease. Gastrointest Endosc 38:172–173, 1991.
11. Wiersema MJ, Kochman ML, Cramer HM, Tao LC, Wiersema LM. Endosonography guided real time fine needle aspiration biopsy. Gastrointest Endosc 40:700–707, 1994.
12. Vilmann P. Hancke S, Henrikson FW, Jacobson GK. Endoscopic ultrasonography-guided fne needle aspiration biopsy of lesions in the upper gastrointestinal tract. Gastrointest Endosc 41(3)230–235, 1995.
13. Chang KJ, Katz KD, Durbin TE, Erickson RA, Butler JA, Lin F, Wuerker RB. Endoscopic ultrasound guided fine-needle aspiration. Gastrointest Endosc 40(5):694–699, 1994.
14. Giovannini M, Seitz JF, Monges G, Perrier H, Rabbia I. Fine needle aspiration cytology guided by EUS. Endoscopy 27:171–177, 1995.
15. Wiersema MJ, Chak A, Kopecky KK, Wiersema LM. Duplex Doppler endosonography in the diagnosis of splenic vein, portal vein and portosystemic shunt thrombosis. Gastrointest Endosc 42:19–26, 1995.
16. Wiersema MJ, Sandusky D, Carr R, Wiersema LM, Erdel WC, Frederick PK. Endosonography-guided cholangiopancreatography. Gastrointest Endosc 43:102–106, 1996.
17. Wiersema MJ, Wiersema LM. Endosonography-guided celiac plexus neurolysis. Gastrointest Endosc 44(6):656–662, 1996.
18. Wiersema MJ. Endosonography-guided cystduodenostomy with a therapeutic ultrasound endoscope. Gastrointest Endosc 44(5):614–617, 1996.
19. Kobayashi H, Danbara T, Tamaki S, Kitamura S, Hata E, Fukushima K, Kira S. Detection of the mediastinal lymph nodes metastasis in lung cancer by endoscopic ultrasonography. Jpn J Med 27(1):17–22, 1988.
20. Schuder G, Isringhaus H, Kubale B, Seitz G, Sybrecht GW. Endoscopic ultrasonography of the mediastinum in the diagnosis of bronchial carcinoma. Thorac Cardiovasc Surgeon 39:299–303, 1991.
21. Kondo D, Imaizumi M, Abe T, Naruke T, Suemasu K. Endoscopic ultrasound examinations for mediastinal lymph node metastases of lung cancer. Chest 98:586–593, 1990.
22. Ferguson MK. A sound idea. Chest 98(3):526–527, 1990.
23. Rosch T, Lorenz R, Von Wichert A, Siewart JR, Claussen M. Endoscopic ultrasonography is not useful in the differential diagnosis of gastric ulcer. Gastrointest Endosc 38(2):241, 1992.
24. Rosch T, Lorenz R, Braig C, Feuerback S, et al. Endoscopic ultrasound in pancreatic tumor diagnosis. Gastrointest Endosc 37(3):347–352, 1991.
25. Wiersema MJ, Villman P, Giovannini M, Chang KJ, Wiersema LM. Endosonography guided fine needle aspiration biopsy: Diagnostic accuracy and complication assessment. Gastroenterology 112: 1087–1095, 1997.
26. Harada N, Wiersema M, Wiersema L. Endosonography guided fine needle aspiration biopsy (EUS FNA) in the evaluation of lymphadenopathy: Staging accuracy of EUS FNA versus EUS alone. Gastrointest Endosc (abstract 1997).
27. Wiersema M, Harada N, Daiehagh P, Beltz HF, Pfeiffer M, Allen K, Griffith G, Wiersema LM. Evaluation of mediastinal lympha-

denopathy with transesophageal endosonography guided fine needle aspiration biopsy. Acta Endoscopia 28(1):7–19, 1998.
28. Foley WD, Erickson SJ. Color Doppler flow imaging. AJR 156:3–13, 1991.
29. Eidt JF, Harward T, Cook JM, Kahn MB, Troillett R. Current status of duplex Doppler ultrasound in the examination of the abdominal vasculature. Am J Surg 160:604–609, 1990.
30. Morton MJ, James EM, Wiesner RH, Krom RAF. Applications of duplex ultrasonography in the liver transplant patient. Mayo Clin Proc 65:360–372, 1990.
31. Flinn WR, Rizzo RJ, Park JS, Sandager GP. Duplex scanning for assessment of mesenteric ischemia. Surg Clin N Am 70(1):99–107, 1990.
32. Tessler FN, Gehring BJ, Gomes AS, Perrella RR, Ragavendra N, Busuttil RW, Grant EG. Diagnosis of portal vein thrombosis: Value of color Doppler imaging. AJR 157:293–296, 1991.
33. Johansen K, Paun M. Duplex ultrasonography of the portal vein. Surg Clin N Am 70(1):181–190, 1990.
34. Perisic-Savic M, Colovic R, Miosavljevic T, Ivanovic L. Splenic vein thrombosis diagnosed with Doppler ultrasonography. Hepato-Gastroenterol 38:557–560, 1991.
35. Strandness DE. Duplex scanning and diagnosis of renovascular hypertension. Surg Clin N Am 70(1):109–117, 1990.
36. Kohler TR, Zierler RE, Martin RL, Nicholls SC, Bergelin RO, Kazmers A, Beach KW, Strandness DE. Non-invasive diagnosis of renal artery stenosis by ultrasonic duplex scanning. J Vasc Surg 4:450–456, 1986.
37. Scoutt LM, Zawin ML, Taylor KJW. Doppler ultrasound part II: Clinical applications. Radiol 174:309–319, 1990.
38. Zierler RE. The role of vascular laboratory in clinical decision-making. Seminars in Roentgenology 27(1):63–77, 1992.
39. Brown DL, Bulley CK, Quiel EL. Neurolytic celiac plexus block for pancreatic cancer pain. Anesth Analg 66:869–873, 1987.
40. Cherny NI, Portenoy RK. This management of cancer pain. CA: A Cancer Journal for Clinicians 44(5):262–303, 1994.
41. De Connon F, Caraceni A, Aldrighetti L, Magnani G, Ferla G, Comi G, Ventafridda V. Paralegia following celiac plexus block. Pain 55:383–385, 1993.
42. Wiersema M, Harada N, Wiersema L. Endosonography guided celiac plexus neurolysis (EUS CPN) for abdominal pain: Efficacy in chronic pancreatitis and malignant disease. Acta Endoscopia 28(1):67–79, 1998.

CHAPTER

4

# Practical Guide to Using the Linear Array Echoendoscope

Marcia Irene F. Canto
Kenneth J. Chang

Endoscopic ultrasound-guided fine-needle aspiration (EUS FNA) is an effective modality for establishing a tissue diagnosis of primary malignant lesions within or adjacent to the gastrointestinal tract as well as documenting malignant spread to lymph nodes, free fluid, and liver (1–6). EUS-guided FNA with Doppler ultrasound is currently possible using the curved linear array echoendoscopes available from the Olympus corporation (Olympus America, Inc., Melville, New York) and the Pentax corporation (Pentax Precision Instruments, Orangeburg, New York). Because many experienced radial endosonographers may not yet be familiar with linear array anatomy, and some novice endosonographers may wish to learn EUS using the linear array echoendoscopes, this chapter will provide a practical "how-to" approach to performing EUS and EUS-guided FNA with these instruments. This chapter will focus on intubation, positioning the echoendoscope, techniques for optimal imaging, introduction to color flow and Doppler ultrasound, and the technique of EUS-guided FNA.

## Preliminaries

It is essential to become familiar with cross-sectional anatomy (7, 8) and the basics of color flow Doppler ultrasound (8, 9). Next, the controls and keyboard of the ultrasound console must be learned. The use of the Pentax linear array echoendoscope (Pentax Precision Instrument Corporation, Orangeburg, New York) will be the paradigm for this chapter. It is most often used in conjunction with the Hitachi EUS-515 ultrasound console. There are many keyboard/control functions that are not required for routine EUS imaging. However, minimally, it is important to be aware of the following function keys (Fig. 4–1):

1. FREEZE: This is the key most often used during endosonography. The EUS console also has cine-loop memory, which stores a series of frames (the number stored is shown on the bottom right of the screen). The best image for storage or hard-copy production can be selected by freezing the image and scrolling through the stored images with the trackball.
2. CHARACTER: To label an image, freeze the image, move the cursor with the trackball to the desired area for labeling the image, and type the label.
3. ***MEASUREMENTS*** (DISTANCE): The DISTANCE key measures the distance between several pairs of points and gives an estimate of width, length, depth, etc. To measure a distance between two points on the image, freeze the image and press the DISTANCE key. Move the cursor until reaching the desired point and press the SET button. This series of maneuvers may be repeated using the remaining sets of cursors to obtain additional series of measurements.
4. PRESET #1: The PRESET key resets the console to it's original/default settings and may be useful after several functions such as measurement, label, color Doppler, magnification, gain, etc., have been used.
5. GAIN: The gain (or amount of echo displayed on the screen) can be adjusted either by using the large GAIN knob on the right lower corner of the keyboard or by moving the series of knobs located on the right upper corner of the console's control panel (DEPTH GAIN CONTROL). The DGC adjusts the gain for a series of specific depths of tissue, or distances from the transducer.
6. COLOR DOPPLER (CFM): The CFM (Color Flow Module) key is located on the second (lower) keyboard and controls the use of color flow and Doppler.
7. DEPTH: The DEPTH buttons (two sets of keys with arrowheads facing toward or away from the other) change the size of the displayed image.
8. CONTROL/5: The ultrasound frequency is displayed on the bottom right corner of the screen. To switch from 7.5 MHz to 5 MHz frequency (to increase penetration depth as in imaging the liver, large pancreatic pseudocysts or tumors), press the CONTROL key at the same time as the number 5 key.
9. ZOOM: This key function allows the selection of a particular area of the EUS image within a box (which appears after the key is depressed) and the magnification of the particular area (after the key is depressed a second time).
10. PRINT: If a thermal printer or mavigraph is connected to the console, an instant "hard-copy" can be obtained. To activate the printer, depress SHUTTER button on the ultrasound console's keyboard.
11. RECORD: If a VCR is connected to the ultrasound console, images can be stored on videotape by depressing the RECORD key under VCR. Depress the PAUSE key to temporarily stop recording.

## Preparing for the Examination

Patient preparation for linear array endosonography and EUS-guided FNA is similar to that for routine upper endoscopy. Patients should avoid aspirin and nonsteroidal anti-inflammatory medications for at least one week prior to the procedure. A complete blood count with platelet count, prothrombin time and partial thromboplastin time may be obtained prior to an FNA procedure, if the patient's coagulation status is in doubt. In pa-

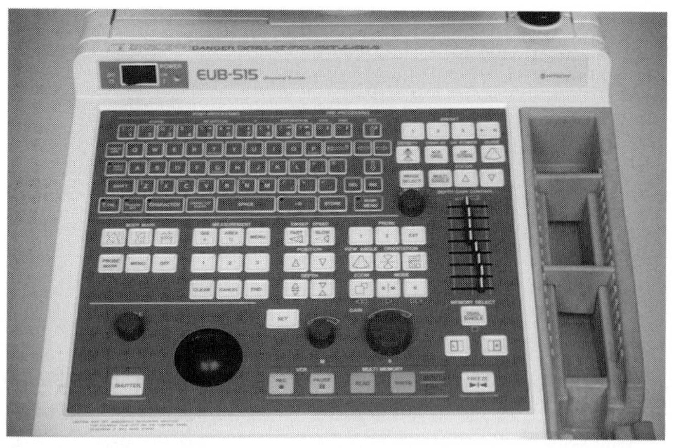


A

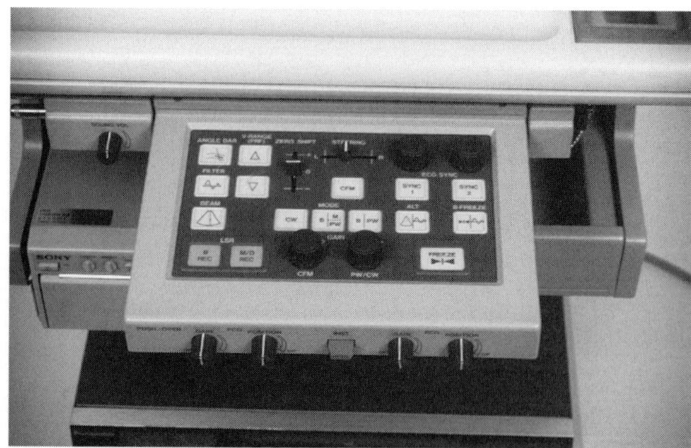


B

**FIGURE 4–1**

Hitachi EUB-515 ultrasound console main/upper keyboard (**A**) and lower keyboard (**B**).

tients with a prolonged prothrombin time (>3 sec), two units of fresh frozen plasma may be administered prior to the procedure. Antibiotic prophylaxis is not required for EUS-guided FNA of the upper gastrointestinal tract unless indicated for bacterial endocarditis prophylaxis. One exception to this is EUS-guided FNA of cystic lesions in the chest or abdomen. Cystic lesions have a significantly higher risk of febrile complications (10). The other indication for antibiotic prophylaxis is EUS-guided FNA through the lower gastrointestinal tract wall. One example of a prophylactic regimen for lower GI FNA is a single dose of IV ciprofloxicin and metronidazole 30 minutes prior to the procedure followed by 3 days of oral antibiotics.

Patients should be positioned in the left lateral decubitus position as for any upper endoscopy procedure. Adding droperidol (2.5–5.0 mg) to meperidine (Demerol) and midazolam (Versed) may provide a more beneficial effect of conscious sedation due to the relatively longer procedure times of EUS and EUS-guided FNA when compared to standard endoscopy.

Prior to intubation, the balloon should be examined for air bubbles and water leakage. If the balloon leaks, suture material or dental floss can be tied over the balloon in the proximal groove (only Pentax FG-32UX) and the groove distal to the transducer. Be certain that the knot is located behind the echoendoscope's optics. Test the balloon by inflating with water before cutting the strings short. Test the water and suction valves. Inability to deflate the balloon can be problematic once the echoendoscope has been inserted into the patient. The inflated balloon may be too large to bring through the esophagus and pharynx and puncture of the balloon with a needle through the biopsy channel would be necessary. If the suction appears does not function properly, make certain that the dial for suction and water is switched to the balloon (B) and not the echoendoscope (E). Assess both the endoscopic and endosonographic images. Ultrasound interference patterns may make EUS imaging difficult and the source of the interference may be elusive. One common source of electrical interference is the pulse oximeter unit. Unplugging the unit and running it on battery power may reduce the interference.

## Intubation

Intubation of the esophagus with an echoendoscope is similar to passing a duodenoscope. Lubricant gel may be avoided as it may interfere with endoscopic or endosonographic imaging. Wetting the tip of the echoendoscope with water just prior to intubation is usually sufficient. If a lubricant gel is used, avoid the latex balloon and optics of the scope. One technique for echoendoscope intubation is as follows: when the tip of the echoendoscope is positioned in the patient's posterior pharynx, rotate the echoendoscope 90° counterclockwise. The endoscopist should lower his/her flexed left elbow towards the left. Next, the echoendoscope tip should be deflected slightly upwards using the left thumb while gently advancing the echoendoscope with the right hand. Alternatively, with the echoendoscope's controls in the neutral position, lock the right/left control, insert the scope tip into the posterior pharynx and deflect downward while advancing the echoendoscope with the right hand as the patient swallows.

## General Considerations in Linear Array EUS

Endosonographers experienced with Olympus radial scanning instruments will notice a difference when handling the Pentax echoendoscope. The direction of the viewing fields for the Pentax FG-32UA and Olympus GF-UM20 are 60° and 70° frontal oblique, respectively (Table 4–1). The air/water and suction valves are also different. The Olympus instruments have two-step valves that toggle between balloon (first step) and lumen (second step) air/water and suction. The Pentax echoendoscope has a one-step valve and a separate switch to select between lumen and balloon and no automatic instillation of water to fill the balloon (FG-32UA). More recent Pentax prototypes have automatic balloon filling, double balloon attachment, a needle elevator (useful for FNA), and conversion to video from fiberoptic imaging (Pentax EG-363).

Radial scanning EUS has a 360° ultrasound field which is oriented perpendicular to the long axis of the

**TABLE 4–1**

Comparison of Radial and Linear Array Echoendoscopes

| | Olympus GF-UM20 | Pentax FG-32UA |
|---|---|---|
| ***Echoendoscope*** | | |
| Viewing direction | 70° forward oblique | 60° forward oblique |
| Viewing field angle | 80° | 105° |
| Up/down angulation | 130° each way | 160° each way |
| Right/left angulation | 90° each way | 100° each way |
| Tip diameter | 13.2 mm | 12 mm |
| Air/water suction | Automatic; 2-step valves for balloon and lumen | Not automatic;1-step valves with separate switch to select balloon or lumen |
| Elevator | 45° range | None |
| ***Ultrasound*** | | |
| Scanning system | Radial | Convex, 100° angle |
| Frequency | 7.5, 12 MHz | 5, 7.5 MHz |
| Color flow/Doppler | Not available | Available |

echoendoscope. Thus, with the probe in the esophagus, images are oriented similarly to those obtained via CT scan or MRI of the chest. Curved linear array EUS has a 100° ultrasound field (wedge-shaped) oriented parallel to the long axis of the echoendoscope. Therefore, B-mode ultrasound images obtained with the curved linear array transducer are generally oriented 90° relative to images obtained with the radial scanner in the same position. Depending on the setting on the ultrasound console, the distal aspect of a longitudinal structure may be located to the left or right of the image. The lower scanning frequency (5 MHz) available on curved linear-array echoendoscopes allows a greater depth of penetration (up to 10 cm) compared to radial echoendoscopes.

## EUS of the Esophagus and Mediastinum

The mediastinum may be imaged by gently advancing the echoendoscope into the distal esophagus. In the mediastinum and the upper abdomen, the descending aorta is the major landmark for orientation. The balloon should be slightly inflated with water (approximately 5 mL). The descending aorta may be located by rotating the shaft of the echoendoscope slightly to the right (clockwise) or left (counterclockwise). Shaft rotation is best accomplished with shoulder rotation or torquing at the level of the echoendoscope handle with the left hand (rather than at the mid-shaft with the right hand). The right hand should remain free to access the ultrasound console's control knobs or to utilize the aspiration needle for FNA. The descending aorta is a large, echopoor, longitudinal structure with a very bright deep wall secondary to the air interface with the left lung (Fig. 4–2).

Rotating to the right of the descending aorta will bring into view sequentially the left lung, left atrium, right lung, azygous vein and spine. The azygous vein can be located by rotating approximately 45° to the left from the descending aorta. It appears as a thin, longitudinal echopoor structure adjacent to the esophageal wall (Fig. 4–3) and can be followed proximally to its

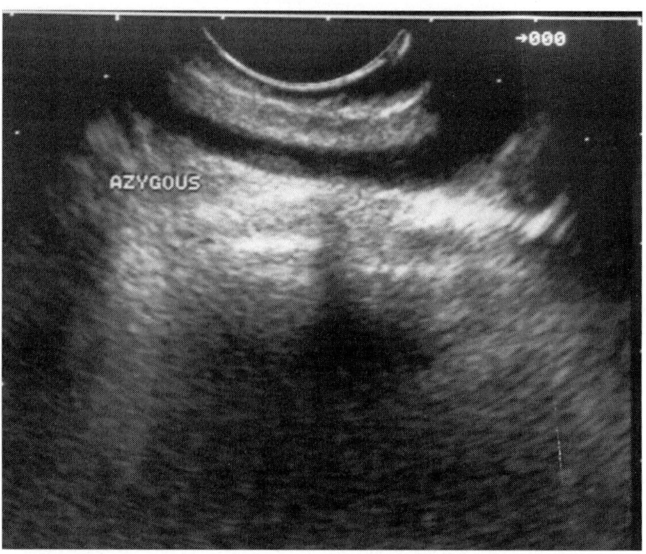


**FIGURE 4–3**

Linear array image (7.5 MHz) of azygous vein from the distal esophagus.

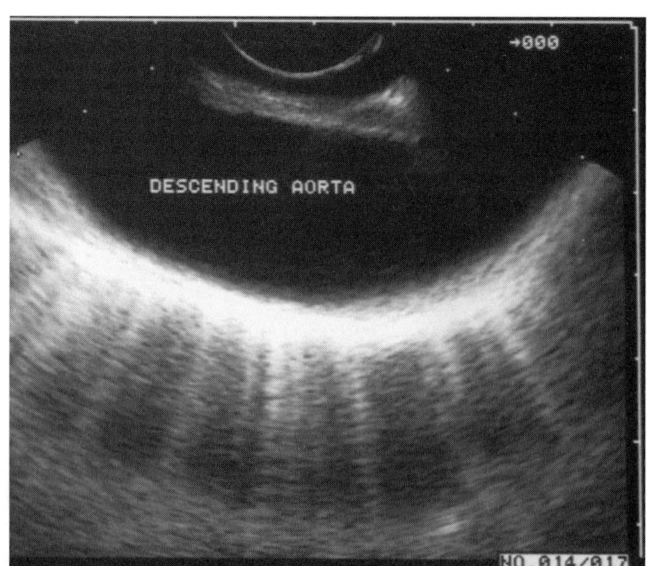


**FIGURE 4–2**

Curved linear array endosonographic view of descending aorta from the distal esophagus at 7.5 MHz.

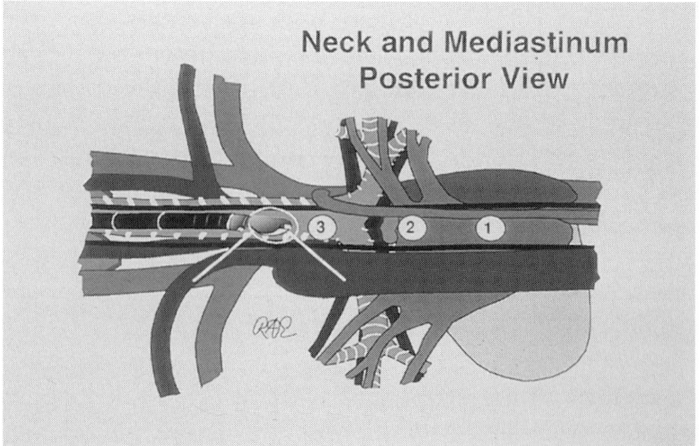


**FIGURE 4–4**

Diagram of echoendoscope imaging positions (stations 1–3) in the esophagus and anatomic relations of the esophagus with mediastinal structures. (*See color insert for color plate.*)

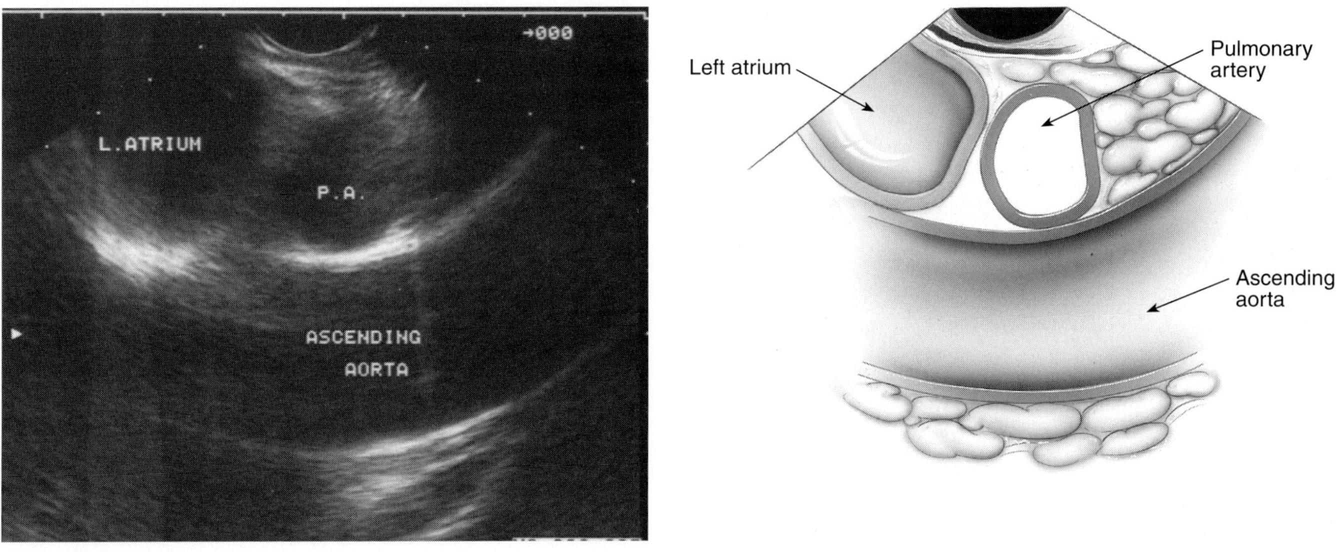


**FIGURE 4–5**

Linear array image of subcarinal region (station 2) with proximal left atrium (L. Atrium), cross section of pulmonary artery (PA), and ascending aorta (7.5 MHz).

union with the superior vena cava. Repositioning the echoendoscope over the mid-left atrium and withdrawing a few centimeters will place the transducer in the subcarinal region (Fig. 4–4, station 2). The large, pulsatile, cephalad portion of the left atrium or upper pulmonary veins can be visualized just distal to a round, cross-sectional view of the pulmonary artery (Fig. 4–5). This is an important location for detecting subcarinal lymph nodes for FNA. Further withdrawal of the echoendoscope will bring the arch of the aorta into view as a large circular structure (Fig. 4–6). By rotating the echoendoscope slightly right and left, the origins of the left subclavian and, occasionally, the left common carotid arteries can be seen above the innominate (brachiocephalic) vein. Just distal to the aortic arch and proximal to the pulmonary artery is the aorto-pulmonary window (Fig. 4–7). The "A-P window" is another important area for fine needle aspiration of mediastinal lymph nodes, especially in staging patients with lung cancer (11).

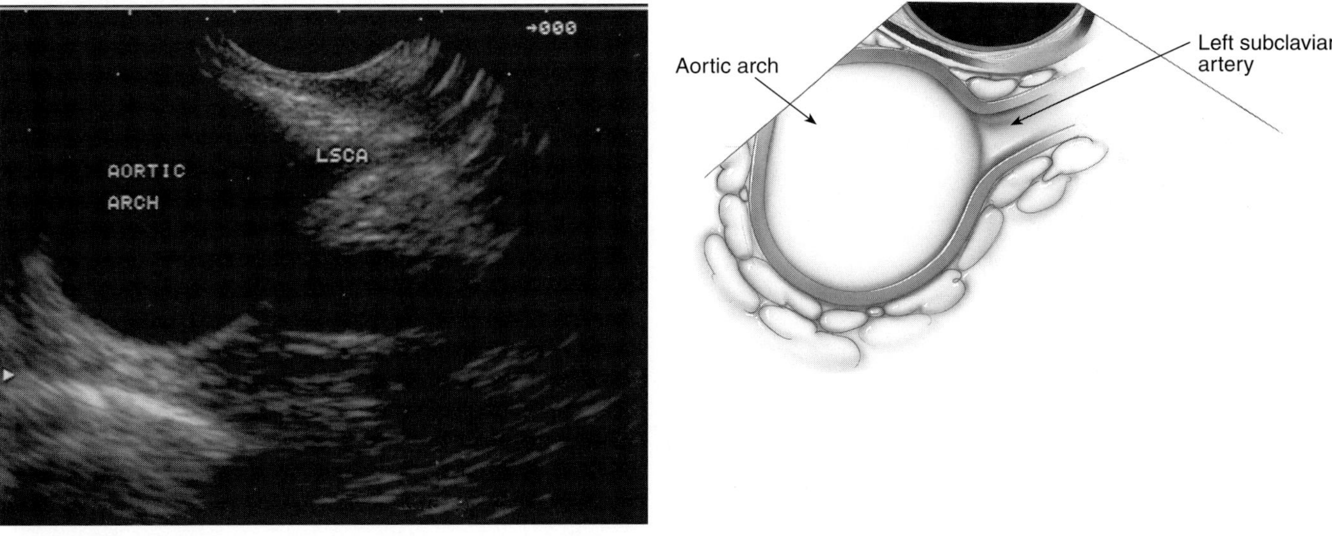


**FIGURE 4–6**

Linear array view (7.5 MHz) of the aortic arch with the origin of the left subclavian artery (LSCA).

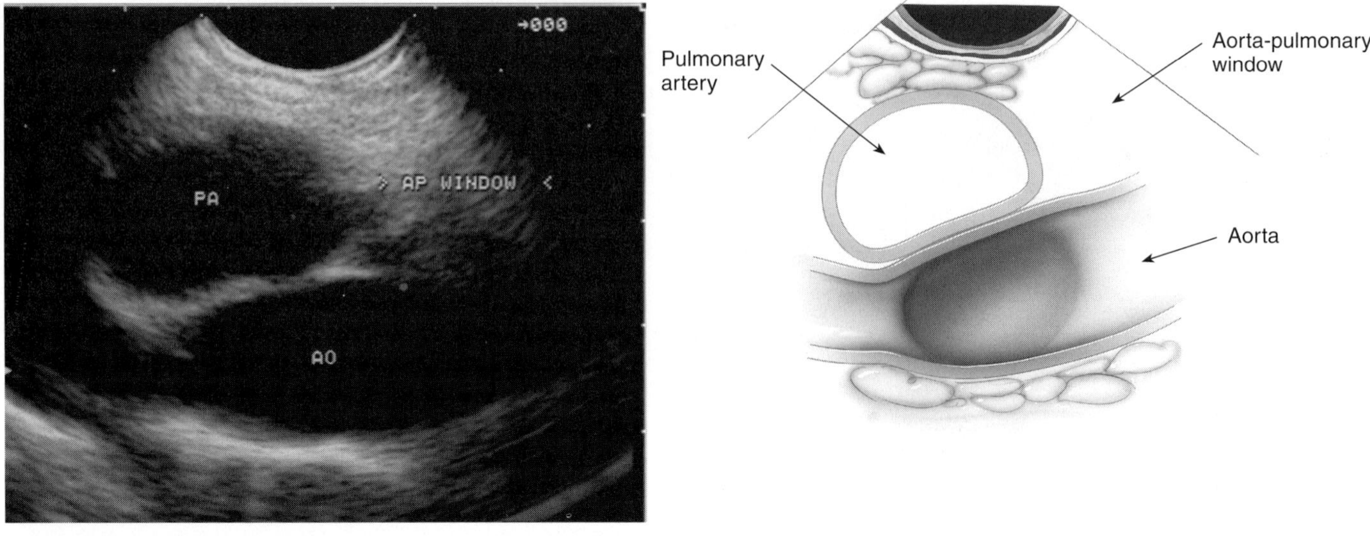


**FIGURE 4–7**

Curved linear array image (7.5 MHz) of aorto-pulmonary window (AP window), located proximal to the pulmonary artery (PA). Scanning from the mid-esophagus. Ascending aorta (AO) shown deep to the PA.

When staging esophageal, gastric, and pancreatic cancers, the celiac axis must be examined for lymphadenopathy. The descending aorta can be located by advancing the echoendoscope past the gastroesophageal junction for a few centimeters. Rotate left and right to examine either side of the celiac trunk which arises at a 45° angle from the aorta (Fig. 4–8). The origin of the superior mesenteric artery from the aorta may also be seen on the same image. The celiac axis is another important area for EUS-guided FNA because metastatic lymph nodes alter the TNM stage of an esophageal cancer to M1.

## Transabdominal EUS

Endosonographic imaging of the abdominal organs and vascular structures is via the stomach and duodenum. The larger capacity, variation in shape, and anatomic relations of the stomach make organ identification more

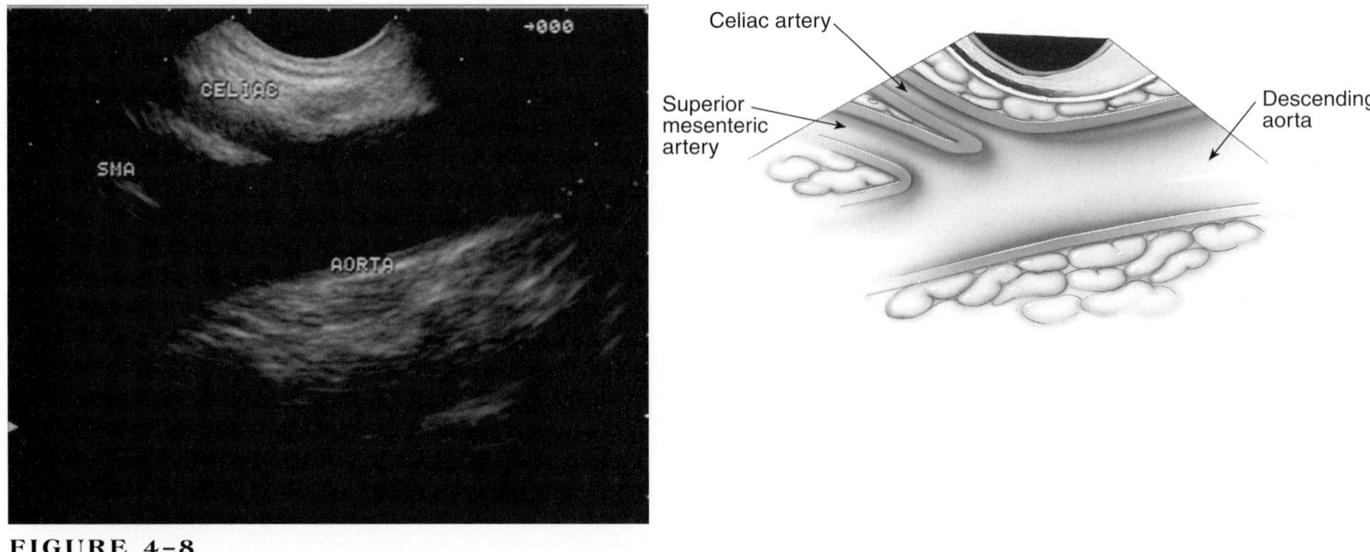


**FIGURE 4–8**

Linear array endosonographic view of the celiac artery and the superior mesenteric artery (SMA) origins from descending aorta; imaging from the proximal stomach.

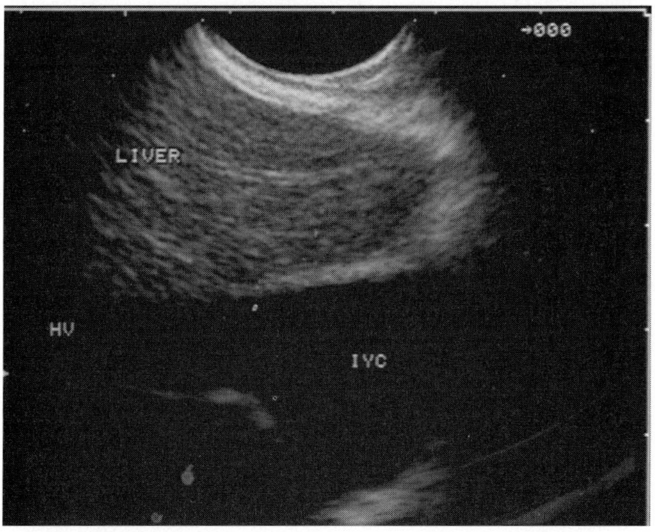


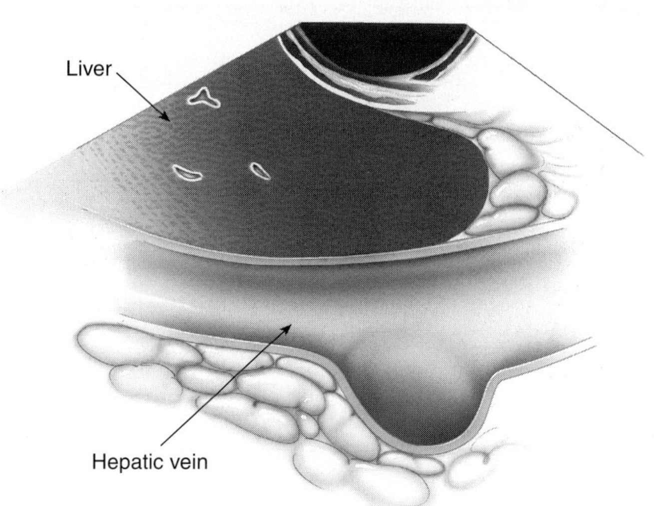


**FIGURE 4–9**

Linear array view (7.5 MHz) of the liver with the hepatic vein (HV) entering the inferior vena cava (IVC); imaging from the gastroesophageal junction.

difficult via transgastric linear array EUS compared to transesophageal EUS. An understanding of the anatomic relationships of major blood vessels and surrounding organs to the extraluminal organs of interest (primarily gallbladder, liver, pancreas, bile duct, adrenal gland, and celiac axis) is essential for linear-array endosonography and EUS-guided-FNA.

## Imaging the Liver

CT scan is more accurate than EUS for diagnosing liver metastases in patients with esophageal cancer (12). However, the endoscopist should examine the liver when staging upper gastrointestinal and pancreatic tumors because suspected liver metastases are amenable to EUS-guided FNA. Confirmation of liver metastases by EUS-guided FNA may impact on patient management (i.e., preclude surgery). The left lobe of the liver can be readily imaged from the proximal stomach by advancing the transducer beyond the gastroesophageal junction into the gastric cardia and rotating left or right. By slightly withdrawing the echoendoscope proximally, the quadrate lobe of the liver may be imaged. The hepatic veins can be readily seen entering the inferior vena cave (Fig. 4–9). To image the hilum of the liver and hepatic parenchyma, the echoendoscope should be advanced into the gastric antrum and distal body of the stomach and rotated anteriorly.

## Imaging the Ampulla and Pancreas

To image the ampulla and pancreas, the transducer should be advanced to the distal descending duodenum past the ampulla of Vater, and the echoendoscope should be maneuvered into the "short" position. As the echoendoscope is withdrawn from the duodenum to the gastric antrum, the uncinate process of the pancreas, and the head and neck of the pancreas will be imaged. Pancreatic imaging is initiated from the duodenum by advancing the transducer to the distal descending duodenum (Fig. 4–10, station 6). Duodenal air should be suctioned from the lumen and the latex balloon partially inflated. The tip of the echoendoscope should be deflected slightly downwards to optimize balloon contact.

Major anatomical landmarks include the inferior vena cava (IVC), abdominal aorta, and often the right

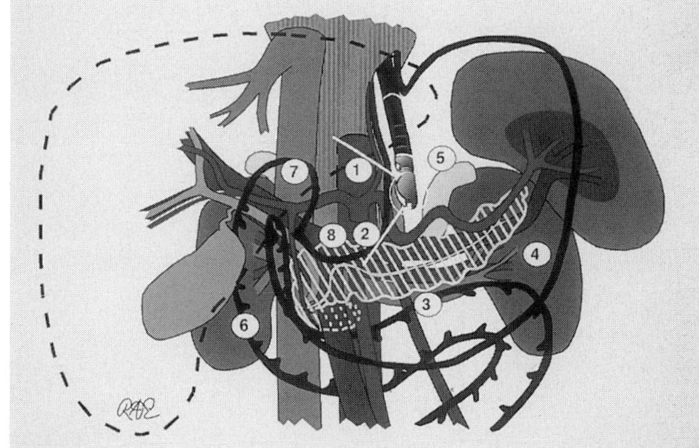


**FIGURE 4–10**

Diagram of linear array echoendoscope positions for imaging abdominal structures. (Reprinted with permission from Chang K. Gastroenterologic Endoscopy. (*See color insert for color plate.*)

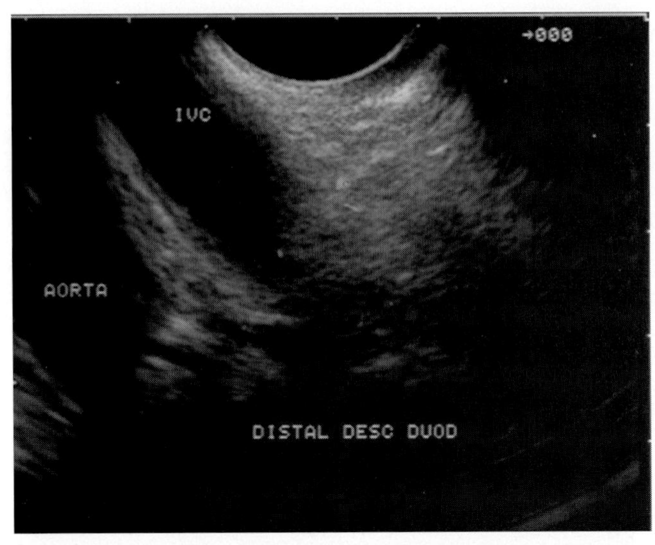


A

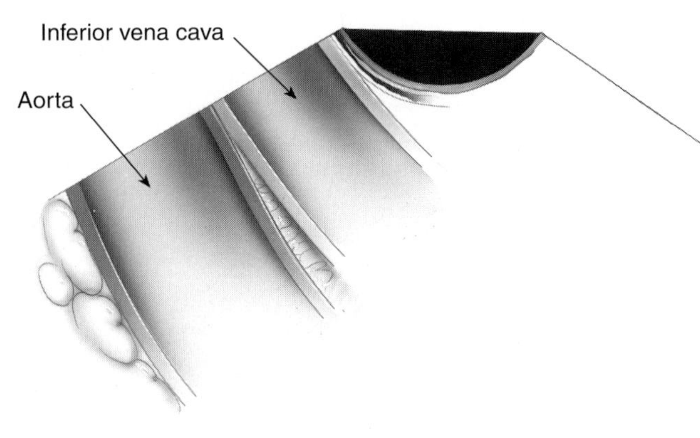


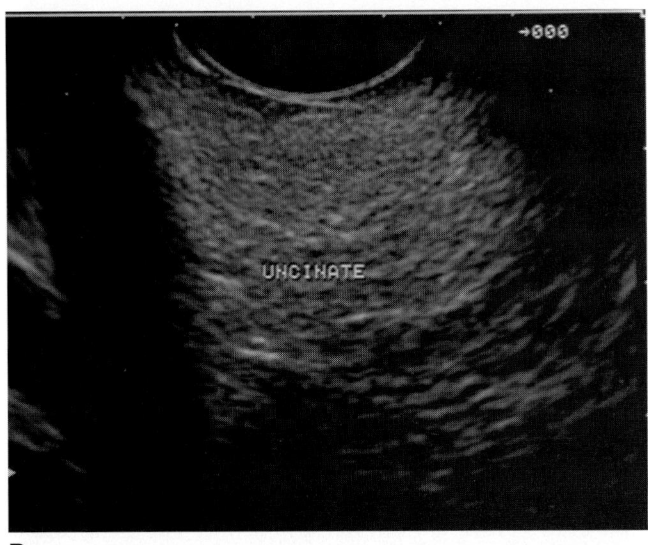


B

**FIGURE 4–11**

Linear array sonographic image from the distal descending duodenum (7.5 MHz). Major landmarks are the inferior vena cava (IVC) and the abdominal aorta (**A**). Uncinate process of the pancreas (**B**).

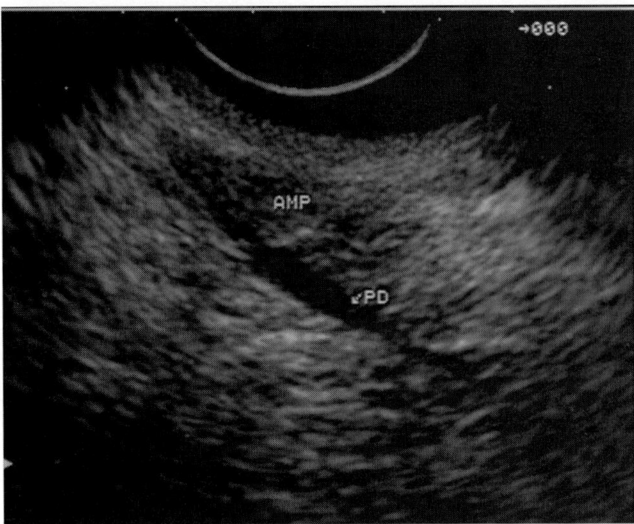


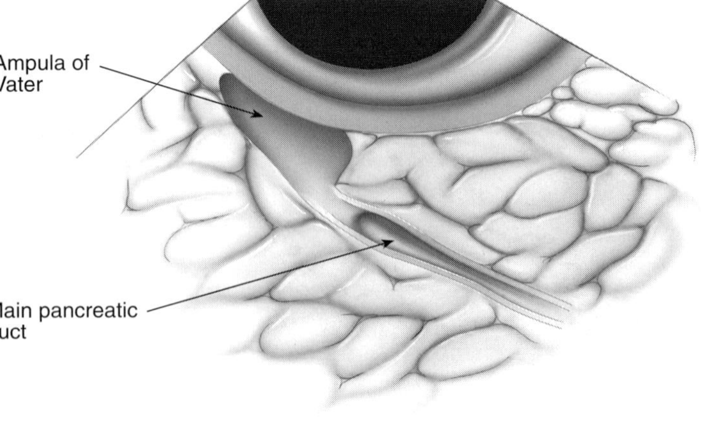


**FIGURE 4–12**

Image from the descending duodenum (7.5 MHz) at the level of the major papilla. Linear array sonographic image of ampulla (AMP) and distal pancreatic duct (PD).

kidney. The appearance of the vascular structures will vary depending on the position of the transducer. In general, the IVC tends to be closer to the transducer than the aorta when the transducer is in the distal descending duodenum (Fig. 4–11A). The orientation may change if the transducer is in the third portion of the duodenum and rotated towards the patient's right and posterior (which will make the aorta appear closer to the duodenal wall). Color flow and Doppler can readily differentiate the aorta from the IVC (see below). The pancreatic head and uncinate process can be visualized adjacent to the ultrasound transducer as echogenic structures with a fine "salt-and-pepper" homogeneous texture. The pancreatic duct is imaged as a transverse or longitudinal ductular structure within the pancreas (Fig. 4–11B). Two distinct areas of the pancreas can be identified due to their differing echogenicities—the dorsal and ventral pancreas. The former may appear hypoechoic and can mimic a "pseudotumor" (13).

As the transducer is withdrawn into the descending duodenum (for beginners, fluoroscopy can assist in identifying transducer position and imaging plane), the major ampulla should be identified endoscopically. The ampulla of Vater is identified endosonographically as an echo-poor fairly well-delineated structure to which a thin longitudinal or oblique structure, the pancreatic duct (PD), can be traced (Fig. 4–12). The ampulla should routinely be evaluated in addition to the bile duct and

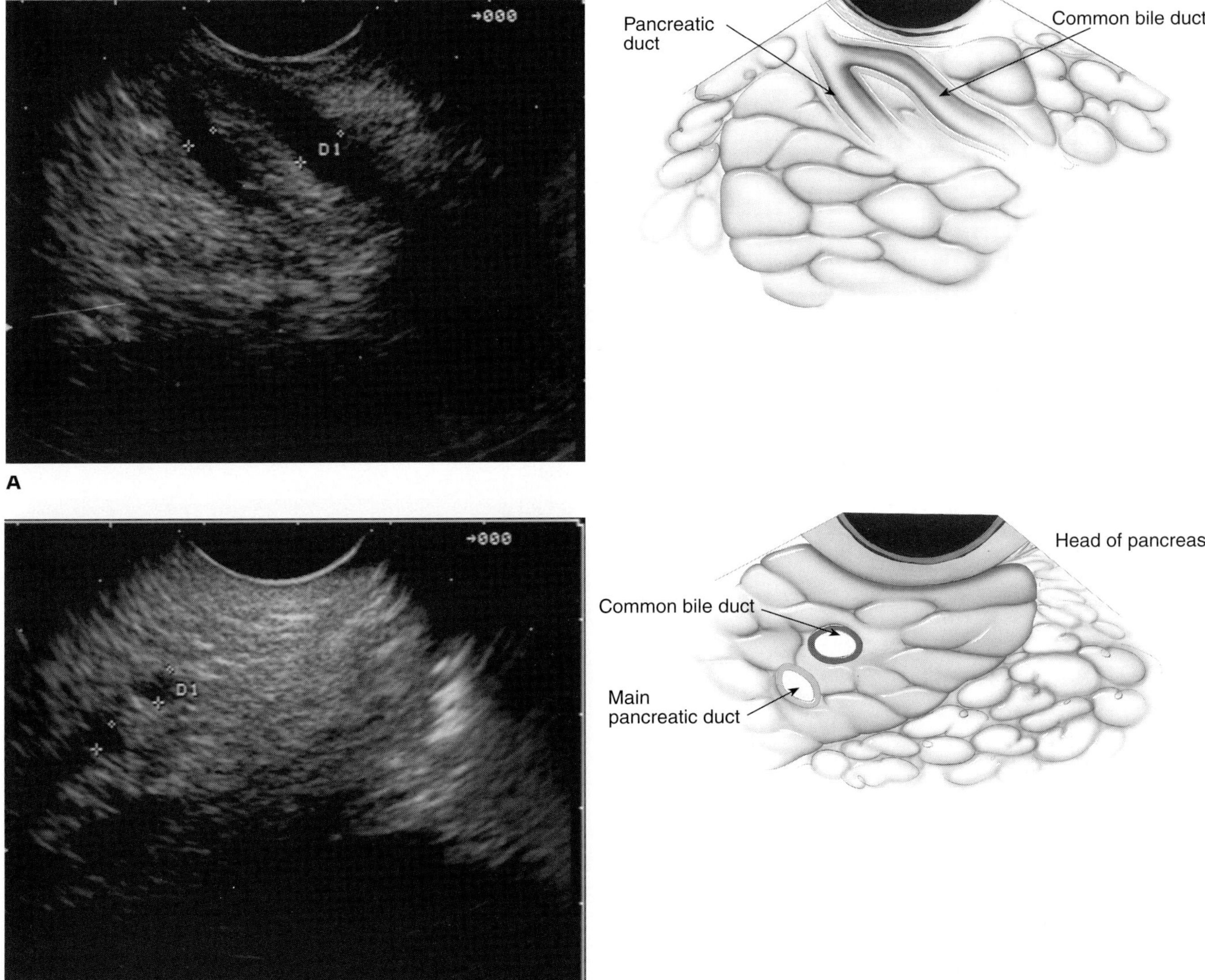


**FIGURE 4–13**

Image of the head of the pancreas from the descending duodenum (7.5 MHz, curved linear array echoendoscope). Longitudinal (**A**) and transverse (**B**) sections of the intrapancreatic common bile duct (CBD) and distal pancreatic duct (PD).

pancreas, in patients with jaundice or cholestasis. Tumors involving the ampulla will appear as hypoechoic lesions, larger than the usual 5 mm diameter of the normal ampulla.

With the transducer in the descending duodenum, withdraw the echoendoscope and rotate the instrument or your body rightwards (clockwise) to visualize a portion of the pancreatic head and longitudinal sections of the common bile duct (CBD) and pancreatic duct (PD) running in parallel (Fig. 4–13A). Transverse sections of the CBD and PD may also be imaged from this location (Fig. 4–13B). Within the pancreatic head, the PD is always located farther away from the transducer than the CBD.

To image the head and neck of the pancreas, withdraw the echoendoscope so that the ultrasound transducer is located in the proximal second portion of the duodenum or duodenal bulb. The neck of the pancreas can be imaged from either from the duodenal bulb or the gastric antrum. Decreasing the amount of water in the balloon will facilitate the transition from the bulb to the antrum and prevent "popping" out of the pylorus into the stomach. From the proximal duodenal bulb or distal antrum, the neck of the pancreas can be imaged with the portal vein (PV) and superior mesenteric artery (SMA) distal to it (Fig. 4–14). The splenic vein–superior mesenteric vein–portal vein confluence may be imaged distal to the pancreas.

The neck and body of the pancreas can also be imaged from the stomach by withdrawing the transducer to the proximal stomach and locating the celiac axis arising from the descending aorta. The echoendoscope should be withdrawn to the level of the gastric cardia and rotated until the abdominal aorta is observed (see Fig. 4–10, station 1). By advancing the echoendoscope a few centimeters along the descending aorta, the celiac trunk can be located emanating from the aorta at a 45° angle (see Fig. 4–8). Examination of the celiac axis is important both for identifying metastatic-appearing celiac lymph nodes for EUS-guided FNA (14) or for performing celiac nerve blocks (15). Next, the echoendoscope should be advanced 2–3 cm distal to the celiac axis to image the SMA, which takes off at a 30° angle (see Fig. 4–8). Between the celiac trunk and the SMA (see Fig. 4–10, station 2), the body of the pancreas can be seen in transverse section (Fig. 4–15) adjacent to the duodenal wall. From this location, the pancreatic duct appears as a small echo-poor circle (Fig. 4–16B). With the ultrasound transducer positioned in the body of the stomach, advance the echoendoscope and rotate slightly to the right to image the body of the pancreas, with the splenic vein and artery just proximal to it (Fig. 4–16A,B). From this imaging position, the splenic artery will always be located more cephalad and anterior (closer to the transducer) than the splenic vein.

To image the pancreatic neck from the gastric body/antrum, advance the echoendoscope further. The SMA will be imaged longitudinally, coursing posterior to the pancreas, parallel and distal to the confluence of the superior mesenteric and splenic veins (Fig. 4–17). Occasionally, the transducer can be oriented to image the pancreas and splenic vein transversely such that

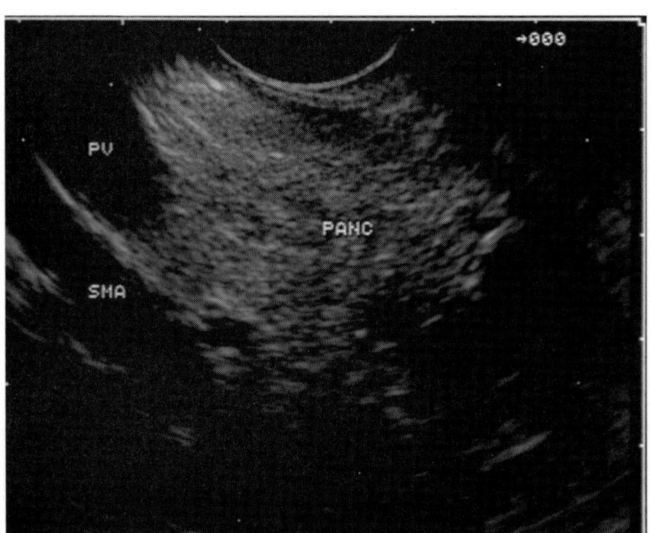


**FIGURE 4–14**

Linear array image of the pancreatic neck (PANC) from the proximal descending duodenum/duodenal bulb (7.5 MHz). Portal vein (PV) and superior mesenteric artery (SMA) are located adjacent and deep to the pancreas.

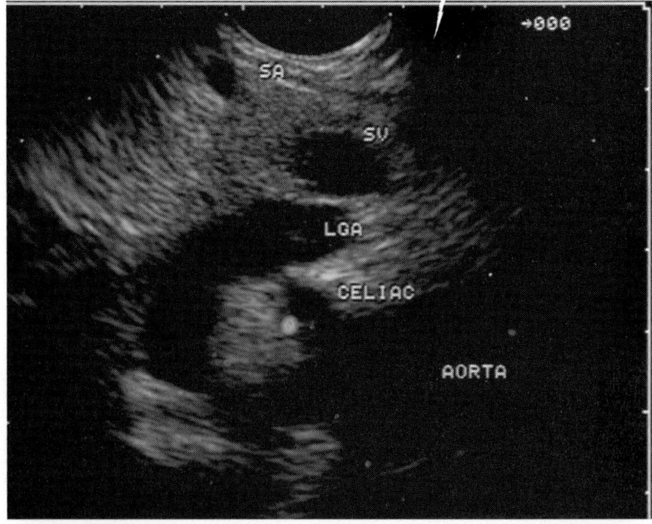


**FIGURE 4–15**

Curved linear array image from the stomach (abdominal echoendoscope, station 1). A transverse section of the body of the pancreas is shown just distal to (to the left of) the splenic artery (SA) and splenic vein (SV). The left gastric artery (LGA) branches from the celiac axis and travels cephalad.

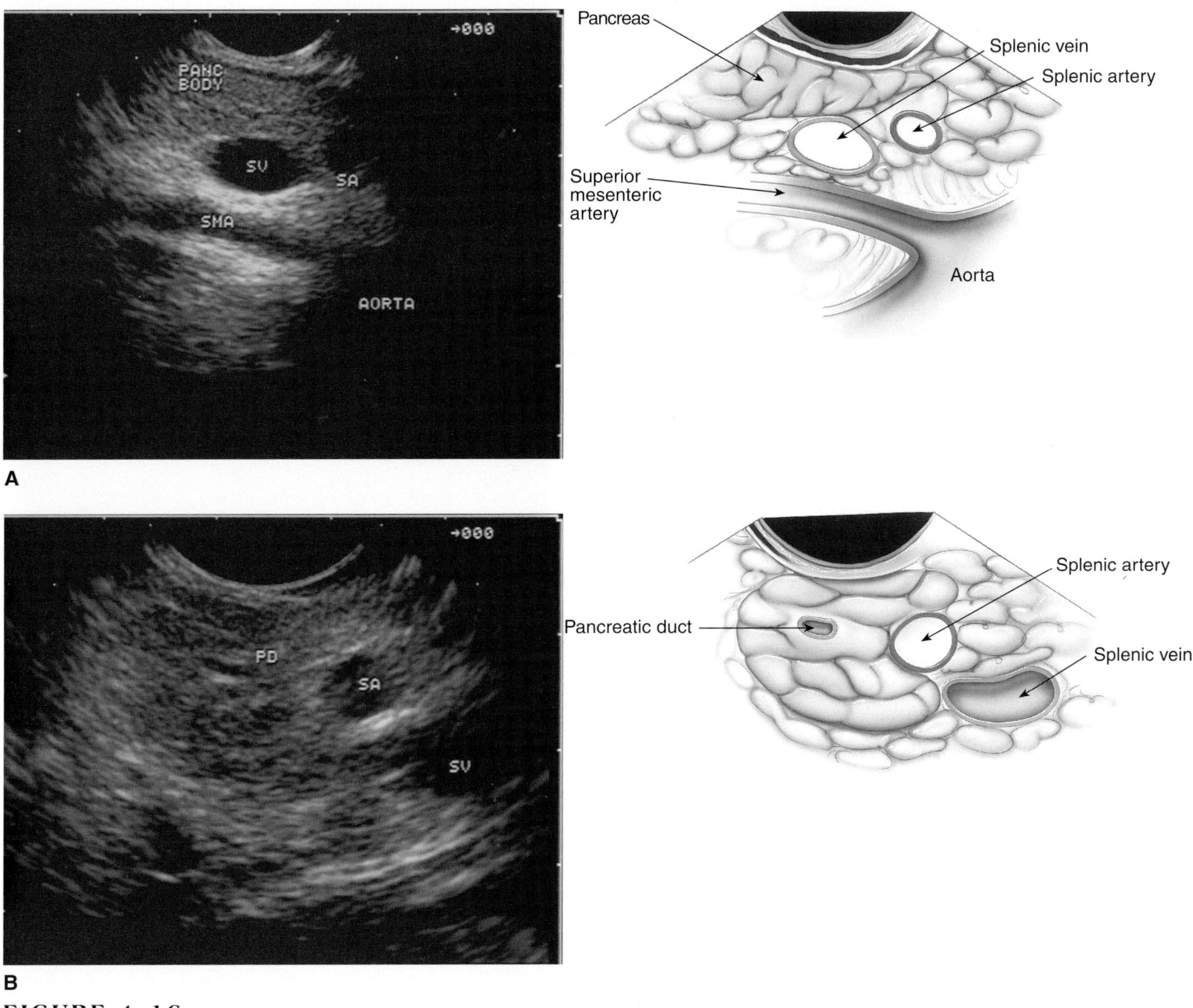


**FIGURE 4-16**

View from the stomach, just distal to celiac axis. (**A**) Origin of the superior mesenteric artery (SMA) from the aorta. The splenic vein (SV) is posterior (deep) to the pancreas and the splenic artery (SA) proximal to the SV. Continuation of the SMA deep to SV, SA, and pancreatic body. (**B**) Closer view of the body of the pancreas with SV and SA and transverse section of normal pancreatic duct (PD).

SMA would appear in cross section (similar to radial scanning). With the SMA longitudinal and deep to the pancreatic neck, the echoendoscope should be rotated left to locate the SV, which may be seen merging into the portal vein deep to the pancreas (Fig. 4–18A). The portal vein confluence is where the splenic vein (which is seen on cross section) and portal vein (which appears as a longitudinal structure just deep to the pancreas) join (Fig. 4–18B). Identification of the portal vein, PV confluence, SMV, and SMA is important for identifying vascular invasion when staging cancers of the pancreas.

To view the distal body and tail of the pancreas, the transducer should be withdrawn into the body of the stomach. Rotating one's shoulders to the right will direct the transducer tip towards the patient's left and into the proximal stomach (see Fig. 4–10, station 4). The tail of the pancreas is located adjacent to the spleen, the splenic vein and artery inferior to the pancreatic tail (Fig. 4–19). The splenic artery can be differentiated from the splenic vein by its serpigenous course, round shape, and cephalad location relative to the pancreas. The splenic vein is typically larger and oval-shaped. The renal

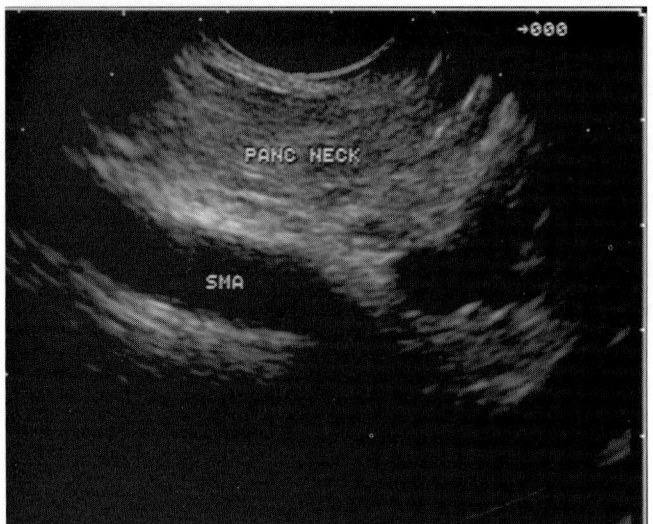


**FIGURE 4–17**

Sonographic image (linear array, 7.5 MHz) of the pancreatic neck from the distal body/antrum of the stomach. The superior mesenteric artery (SMA) is shown positioned longitudinally and deep to the pancreas.

vein and artery are located deep to the splenic artery and vein and can be imaged in thin individuals or at 5 MHz. The renal vein is larger and located closer to the transducer.

## Imaging the Spleen, Left Kidney, and Left Adrenal Gland

With the transducer tip in the proximal stomach positioned to image the pancreatic tail, the spleen is seen as an echogenic structure with a fine, homogeneous texture. Occasionally, the left adrenal gland can be visualized cephalad to the left kidney (see Fig. 4–10, station 5) as a thin, seagull-shaped structure (Fig. 4–20). Alternatively, the left adrenal gland can be located from station 1 (see Fig. 4–10) in the proximal stomach by locating celiac axis, and by rotating to the right and slightly withdrawing the echoendoscope.

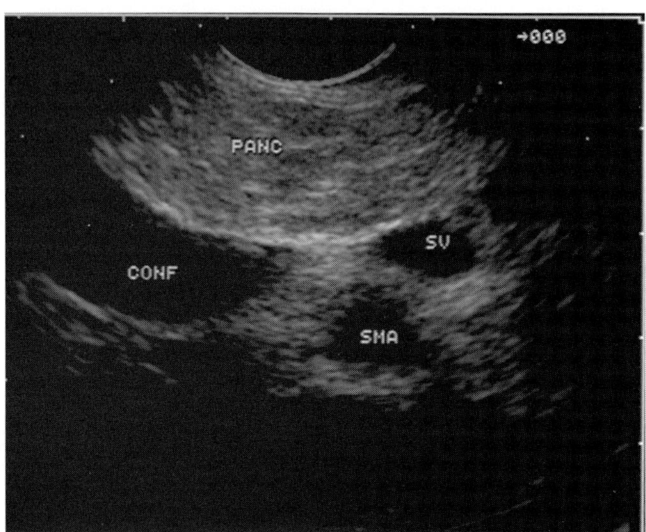


A

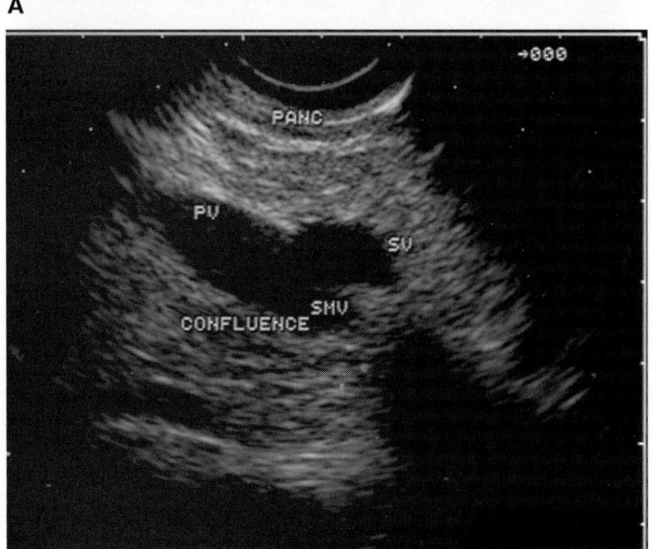


B

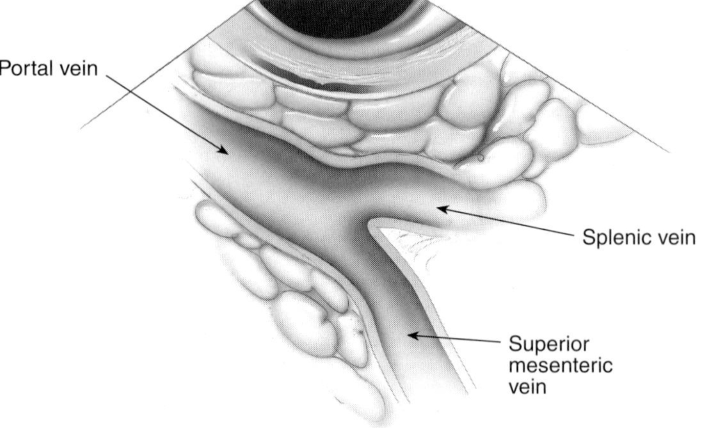


**FIGURE 4–18**

Linear array image (7.5 MHz) of the pancreatic neck from the distal body/antrum of the stomach. (**A**) The superior mesenteric artery (SMA) is located deep to (below) the portal vein–superior mesenteric vein confluence (CONF) and splenic vein (SV). (**B**) Portal vein (PV), superior mesenteric vein, and splenic vein (SV) confluence.

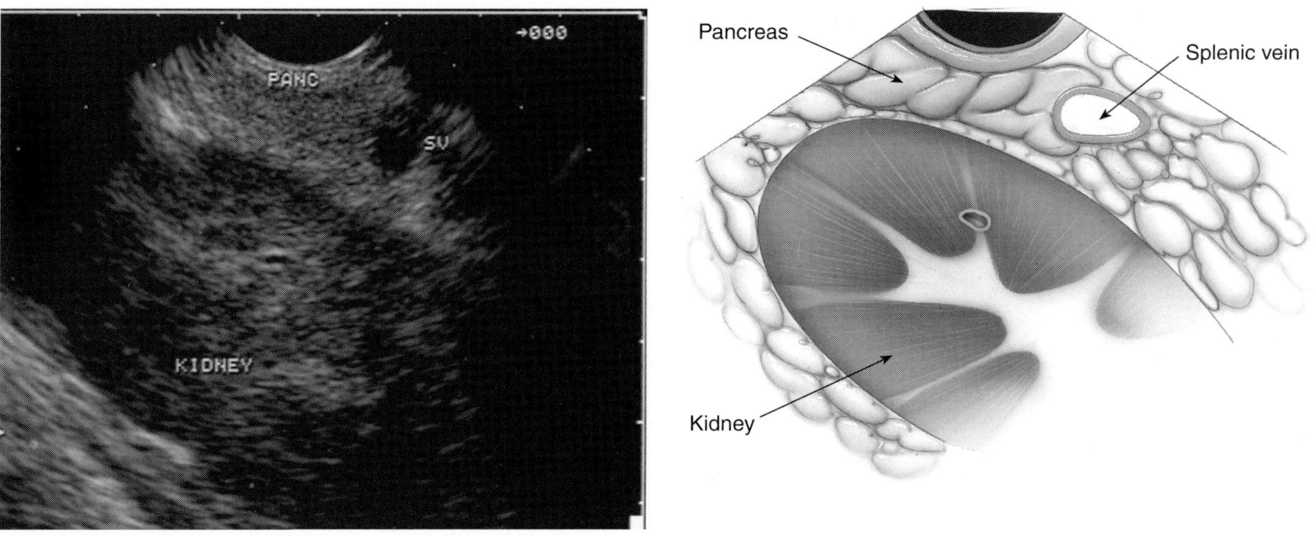


**FIGURE 4–19**

Linear array image (7.5 MHz) of a transverse section of the tail of the pancreas (PANC) from the body of the stomach. Cross sections of the splenic vein (SV) and left kidney are shown posterior (deep) to the pancreas.

## Imaging the Extrahepatic Bile Duct

EUS readily provides excellent images of the extrahepatic bile duct. Such images are useful for detecting common bile duct stones (16, 17) as well as for diagnosing and staging bile duct tumors (18). Imaging the CBD is best accomplished by placing the ultrasound transducer in the descending duodenum at the level of the ampulla of Vater. The intrapancreatic CBD can be imaged in longitudinal section adjacent to the pancreatic duct (Fig. 4–21A). Withdrawing the transducer while rotating to the right will provide images of the remainder of the CBD (Figure 4–21B). Withdrawing the transducer into the proximal descending duodenum and distal duodenal bulb will permit the identification of the extrapancreatic CBD and the PV deep to it (Fig. 4–22A). The extrapancreatic CBD can be tracked by slowly withdrawing the echoendoscope. From this location, it will be imaged coursing proximally towards the liver (Fig. 4–22B). This is an ideal location for injecting contrast through the duodenal wall into the CBD under EUS guidance (endoscopic ultrasound retrograde cholangiography) in patients with difficult ERCP cannulation (19). The gastro-

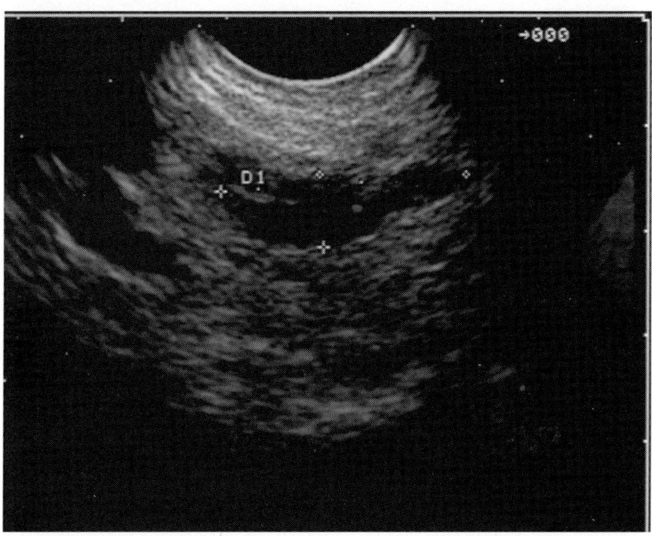


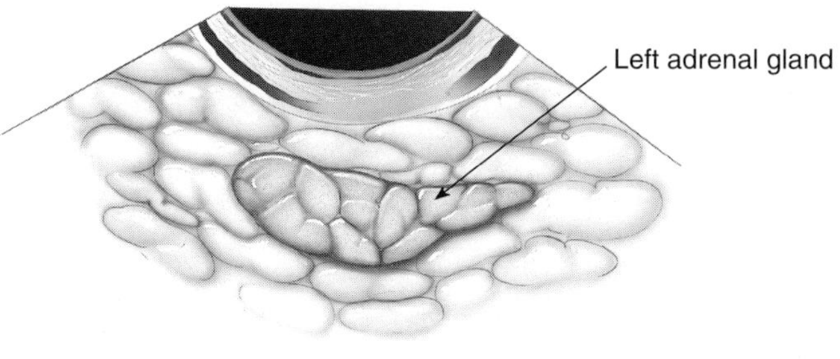


**FIGURE 4–20**

Curved linear array view (7.5 MHz) of the left adrenal gland imaged from the stomach.

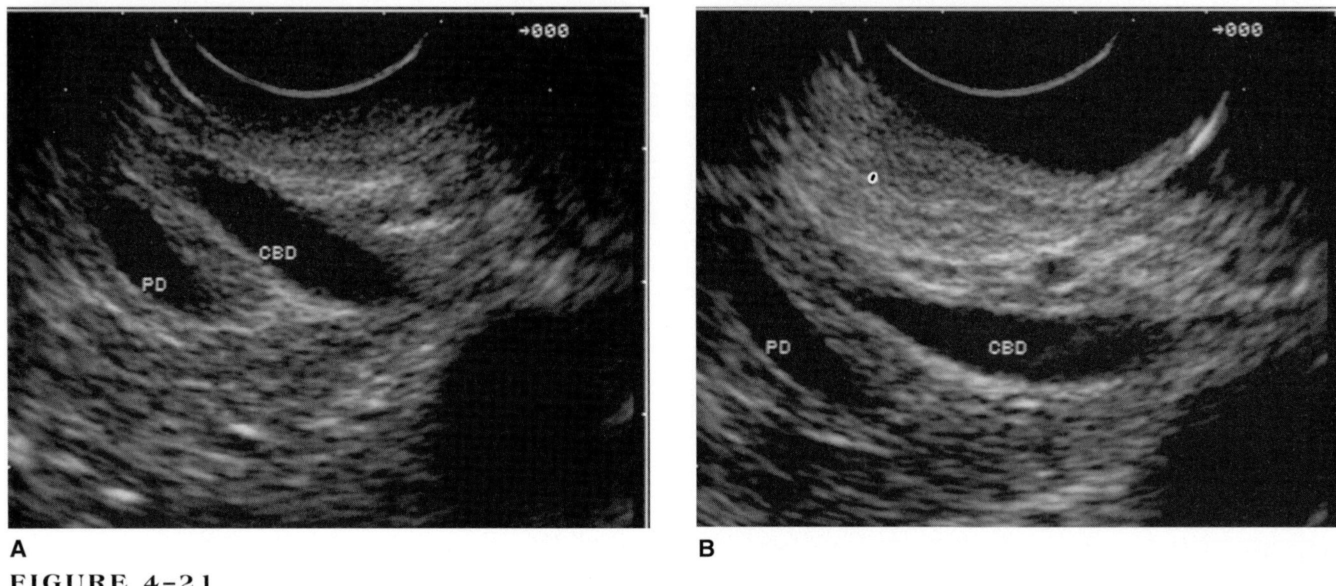


FIGURE 4–21

(**A**) Close-up linear array images (7.5 MHz) of the common bile duct (CBD) and the distal pancreatic duct (PD) in the pancreatic head from the descending duodenum. (**B**) CBD and PD shown in longitudinal section after slightly withdrawing the transducer.

duodenal artery may appear adjacent to the CBD and duodenal wall (Fig. 4–23).

## Imaging the Gallbladder

Transabdominal ultrasound (US) is the safest, easiest, and least expensive method of imaging the gallbladder. However, preliminary data suggest that EUS provides additional diagnostic yield over US. When abdominal US of the gallbladder is normal, EUS can detect gallstones in obese patients (20) and in patients with biliary-type pain (21). The gallbladder is best imaged from the duodenum or gastric antrum. From a position within the duodenal bulb, and with the pancreatic head/neck in

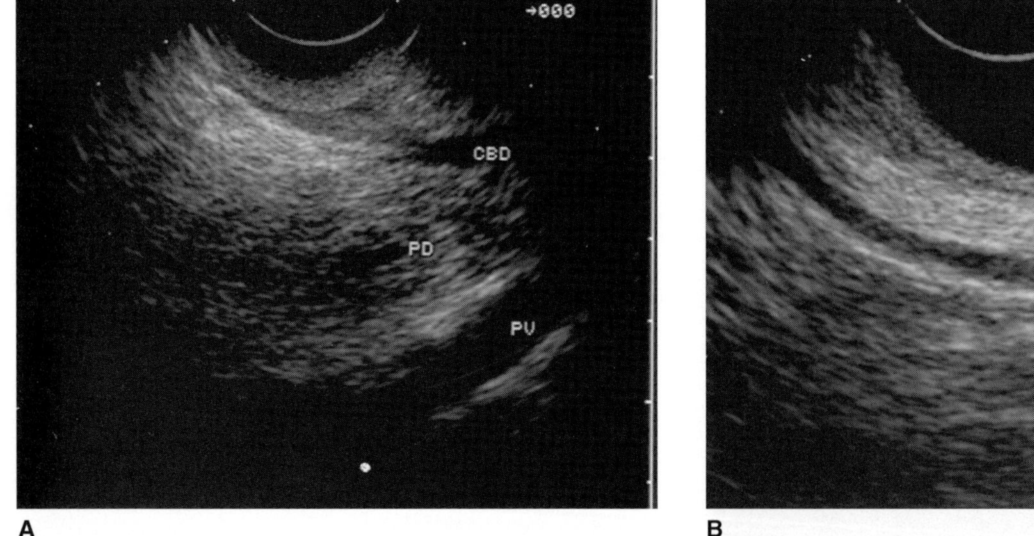


FIGURE 4–22

Close-up linear array images (7.5 MHz) of the common bile duct (CBD) and the distal pancreatic duct (PD) from the proximal descending duodenum. (**A**) Longitudinal section of the common bile duct entering the head of the pancreas. The portal vein (PV) is shown posterior (deep) to the pancreas. (**B**) Extrapancreatic CBD moving cephalad toward the liver (not shown).

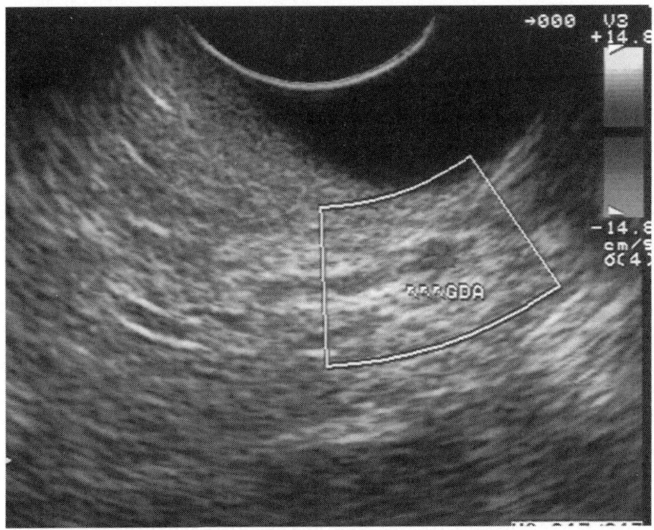


**FIGURE 4–23**

Color flow image of the gastroduodenal artery (GDA) just outside the duodenal wall. (*See color insert for color plate.*)

view, the gallbladder can be seen after rotating the echoendoscope to the left and locating the liver. Rotating the echoendoscope in a leftward rotation to a position nearly 180° from the pancreas will bring the gallbladder into view (Fig. 4–24). From the gastric antrum, the gallbladder can be imaged by endoscopically placing the transducer proximal to the pylorus and rotating right to face the transducer anteriorly.

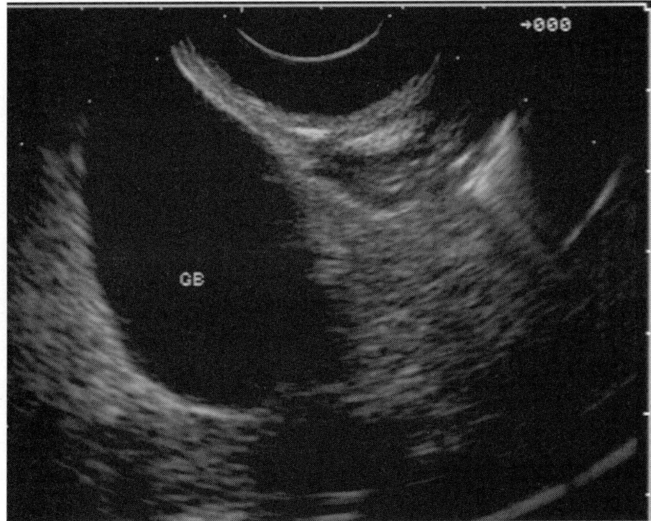


**FIGURE 4–24**

Curved linear array image (7.5 MHz) of the gallbladder from the duodenal bulb.

## Color Flow and Doppler Endosonography

The principles of Doppler endosonography are as follows (9): If an object is moving at a 90° angle to the ultrasound beam, no motion away from the beam is detected; thus the transmitted and reflected sound frequencies are equal. Objects moving toward an ultrasound transducer augment the reflection of sound waves from their surface; hence, the sound frequency increases. Objects moving away from an ultrasound transducer produce a soft reflection of sound, and a low-frequency sound is returned from the object to the transducer. The difference between the frequency of transmission ($F_t$) and the frequency of reflection ($F_r$) is measured by the ultrasound device and represents the Doppler (or frequency) shift. The velocity of the object is directly proportional to the detected frequency shift (9). Hence, Doppler is an excellent method of detecting movement, such as blood flow in blood vessels.

With the Pentax echoendoscope and Hitachi EUB-515 ultrasound unit (see Fig. 4–1), there are three ways of using color flow and Doppler. The function keys are located on the lower keyboard. The BEAM key, which places the gate on the structure of interest, is used to hear the reflected Doppler signals. Color Doppler is obtained by pressing the CFM key. By doing so, a window appears, which can be positioned over the structure(s) of interest using the track ball. The size of the window can be changed by pressing the CANCEL key, adjusting the window, then pressing the CANCEL to move the track ball over the figure(s) of interest. The color red arbitrarily indicates that movement or flow is directed towards the ultrasound transducer. The color blue indicates the movement or flow is directed away from the ultrasound transducer. If there is no color, either there is no flow (the structure is not a blood vessel) or the flow is at right angles to the ultrasound beam. Dark colors indicate slow flow and light colors represent higher velocity (9). The PULSED WAVE GRAPH key (the rightmost key under CFM MODE, labeled B/PW) allows duplex ultrasonography and combines two-dimensional gray scale imaging with pulsed-wave Doppler techniques. The ultrasound console displays the EUS image with color flow on the left of the screen. By depressing the B FREEZE key, the transmitted sound waves become audible and can be heard as the Doppler waveform can be seen on the right of the screen.

Color flow and Doppler are helpful in differentiating blood vessels from ductular structures and cystic lesions (which can both appear as anechoic roundish structures) and lymph nodes at the time of EUS-guided FNA. Doppler can also identify major blood vessels, which serve as important anatomical landmarks during

EUS imaging. For example, the PD and CBD can be differentiated from the adjacent portal vein and SMA when imaging from the duodenum (Fig. 4–25A,B). The dilated PD and CBD have no color or Doppler waveform in contrast to the adjacent blood vessels. Color flow and Doppler may enhance the ability to assess PV invasion in patients with a pancreatic head cancer. The PV has a predominantly blue color (Fig. 4–26A) and a typical waveform characterized by a continuous venous hum that extends throughout systole and diastole (Fig. 4–26B). The SMV has a similar Doppler waveform to that of the PV (Fig. 4–26C) in contrast to the arterial waveform of the SMA.

The splenic vein can be differentiated from the splenic artery by color flow and Doppler when imaging the body and tail of the pancreas. The former has a Doppler waveform similar to that of the portal vein (Fig. 4–26D), while the splenic artery has an arterial Doppler waveform (see below). The IVC can also readily be distinguished from the abdominal aorta using color flow and Doppler imaging. The IVC has a typical pulsatile "sawtooth" waveform with some reversal of flow due to right atrial contraction (Fig. 4–27). In contrast, the aorta is displayed as predominantly red (Fig. 4–28A) and has a characteristic arterial velocity waveform with a sharp upstroke, a slower downstroke, and substantial diastolic flow (Fig. 4–28B).

Color flow and Doppler ultrasound can be used to verify the celiac artery at the time of FNA of lymph nodes in the celiac axis. The celiac artery is predominantly red (Fig. 4–29) and has a typical mesenteric arterial Doppler waveform with a sharp upstroke followed by a substantial diastolic flow from the low resistance of the mesenteric vascular bed.

## Technique of EUS-Guided FNA

The lesion of interest is typically located prior to EUS-FNA using radial scanning EUS. For mediastinal lesions such as lymph nodes, the distance to the target is noted in centimeters from the incisor teeth and the relationship of the lesion to major blood vessels, such as the aorta. When the linear array echoendoscope is passed, the lesion will readily be located by advancing to the previously-noted distance and rotating left or right from the aorta. For example, if the lesion is located to the patient's left and to the left of the aorta (counterclockwise), the echoendoscope should be rotated right or clockwise.

To date, the best commercially available needle is the GIP/Mediglobe 22 gauge steel needle (Fig. 4–30A). The assembly consists of a metal spiral sheath and an aluminum handle (GIP-Medizin Technik, Grassau, Germany) (Fig. 4–30B) that can be luer-locked onto the biopsy channel of the echoendoscope. The needle has a round or beveled stylet, which is also Luer-locked onto the needle shaft. The needle allows puncture of the gastrointestinal wall and sampling of extraluminal lesions, while the needle's stylet minimizes

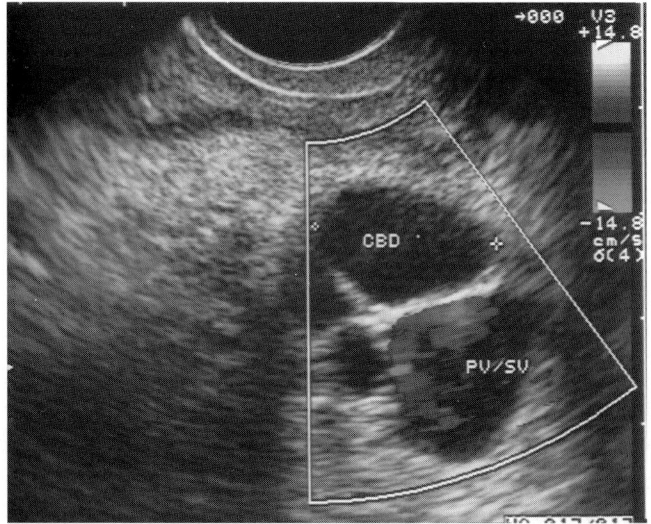


B

PD
CBD
SMA

**FIGURE 4–25**

Color flow images from the duodenum. (**A**) A dilated common bile duct (CBD) and portal vein (PV) deep to it. The portal vein has color, which is absent in the CBD. (**B**) A dilated pancreatic duct (PD) and common bile duct (CBD) without color flow, unlike the superior mesenteric artery (SMA) and portal vein. (*See color insert for color plate.*)

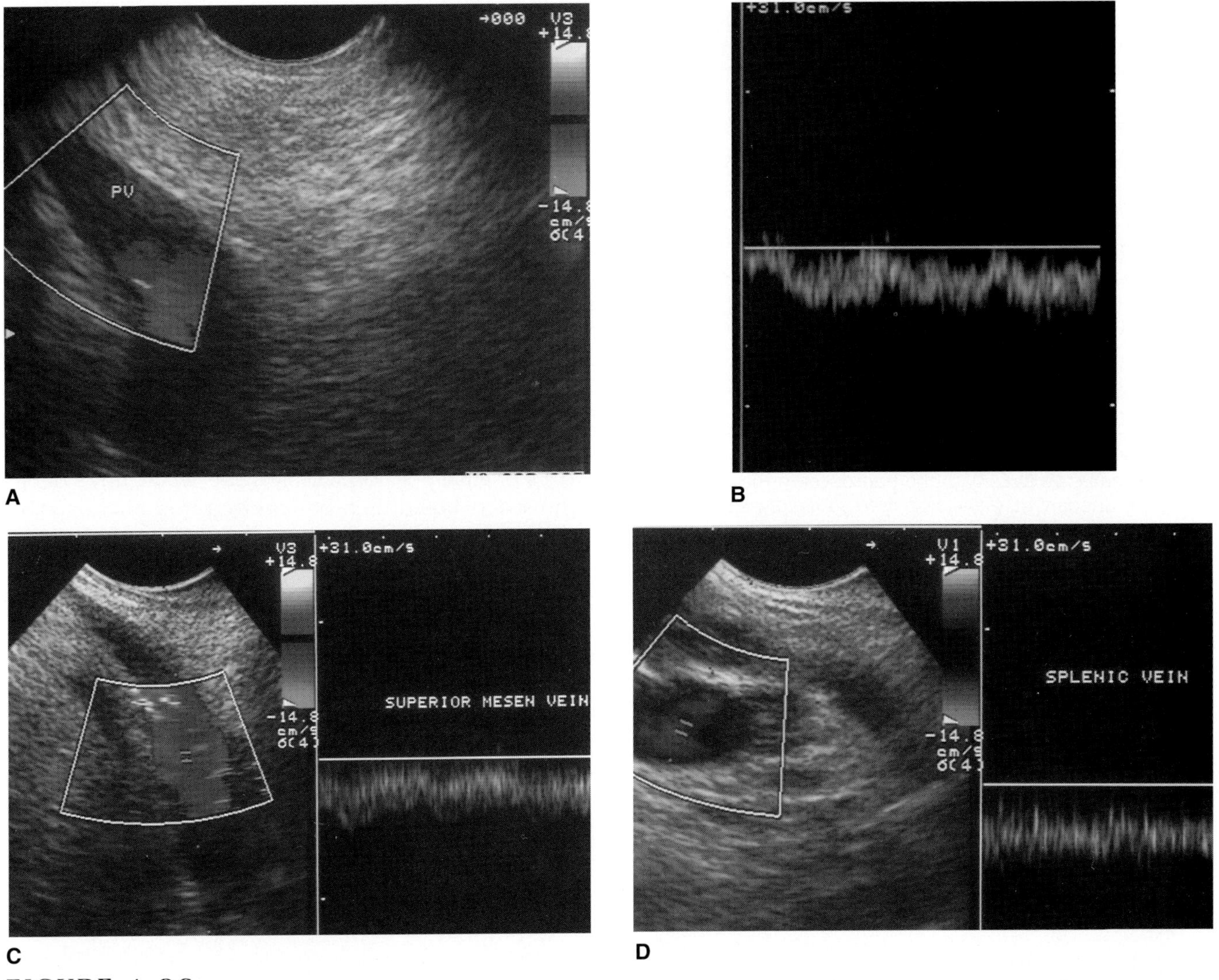


**FIGURE 4–26**

Color flow image (**A**) and Doppler (**B**) waveform of the portal vein from the duodenum. The superior mesenteric vein (SMV) has a similar color flow and Doppler waveform (continuous venous hum). (**C**) Color flow and Doppler waveform of the splenic vein imaged from the stomach at the level of the pancreatic body (**D**). (*See color insert for color plates of* ***A, C, and D.***)

contamination of the specimen with normal gastrointestinal tract wall cells. The round stylet can be advanced to the GI tract wall with the needle tip inside it to allow targeting of the lesion without puncture. Multiple passes are more readily performed with the needle and round stylet compared to the beveled stylet. The GIP/Mediglobe needle is endosonographically imaged as a hyperechoic line (Fig. 4–31) The tip of the needle (which has been sandblasted for enhanced endosonographic visualization) also images well. It is the excellent visualization of the needle and tip under real time endosonography that allows safe and effective tissue sampling.

Prior to initiating EUS-guided FNA, the target lesion should be identified endosonographically and the echoendoscope positioned such that the lesion appears in the center or slightly to the left of center on the EUS image. Color flow and Doppler imaging of the lesion and surrounding structures may be used to distinguish vascular structures from the target lesion. Contols on the echoendoscope should be in the locked position. The needle and stylet should be assembled and inserted through the uncapped accessory channel of the echoendoscope. The handle should be locked into position in the inlet of the accessory channel. While depressing the small knob on the assembly handle, advance the needle (with stylet inside) beyond the tip of the echoendoscope until it appears in the ultrasound field by pushing the handle's center piston into the handle. Continue to advance the needle until the stylet abuts

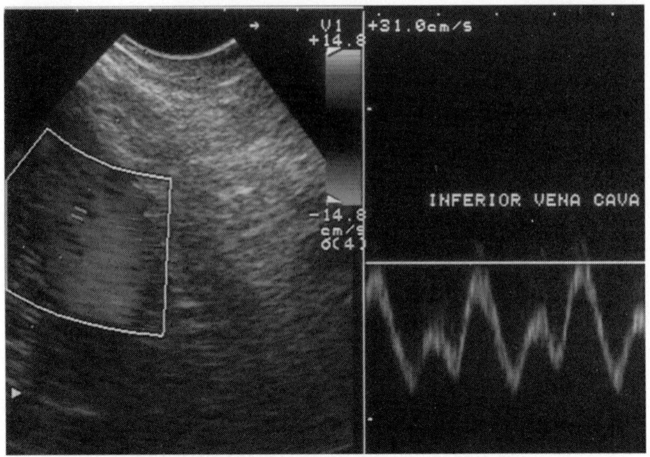


**FIGURE 4–27**

Color flow image and typical sawtooth Doppler waveform of inferior vena cava (IVC) with the transducer in the distal descending duodenum. (*See color insert for color plate.*)

the gastrointestinal tract wall. Assess the potential trajectory of the needle before advancing it into the lesion. Sampling the periphery of the target lesion where the tumor is less necrotic or fibrotic may result in an improved yield in some instances.

Withdrawing the stylet 5 mm will sharpen the needle. The needle should be advanced under EUS guidance into the lesion. Constant pressure on the echoendoscope's up/down control knob will maintain the position of the echoendoscope tip against the gastrointestinal tract wall and the target lesion in focus. This is particularly important for very firm or fibrotic tumors. The endosonographer typically feels the tip of the needle penetrate the mass or lymph node as there is a sudden motion or "pop" that is transmitted throughout the length of the needle to the endosonographer's hand. The lesion may disappear from view momentarily as the needle sinks into the tissue. Withdrawing the needle slightly and readjusting the image focus will bring the lesion and needle tip back into view (Fig. 4–31). Once the needle is located within the lesion, advancing the stylet to it's original position will clear the needle tip of debris. The stylet should then be removed from the assembly. The needle can be advanced up to 10 cm beyond the catheter.

A 10-mL syringe should be Luer-locked to the proximal end of the needle 5–7 mL of constant suction should be applied. Advancing the needle under EUS guidance back and forth into the lesion five or six times under

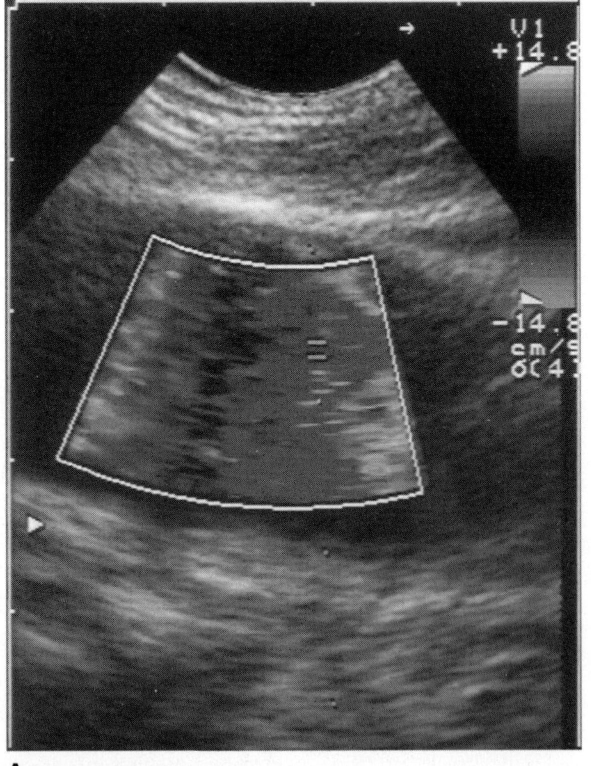


A

B

**FIGURE 4–28**

Color flow (**A**) and Dopper waveform (**B**) of the aorta, showing characteristic arterial pattern—sharp upstroke, slower downstroke, and substantial diastolic flow. (*See color insert for color plate of **A**.*)

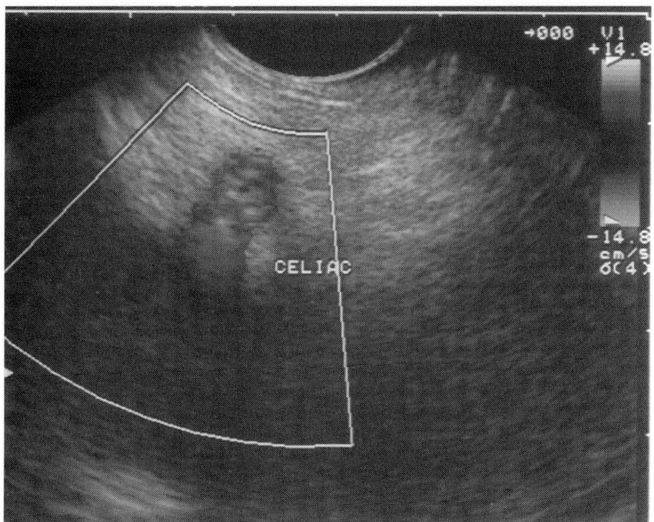


**FIGURE 4–29**

Color flow of the celiac artery; scanning from the stomach. (*See color insert for color plate.*)

constant suction will draw the aspirate into the needle and sometimes the syringe. Releasing the suction on the syringe will allow the vacuum to equilibrate. This should occur while the needle tip is still within the lesion. Finally, the needle should be withdrawn into the steel sheath and the entire assembly removed from the echoendoscope.

Slides are prepared by advancing the needle slightly beyond the catheter and using the syringe to expel one large drop of specimen onto each of two glass slides. Adequate cellular specimens generally appear to contain gelatinous and/or particulate material and little blood. Remaining cellular material should be placed onto another slide or in formalin for cell block. Reinserting the stylet removes any remaining portion of the specimen. Quickly smear the specimen evenly on each slide before it dries by placing one on top of the other completely then pulling in opposite directions. Place the slides in alcohol immediately. Process the slides with either modified Papanicolaou or Diff-Quick stain for review by the cytopathologist.

Having a cytopathologist or cytology technician present at the time of the procedure to review the slides and determine the adequacy of the specimen improves the diagnostic yield and minimizes the number of inconclusive diagnoses from inadequate sampling (1,4). The cytopathologist can often provide a preliminary diagnosis at the time of EUS-guided FNA. If all the passes are negative for malignancy or nondiagnostic, the cell block may still provide a positive (although delayed) diagnosis. Aspirated ascitic/pleural fluid or pancreatic cyst/pseudocyst fluid should immediately be sent to the pathology laboratory in a vial or syringe for cytospin and cytological examination. Extra fluid may be sent for CA 19-9, amylase, culture, and other special studies.

If more than one pass is required, sterile normal saline should be flushed through the needle and the needle wiped down with alcohol to remove any blood or other material. Flushing the needle with alcohol followed by saline is suggested when performing multiple passes for cystic pancreatic lesions.

## Conclusions

Linear array endosonography with EUS-guided fine-needle aspiration and fine-needle injection, with and

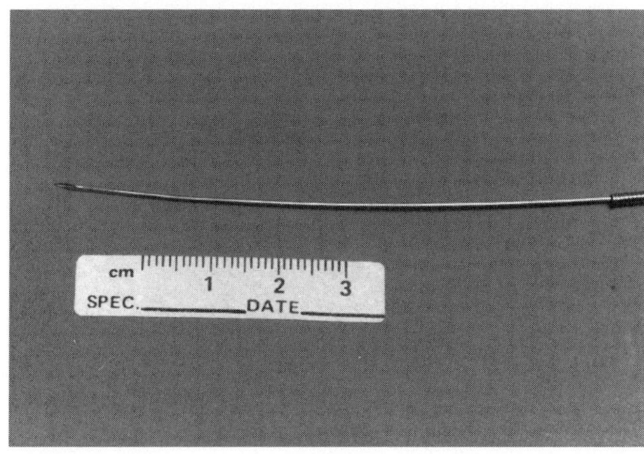


A

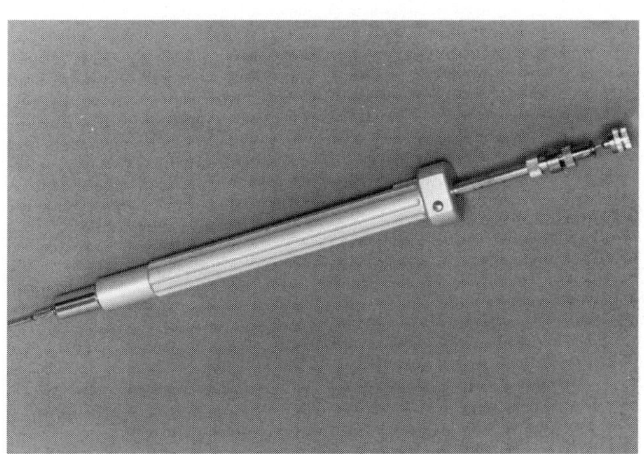

B

**FIGURE 4–30**

GIP/Mediglobe needle (**A**) with Vilmann handle (**B**).

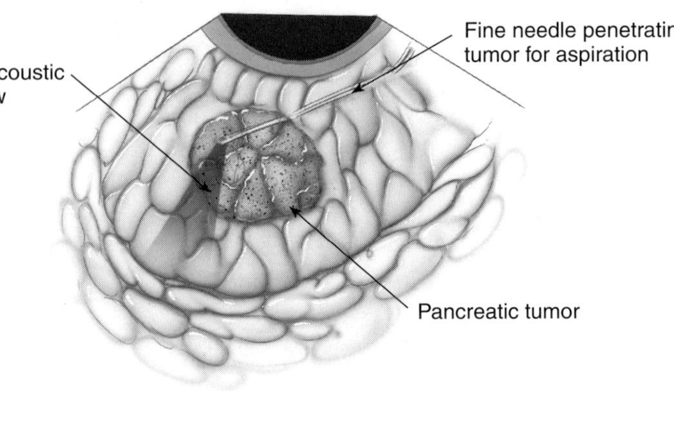


**FIGURE 4–31**

EUS FNA of a tumor in the head of the pancreas. The hyperechoic Vilmann needle is clearly seen with the needle tip within the target.

without color flow mapping and Doppler ultrasound capabilities (22–26), has become an essential diagnostic and therapeutic modality. It can provide unparalleled images of the gastrointestinal wall and surrounding structures for tumor staging and other indications, as well as furnish material for cytological diagnoses for a variety of disorders. EUS-guided FNA of mediastinal and abdominal lymph nodes, free fluid, and metastatic liver lesions can stage pulmonary and gastrointestinal malignancies accurately. EUS-guided injection may also provide therapeutic benefit. An understanding of linear array anatomy, familiarity with linear EUS instruments, and comprehension of the technique of FNA comprise the essential foundation upon which these diagnostic and therapeutic procedures can be performed safely and effectively.

## References

1. Chang KJ, Katz KD, Durbin TE, Erickson RA, Butler JA, Lin F. Endoscopic ultrasound guided fine needle aspiration. Gastrointest Endosc 40(6):694–699, 1994.
2. Wiersema MJ, Kochman ML, Cramer HM, Tao LC, Wiersema LM. Endosonography-guided real-time fine-needle aspiration biopsy. Gastrointest Endosc 40(6):700–707, 1994.
3. Wegener M, Adamek RJ, Wedmann B, Pfaffenbach B. Endosonographically guided fine-needle aspiration puncture of paraesophagogastric mass lesions: preliminary results. Endoscopy 26:586–591, 1994.
4. Vilmann P, Hancke S, Henriksen FW, Jacobsen GK. Endoscopic ultrasonography-guided fine-needle aspiration biopsy of lesions in the upper gastrointestinal tract. Gastrointest Endosc 41(3): 230–235, 1995.
5. Giovannini M, Seitz JF, Monges G, Perrier H, Rabbia I. Fine-needle aspiration cytology guided by endoscopic ultrasonography: Results in 141 patients. Endoscopy 27(2):171–177, 1995.
6. Chang KJ, Albers CG, Nguyen P. Endoscopic ultrasound guided fine needle aspiration of pleural and ascitic fluid. Am J Gastroenterol 90(1):148–150, 1995.
7. Chang KJ, Erickson RA. A primer on linear array endoscopic anatomy. Gastrointest Endosc 43(2 suppl):S43–S47, 1996.
8. Kremkau F. Doppler ultrasound: Principles and instruments. Philadelphia: W.B. Saunders, 1990.
9. Stewart JH, Grubb M. Understanding vascular ultrasonography. Mayo Clin Proc 67:1186–1196, 1992.
10. Wiersema M, Vilmann P, Giovannini M, Chang K. Prospective multicenter evaluation of EUS guided fine needle aspiration biopsy (FNA): Diagnostic accuracy and complication (CX) Assessment. Gastrointest Endosc 1996 (abstract in press).
11. Gress F, Savides T, Ikenberry S, et al. A prospective comparison study of endoscopic ultrasound (EUS), computed tomography (CT) and EUS directed fine needle aspiration biopsy (EUS/FNA) of the mediastinum in the preoperative staging of non-small cell lung cancer (NSCLCA). Gastrointest Endosc 41:304, 1995.
12. Botet J, Lightdale C, Zauber A, et al. Preoperative staging of esophageal cancer: Comparison of endoscopic US and dynamic CT. Radiology 181:419–425, 1991.
13. Savides TJ, Gress FG, Zaidi SA, Ikenberry SO, Hawes RH. EUS detects the pancreatic ventral anlage. Gastrointest Endosc 41:312, 1995.
14. Chang K, Durbin T, Katz K, Lin F, Wuerker R. Endoscopic ultrasound (EUS) guided fine needle aspiration (FNA) of upper gastrointestinal peri-luminal and celiac lymph nodes (LN). Gastrointest Endosc 40(part 2):62, 1994.
15. Wiersema M, Sandusky D, Carr R, Erdel W, Frederick P, Wiersema L. Endosonography guided celiac plexus neurolysis (EUS CPN) in patients with pain due to intra-abdominal (IA) malignancy. Gastrointest Endosc 41(4):315, 1995.
16. Amouyal P, Amouyal G, Levy P, et al. Diagnosis of choledocholithiasis by endoscopic ultrasonography. Gastroenterology 106: 1062–1067, 1994.
17. Canto M, Chak A, Sivak MV. Endoscopic ultrasonography (EUS) versus cholangiography for diagnosing extrahepatic biliary stones: A prospective, blinded study in pre- and post-cholecystectomy patients. Gastrointest Endosc 41(4):391, 1995.
18. Rösch T, Lorenz R, Braig C, et al. Endoscopic ultrasonography in diagnosis and staging of pancreatic and biliary tumors. Endoscopy 24(suppl 1):304–308, 1992.
19. Wiersema M. Clinical applications of endosonography guided cholangiopancreatography. Gastrointest Endosc 1995. (submitted).

20. Peikin S, Feld R, Kastenberg D, et al. Role of endosonography in the diagnosis of gallstone disease in obese patients. Gastroenterology 104:A328(abstract), 1992.
21. Dill J, Callis J, Hill S, Evans P. Combined endoscopic ultrasound and endoscopic Meltzer-Lyon testing in the diagnosis of cholelithiasis. Am J Gastroenterol 89(6):956–957, 1994.
22. Binmoeller KF, Brand B, Thul R, Rathod V, Soehendra N. EUS-guided, fine needle aspiration biopsy using a new mechanical scanning puncture echoendoscope. Gastrointest Endosc 47:335–340, 1998.
23. Tio TL. EUS-guided FNA: A few caveats. Gastrointest Endosc 47:421–422, 1998.
24. Kulling D, Sahai AV, Knapple WL, Cunningham JT, Hoffman BJ. Diagnostic endoscopic ultrasound of the pancreas may cause acute pancreatitis. Endoscopy 30:S7–S8, 1998.
25. Hunerbein M, Dohmoto M, Haensch W, Schlag PM. Endosonography-guided biopsy of mediastinal and pancreatic tumors. Endoscopy 30:32–36, 1998.
26. Binmoeller KF, Thul R, Rathod V, Henke P, Brand B, Jabusch HC, Soehendra N. Endoscopic ultrasound-guded, 18 guage, fine needle aspiration biopsy of the pancreas using a 2.8 mm channel convex array echoendoscope. Gastrointest Endosc 47:121–127, 1998.

CHAPTER

# High-Resolution Endoluminal Sonography of the Upper Gastrointestinal Tract: THE LINEAR SCANNING ULTRASOUND PROBE

Michael B. Kimmey
Svein Ødegaard

The concept of using an ultrasound transducer on an endoscopically passable probe at the time of routine endoscopy is appealing. Potentially, the endoscopist could obtain information about the depth of a mucosal lesion as well as elucidate the cause of impressions on the normal mucosa created by lesions within or adjacent to the gastrointestinal wall. If an ultrasound probe device were effective, it would minimize the necessity for additional procedures using combined ultrasound endoscopes and other imaging tests such as computed tomography.

Several attempts have been made to develop this type of miniature ultrasound instrument. The resulting devices can be classified according to the type of scanning—radial or linear—and the ultrasound frequency used. Two types of radial scanning probes are reviewed in Chapters 6 and 7. This chapter deals with the development and clinical application of a mechanical linear scanning ultrasound probe.

## Physics of Small-Aperture Ultrasound Transducers

Imaging with all miniature ultrasound probes is constrained by the physical limitations imposed by the small diameter, *aperture,* of the ultrasound transducers (1). Knowing the physics of ultrasound helps us understand these imaging limitations.

Both the axial and lateral resolution of the ultrasound beam are critical to the quality of the image obtained with a miniature probe. The *axial resolution* is the ability of the system to distinguish between two points in a plane lying in the same direction as the ultrasound beam. The magnitude of the axial resolution is determined by (a) the duration of the ultrasound pulse and (b) the frequency of the ultrasound wave. In general, the higher the ultrasound frequency, the shorter the ultrasound pulse and the smaller (better) the axial resolution. Higher ultrasound frequencies are limited, however, because they are more attenuated by tissue and therefore penetrate less deeply (2).

*Lateral resolution* is the ability to distinguish between two points in a plane lying transverse to the direction of the ultrasound beam (Fig. 5–1). The magnitude of the lateral resolution depends on the diameter and frequency of the transducer, and on how it is focused. Adjacent to the transducer, the lateral resolution is similar to the diameter of the transducer. The lateral resolution improves as the ultrasound beam propagates until it reaches a transition point—termed the near–far field transition point—after which the beam diverges and the lateral resolution worsens (Fig. 5–2). For a transducer of given diameter, the near–far transition point approaches the transducer and the beam diverges away from this point more rapidly for lower compared to higher ultrasound frequencies.

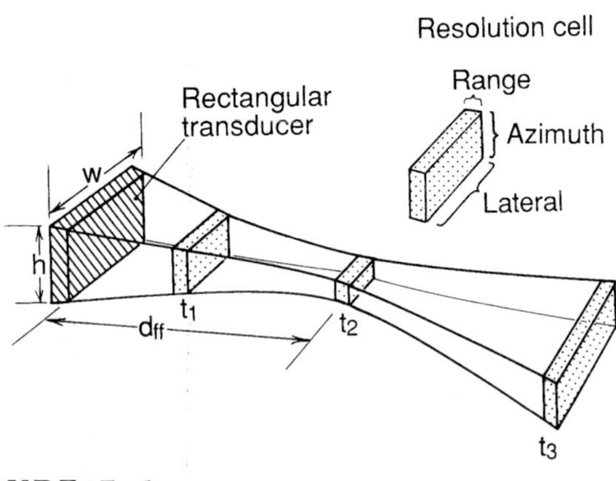


**FIGURE 5–1**

The resolution of a rectangular ultrasound transducer of specified height ($h$) and width ($w$) in three dimensions is illustrated at three points in time ($t_1$, $t_2$, and $t_3$). The resolution types include axial (also termed range), lateral, and azimuthal. The axial resolution, determined by the ultrasound pulse length, remains constant at all points. However, lateral and azimuthal resolution varies according to time or distance from the transducer. The best overall resolution is found at the near–far field transition point ($d_{ff}$) at time $t_2$. (Reprinted with permission from GI Endoscopy Clinics of North America 2:560, 1992, W.B. Saunders.)

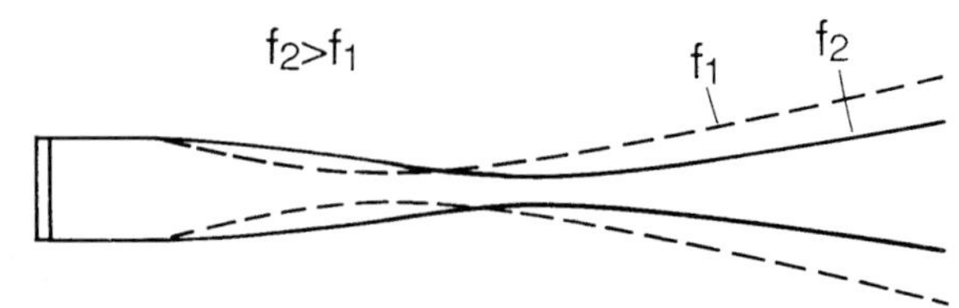


**FIGURE 5–2**

The ultrasound beam patterns for a given size transducer and two different ultrasound frequencies $f_2$ and $f_1$ are plotted. The higher frequency ($f_2$) transducer has a near–far field transition point that is farther from the transducer, exhibiting less beam divergence in the far field than the lower frequency ($f_1$) transducer. (Reprinted with permission from GI Endoscopy Clinics of North America 2:561, 1992, W.B. Saunders.)

Given these limitations, several conclusions can be reached about imaging with miniature ultrasound probes. In most cases, little useful information can be obtained from tissue more than 2–3 cm from the transducer. Even if lower frequency transducers (7.5 MHz) are used, the divergence of the lateral resolution in the far field produces unclear details in the deeper areas of the image (3). Placing the transducer at the appropriate distance from the target tissue is also very important, especially with lower frequency transducers whose optimum zone of lateral resolution or focus may be quite narrow. Ideally, a balloon placed around the transducer can be filled to a variable degree with water, thus allowing changes to be made in this distance. Practically, this has been difficult to achieve as the diameter of the probe catheter that will fit down the endoscope channel is severely limited.

## Linear Probe Development and Description

With the goal of developing a catheter probe that could be used to image the gastrointestinal wall, prototype ultrasound catheters were developed using an ultrasound frequency of 20 MHz and a transducer diameter of 1.8 mm (4,5) (Fig. 5–3A). These prototype probes had an axial resolution of 0.21 mm and a lateral resolution of 0.65 mm. The optimum lateral resolution was achieved at a distance of 5 mm from the transducer. (Current manufactured probes have a similar design and scanning characteristics, as shown in Figure 5–3A.)

Scanning with this device is accomplished by moving the probe in and out of the biopsy channel to create a linear compound B mode scan (6). Echoes from the tissue scanned are displayed on the vertical axis of the image, and the distance that the probe moves is recorded on the horizontal axis. Mechanical movement

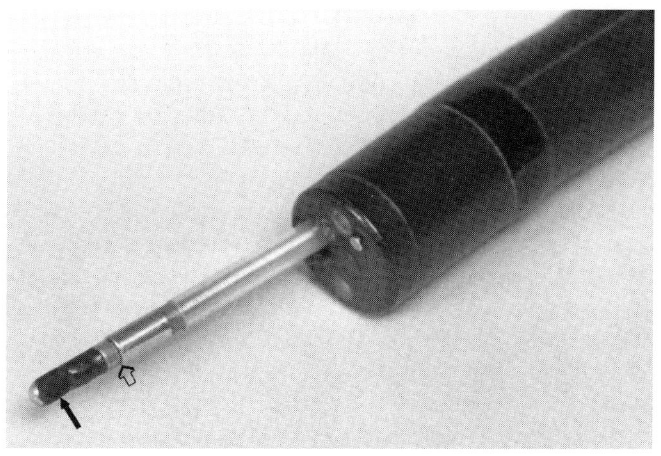

A

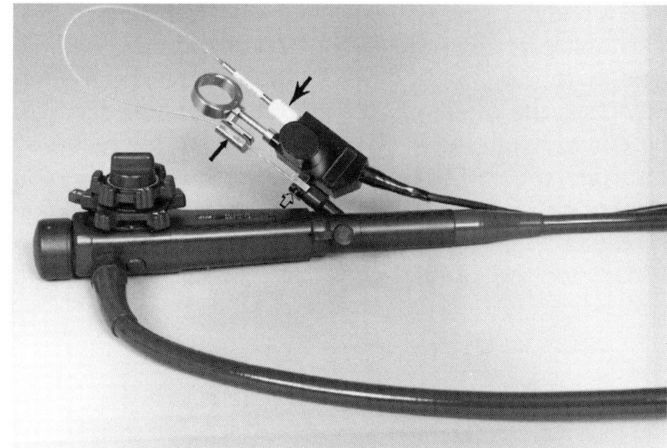

B

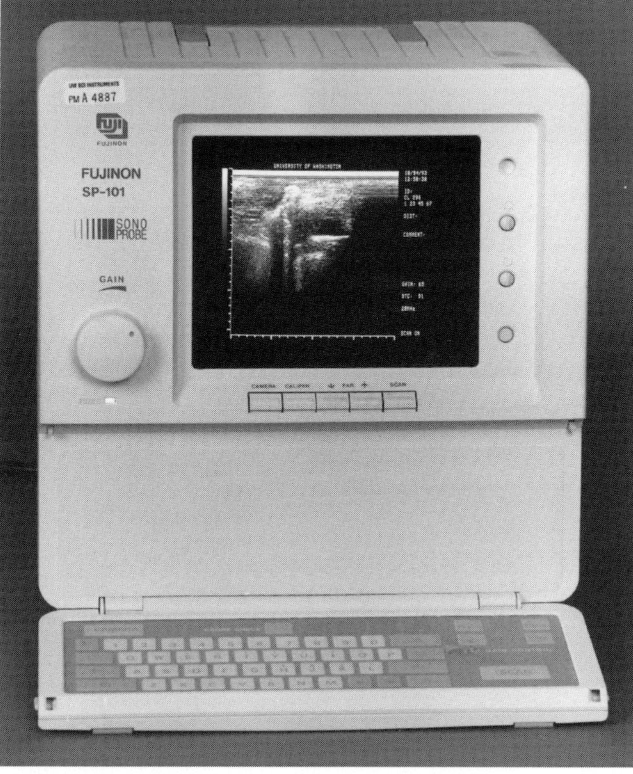


C

**FIGURE 5–3**

(**A**) The linear ultrasound catheter with the probe tip protruding from the biopsy channel of an endoscope. The probe tip distal to the open arrow rotates to allow alignment of the transducer (solid arrow) with the target. (**B**) The translator assembly is attached by a clamp to the biopsy channel entrance (open arrow). A probe is then passed down the channel and clamped to the thumb ring (solid arrow), which is manually pushed in and out to achieve linear scanning. The probe end is connected to the translator by a rotatable screw (arrowhead) which is turned to rotate the transducer. (**C**) The ultrasound processor for the linear probe has a built-in monitor and keyboard for data entry.

of the probe is translated electronically to the image using a potentiometer in the scanning apparatus attached to the biopsy channel entrance (Fig. 5–3B).

The transducer must be manually rotated within the probe catheter so that it is aligned with the area of the gastrointestinal wall being imaged. This alignment is also critical for ensuring that the ultrasound beam is perpendicular to the underlying wall. Nonperpendicular scan planes produce tangential scanning artifacts and image distortion. An outer sheath on the probe allows turning of an inner torque stable catheter attached to the transducer (5). The endoscopist controls the rotation of the transducer by turning the proximal end of the probe where it inserts into the translator assembly. A short colored line is marked on the probe tip exactly 180° opposite the transducer to facilitate alignment of the transducer with the underlying wall.

The mechanical linear ultrasound probe has been developed further by the Fujinon Corporation. 15-Megahertz transducers have been developed but appear to offer no significant advantage over the 20-MHz probes. The ultrasound processor and monitor have been combined into a portable unit with attached keyboard (Fig. 5–3C). This unit contains controls for overall and time variable gain as well as an electronic caliper for direct measurements on the monitor. Patient and procedure data can be entered with the keyboard. Images can be recorded on videotape and hard copies made by using a thermal printer or with color heat transfer technology. The endoscope's video processor can be configured to allow printing of the ultrasound image next to the endoscopic image (Fig. 5–4).

## Technique of Linear Probe Application

The linear ultrasound probe can be passed through the channel of any endoscope with a standard or therapeutic channel (≥2.8 mm). Therapeutic endoscopes provide the additional flexibility of having an auxiliary wash channel for introducing water into the lumen. Video endoscopes are favored because they allow a side-by-side comparison of the endoscopic and ultrasound images. There are three lengths of probes available, one for use with a flexible sigmoidoscope (120 cm), a gastroscope (160 cm), or a colonoscope (220 cm) (7). When a lesion is encountered at endoscopy, the biopsy channel cover is removed and the translator apparatus is attached to the biopsy channel entrance. Adapters are available for attaching the translator to endoscopes manufactured by companies other than Fujinon. The probe is passed through the translator and down the channel until it is visible on the endoscopic image. The proximal end of the catheter is then attached to the translator in two locations (see Fig. 5–3B).

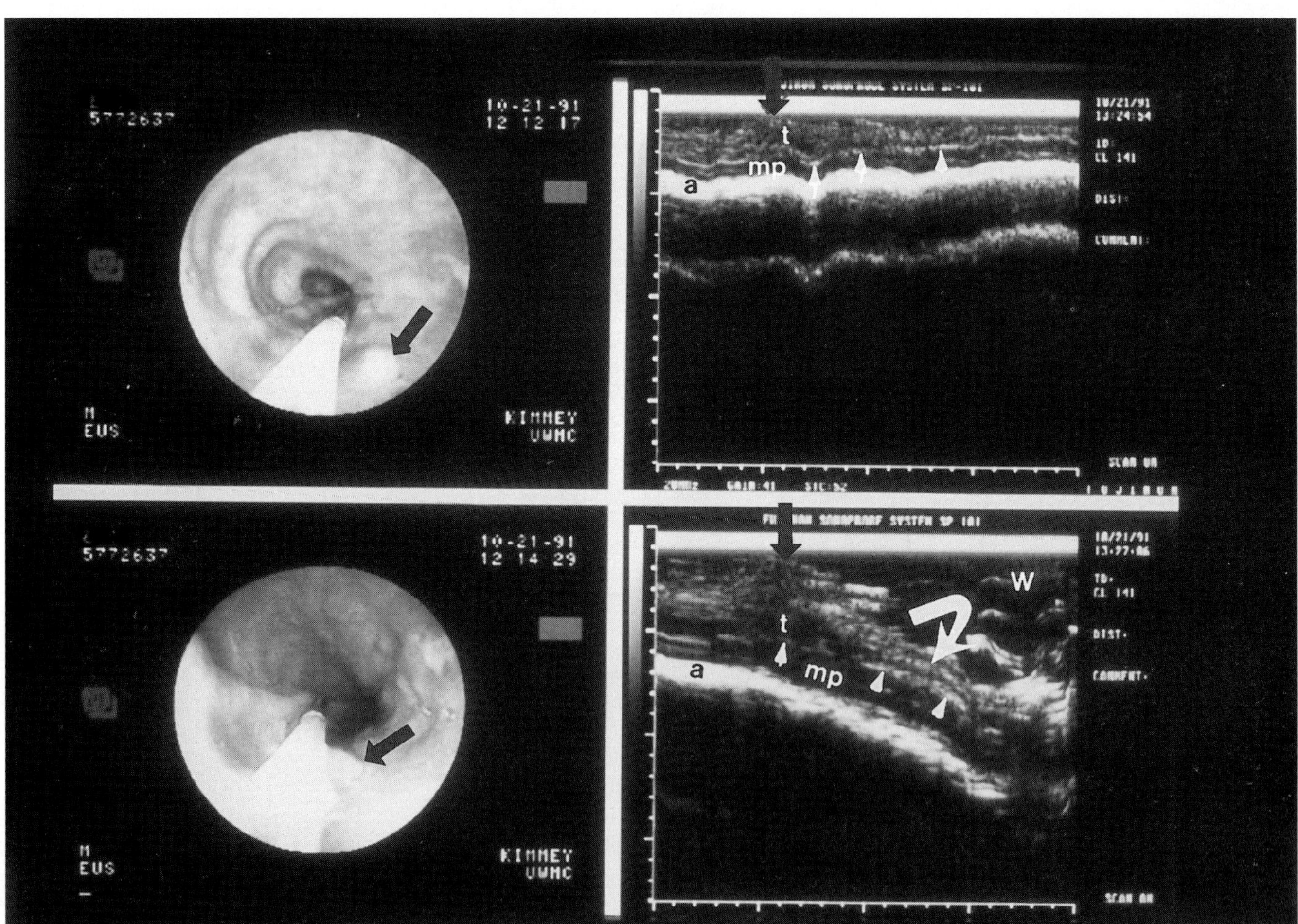


**FIGURE 5–4**

A nodule in Barrett's esophagus (large straight black arrow) is seen on both endoscopic and ultrasound images. The ultrasound image corresponds to the endoscopic image on the left in this four-on-one format. The hypoechoic expansion of the second ultrasound layer is due to an area of intramucosal carcinoma (t). Layers corresponding to the interface between the lamina propria and muscularis mucosae (large curved white arrow), submucosa (small white arrowheads), muscularis propria (mp), and adventitia (a) are also shown in these images made by scanning through water (W). (*See color insert for color plate.*)

The endoscope must be maneuvered so that the tissue of interest is endoscopically visible. Imaging can be accomplished with the endoscope tip straight or retroflexed. The ultrasound transducer is then rotated within the probe catheter to align the transducer directly over the lesion. Optimal images are obtained when the ultrasound beam is orthogonal to the tissue. The endoscopist then begins imaging by moving the probe in and out of the channel. The speed of probe movement is not critical. Images are updated on the screen with each movement of the probe. Better images are sometimes obtained with reverse scanning, especially when forward probe movement results in tissue contact.

The placement of the transducer at the proper distance from the target tissue is also critical. The probe tip can be moved back and forth directly on tissue with a smooth surface, resulting in resolution of the deeper gastrointestinal wall layers and immediately surrounding tissues. But irregular and polyploid lesions cannot be imaged in this way. Moreover, with this direct scanning technique image interpretation can be difficult. The most superficial two or three layers are obscured by the excitation artifact from the transducer, resulting in loss of mucosal and submucosal details and loss of a frame of reference to identify the underlying layers (Fig. 5–5).

Whenever possible, imaging should be performed through water instilled into the lumen and gravitated over the area of interest. This allows optimal imaging of superficial lesions and the display of all wall layers for easier image interpretation. Polyploid and irregular-surfaced tissue should also be imaged through water. Furthermore, the wall can be moved into the optimum

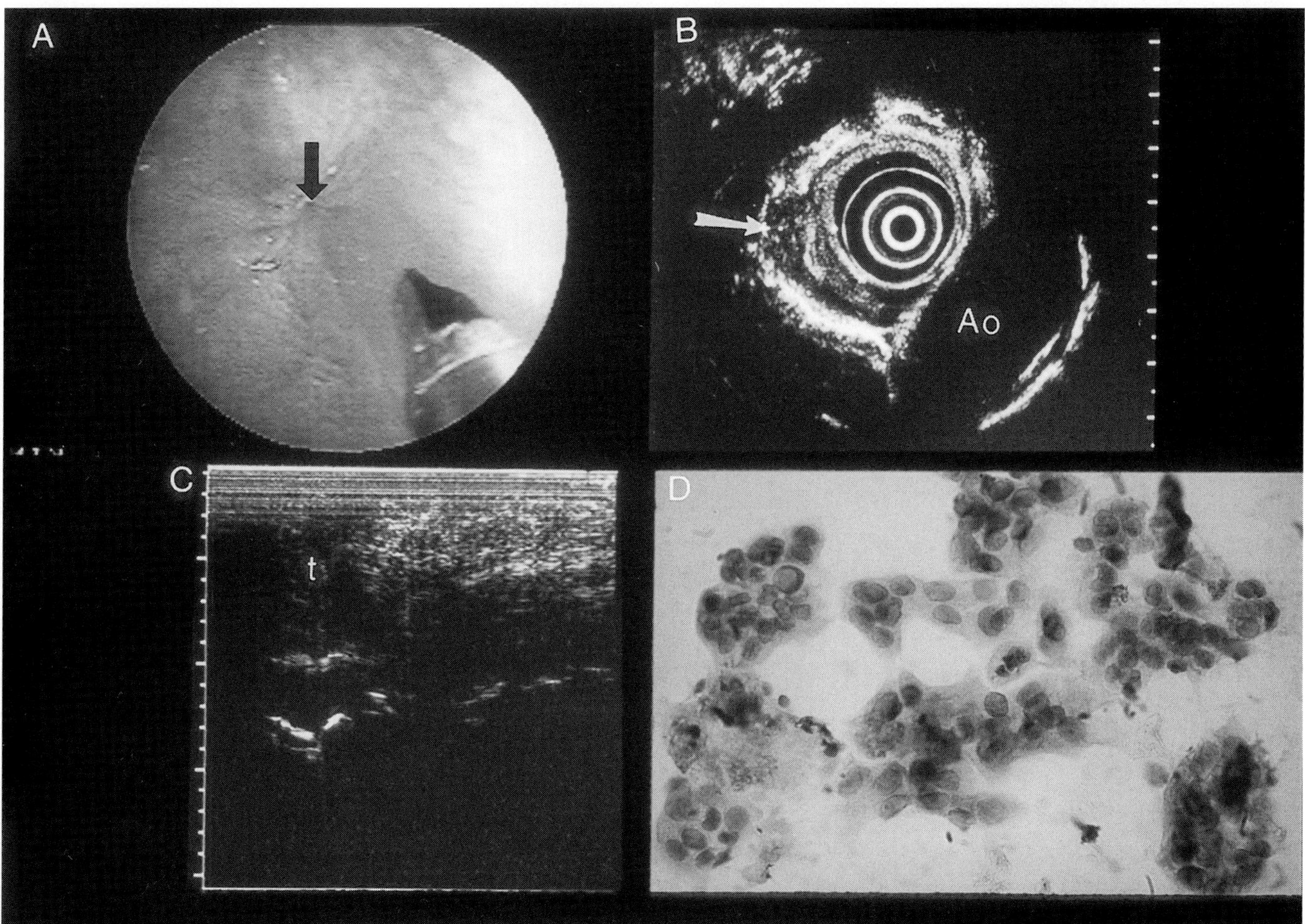


**FIGURE 5–5**

(**A**) Extrinsic invasion of the esophagus produced a tight, impassable stricture (arrow) as shown on the endoscopic image. (**B**) Conventional endosonography from above the stricture also showed a mass (arrow) invading the esophageal wall opposite from the descending aorta (Ao). (**C**) Imaging from within the stricture with a linear probe showed the quadrant containing the tumor mass (t). (**D**) Immediately following probe imaging an aspirating needle was directed into the area of thickened esophagus, revealing these malignant cells. (*See color insert for color plate.*)

focal zone of the transducer, which is approximately 5 mm away.

It can be difficult to maintain a pool of water over the area of interest. Rotation of the patient is helpful to move the lesion to a dependent position. Elevating the head of the patient's bed allows instillation of more water in the esophagus. The stomach can be filled with water, residual air suctioned, and imaging performed with the endoscope in any configuration. Imaging within the duodenum and colon sometimes requires repetitive water instillation followed by imaging before the water flows away. A few drops of simethicone in the water speeds dissipation of bubbles that form during rapid water instillation.

Occasionally it is helpful to observe a point in the image over time. This is termed M-mode imaging and is accomplished by pushing the PROBE CHECK function on the keyboard. This converts the horizontal axis from translational distance to a time-based function. When the probe tip is held over a target selected on B-mode imaging, the M-mode function displays changes in the target with time (8). This technique can be useful for detecting arterial pulsation in a vessel when it is not clearly transmitted to the mucosal surface (Fig. 5–6).

## Image Interpretation

The gastrointestinal wall is imaged as a five-layered structure with this and other ultrasound devices having frequencies between 5 and 20 MHz (Figs. 5–7, 5–8) (9). When imaging is performed through water, the mucosa is visualized as a thin echoic layer with thicker under-

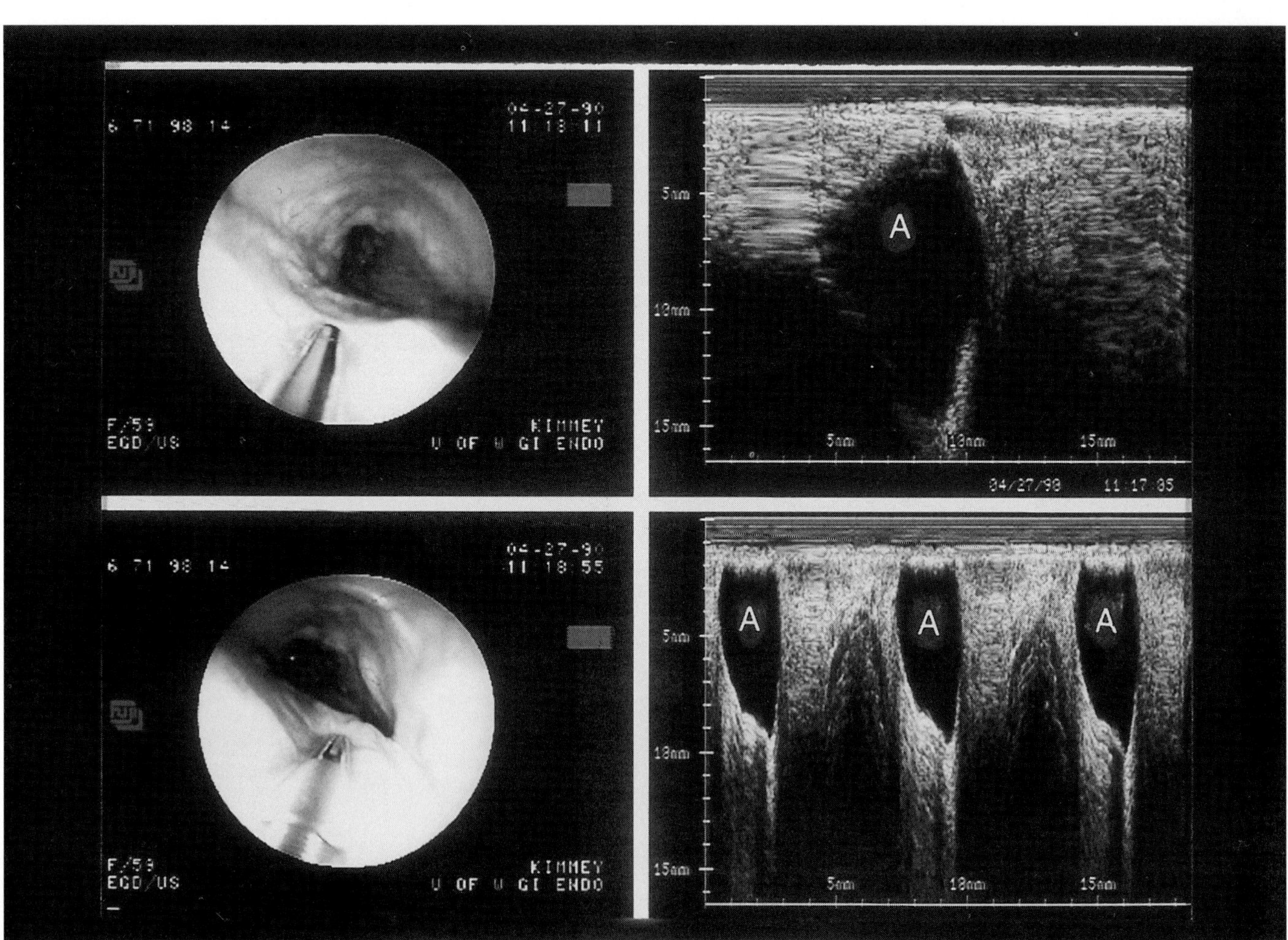


**FIGURE 5–6**

A large anechoic vessel (A) is imaged adjacent to the esoph-ageal wall on B mode scanning (upper two pictures). The horizontal axis represents mechanical movement of the probe over the esophageal wall. When the probe is held in one position over the vessel and the horizontal axis is changed to time, an M mode image is produced (bottom right image) and the vessel (A) can be seen to have arterial pulsation. (*See color insert for color plate.*)

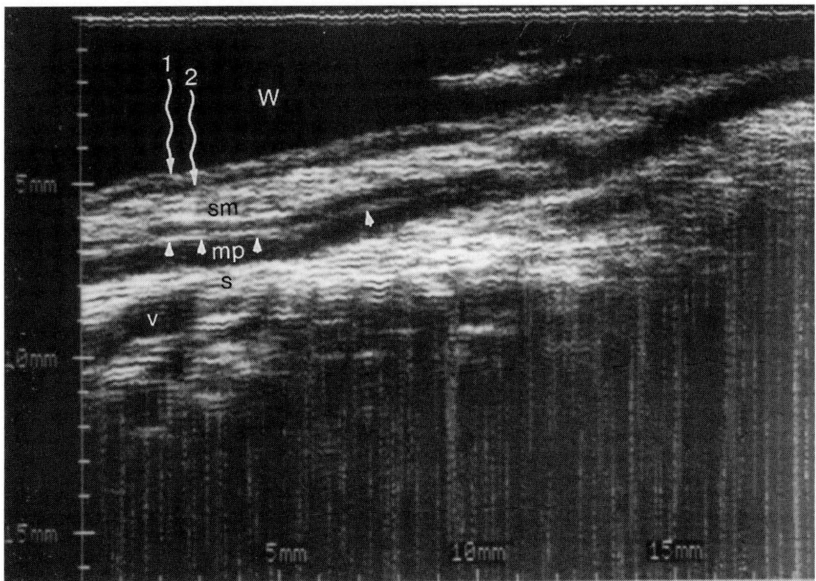


**FIGURE 5–7**

The 20-MHz linear probe image of normal rectum imaged through luminal water (W) is shown. Mucosa (crooked arrows), submucosa (sm), muscularis propria (mp), and serosa and subserosal fat(s) containing a small vein (v) are easily distinguished. The area of connective tissue between the inner circular and outer longitudinal components of the muscularis propria is imaged as a thin echoic line (arrowheads). The horizontal and vertical scale is in millimeters.

lying hypoechoic layers (10). A separate echoic line is sometimes imaged in the deep aspect of the second layer (see Fig. 5–4). This line, caused by the interface between the lamina propria and the muscularis mucosae, can be seen separate from the underlying submucosal layer when the muscularis mucosae is thickened (11). The prominent central echoic layer is due to the submucosa and adjacent interfaces. The muscularis propria accounts for the fourth layer; it is hypoechoic and usually divided by an echoic line caused by connective tissue between the inner circular and outer longitudinal muscular components. The outer layer is echoic and caused by subserosal or adventitial fat and connective tissue. The serosa itself is too thin to be resolved.

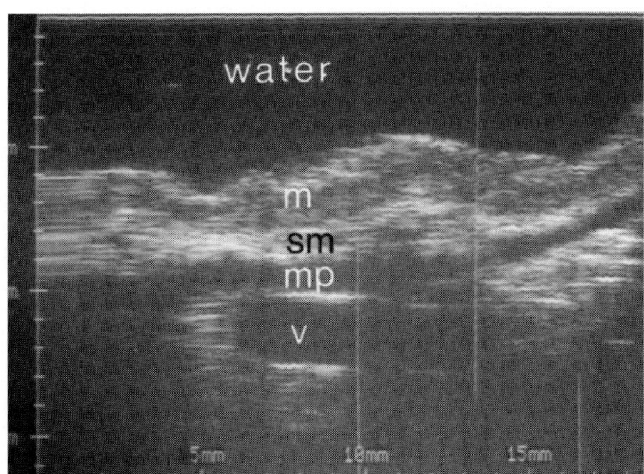


**FIGURE 5–8**

The 20-MHz linear probe image of normal stomach imaged through luminal water is shown. Mucosa (m), submucosa (sm), muscularis propria (mp), and subserosal tissue containing a small vein (v) are easily distinguished. The deep mucosal layer of the normal stomach is thicker than the corresponding layer of the rectum (see Fig. 5–7). The horizontal and vertical scale is in millimeters.

Fat and connective tissue around the esophagus and rectum produce very bright echoes. This is very helpful when interpreting images made by placing the probe directly against the tissue. In this situation, superficial layers are obscured by transducer excitation artifact so wall layers must be identified in relationship to the bright outer or fifth layer. This bright outer layer also provides an important landmark for the detection of malignant invasion outside the gastrointestinal wall.

High frequencies are subject to a greater degree of attenuation by tissue than are lower frequencies (2). This reduces overall penetration through normal and abnormal tissue. Fat attenuates the US beam to a greater extent than lean tissue, thereby aiding in the diagnosis of lipomas. Carcinomas are often associated with a desmoplastic response containing collagen and other fibrous tissue, which is also highly attenuating. This property of malignant tissue may help the alert sonographer to recognize lateral tumor spread. More often, however, it is an impediment to detecting the full extent of the depth of invasion (Fig. 5–9).

## Specific Applications

Small subepithelial masses are the ideal imaging targets for the mechanical linear probe. These masses are detected as an endoscopically visible inward bulge on the mucosa, allowing the endoscopist to direct the probe over their surface. When an ultrasound probe is

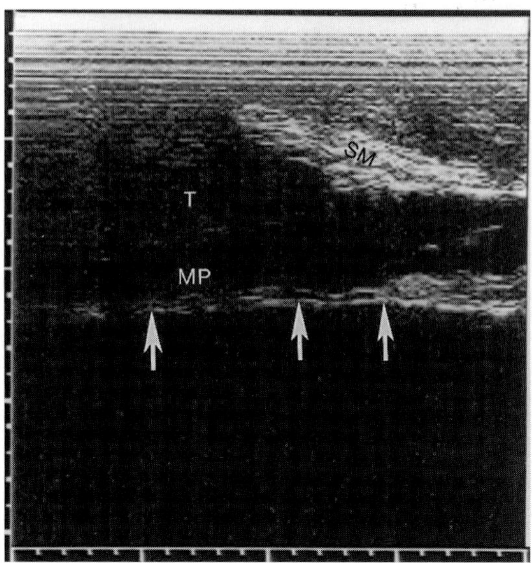


**FIGURE 5–9**

A 20-MHz ultrasound image of one area of a malignant esophageal stricture is shown. The tumor (T) disrupts the echoic submucosa (SM). Invasion of the muscularis propria (mp) is also likely, but is difficult to appreciate on this image. The peri-esophageal fat stripe (arrows) is intact. The horizontal lines at the top of the image are an artifact of transducer excitation. The scale is in millimeters, indicating a penetration of the ultrasound beam of 12 mm.

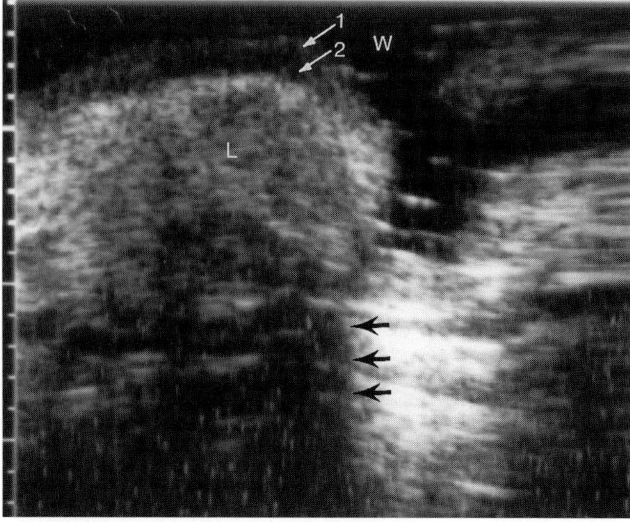


**FIGURE 5–10**

A lipoma (L) in the duodenum is imaged through water (W) as an echoic mass below the mucosal layers (1 and 2). An acoustic shadow (arrows) is produced by the highly attenuating fat of the lipoma.

available, the mass can be imaged directly at the time of the index endoscopy, often obviating the need for further testing (12). Subepithelial masses are characterized by their relationship to the wall layers and by their intrinsic echogenicity (13). Lesions more than 3 cm in diameter and extramural structures are more difficult to image with the linear probe because of the limited penetration of the ultrasound beam.

Cysts, which may be found anywhere within the gastrointestinal tract, are easily recognized by their rounded appearance and absence of internal echoes. They can usually be distinguished from blood vessels because they neither pulsate nor demonstrate tubular extension. Although cysts are most commonly seen within the central submucosal layer, they sometimes have a complex layered structure suggestive of a congenital gastrointestinal duplication (14). Varices may look like cysts on EUS images, but are usually distinguished by their multiplicity and characteristic endoscopic features (15).

Lipomas are often suspected based on their endoscopic appearance as smooth, slightly yellowish masses that push up the mucosa. They are soft and may be indented by a probing forceps. They are imaged within the submucosal layer as a dense collection of echoes that highly attenuate the high-frequency ultrasound beam (Fig. 5–10). The underlying muscularis propria layer cannot usually be imaged when the lipoma is more than 1 cm thick because of this characteristic attenuation.

Leiomyomas are usually imaged as hypoechoic expansions of the fourth ultrasound layer corresponding to the muscularis propria (Fig. 5–11). It is often possible to detect whether the leiomyoma arises from the inner circular or outer longitudinal component of this

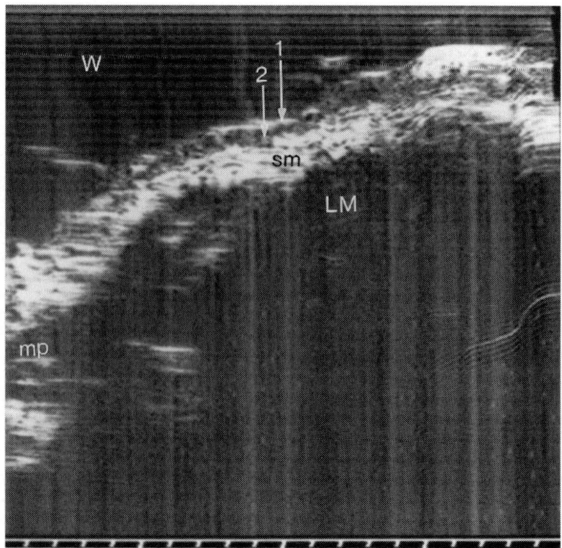


**FIGURE 5–11**

A leiomyoma (LM) in the sigmoid colon is shown as a hypoechoic expansion of the muscularis propria (mp). The mucosa (layers 1 and 2) and submucosa (sm) are shown over the leiomyoma in this image made through luminal water (W).

muscular layer. Rarely, they may occur within the muscularis mucosae and be imaged as an expansion of the second layer. Large leiomyomas are not completely imaged, making linear probe ultrasonography unreliable in predicting whether a leiomyosarcoma or leiomyoblastoma is present (Fig. 5–12).

There are several other causes of subepithelial, intramural masses that we have imaged. Pancreatic rests are usually found in the gastric antrum and have a central crater. On ultrasonography, there is a dense homogeneous collection of submucosal echoes with a texture reminiscent of the pancreatic parenchyma. Brunner's gland polyps within the proximal duodenum reveal a hypoechoic expansion of the second layer, sometimes with deep extension into the submucosal layer. Tiny hypoechoic lines are seen that correspond to the gland openings. Endometrial implants can be seen in any layer or outside the bowel wall and are of variable, often mixed, echo pattern.

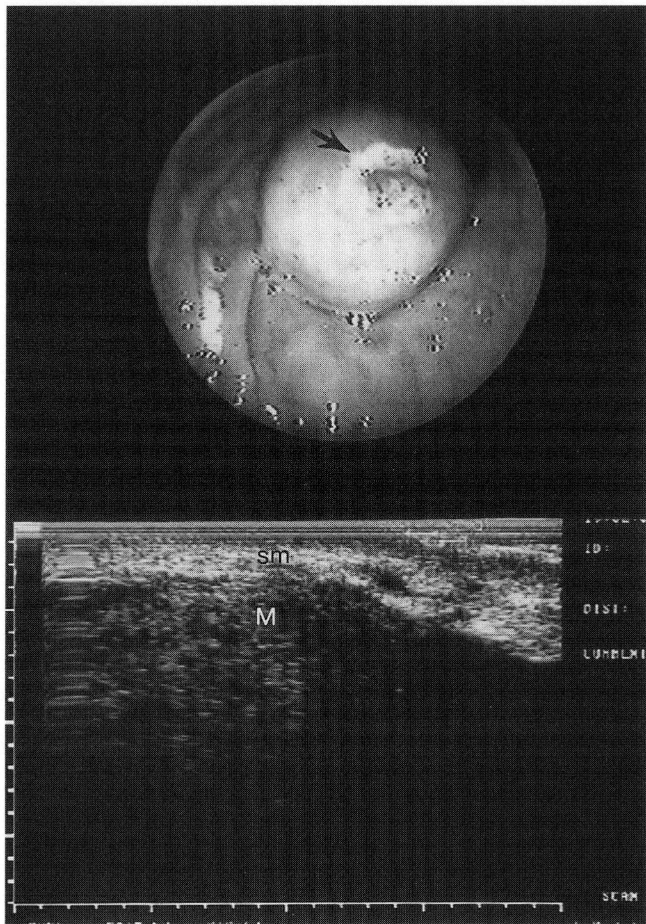


**FIGURE 5–12**

This ulcerated (arrow on top photo), polyploid subepithelial mass in the stomach was found at surgery to be a leiomyosarcoma. The linear probe image (bottom) shows a hypoechoic mass (M) below the submucosa (sm), but incomplete tissue penetration does not allow full evaluation of the size, extent, and presence of lobulation of the mass, which might suggest the presence of a malignant neoplasm. (*See color insert for color plate.*)

It is usually possible to determine whether a bulge into the gastrointestinal lumen is caused by a structure outside the gastrointestinal wall. The intact five-layered wall is imaged over the mass. It is more difficult, and often impossible, to determine what the extramural structure is. Liver and spleen have similar appearances when incomplete penetration prevents the imaging of bile ducts and portal vessels within the liver. Cystic structures adjacent to the gastric wall may be due to the gallbladder, hepatic cysts, or pancreatic pseudocysts. Vessels in the splenic hilum are usually distinguishable by their location along the greater curvature of the gastric fundus and their tubular, anechoic images.

The linear probe is occasionally helpful in directing fine needle aspiration of masses that are adjacent to the gastrointestinal tract. When a mass has been confirmed by CT scanning or standard endosonography, the linear probe can direct the endoscopist to the appropriate quadrant just before use of an aspirating needle (see Fig. 5–5).

Endosonography with combined ultrasound endoscopes has proved most useful in the staging of gastrointestinal malignancies. These instruments are more accurate than CT scanning for detecting the depth of invasion within the GI wall and for detecting regional lymph node involvement (16). It can be difficult to image early, superficially invasive neoplasms with these instruments, however, because it is not always possible to place the transducer directly over a small lesion. In the esophagus, compression with the transducer and the surrounding balloon can also compress layers and distort the image (17).

The linear probe is not useful in staging most gastrointestinal neoplasms. Limited tissue penetration may prevent detection of the full depth of a neoplasm (see Fig. 5–9). While it may be possible to see extension outside the gastrointestinal wall, the detection of adjacent organ involvement is usually impossible. Detection of regional lymph node involvement is also limited both by tissue penetration and by the lack of comprehensive scanning of surrounding tissue afforded by the linear scanning technique (18). Lymph nodes are imaged only if they are adjacent to the muscularis propria when the wall is not very thick and when the node is within the scan plane of the probe (Fig. 5–13).

Linear probe imaging can be complementary to conventional endosonography for detecting the depth of invasion of small, superficial neoplasms (Figs. 5–14, 5–15) (19). The absence of submucosal invasion is reassuring when attempting endoscopic resection of gastric

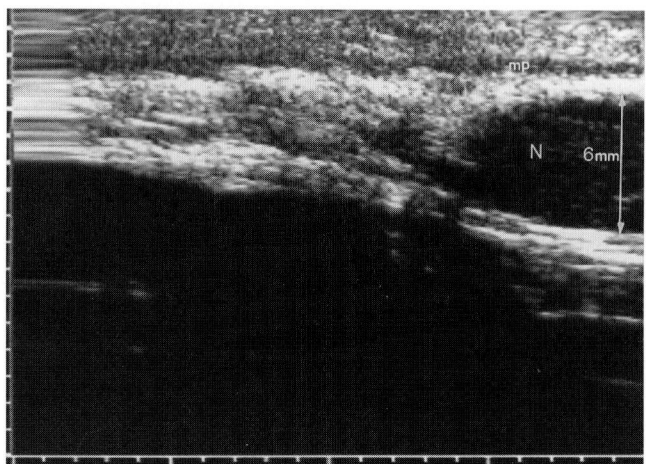


**FIGURE 5–13**

This 6-mm-thick, benign lymph node (N) adjacent to a peptic esophageal stricture is imaged with the linear probe because it is immediately adjacent to the muscularis propria (mp) of a normally thick esophageal wall. Lymph nodes under thickened tissue, as in malignant strictures, are not as easily imaged because the high-frequency ultrasound beam does not penetrate the tissue completely.

or colorectal polyps. It may be necessary to debulk large polyps with piecemeal polypectomy prior to performing endosonography. As with conventional endosonography, high-frequency probe endosonography cannot distinguish persistent neoplasm from scar following chemoradiation therapy (Fig. 5–16).

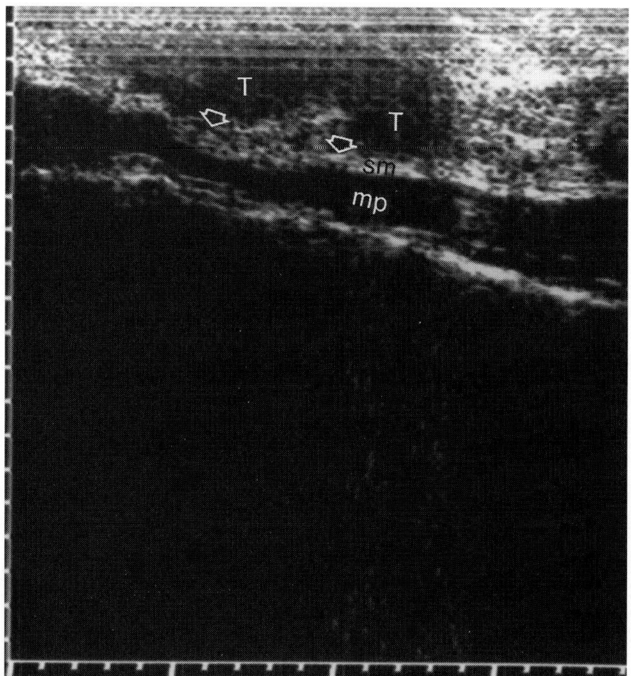


**FIGURE 5–14**

An early esophageal cancer (T) with submucosal (sm) invasion (open arrows) is shown. The muscularis propria (mp) is intact.

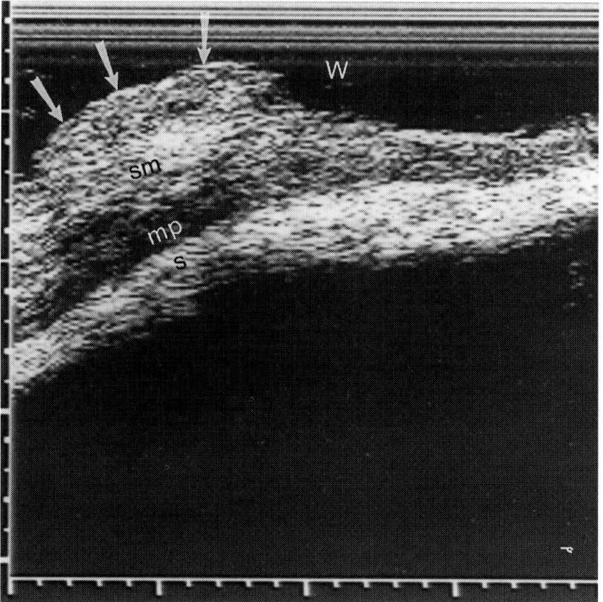


**FIGURE 5–15**

This image made through luminal water (W) of a gastric adenomatous polyp (arrow) shows an intact underlying submucosa (sm), muscularis propria (mp), and serosa (s).

Depth of invasion of intramucosal and T1 cancers (submucosal invasion) is readily detected with the linear probe when it is possible to image through water. We have not been able to distinguish high-grade dysplasia from intramucosal carcinoma in Barrett's esophagus unless an endoscopically visible nodule is present. When submucosal invasion is found with any cancer, conventional endosonography should also be done to search for regional lymph node metastases that are not reliably detected with probe imaging.

The measurement of gastrointestinal wall layer thickness on EUS images is possible, but has not proved clinically useful. A thickened muscularis propria can be imaged in patients with colonic diverticular disease and proximal to obstruction of the stomach or esophagus. We and others have found a thickened muscularis propria in patients with achalasia, especially the vigorous form of this disease (20).

There is little reported experience of this linear probe's use within the pancreatic or bile ducts. However, the catheter is small and flexible enough for this application. It must be introduced through a sheath that has been previously placed through a stricture. Imaging is possible when the sheath is withdrawn (Fig. 5–17). The linear scanning technique is less conducive than radial scanning to fluoroscopically con-

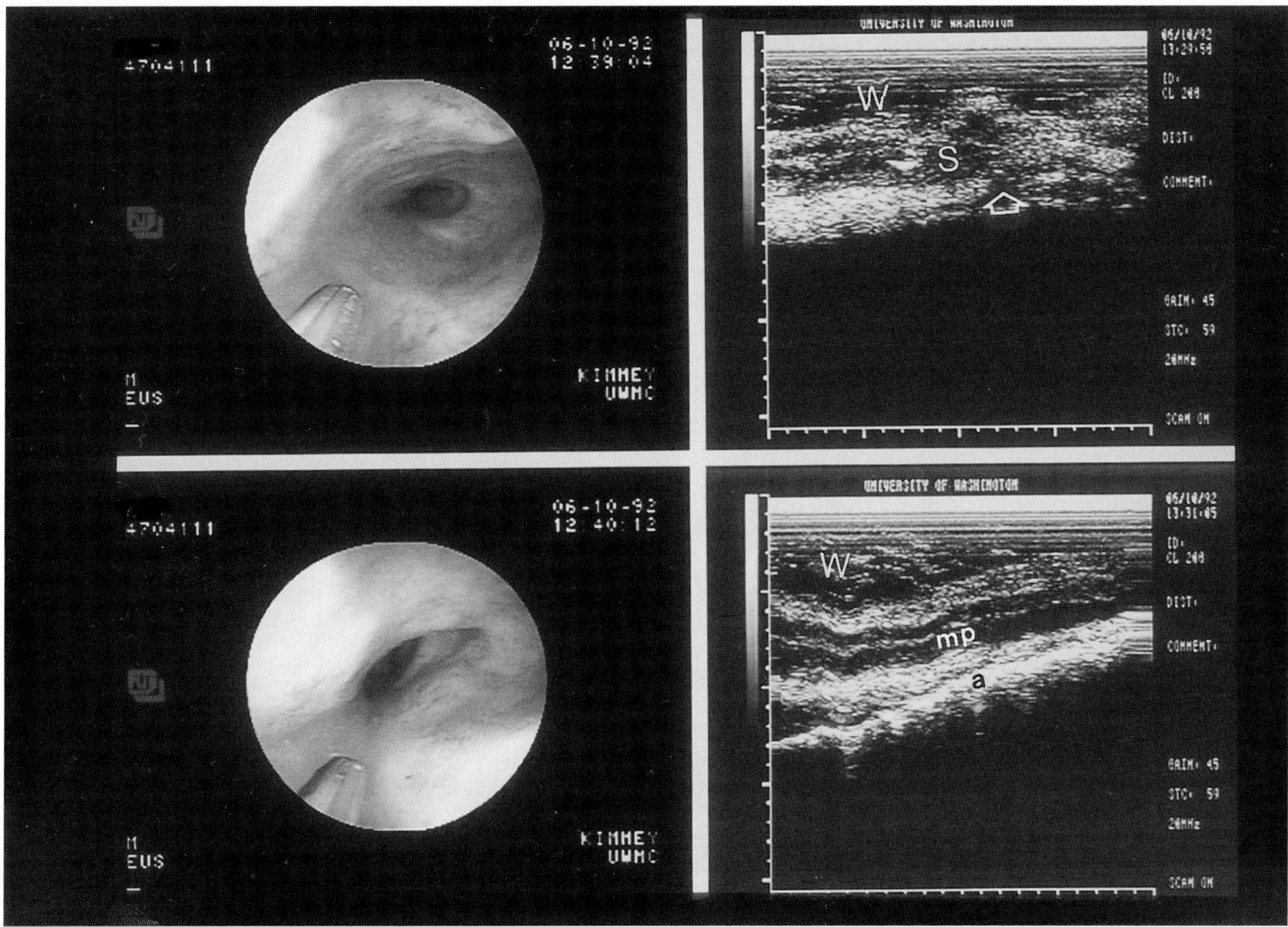


**FIGURE 5–16**

A slightly depressed area of the esophagus (upper left) where a T3 squamous cell carcinoma had been treated with chemo-therapy and radiation therapy without resection two years previously. The image reveals persistent disruption of the normal wall layers (upper right image). Wall detail is shown by imaging through a small amount of water (W) in the lumen.
A hypoechoic area extends through into the adventitia (open arrow) and is caused by scar (S) at the location of the previous tumor. Normal wall layers are shown from imaging an area of esophagus distal to the scar (bottom left and right). (*See color insert for color plate.*)

trolled imaging because it is difficult to determine the direction of the ultrasound beam. In vitro studies have shown the bile duct to be a three-layered structure when imaged with this probe, corresponding to the inner luminal interface and epithelium, the middle bile duct fibromuscular wall, and the outer subserosal and surrounding tissue (21).

## Summary and Future Prospects

The mechanical linear ultrasound probe (Fujinon Sonoprobe) is an auxiliary endoscopic ultrasound device for use in select situations. The device is useful in imaging small intramural masses and small superficial neoplasms where endoscopic vision can direct imaging. It is not useful in larger and deeper lesions or for imaging the tissue or other organs surrounding the gastrointestinal wall. Therefore, it is not sufficient for many standard applications of conventional endosonography.

The Sonoprobe system is under further development. We have preliminary experience with a new prototype system that allows both linear and radial scanning with the same probe. This should simplify imaging of some structures and expand the range of applications of this system. Combining this imaging probe with a Doppler probe has also been discussed. If engineering requirements can be met, this type of device may also enhance detection of hidden arteries responsible for ulcer bleeding.

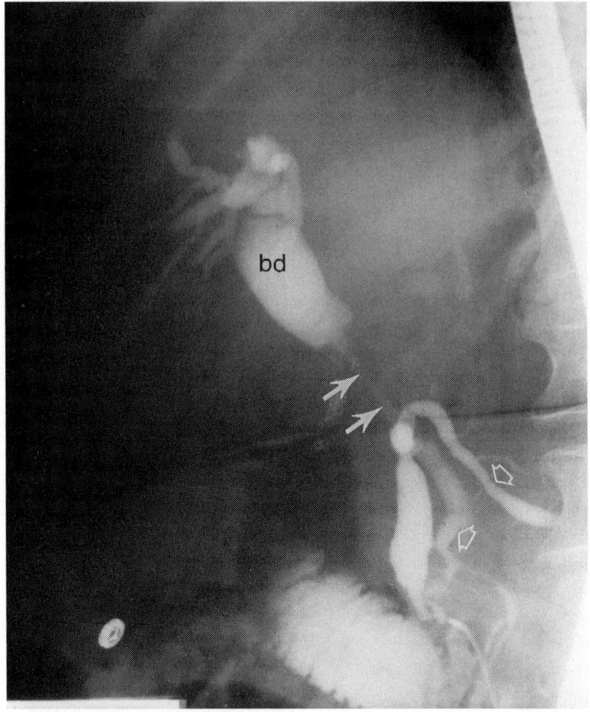

A

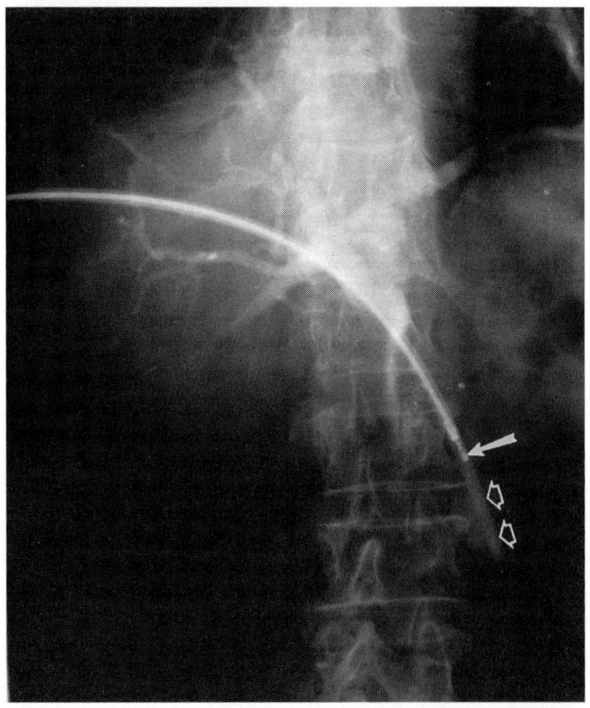

B

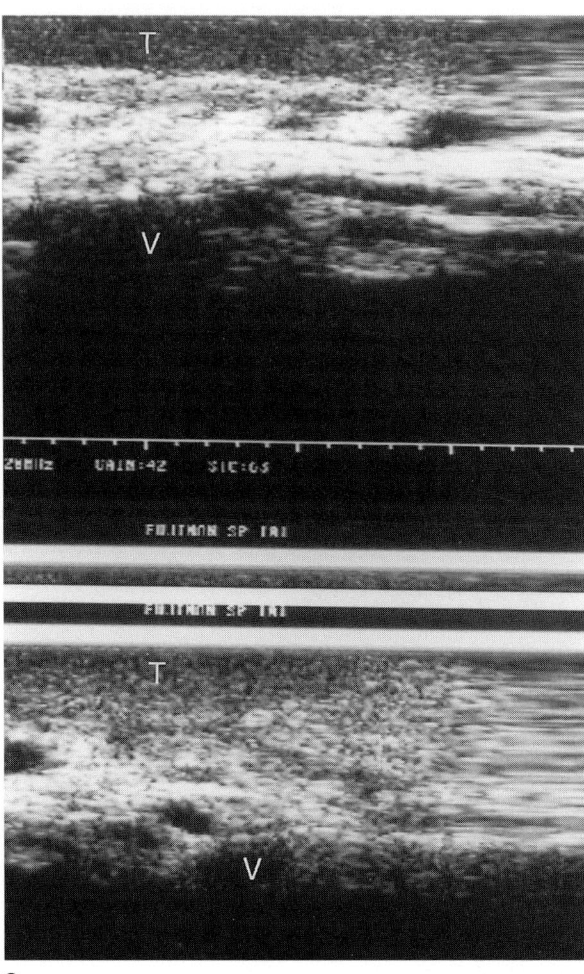


C

**FIGURE 5–17**

(**A**) Retrograde cholangiography reveals a mid–common bile duct stricture (closed arrows), dilated proximal bile duct (bd), and normal pancreatic duct (open arrows) suggestive of a cholangiocarcinoma. (**B**) A 20-MHz linear probe (arrow) has been placed into the stricture through a sheath (open arrows) placed by a transhepatic approach. (**C**) These two linear probe images of the biliary stricture reveal hypoechoic thickening of the bile duct wall (T) without clear extension of the tumor into the underlying vessel (V).

## References

1. Kimmey MB, Martin RW. Fundamentals of endosonography. Gastrointestinal Endoscopy Clinics of North America 2:557–573, 1992.
2. Kimmey MB, Martin RW, Mack LA, Franklin DW. Endoscopic ultrasound (EUS): What US frequency is best? Gastroenterology 94:A226, 1988.
3. Rösch T, Classen M. A new ultrasonic probe for endosonographic imaging of the upper GI tract. Endoscopy 22:41, 1990.
4. Martin RW, Silverstein FE, Kimmey MB. A 20 MHz ultrasound system for imaging the intestinal wall. Ultrasound Med Biol 15: 273–280, 1989.
5. Martin RW, Silverstein FE, Kimmey MB, Jiranek GC, Proctor A. B mode imaging and Doppler ultrasonic catheters for use with

fiberoptic endoscopes. SPIE Vol. 904- Microsensors and Catheter Based Imaging Technology:121–126, 1988.

6. Silverstein FE, Martin RW, Kimmey MB, Jiranek GC, Franklin DW, Proctor A. Experimental evaluation of an endoscopic ultrasound probe: In vitro and in vivo canine studies. Gastroenterology 96: 1058–1062, 1989.
7. Ødegaard S, Kimmey MB. Colorectal endoscopic ultrasonography using a transendoscopic linear probe system. Endoscopy 24(suppl 1):387, 1992.
8. Kimmey MB, Martin RW, Jiranek GC, Myers J, Silverstein FE. Modification of a 20 MHz endoscopic ultrasound probe imaging system to allow real time imaging with M mode. Gastrointest Endosc 36:219, 1990.
9. Kimmey MB, Martin RW, Haggitt RC, Wang KY, Franklin DW, Silverstein FE. Histological correlates of gastrointestinal endoscopic ultrasound images. Gastroenterology 96:433–441, 1989.
10. Kimmey MB, Silverstein FE, Jiranek GC, Proctor A, Martin RW. High resolution imaging of the normal gastrointestinal tract using a 20 MHz endoscopic ultrasound probe. Gastrointest Endosc 36:219, 1990.
11. Ødegaard S, Kimmey MB. Location of the muscularis mucosae on high frequency gastrointestinal ultrasound image. Eur J Ultrasound 1:39–50, 1994.
12. Ødegaard S, Nesje LB, Kimmey MB, Matre K. Transendoskopische Ultraschalldiagnostik bei Lasionen im oberen Verdauungstrakt im Rahmen der Routineendoskopie. Ultraschall Klin Prax 7:99–103, 1992.
13. Kimmey MB, Silverstein FE, Jiranek GC, Sillery J, Martin RW. Imaging of gastrointestinal mural lesions with a 20 MHz endoscopic ultrasound probe: Advantages and limitations. Gastroenterology 98:A289, 1990.
14. Kimmey MB. Endoscopic ultrasound probes. Endoscopy Review 8:8–31, 1991.
15. Kimmey MB, Martin RW, Silverstein FE. Clinical applications of linear ultrasound probes. Endoscopy 24(suppl 1):364–369, 1992.
16. Kimmey MB, Yasuda K, Kawai K. Endoscopic ultrasonography. In Yamada T (ed): Gastroenterology. Philadelphia: Lippincott, 1991, pp 2343–2360.
17. Ødegaard S, Kimmey MB, Martin RW, Yee HC, Cheung AGS, Silverstein FE. The effects of applied pressure on the thickness, layers, and echogenicity of gastrointestinal wall ultrasound images. Gastrointest Endosc 38:351–356, 1992.
18. Kimmey MB, Wang KY, Jiranek GC, Ødegaard S, Silverstein FE, Martin RW. Staging of esophageal carcinoma using a linear endoscopic ultrasound probe. Gastroenterology 100:A375, 1991.
19. Kimmey MB, Martin RW, Silverstein FE. Endoscopic ultrasound probes. Gastrointest Endosc 36:S40–46, 1990.
20. Trowers EA, Kimmey MB, Yee HC, Martin RW, Taniguchi D, Silverstein FE. Assessment of esophageal muscle thickness in achalasia using a high frequency linear endoscopic ultrasound probe. Gastrointest Endosc 38:244, 1992.
21. Ishihara A, Tsukamoto Y, Naitou Y, Mitake M, Yamada M, Nakgawa H, Hirooka Y, Kimoto E. An ultrasonographic study of bile duct wall and carcinoma of the extrahepatic bile duct by 20-MHz ultrasound probe system (Sonoprobe system). Gastroenterology 100:1320, 1991.

CHAPTER

# 6

# High-Resolution Endoluminal Sonography of the Upper Gastrointestinal Tract

## THE RADIAL SCANNING ULTRASOUND PROBE: PART I

Larry S. Miller
Ji-Bin Liu

Ultrasound transducers have been placed in the gastrointestinal tract for imaging of mural and extramural structures. The most common transducer frequency used clinically ranges from 7.5 to 12 MHz. Placement of an endoluminal ultrasound transducer was first reported by Wild and Reid (1) in 1956. They used an ultrasound transducer in the rectum to evaluate the wall of the bowel in an attempt to identify malignant tumors. Since that time a number of researchers have been working on the further development of endoluminal sonography. In 1976 Lutz and Rosch (2) reported using an ultrasound probe passed through the accessory channel of an endoscope. They obtained an A-mode image to evaluate the cystic versus solid characteristics of lesions deforming the gastric wall. In the early 1980s the concept of combining a flexible endoscope with an ultrasound transducer to image the gastrointestinal tract wall was developed; results were published by Fukuda et al. (3) and DiMagno et al. (4) with the use of 7.5- to 12.5-MHz transducers. Using these transducers, it was possible to image both the mural structures of the gastrointestinal tract and structures adjacent to the gastrointestinal tract wall (5). This approach proved useful in the preoperative diagnosis and staging of esophageal and gastric cancers (6,7). Using this type of transducer, the normal and abnormal endoluminal anatomy was defined. In 1989 Silverstein et al. (8) used a 20-MHz linear array ultrasound probe that could be passed through the biopsy channel of a flexible endoscope to evaluate the gastrointestinal tract wall. Later, Rosch and Classen (9) used a 7.5-MHz 3.7-mm (diameter) ultrasound probe to image the esophagus, stomach, and duodenum by means of the working channel of a gastroscope.

Over the past several years flexible ultrasound transducer containing catheters (4.8–9 French) originally designed for intravascular ultrasound applications have become available to investigators studying other structures (10,11). These miniature catheter-based transducers have been used to evaluate nonvascular lumina, including the genitourinary tract, endometrial canal, bile ducts, and bronchial trees (12–16). In this chapter we report the use of these high-frequency, high-resolution ultrasound transducers in the gastrointestinal tract with particular attention to their use in the esophagus and stomach.

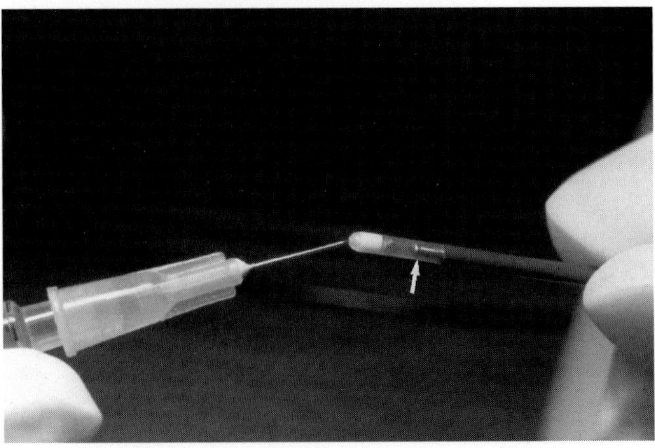

**FIGURE 6–1**

The endoluminal ultrasound transducer (arrow) is mounted on the end of a drive wire (core), which is housed in a 6.2 French catheter. Sterile water (0.5–1.0 mL) is injected with a 27-gauge needle through the sealed catheter tip to eliminate any air around the transducer. (Reproduced with permission from Liu JB, et al. Radiology 184:721–727, 1992.)

## Preliminaries

The ultrasound imaging system used in all of the following studies is available commercially from IVUS, Diasonics (Milpitas, California). (However, both Fuginon and Olympus have developed such probe systems: Olympus OM-2R/3R and Fuginon SP-501.) Specially developed 6.2 French catheters (2 mm in diameter, 95 cm in length) containing 20-MHz transducers were used (Sonocath™, Microvasive/Boston Scientific; Watertown, MA) (Fig. 6–1). The single-element ultrasound transducer is mounted on the end of a wire (core), which is connected to a motor on the ultrasound instrument. The 1.35-mm–diameter core is inserted into the flexible catheter, and the motor is rotated to produce a 360° transaxial real-time image. Sterile water (0.5–1.0 mL) is introduced between the core and the catheter to eliminate air, which can interfere with the transmission of the ultrasound beam. The transducer sends and receives the ultrasound signal at an angle 10° from the perpendicular to the long axis of the catheter. The operating frequency of 20 MHz results in an axial resolution of 0.1 mm and a penetration of about 2 cm. Real-time images are recorded on videotape for later evaluation, and individual frozen images can be stored on a digital imager disk system (3M Medical Imaging Systems; St. Paul, Minnesota).

These ultrasound transducers differ from the routinely used clinical ultrasound scopes in a number of ways. First, the ultrasound catheter is much smaller than that in the dedicated scopes. The catheters are so small that they fit easily through a nasogastric tube or the biopsy channels of colonoscopes and upper gastrointestinal endoscopes. In addition, their small size permits these catheters to be used through strictured areas that dedicated endosonoscopes cannot go through. Second, the 20-MHz frequency is much higher than the frequency currently used clinically, which ranges from 7.5 to 12 MHz. This higher frequency increases the axial resolution of the image so that mural gastrointestinal structures can be seen with much greater resolution. However, the penetration of the ultrasound waves is limited by the higher frequency, so that, structures surrounding the gastrointestinal tract are often not imaged. Thus the ability of these transducers to stage large or advanced carcinomas is limited. Third, these transducers are not surrounded by a latex water-filled balloon as are the lower frequency transducers in the dedicated endosonoscopes. There are certain advantages and disadvantages to this. The major advantage is that there is no compression effect on mural structures. Because of the smaller size and the lack of compression, small mural structures such as esophageal and gastric varices are much less distorted. The disadvantage is a possible loss of acoustic coupling in air-filled organs such as the stomach and the small intestine. This leads to distortion and sometimes total inability to image certain areas.

Using a 7.5- or 12-MHz endoscopic ultrasound transducer, the gastrointestinal tract wall appears as five ultrasonic layers of different echogenicities. These layers, parallel to the mucosal surface, are distinguished by their different echotexture and echogenicity. The first or innermost is hyperechoic (bright or white), the second is hypoechoic (dark), the third is hyperechoic, the fourth hypoechoic, and the fifth or outermost layer is hyperechoic. All of these sonographic layers have approximately the same thickness. Kimmey et al. (17) hypothesize that the overall appearance of the ultrasound image is determined by a combination of echoes from two sources—(1) those created at interfaces between tissue layers with different acoustic impedances, and (2) those created within the internal structure of the tissue layers. The five major echo layers seen on sonographic imaging of the esophagus, stomach, colon, and rectum represent the following structures:

First hyperechoic layer—the superficial mucosa
Second hypoechoic layer—the deep mucosa
Third hyperechoic layer—the submucosa plus the acoustic interface between the submucosa and the muscularis propria
Fourth hypoechoic layer—the muscularis propria minus the acoustic interface between the submucosa and the muscularis propria
Fifth hyperechoic layer—the serosa and subserosal fat

Kimmey also noted that, in vitro, the esophageal and colonic walls may occasionally separate into six layers, provided the ultrasound transducer is at the correct distance from the mucosa. In the laboratory the fourth layer is separated by a thin hyperechoic layer into two hypoechoic layers. This thin echogenic line is produced by connective tissue between the inner circular and outer longitudinal components of the muscularis propria (19).

## In Vitro Studies

### Sheep Esophagus

The initial gastrointestinal studies done using the 20-MHz catheter-based ultrasound transducer were animal studies in sheep esophagi. Whole esophageal specimens were studied in vitro. The fresh specimens were placed in a water bath and the transducer-containing catheter was inserted into the lumen of the esophagus. To eliminate near-field transducer artifact, 15 mL of saline was injected into the lumen of the esophagus. After sonographic imaging, the specimens were fixed in 10% formalin, embedded in paraffin, and histologic cross sections were prepared. These cross sections corresponded to the ultrasound imaging planes. In the sonographic images it was possible to delineate seven layers of the esophageal wall (18). Correlation of the histologic findings with ultrasound images showed that the innermost layer (hyperechoic) represented the squamous epithelium and lamina propria, the second layer (hypoechoic) the deep mucosa and muscularis mucosa, the third layer (hyperechoic) the submucosa, the fourth layer (hypoechoic) the circular muscle, the thin fifth layer (hyperechoic) the intermuscular connective tissue, the sixth layer (hypoechoic) the longitudinal muscle, and the seventh layer (hyperechoic) the adventitia (Fig. 6–2).

Although five layers have been described in the human gastrointestinal tract, it is usually possible to see only three sonographic layers in the human esophagus using existing endoscopic ultrasound technology.

A

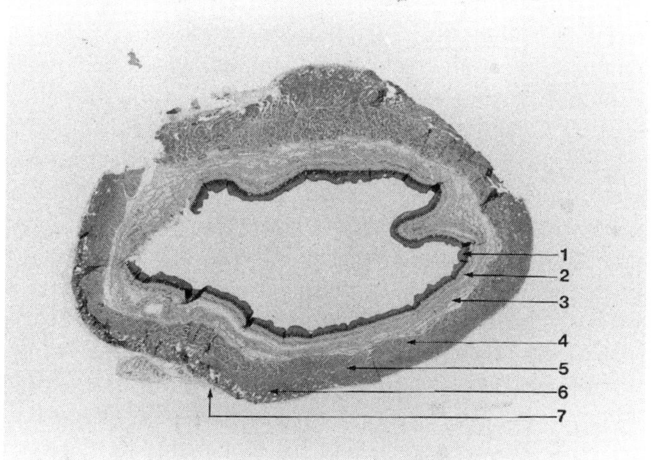


B

**FIGURE 6–2**

(**A**) The 20-MHz ultrasound transducer (T) located within the saline-distended sheep esophagus delineates seven layers of the esophageal wall. (**B**) Close correlation between the cross-sectional histologic slice and the ultrasound imaging in (**A**) can be seen: (1) Mucosa, (2) muscularis mucosa, (3) submucosa, (4) circular muscle, (5) intermuscular connective tissue, (6) longitudinal muscle, (7) adventitia. (Reproduced with permission from Liu JB, et al. Radiology 184:721–727, 1992.)

This is probably because of the difficulty in focusing the ultrasound beam on the esophageal wall when the wall is in direct contact with the ultrasound transducer and because of compression by the water-filled latex balloon on the esophageal wall. The three layers normally seen in the esophagus are as follows: the first hyperechoic layer, which corresponds to the balloon mucosa/submucosa together with the submucosa/muscularis propria interface; the second hypoechoic layer, which corresponds to the muscularis propria; and the third hyperechoic layer, which represents the interface between the muscularis propria and the surrounding tissue (19).

## Human Esophagus

A number of human autopsies were done in which the esophagus was evaluated with the 20-MHz ultrasound transducer. In this study the chest and abdominal cavities of the human cadaver were opened and the esophagus was removed along with the gastric cardia. The stomach was ligated just distal to the gastroesophageal junction and the esophagus was suspended from a tripod stand with silk sutures. The esophagus was then placed in a water bath, the catheter containing the ultrasound transducer was introduced into the proximal esophagus, and an image of the esophagus was obtained. The catheter was then advanced distally to image the entire length of the esophagus. After the initial imaging, the esophagus was infused with various volumes of water and reimaged at the same locations. Silk sutures were placed in the adventitial surface of the esophagus at various imaging locations. The esophagus was then fixed in 4% buffered formalin, and sections for histologic evaluation were taken at the levels of the sutures. Histologic examination was performed on standard paraffin-embedded specimens, stained with hematoxylin–eosin and Masson's trichrome. The histologic observations on cross-section were compared with the cross-sectional endoluminal sonography at the corresponding levels.

Analysis of cross-sectional images obtained in the in vitro non–fluid-filled esophagus revealed six alternating echo layers. Analysis of images obtained in the in vitro fluid-filled esophagus revealed seven reproducible and distinct alternating hyper- and hypoechoic layers in the esophageal wall. Each of these seven layers corresponded to distinct histologic structures. From medial (closest to the transducer) to lateral (farthest from the transducer), the first hyperechoic layer corresponds to the mucosa (squamous epithelium and lamina propria), the second thin hypoechoic layer to the deep mucosa and muscularis mucosae, the third very bright hyperechoic layer to the submucosa, the fourth hypoechoic layer to the circular smooth muscle, the fifth thin hyperechoic layer to the intermuscular connective tissue, the sixth hypoechoic layer to the longitudinal smooth muscle, and the seventh hyperechoic layer to the adventitia.

The difference between the non–fluid-filled and the fluid-filled esophagus is that the first layer in the non–fluid-filled esophagus (the layer closest to the transducer) appears as a mixed echoic layer corresponding to the squamous epithelium, lamina propria, and muscularis mucosae. Therefore, the squamous epithelium, lamina propria, and muscularis mucosae cannot be clearly distinguished from each other in the non–fluid-filled esophagus. This is because the first three histologic layers (squamous epithelium, lamina propria, and muscularis mucosae) are folded and contracted around the transducer: Thus the sound waves pass through redundant layers of tissue and the summation effect is a relatively hypoechoic or mixed echoic pattern. But when filled with fluid, the first three histologic layers distend so that the sound waves pass through each layer in an orderly sequence. Additionally, the near field of the ultrasound image has lower resolution than the mid field of ultrasound image. Therefore, when fluid within the lumen pushes the mucosal layer away from the transducer, the resolution is better and the mucosal layer can be separated into two distinct echo structures (Fig. 6–3). The squamous epithelium and lamina propria cannot be separated into two distinct layers, probably because these two layers possess similar acoustic properties.

# In Vivo Studies

## Normal Anatomy of the Esophagus

Since the miniature ultrasound transducers demonstrated a very high resolution in both in vitro animal esophagi and in human esophageal autopsy specimens, it was decided to test these transducers in normal human volunteers to see if these findings could be reproduced in vivo. The initial prototype ultrasound transducers were only 95 cm long and therefore could not be passed through a standard upper endoscope for visualization of the esophagus. Therefore, a method of passage was developed in order to visualize the human esophagus in vivo. The method used to introduce the 6.2 French ultrasound catheters into the human stomach and esophagus was to place a 16 French nasogastric tube transnasally into the stomach. The nasogastric tube placement was confirmed by aspiration of gastric contents. The 6.2 French ultrasound catheter was then placed through the lumen of the nasogastric tube and placement was confirmed by imaging in the stomach. The ultrasound transducer could then be pulled up into the esophagus and the esophagus imaged. By manipulating the nasogastric

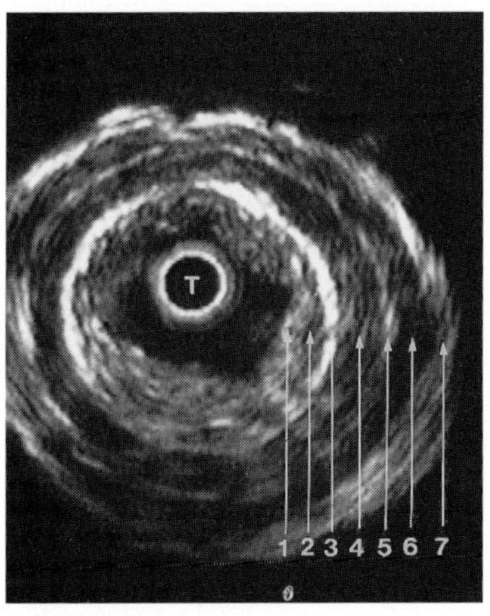


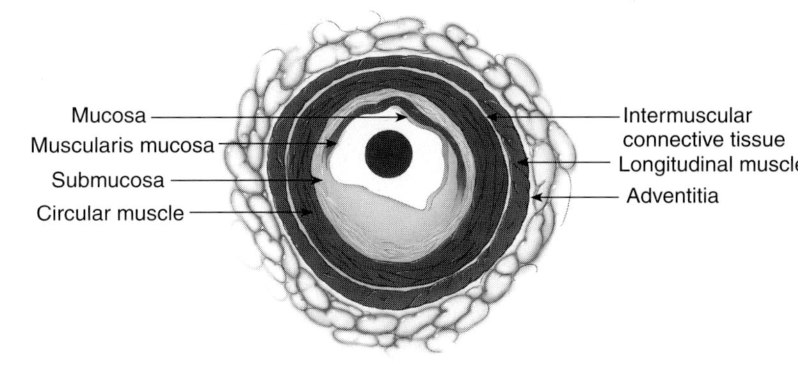


**FIGURE 6–3**

Seven layers of esophageal wall in a human autopsy specimen (water fills the lumen around the transducer).(1) Mucosa, (2) muscularis mucosa, (3) submucosa, (4) circular muscle, (5) intermuscular connective tissue, (6) longitudinal muscle, (7) adventitia.

tube and the ultrasound catheter it was possible to image the entire esophagus from the lower esophageal sphincter to the upper esophageal sphincter.

Studies in normal volunteers were performed in order to correlate the echo layers seen in vitro with echo layers seen in vivo in the human esophagus. It was found that in normal volunteers all the echo layers seen in the autopsy esophageal specimens were also seen in the in vivo human esophagus. In the esophagus at rest, six echo layers were seen, similar to the non–fluid-filled autopsy specimens. During swallowing of a 5–10 mL water bolus, seven echo layers were seen, similar to the water-filled autopsy esophageal specimen. A number of other findings were also consistently seen on imaging of the normal volunteers' esophagi. First, in the area of the lower esophageal sphincter the muscle layers were found to be significantly thicker than in areas above the lower esophageal sphincter (Fig. 6–4). Second, the area of the lower esophageal sphincter was consistently round and symmetric and the diaphragm was consistently visualized as thick hypoechoic bands (Fig. 6–5). However, in areas of the mid and upper esophagus, the

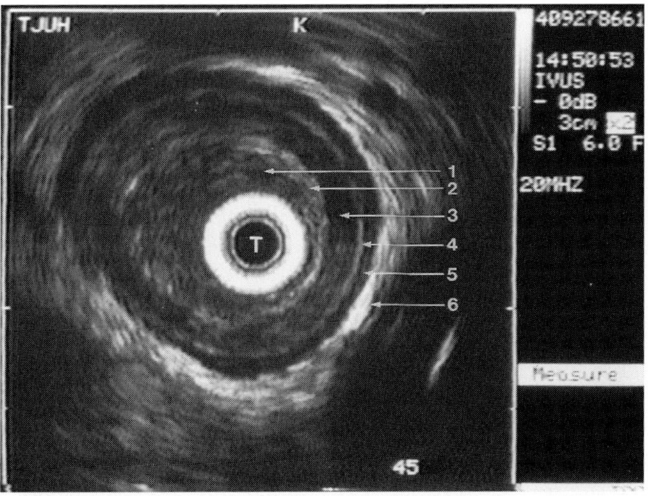


A

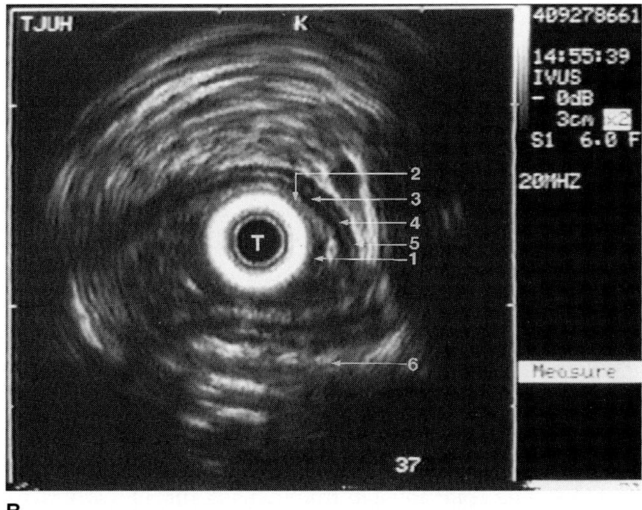


B

**FIGURE 6–4**

The catheter-based transducer (T) positioned within the LES region (**A**) and 8 cm above the LES (**B**) in a normal volunteer delineates the various normal layers of the esophageal wall. Note that the thickness of the muscular layers in the LES region is greater than that in the body of the esophagus. (1) Mucosa, (2) submucosa, (3) circular muscle, (4) intermuscular connective tissue, (5) longitudinal muscle, (6) adventitia. (Reproduced with permission from Liu JB, et al. Radiology 184:721–727, 1992.)

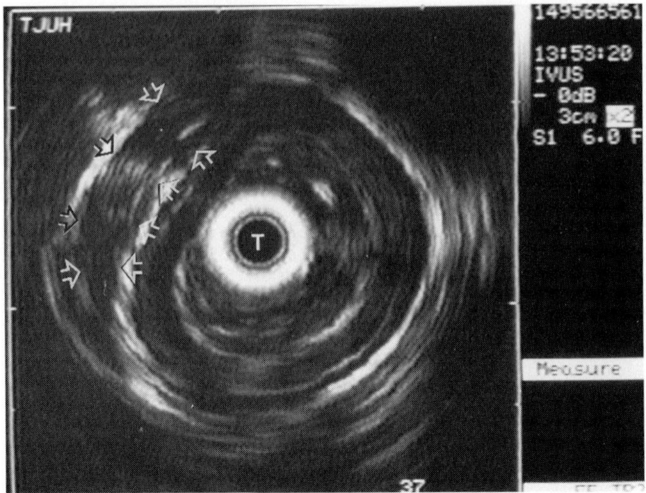


**FIGURE 6–5**

The cross-sectional ultrasound image obtained from the gastroesophageal junction shows a hypoechoic region (open arrows) adjacent to the esophageal wall representing the diaphragm. (Reproduced with permission from Liu JB, et al. Radiology 184:721–727, 1992.)

**TABLE 6–1**

Mean Muscle Thickness at and above the LES (n=17)

| | Circular Smooth Muscle | Longitudinal Smooth Muscle | Total Width of Muscle |
|---|---|---|---|
| At LES | .134 cm ± .034 cm | .079 cm ± .013 cm | .236 cm ± .046 cm |
| 5–10 cm above LES | .072 cm ± .026 cm | .051 cm ± .011 cm | .130 cm ± .039 cm |

esophagus was asymmetric, probably owing to compression from extraesophageal structures. Third, the submucosa was consistently brighter (more hyperechoic) in the area just below the upper esophageal sphincter than in the body or the lower esophageal sphincter area. This may be due to the number of glands found in the submucosa in that area. Fourth, the upper esophageal sphincter was demonstrated in every subject. Although the penetration of the transducer was only 2 cm, the penetration was deep enough—and the esophageal wall thin enough—to image some peri-esophageal structures, including lymph nodes and blood vessels.

A digital computer analysis system permitted repetitive measurements to be made of the circular smooth muscle, longitudinal smooth muscle, and total muscle width of the muscularis propria in each volunteer subject. The various muscle widths at the lower esophageal sphincter (LES) were compared to the muscle widths 5–10 cm above the LES in the body of the esophagus. Each muscle layer at the LES was found to be significantly thicker when compared to its counterpart 5–10 cm above the LES. In addition, the circular smooth muscle was significantly thicker than the longitudinal smooth muscle both at the level of the LES and 5–10 cm above the LES. The total muscle thickness at the LES (the total thickness of the muscularis propria) was almost twice the total muscle thickness 5–10 cm above the LES (Table 6–1) (20).

Sequential ultrasound imaging was obtained both at the level of the LES and in the body of the esophagus during swallowing of 5–10-mL boluses of water in each healthy volunteer. The stages of swallowing correspond to the following figures (Fig. 6–6). Figure 6–6A represents a cross-sectional image of the esophagus during its resting state. Figure 6–6B is an image obtained after the lumen of the esophagus was distended by the swallowing of 10 mL of water. Note that the two muscle layers become thinner and that all seven layers of the esophageal wall can be demonstrated, as opposed to the six layers of the esophageal wall shown in Figure 6–6A. Figure 6–6C is an image of the contraction of the muscular layers associated with increased wall thickness. It was also found that during peristaltic contractions the circular muscle layer increased in echogenicity. Finally, Figure 6–6D shows the esophagus returning to its resting or basal state.

## Esophageal Disorders

### Achalasia

Once the normal sonographic anatomy of the esophagus was defined in vivo using the 20-MHz ultrasound transducer, it was possible to look for abnormalities in patients with various esophageal disorders. Miller et al. (25) used the Endosound 20-MHz transducer to evaluate the width of various muscle layers at the gastroesophageal junction in normal volunteers and patients with achalasia. The resolution achieved with this 20-MHz ultrasound transducer is superior to that obtained with the other transducers. The ultrasound transducer makes contact with the mucus and water layer on the mucosal surface at the LES; therefore, acoustic coupling is accomplished without a water-filled balloon around the transducer which can distort the native anatomy of the esophagus. Because the esophagus above the LES is usually markedly dilated, acoustic coupling can be accomplished only in the area of the LES. To perform this high-frequency endoluminal sonography (HRES) above the LES, water was placed into the esophageal lumen. With the relatively high resolution of these HRES transducers, each component muscle layer at the LES could be imaged and measured quite accurately.

The purpose of the study was to resolve the issue of whether or not the muscularis propria layer at the

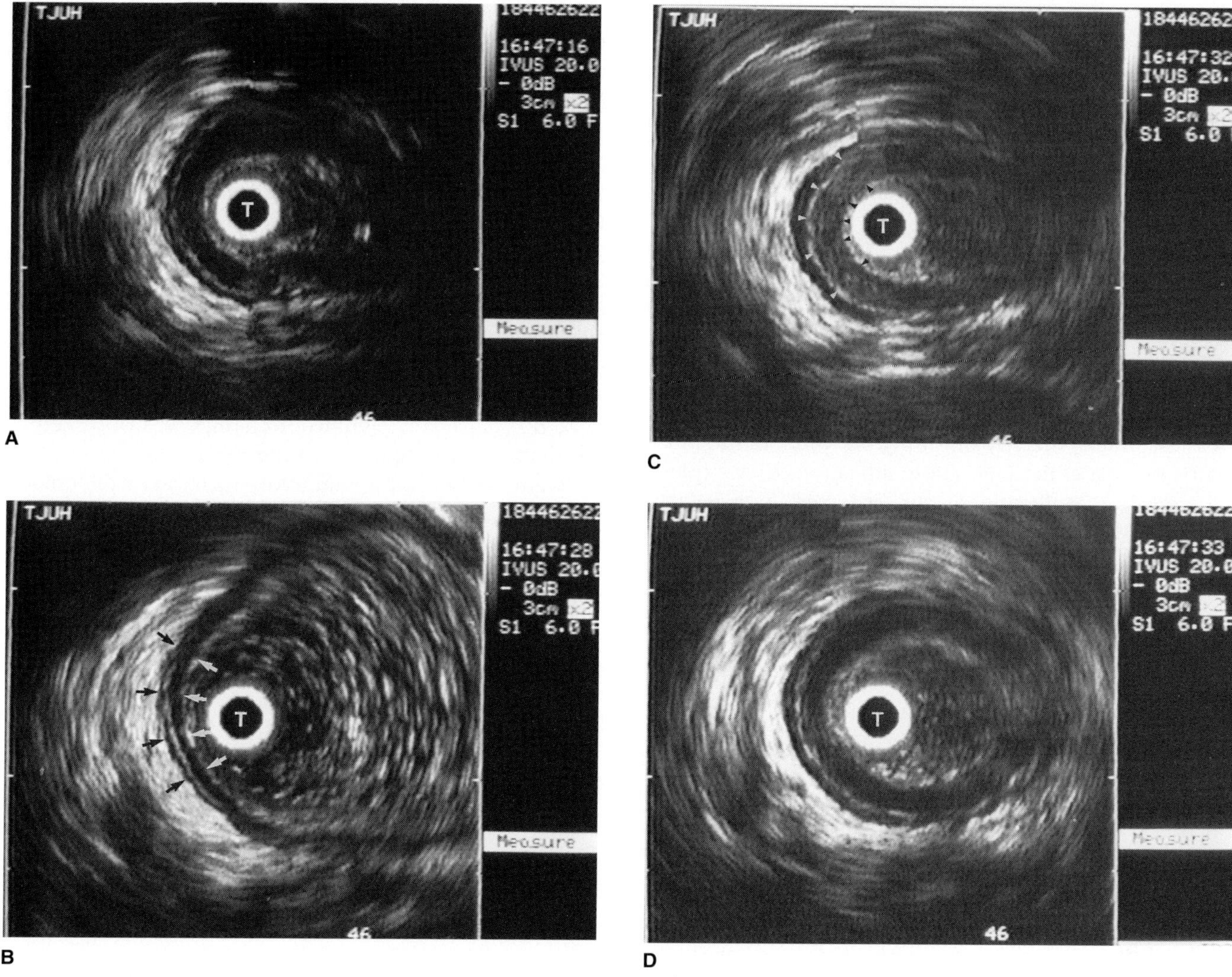


**FIGURE 6–6**

Sequential ultrasound images, obtained at the level of the LES, demonstrate the swallowing process in a normal volunteer. (**A**) The cross-sectional image of the esophagus during its resting state. (**B**) The lumen of the esophagus distended by swallowing 10 mL of water. Note that the two muscle layers have become thinner (arrows) and that all seven layers of the esophageal wall are demonstrated. (**C**) Peristaltic contraction of the muscular layers associated with increased wall thickness can be seen. During peristaltic contraction the circular muscle layer increases in echogenicity (arrowheads) while the longitudinal muscle layer does not change. (**D**) The esophagus has returned to its resting state. (Reproduced with permission from Liu JB, et al. Radiology 184:721–727, 1992.)

LES is thickened in achalasia patients. The muscle width was measured at a baseline resting state at the LES. This was accomplished by leaving the transducer at the level of the LES for a considerable length of time, making sure that the patient didn't swallow during this period. Tangential artifacts were excluded by moving the transducer within the LES to a position where the thickness of the muscularis propria layers was symmetrically equal circumferentially around the transducer.

This in vivo study (25) demonstrated that the mean width of the muscle layers is in fact increased in achalasia patients when compared to normal controls (Table 6–2). However, despite the statistically significant thickening, there was also an overlap in the muscle width thicknesses between these groups. Therefore, a thickened muscularis propria cannot be used to clinically diagnose achalasia. Upon retrospective review of clinical, manometric, and radiographic data, achalasia patients with marked thickening of the muscularis propria could not be differentiated from achalasia patients without this muscular thickening (Fig. 6–7).

Esophageal imaging with lower-frequency, lower-resolution transducers does not allow for precise measurements of the width of the muscularis propria layer. Moreover, component muscle layers cannot be differentiated and measured individually. The larger size of the

**TABLE 6–2**

Muscle Thickness Measurements at the LES in Achalasia Patients (n=8)*

| | Maximum (cm) | Minimum (cm) | Mean + SD (cm) |
|---|---|---|---|
| CSM | 0.600 | 0.187 | 0.339 ± 0.161 |
| LSM | 0.145 | 0.092 | 0.119 ± 0.020 |
| TM | 0.783 | 0.333 | 0.496 ± 0.180 |

*SD = Standard deviation; LES = lower esophageal sphincter; CSM = circular smooth muscle; LSM = longitudinal smooth muscle; TM = total muscle.

Reproduced with permission from Liu JB, et al. Radiology 184:721–727, 1992.

lower-frequency transducers and the fact that they are surrounded by a water-filled balloon can cause compression artifact, thereby distorting the width of the muscularis propria at the LES. These limitations may explain the previous conflicting results observed in achalasia patients. The fact that a 20-MHz catheter is so small, is not surrounded by a balloon, and has much better resolution allows for more precise measurement of the layers of the muscularis propria at the LES in achalasia.

Schiano et al. (26) have employed HRES to determine how much wall damage occurs at the GE junction after both pneumatic dilatation and injection of botulinum toxin in the treatment of achalasia. The HRES transducer was passed through the biopsy channel of a standard 34 French endoscope to the level of the GE junction. The layers of the esophageal wall were imaged before, immediately after, and 24 hours after pneumatic dilatation or intrasphincteric injection of botulinum toxin. The thicknesses of the mucosa–submucosa and the CSM and LSM layers at the level of the diaphragm were measured before and after treatment.

HRES revealed similar pretreatment mucosa–submucosa diameter thicknesses for botulinum toxin injection and pneumatic dilatation patients. This was similar to that seen in normal controls. The mucosa–submucosa diameter significantly increased immediately after pneumatic dilatation whereas no significant difference was observed in the mucosa–submucosa diameter after botulinum toxin injection. The increase in mucosa– submucosa diameter was diffuse after pneumatic dilatation, consistent with edema and/or hematoma formation. The twofold increase in the mucosa–submucosa diameter and cross-sectional surface area in pneumatic dilatation patients normalized within 24 hours, indicating a transient traumatic insult. In addition, no statistically significant change was observed in the thickness or character of the muscle layers immediately after either botulinum toxin injection or pneumatic dilatation, or at 24 hours post-treatment. In comparing the subjective symptomatic response to the objective HRES measurements, no correlation was found between the improvement in symptoms and the change in the submucosal thickness of the esophageal wall post-pneumatic dilatation.

Muscle fibrosis and other postoperative changes can be seen in achalasia patients after Heller cardiomyotomy. The mucosa–submucosa appears normal, but the muscle layers are disrupted by hyperechogenicity consistent with scar tissue formation from the myotomy.

## Esophageal and Gastric Varices

High-frequency endoluminal sonography was also used in the evaluation of esophageal and gastric varices.

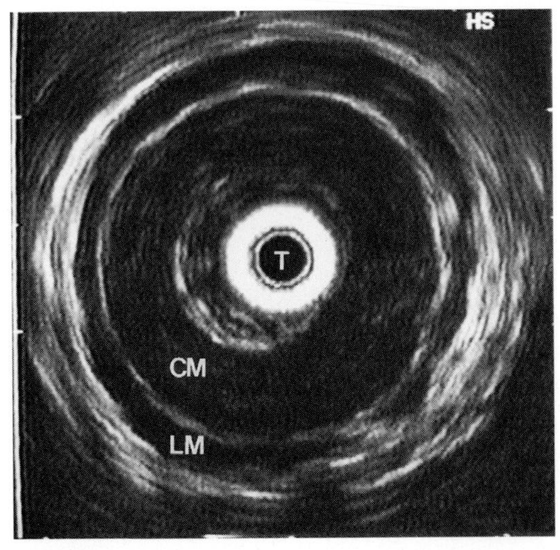


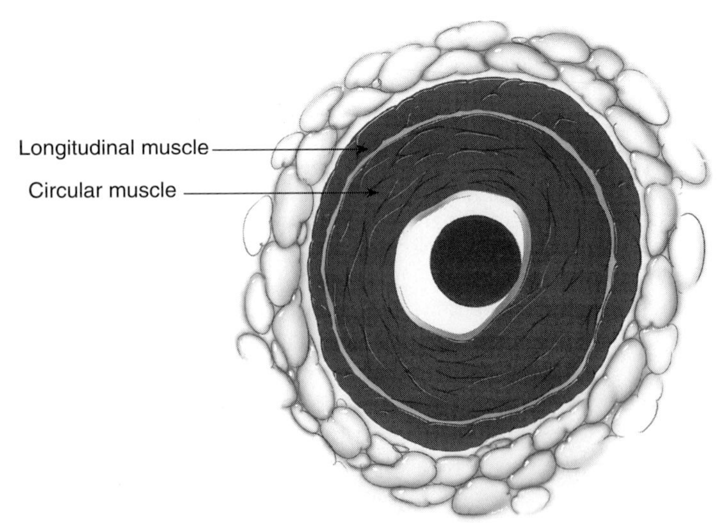


**FIGURE 6–7**

In a patient with achalasia, endoluminal ultrasound demonstrates an increased thickness of the two muscular layers in the LES region. Note the circular muscle layer (CM) is much thicker than the longitudinal muscle layer (LM). T: transducer. (Reproduced with permission from Liu JB, et al. Radiology 184:721–727, 1992.)

Prior studies using low-frequency transducers (21) found that esophageal varices, when displayed in transverse section, appear as round anechoic structures just beneath the mucosal layer. In these prior studies, however, endoscopic ultrasound revealed esophageal varices in only 50% of the patients in which varices were demonstrated by endoscopy. Endoscopic ultrasound demonstrated varices in 14% of the patients with endoscopic grade 1 esophageal varices, 78% of patients with endoscopic grade 2 varices, and 50% of patients with endoscopic grade 3 varices. Peri-esophageal collateral veins appeared in transverse section as echo-free structures outside the esophageal wall in 80% of the patients. Caletti (21) was able to demonstrate peri-esophageal collateral vessels by endoscopic ultrasound in 57% of grade 1 varices, 89% of endoscopic grade 2 varices, and all patients with endoscopic grade 3 varices. Endoscopic ultrasound was deemed significantly inferior to endoscopy in detecting and grading esophageal varices ($p < .0005$). However, endoscopic ultrasound was superior to the detection of varices in the fundus of the stomach ($p < .0005$).

With the 20-MHz ultrasound transducer, esophageal and gastric varices as well as peri-esophageal and perigastric varices also appear as anechoic structures (Figs. 6–8 to 6–10). Because of the higher resolution and lack of compression of the varices by the transducer, submucosal varices in the esophagus are well delineated and their size can be precisely measured. In comparing videoendoscopy to HRES evaluation for the size of esophageal varices, a poor correlation is found. We believe HRES to be a precise and reproducible way of evaluating the presence and size of esophageal varices. Compared to HRES, endoscopy for the evaluation of the presence or absence of gastric varices appears to be imprecise. We feel that this inability to define the presence or absence of gastric varices is due to the endoscopists' inability to discriminate between varices and normal gastric folds (22).

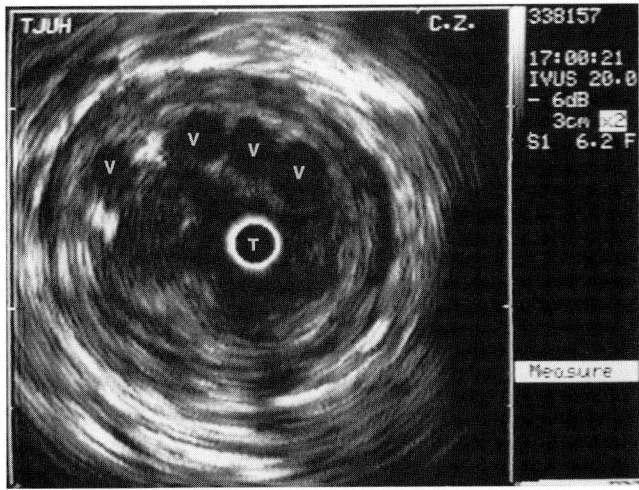


**FIGURE 6–8**

In a patient with documented cirrhosis and portal hypertension anechoic round areas (V) representing varices can be seen in the submucosa of the distal esophagus. T: transducer.

High-resolution endoluminal sonography appears to be better at quantitating the size of esophageal varices than conventional endoscopic ultrasound for three reasons: (1) The higher frequency (20-MHz) allows for improved resolution of submucosal structures; (2) no water-filled balloon around the transducer distorts the native anatomy of the esophagus and varix; (3) the transducer itself is so small that it does not interfere with the size or shape of the varix. In addition, HRES gives additional valuable information that cannot be obtained endoscopically, including the exact size of the varices, the presence or absence of perigastric and peri-esophageal varices, and the presence or absence of perforating veins and ascites.

In six patients (17%), no varices were imaged at the high-pressure zone, but varices were imaged in the distal esophagus. The mean cross-sectional surface area per varix at the high-pressure zone was much less than that in the area 5 cm above it. Similarly, The average total cross-sectional surface area occupied by varices at the high-pressure zone was significantly less than that of the area 5 cm above it. Moreover, the mean percent esophageal wall cross-sectional surface area occupied by varices at the high-pressure zone was significantly less than that of the area 5 cm above it. These findings suggest that HRES may be used to observe modifications of variceal size with pharmacologic intervention directed at the esophageal high-pressure zone.

Several clinical and endoscopic parameters have been associated with the identification of patients at risk for variceal bleeding. It has been suggested that the risk of variceal bleeding increases with variceal size, and that the actual rupture of a varix depends on its wall tension. Theoretically, a Laplace equation, $T = p_t(r/w)$, can be used to determine the wall tension of a varix in the esophagus based on the measurement of three separate variables ($p_t$, $r$, $w$): Here $T$ = wall tension, $p_t$ = transmural pressure between the varix and the esophageal lumen, $r$ = the radius of the varix, and $w$ = the wall thickness of the varix. To date, only $p_t$ has been measured in vivo and no method has been found to accurately measure or calculate $r$ or $w$.

Miller et al. (27) sought to evaluate esophageal variceal radius and wall thickness in an attempt to derive and correlate the two previously undetermined variables to the Laplace equation. Water was instilled into the esophageal lumen through the biopsy channel of an endoscope to distend the esophagus. Using HRES, all measurements were made at a cross section of the varix where the varix appeared circular, in order to

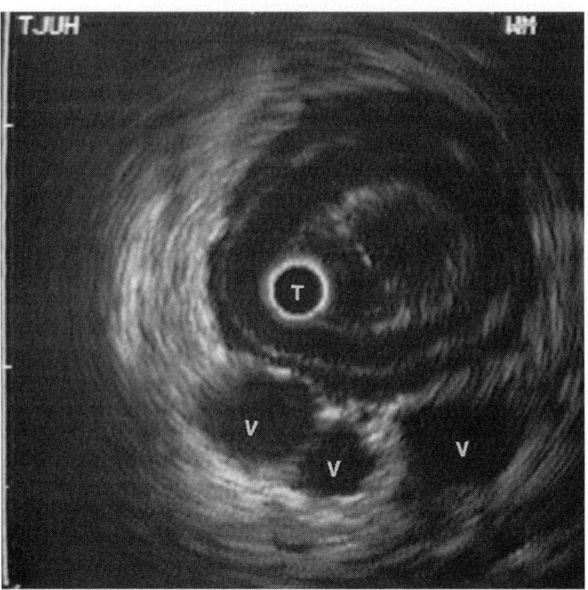


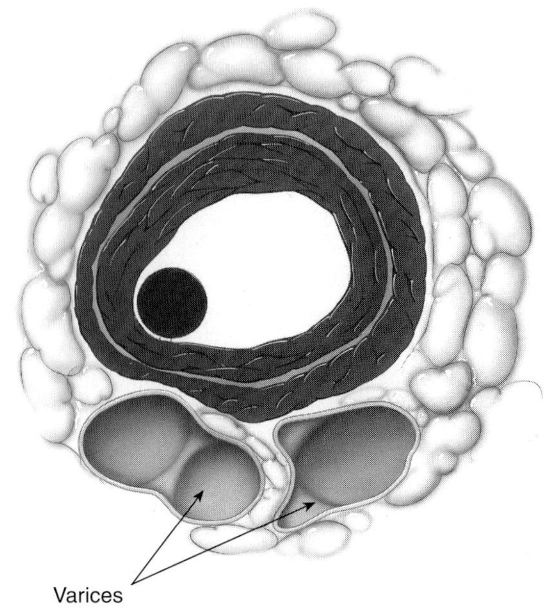


**FIGURE 6–9**

Peri-esophageal varices (V) can be seen adjacent to the esophagus in a patient with portal hypertension. T: transducer.

avoid trangential imaging. Multiple varices were imaged at different levels of the esophagus in each of 36 patients. Measurement of the outer ($C_o$) and inner ($C_i$) circumference of the varices was made. The outer circumference was measured at the border between the hypoechoic fluid-filled esophageal lumen and hyperechoic mucosa where the varix protruded into the esophageal lumen. In the intramural portion of the varix, the outer circumference was measured at the border between the hyperechoic submucosa and hypoechoic muscularis propria. The inner circumference was measured at the border of the hypoechoic blood-filled variceal lumen and hyperechoic inner wall of the varix. The inner and outer radii of each varix ($r_i$,$r_o$) were calculated using the formulas $r_i = C_i/2\pi$ and $r_o = C_o/2\pi$. The variceal wall thickness *(w)* was then calculated using the formula $w = (C_o - C_i)/2\pi$.

**FIGURE 6–10**

Gastric varices (V) are seen in the submucosa of the fundus of the stomach. T: transducer.

All normal controls were identified by HRES as lacking in varices. Varices in the patients with portal hypertension appear as hypoechoic fluid-filled round structures within the hyperechoic submucosa. The varices protrude into the hypoechoic fluid-filled esophageal lumen.

This study demonstrated that variceal size (radius) and variceal wall thickness could be measured directly using HRES. Furthermore, there was no direct correlation between variceal size and variceal wall thickness. This lack of correlation implies that variceal wall tension cannot be accurately estimated by endoscopic observation of variceal size alone, or even by size measurements combined with intravariceal pressure measurements. These findings have important clinical implications. The direct measurement of variceal wall tension may allow for the prediction of impending variceal bleeding and thus allow for nonemergent intervention. Endoscopic sclerotherapy or band ligation can be undertaken, β-blockers and/or nitrates can be started, or their pre-existing doses can be increased.

Miller et al. (28) used HRES to image and measure esophageal varices in patients with known cirrhosis, then correlated the images with endoscopic findings using predefined quantitative criteria. Nine normal controls and 68 cirrhotics underwent videotaped HRES and EGD. A blinded reviewer graded the largest varix in each patient based on a 5-point grading system: Grade I—no varices; Grade II—varices flattened with air insufflation; Grade III—varices 0–30% of the radius of the esophageal lumen; Grade IV—varices 30–60% of the radius of the lumen; Grade V—varices 60–100% of the radius in the lumen. All nine control patients were correctly identified by EGD and HRES as Grade I (no varices). The correlation between HRES and EGD was $r = .5$. This poor correlation was due to the enormous overlap in HRES size measurements for each EGD variceal guide. EGD failed to identify eight of ten patients with varices that were identified by HRES.

The variability in HRES size measurement among EGD grade categories may be a reflection of the intrinsic subjectivity and inaccurancy of EGD grading. It is likely that HRES size measurements more accurately reflect true variceal size. Thus, HRES is more capable than EGD of detecting esophageal varices at an earlier stage of development. This information can allow for the earlier initiation of prophylactic β-blocker therapy and for a more accurate assessment of objective response to other treatments undertaken to decrease variceal size [e.g., transjugular intrahepatic portosystemic shunts (TIPS)]. There are many potential clinical applications using HRES in the setting of portal hypertension. This technology may be used in the future to determine the size of esophageal varices pre- and post-TIPS, to follow patients during sclerotherapy to determine the patency of the varices, and to image the stomach for the presence or absence of gastric varices when endoscopy is equivocal.

## Scleroderma

A three-part study evaluating esophageal involvement by scleroderma was also undertaken (23). In the first part, esophageal autopsy specimens were compared histologically and sonographically; these specimens were taken from patients with scleroderma and patients who died of diseases unrelated to the esophagus. In the second part, the esophagi of normal controls and scleroderma patients were evaluated in vivo using the high-frequency ultrasound technology. This was done to determine whether or not there were sonographic abnormalities consistent with the sonographic abnormalities seen on autopsy specimens. In the third part, the degree of sonographic abnormality seen in the scleroderma patients was quantitated and compared to various esophageal functional studies, including measurements of upright, supine, and total reflux as well as esophageal manometry looking at peristaltic contraction and lower esophageal sphincter pressure.

The first part of the study revealed a hyperechoic abnormality in the normally hypoechoic muscularis propria in patients with scleroderma. This hyperechoic abnormality, which was not evident in patients who died of nonesophageal-related diseases, seemed to correlate with the presence of fibrosis on histologic sections from these autopsy specimens. The second part of the study revealed similar hyperechoic abnormalities in many of the patients with scleroderma and no hyperechoic abnormalities in any of the normal volunteer subjects. It was found that the difference between the presence of these hyperechoic abnormalities in scleroderma patients and the absence of these hyperechoic abnormalities in the normal control population was significant ($p < .001$) (Fig. 6–11).

Finally, these hyperechoic abnormalities were graded using the following system: Grade 1—normal appearing, no hyperechoic abnormality of the muscularis propria; grade 2—hyperechoic abnormality into but not obliterating the inner circular smooth muscle; grade 3—hyperechoic abnormality obliterating the circular smooth muscle but not encroaching in the outer longitudinal smooth muscle; grade 4—hyperechoic abnormality obliterating the circular smooth muscle and into the longitudinal smooth muscle but not obliterating the longitudinal smooth muscle; grade 5—complete replacement of the entire muscularis propria with the hyperechoic abnormality. These sonographic abnormalities were correlated with an evaluation for peristaltic contractions using the

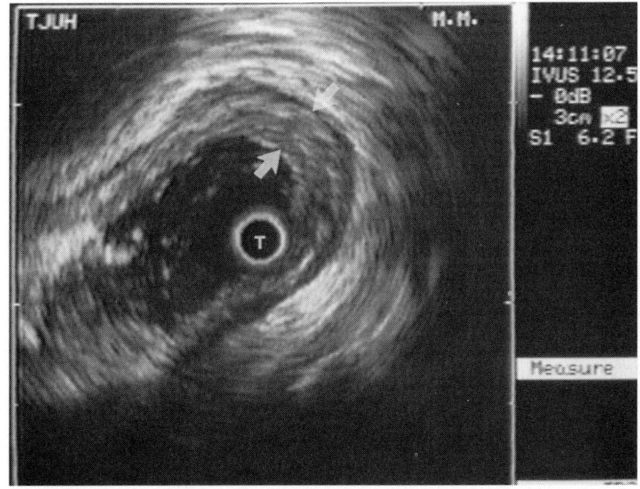


**FIGURE 6–11**

Endoluminal catheter-based transducer (T) located in the distal esophagus in a patient with scleroderma shows a diffusely increased echogenicity of the esophageal wall (arrows). The normal delineation of the various wall structures has disappeared and the esophageal lumen remains slightly dilated in the resting state. T: transducer.

following criteria: Grade 1—normal peristaltic contraction; grade 2—less than 50% nontransmitted waves of low amplitude pressures (<35 mm Hg); grade 3—absent peristalsis. A significant correlation was found between the grade of manometric abnormality and degree of hyperechoic abnormality ($r$ = .89, $p$ < .001). There was also a good correlation between 24-hour pH monitoring, percent supine, and total acid reflux with the degree of hyperechoic abnormality. However, no correlation was found between the hyperechoic abnormality and the percent upright reflux or LES pressure. The hyperechoic abnormality represents fibrosis in the muscularis propria and the degree of fibrosis can be accurately quantitated by evaluating the hyperechoic abnormality in the muscularis propria according to the grading system described.

## Other Abnormalities

Due to the high frequency and high resolution of HRES, imaging of gastrointestinal tract structures for submucosal lesions, particularly in the esophagus, is exquisitely sensitive. As with the lower frequency endoscopic ultrasound transducers, various submucosal lesions have characteristic echodensities and echotextures arising from characteristic areas of the gastrointestinal tract wall. High-frequency endoluminal ultrasound technology allows very small lesions to be imaged with high resolution and without the compression artifacts engendered by a water-filled latex balloon or a large transducer. Leiomyomas appear as hypoechoic masses contiguous with the muscularis propria. They have a smooth outer margin. Lipomas appear hyperechoic and arise from the submucosa. Hemangiomas appear as hyperechoic lesions. Esophageal varices and gastric varices appear as multiple anechoic lesions.

In addition to imaging submucosal lesions, HRES is also a sensitive technology for imaging lymph nodes in the peri-esophageal area. Small lymph nodes can be imaged using this technology, and abnormally large lymph nodes can be imaged with a great deal of definition. One-third of the patients with scleroderma imaged with HRES were found to have peri-esophageal lymph nodes. Comparison of chest CT scan to HRES for the detection of lymph nodes in the peri-esophageal area demonstrates that endoluminal ultrasound is far superior. However, a major disadvantage in imaging peri-esophagal structures with HRES is the limited penetration of the transducer: If the abnormality exceeds 2 cm in the axial plain perpendicular to the transducer, the distal borders of the lesion will not be imaged.

A number of patients with acute esophagitis and Barrett's esophagus, as documented by endoscopy and endoscopic biopsy, have been imaged with HRES. Imaging of patients with acute esophagitis reveals specific abnormalities: thickening in the area of the submucosa, often three to four times the normal thickness, with small dilated vessels within this region (Fig. 6–12). In investigating Barrett's esophagus, we hoped: (1) to define a specific abnormality consistent with Barrett's esophagus by looking at thickening of the mucosa or the abnormal echotexture of the mucosa; (2) to localize areas of dysplasia or premalignant areas by evaluating the echogenicity of these various areas. Barrett's metaplasia appears as a thickening of the second hypoechoic layer of the mucosa. Unfortunately, dysplasia cannot be diagnosed using HRES. It was also our hope that HRES would be of value in staging esophageal and gastric malignancies. Esophageal and gastric malignancies appear as either hypo- or hyperechoic masses on HRES (Fig. 6–13). Early-stage lesions can be detected and staged with great accuracy because the high resolution of the transducer provides great definition in the evaluation of the gastrointestinal tract wall. However, the low penetration (2 cm) limits the direct application of these ultrasound transducers in higher stage malignancies since advanced malignancies or lymphadenopathy will be out of the range of ultrasound beam penetration.

## HRES Swallowing Studies

Miller et al. (29) have developed a method to quantitate the changes in esophageal wall motion by measuring the width of the muscularis propria during swallowing in the esophageal body. They have correlated these changes in

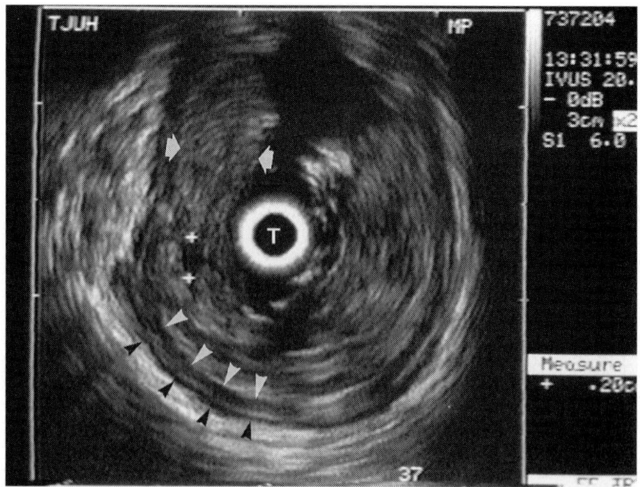


**FIGURE 6–12**

In a patient with ulcerative esophagitis, the cross-sectional endoluminal ultrasound image demonstrated loss of the mucosa and thickening of the submucosa (arrows) in the lower portion of the esophagus. Dilated vessels (+) within the submucosa can be seen. Note that the two muscular layers (arrowheads) are not involved. T: transducer. (Reproduced with permission from Liu JB, et al. Radiology 184:721–727, 1992.)

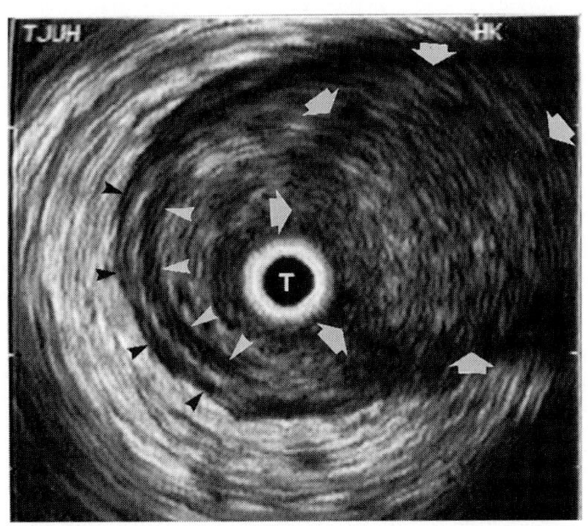


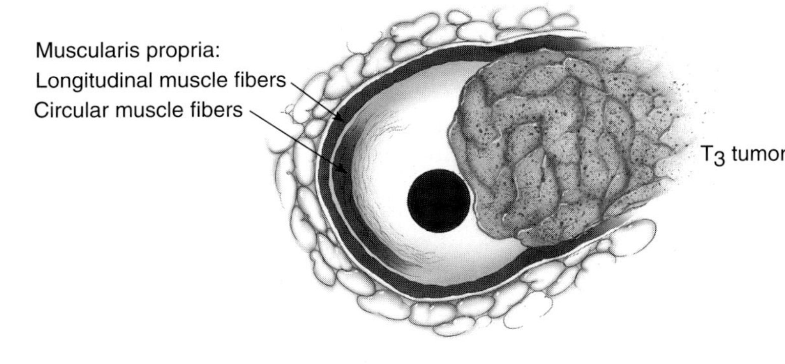


**FIGURE 6–13**

Cross-sectional endoluminal ultrasound image of a 1.6 × 1.3 cm hyperechoic mass (arrows) located in the lower portion of the esophageal wall. The normal muscular layers of the esophagus (arrowheads) can still be seen in the noninvolved portion. Biopsy of the region confirmed presence of an esophageal carcinoma. T: transducer. (Reproduced with permission from Liu JB, et al. Radiology 184:721–727, 1992.)

muscle width and lumen circumference to changes in intraluminal pressure and defined various HRES phases of the swallowing sequence based on manometrically defined pressure changes in the esophageal lumen.

Liu et al. (18) utilized HRES in human subjects to examine wall motion of the body of the esophagus during deglutition. Taniguchi et al. (30) used HRES to evaluate swallowing in the sheep esophagus. Using a 20-MHz M-mode suction ultrasound probe, they observed thickening of the circular smooth muscle but none in the longitudinal smooth muscle during occlusive contractions.

Miller et al. (29) demonstrated four phases of the peristaltic sequence: Phase I—resting state; Phase II—passive distension; Phase III—contraction; Phase IV—relaxation. During Phases I and II esophageal pressure did not change, nor did lumen circumference or muscle thickness. However, the passage of a bolus forced the esophageal lumen to open and the muscle to thin during Phase III. Phase III began with the upstroke of the pressure recording and continued until peak pressure was attained. During this phase there was a rapid decrease in the esophageal lumen circumference, and a progressive increase in the muscle width of all of the muscular layers was observed as the lumen pressure increased. Phase IV began as the pressure started to decline from its maximum and concluded when it reached baseline resting pressure. During Phase IV a marked decrease in muscle width was observed in all the layers of the muscularis propria and the esophagus reverted to its resting configuration.

Increasing muscle width was found to be the sonographic correlate of increasing luminal pressure as measured by manometry, while decreasing muscle width was the sonographic correlate of decreasing luminal pressure. The inner circular smooth muscle is thought to be the main contributor to the amount of intraluminal pressure generated during a contraction.

Miller's study demonstrated a number of previously unrecorded rates of phenomena in the human esophagus: the rate of esophageal muscular wall thickening and thinning during the peristaltic sequence, the rate of luminal opening and closing during esophageal peristalsis, the maximum and minimum muscle thickness and lumen circumference during the peristaltic sequence, and the manometric correlation. With this technique, it may be possible to study esophageal motor disorders in the skeletal and smooth muscle segments of the esophagus and the LES before, during, and after swallowing in normal controls and in patients with various motility disorders.

We have also found miniature transducer-containing catheters useful for ultrasound imaging of abdominal and pelvic structures during laparoscopy (24). Ultrasound transducers are advanced through established laparoscopic openings to the area of interest in the abdomen and pelvis. We have reported on fifteen patients, ten of whom were undergoing laparoscopic cholecystectomy; one, exploratory laparoscopy; and four, pelvic laparoscopy. Normal structures were imaged including the liver, gallbladder, cystic and common bile ducts, blood vessels, ovaries, and fallopian tubes. A variety of abnormalities were also imaged using these miniature transducer-containing catheters, including gallstones, polyps, cysts, and lymphadenopathy. In two cases, this approach was used to successfully guide needles laparoscopically for aspiration and biopsy. Miniature transducers can easily be passed through standard laparoscopic openings and guided to areas of interest, providing information not available with other imaging approaches. As a result it is possible to evaluate the biliary system and pelvic organs for the presence of a variety of abnormalities, to detect masses in such areas as the liver and ovaries, and under ultrasound guidance to laparoscopically biopsy or aspirate lesions.

Use of high-resolution endoluminal sonography in the gastrointestinal tract has not been limited to the esophagus and stomach. We have also imaged the duodenum, sigmoid colon, rectum, and the anal canal.

In summary, HRES appears to be a promising imaging modality in the investigation of the gastrointestinal tract. The major advantages of HRES are increased resolution and the ability to image mural structures without distortion of those structures. Its major limitation appears to be inadequate penetration for staging of gastrointestinal malignancies and for evaluation of structures not within the immediate vicinity of the luminal GI tract (e.g., pancreas, liver). We believe that the technology will progress so that catheters with various ultrasound frequencies will become available for imaging various lesions, thereby eliminating many of the problems with penetration. In addition, we believe that this technology will be used routinely through endoscopes for the sonographic imaging of lesions found at endoscopy.

## References

1. Wild JJ, Reid JM. Diagnostic use of ultrasound. Br J Phys Med 19:248–257, 1956.
2. Lutz H, Rosch W. Transgastroscopic ultrasonography. Endoscopy 8:203–205, 1976.
3. Fukuda M, Hirata K, Saito K, et al. On the diagnostic use of echoendoscope in abdominal diseases. I. Diagnostic experiences with a new type echoendoscope on gastric diseases. Proc Jpn J Med Ultrasonography 37:409–410, 1980.
4. DiMagno EP, Regan PT, Clain JE, James EM, Buxton JL. Human endoscopic ultrasonography. Gastroenterology 83:824–829, 1982.
5. Rifkin MD, Gordon SJ, Goldberg BB. Sonographic examination of the mediastinum and upper abdomen by fiberoptic gastroscope. Radiology 151:175–180, 1984.
6. Bótet JF, Lightdale CJ, Zauber AG, Gerdes H, Urmacher C, Brennan MF. Preoperative staging of esophageal cancer: Comparison of endoscopic US and dynamic CT. Radiology 181:419–425, 1991.
7. Bótet JF, Lightdale CJ, Zauber AG, et al. Preoperative staging of gastric cancer: Comparison of endoscopic US and dynamic CT. Radiology 181:426–432, 1991.
8. Silverstein FE, Martin RW, Kimmey MB, Jiranek GC, Franklin DW, Proctor A. Experimental evaluation of an endoscopic ultrasound probe: In vitro and in vivo canine studies. Gastroenterology 96:1058–1062, 1989.
9. Rösch TH, Classen M. A new ultrasonic probe for endosonographic imaging of the upper GI tract. Endoscopy 22:41–46, 1990.
10. Isner JM, Rosenfield K, Losordo DW, et al. Percutaneous intravascular US as adjunct to catheter-based interventions: Preliminary experience in patients with peripheral vascular disease. Radiology 175:61–70, 1990.
11. Yock PG, Linker DT, White NW, et al. Clinical applications of intravascular ultrasound imaging in atherectomy. Int J Cardiac Imaging 4:117–125, 1989.
12. Goldberg BB, Liu JB, Merton DA, Kurtz AB. Endoluminal US: Experiments with nonvascular uses in animals. Radiology 175:39–43, 1990.
13. Goldberg BB, Bagley D, Liu JB, Merton DA, Alexander A, Kurtz AB. Endoluminal sonography of the urinary tract: Preliminary observations. Am J Radiol 156:99–103, 1991.
14. Goldberg BB, Liu JB, Kuhlman K, Merton DA, Kurtz AB. Endoluminal gynecologic ultrasound: Preliminary results. J Ultrasound Med 10:583–590, 1991.
15. Engstrom CF, Wiechel KL. Endoluminal ultrasound of the bile ducts. Surg Endosc 4:187–190, 1990.
16. Hurter TH, Hanrath P. Endobronchial sonography in the diagnosis of pulmonary and mediastinal tumours. Dtsch Med Wochenschr 115:1899–1905, 1990.
17. Kimmey MB, Martin RW, Hagitt RC, Wang KY, Franklin DW, Silverstein FE. Histologic correlates of gastrointestinal ultrasound images. Gastroenterology 96:433–441, 1989.
18. Liu JB, Miller LS, Goldberg BB, Feld RI, Alexander AA, Needleman L, Castell DO, Klenn PJ, Millward CL. Transnasal US of the esophagus: Preliminary morphologic and function studies. Radiology 184:721–727, 1992.
19. Caletti G, Ferrari A, Brocchi E, Bonora G, Carfagna L, Barbara L. Normal EUS anatomy: The gut wall. In Endoscopic Ultrasonography: A Tutorial. Course Syllabus for Symposium sponsored by the Cleveland Clinic Foundation, March 21–22, 1992, pp 35–42.
20. Miller L, Liu JB, De Vault K, Feld R, Alexander A, Goldberg B, Castell D. In vivo quantitative measurement of the human lower esophageal sphincter (LES) using a high frequency (20 MHz) ultrasound transducer. (Abstract) Am J Gastroenterol 86:1299, 1991.
21. Caletti G, Brocchi E, Baraldini M, Ferravi A, Gibilaro M, Barbara L. Assessment of portal hypertension by endoscopic ultrasonography. Gastrointest Endosc 36(2 suppl):S21–27, 1990.
22. Miller LS, Liu JB, Newman M, DeVault K, Patel K, Lynn R, Goldberg BB. High frequency endoluminal sonography of esophageal varices using a 20 MHz ultrasound transducer compared to endoscopic grading of the size of esophageal varices. (Abstract) Gastroenterology 102:A853, 1992.
23. Miller LS, Liu J-B, Klenn PJ, Holahan MP, Varga J, Feld RI, Troshinsky M, Jimonez SA, Castell DO, Goldberg BB. Endoluminal ultrasonography of the distal esophagus in systemic sclerosis. Gastroenterology 105:3109, 1993.
24. Goldberg BB, Liu JB, Barbot DI, Miller LS, Winkel CA, Merton DA, Feld RI. Endoscopic laparoscopic ultrasound. (Abstract) J Ultrasound Med 11:S16, 1992.
25. Miller LA, Liu JB, Christopher BA, Barkowski RJ, Dhuria M, Schiano TD, Goldberg BB, Fisher RS. High-Resolution endoluminal sonography in achalasia. Gastrointest Endosc 42:545–549, 1995.
26. Schiano TD, Fisher RS, Parkman HP, Cohen S, Dabezies M. Miller LS. Use of high-resolution endoscopic ultrasonography to assess esophageal wall damage after pneumatic dilatation and botulinum toxin injection to treat achalasia. Gastrointest Endosc 44:151–157, 1996.
27. Schiano TD, Adrian AL, Cassidy MJ, McCray W, Liu JB, Baranowski RJ, Bellary S, Black M, Miller LS. Use of high-resolution endoluminal sonography to measure the radius and wall thickness of esophageal varices. Gastrointest Endosc 44:425–428, 1996.
28. Miller LS, Schiano TD, Adrian A, Cassidy M, Liu JB, Ter H, Bellary SV, Dabezies MA, Black M. Comparison of high-resolution endoluminal sonography of video endoscopy in the detection and evaluation of esophageal varices. Hepatology 24:552–555, 1996.
29. Miller LS, Liu JB, Golizzo FP, Ter H, Marzano J, Barbavevech C, Hedwig K, Leung L, Goldberg BB. Correlation of high frequency esophageal ultrasound and manometry in the study of esophageal motility. Gastroenterology 109:832–837, 1995.
30. Taniguchi DK, Martin RW, Trowers EA, Dennis MB, Odegaard S, Silverstein EE. Changes in esophageal wall layer during motility; measurements with a new miniature ultrasound device. Gastrointest Endosc 39:149–152, 1993.

CHAPTER

# High-Resolution Endoluminal Sonography of the Upper Gastrointestinal Tract

## THE RADIAL SCANNING ULTRASOUND PROBE: PART II

Kenjiro Yasuda

Although endoscopic ultrasonography (EUS) has become an accepted part of gastrointestinal imaging, the standard endoscope-based system (echoendoscope) is limited by virtue of its size and inability to gain access to ductal (common bile duct or pancreatic duct) or stenotic (malignant esophageal strictures) spaces. It is also limited by its relatively low ultrasound frequency (7.5 MHz and 12.0 MHz). Ultrasound (US) probes offer greater access to narrow intraluminal spaces than does the echoendoscope. Moreover, US probes image at higher ultrasound frequencies providing higher resolution imaging.

Progress in industrial technology has provided smaller ultrasound transducers (1–4). Ultrasound probes with a 3.4-mm diameter containing 7.5-MHz radial scanning transducers were developed in 1989 (Fig. 7–1A). But ultrasonic images were inferior to those of conventional echoendoscopes in their depth of penetration, image quality, and durability. In addition, a large-channel endoscope was required for the larger ultrasound probes. As is true with all ultrasound imaging, the best imaging is obtained when a water interface is used between the ultrasound probe and the target structure. Nevertheless, the prototype probes did not employ a balloon attachment.

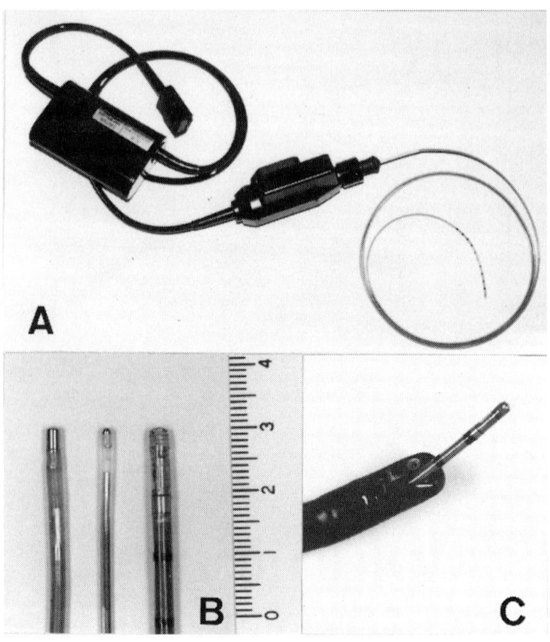


**FIGURE 7–1**

Ultrasound probes: (**A**) First-generation Olympus ultrasound probe. (**B**) Distal tip of prototype Olympus ultrasound probes (from left to right: 2.5-mm probe, 1.7-mm probe, UM-1W). (**C**) UM-1W exiting the accessory channel of a duodenoscope.

Newer ultrasonic probes have tip diameters of 2.5 mm and 1.7 mm with 12-MHz and 20-MHz radial scanning transducers (Fig. 7–1B–C). These probes may be passed via the accessory channel of standard (non-therapeutic) endoscopes. As with all endoscopic ultrasound probes, the depth of ultrasound penetration depends on the frequency of the probe. Thus, a 2.5-mm probe with a 12-MHz ultrasound transducer offers deeper penetration with better quality images than those obtained using the UM-1W. In contrast, the 20-MHz ultrasound probe provides poor penetration but high resolution of images.

The specifications of Olympus ultrasonic probes are listed on Table 7–1 together with the useful ultrasound penetration range of each probe. Figure 7–2 shows the ultrasonic images of resected gastric wall obtained by each probe compared with images obtained using a conventional echoendoscope.

## Clinical Application of Ultrasonic Probe

Because of the small diameter of the ultrasound probe, endosonographic examination may be performed via the accessory channel of a standard endoscope (5). This technique permits direct visualization of gastrointestinal lesions such as subepithelial lesions. It also allows one to obtain endosonographic images of stenotic lesions of such malignant tumors as advanced esophageal carcinoma. Furthermore, new approaches are possible. That is, intra-choledochal or intra-pancreatic ductal scanning may be accomplished via the accessory channel of a duodenoscope or via the percutaneous route. Intra-biliopancreatic ductal endosonographic imaging is impossible with standard echoendoscopes.

### Gastrointestinal Tract Lesions

The ultrasound probe may be used to examine the esophagus when the echoendoscope is not capable of reaching the target lesion (6–8). It may also be useful in specialized cases, such as patients presenting with Barrett's esophagus (9). Sometimes, one can insert the ultrasound probe into a narrowed lumen. However, a complete examination of the esophageal or gastric wall through all 360° simultaneously is not always possible owing to the large volume of the organ. An endosonograph of an advanced esophageal carcinoma is shown in Figure 7–3A. The endosonograph demonstrates the tumor mass, an enlarged regional lymph node, and adjacent organs such as a bronchus and the aorta. An endosonograph could not be obtained from this position, deep within the lesion, using the standard echo-

**TABLE 7–1**

Specifications of Ultrasound Probes

| | UM-1W | RUM-2 (2.5/12) | RUM-3 (2.5/20) | RUM-4 (1.7/20) |
|---|---|---|---|---|
| ***Instrument*** | | | | |
| Diameter of tip (mm) | 3.4 | 2.5 | 2.5 | 1.7 |
| shaft (mm) | 3.0 | 2.4 | 2.4 | 1.6 |
| Working length (mm) | 2500 | 2050 | 2050 | 2050 |
| ***Ultrasound*** | | | | |
| Method of scanning | mechanical/radial | mechanical/radial | mechanical/radial | mechanical/radial |
| Transducer frequency (MHz) | 7.5 | 12.0 | 20.0 | 20.0 |
| Scanning angle (degrees) | 360 | 360 | 360 | 360 |
| Contact method | water | water | water | water |
| Range of scanning (mm) | 15–25 | 15–20 | 10–15 | 5–8 |

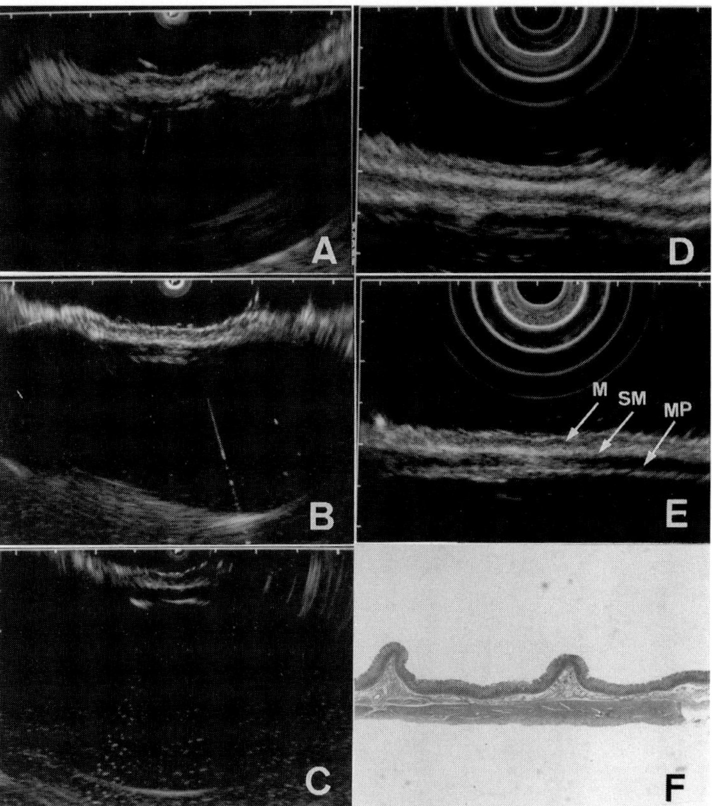


**FIGURE 7–2**

Ultrasound images of the resected (in vitro) gastric wall obtained using each type of ultrasonic probe and echoendoscope: (**A**) 2.5 mm, 12 MHz; (**B**) 2.5 mm, 20 MHz; (**C**) 1.7 mm, 20 MHz; (**D**) XGF-UM200, 7.5 MHz; (**E**) XGF-UM200, 20 MHz. (**F**) Pathologic section of the gastric wall.

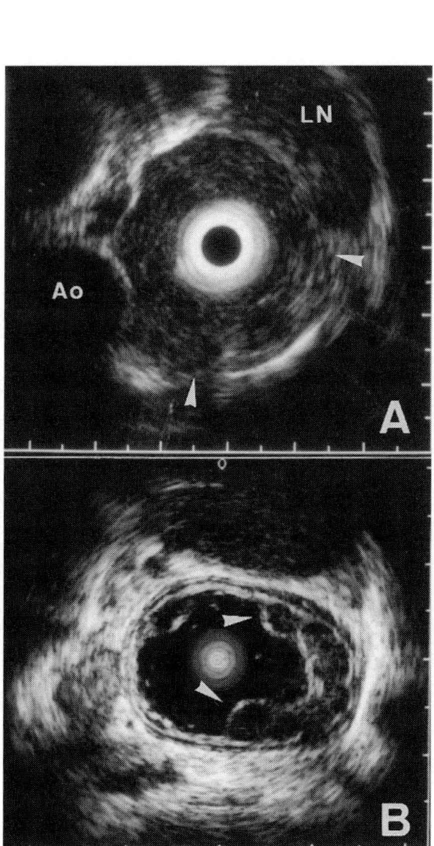


**FIGURE 7–3**

Esophageal endosonographs obtained using the EUS probe. (**A**) Endosonograph of an advanced esophageal carcinoma demonstrated by the UM-1W. The tumor mass (arrow) with enlarged regional lymph nodes (LN) is demonstrated. The aorta (Ao) is also demonstrated. (**B**) Esophageal varices, showing the honeycomb shape observed by the 2.5-mm, 20-MHz probe (arrow).

endoscope, owing to the stenotic nature of the lesion. Esophageal varices are also clearly demonstrated by this procedure (Fig. 7–3B) showing the echo-free vascular structures characteristic of esophageal varices.

An example of an early gastric carcinoma is shown in Figure 7–4. The stomach is filled with de-aerated water. The lesion is polypoid and the cancer is limited to the mucosa, as demonstrated by 12- and 20-MHz ultrasonic probes of diameter 2.5 mm and by the 20-MHz XGF-UM200. However, the depth of penetration of such high-frequency ultrasound probes is limited, therefore, the deeper aspects of the lesion may be less well visualized (Fig. 7–5). The diagnostic accuracy of the depth of gastric cancer invasion was 76.5% using these probes in 34 patients with early gastric cancer, while the accuracy rate by standard echoendoscopes was 78.6% in 500 cases in our study.

## Pancreaticobiliary Tract Diseases

Ultrasound probes have been used for imaging pancreaticobiliary diseases and have thus provided additional information hitherto unobtainable preoperatively (10–11). To perform endosonographic imaging in the bile duct or pancreatic duct, the EUS probe is introduced into the duct via the accessory channel of a duodeno-

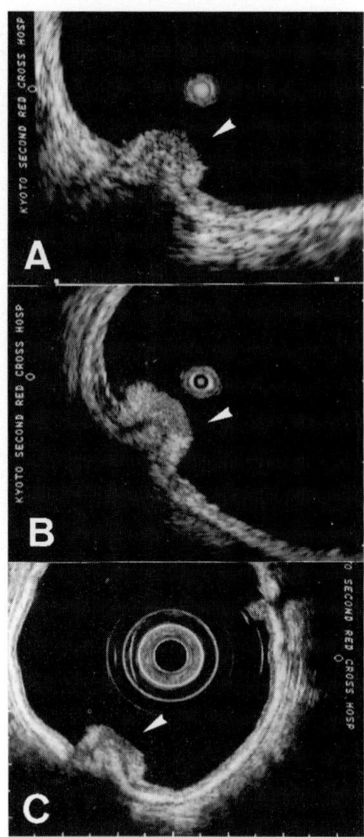


**FIGURE 7–4**

Endosonograph of an early gastric cancer (polypoid type) limited to the gastric submucosa. The endosonograph demonstrates the normal layered mural structure beneath the submucosal layer observed by different types of instruments: (**A**) 2.5 mm, 12 MHz; (**B**) 2.5 mm, 20 MHz; (**C**) XGF-UM200, 20 MHz.

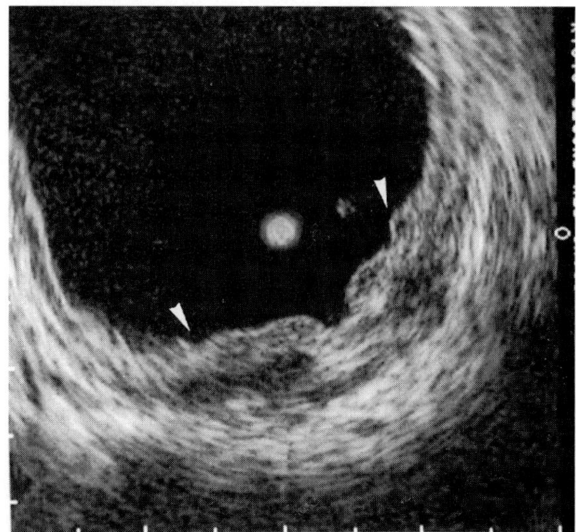

**FIGURE 7–5**

Advanced gastric cancer obliterating the layered structure of the gastric wall by tumor invasion (arrow) as demonstrated using the 2.5-mm, 12-MHz ultrasound probe.

scope after ERCP. After the probe is inserted as proximally into the duct as possible (or to the level of the target lesion), ultrasound scanning is performed as the probe is withdrawn. Retracting the probe to the papilla of Vater, ultrasonic images are observed continuously and recorded by still endosonographs or videotape recording. By inserting the ultrasound probe into the choledochus, one can also use a percutaneous approach. Using the smallest probe (diameter 1.7 mm), we have performed the intracholedochal ultrasonic scanning under direct visualization of percutaneous choledochoscopy. At present, we confirm the scanning position fluoroscopically. From these procedures, we can obtain EUS images of the common bile duct and adjacent organs and pancreas that are more precise than transduodenal ultrasonic scanning images obtained by conventional echoendoscopy.

Figure 7–6 shows the intraductal ultrasound image of cholangiocarcinoma demonstrating papillary growth

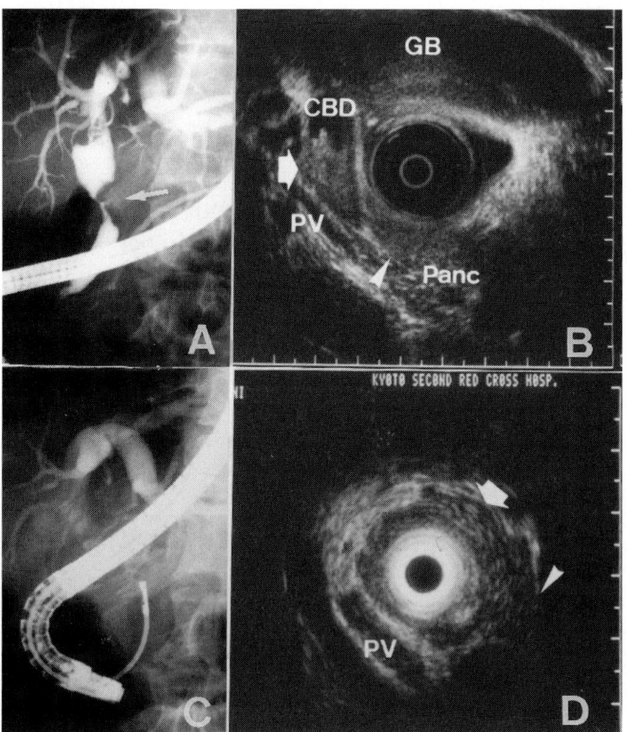


**FIGURE 7–6**

Cholangiocarcinoma in the middle common bile duct showing the duct wall thickened by the tumor invasion. The images are compared with images obtained by a conventional echoendoscope GF-UM20. (**A**) ERCP finding shows a malignant stricture in the middle common bile duct (arrow). (**B**) Endosonograph of the tumor (arrow) observed via the second portion of the duodenum. (**C**) Radiograph showing the insertion of the UM-1W via the papilla of Vater under direct endoscopic and fluoroscopic guidance. (**D**) Endosonograph of the tumor showing the thickened wall of the common bile duct.

and tumor extension into the common bile duct. The transpapillary approach of ultrasonic probe was technically difficult when we used the UM-1W, even after sphincterotomy. With the later prototype probes (diameter 2.5 mm and 1.7 mm), insertion of the ultrasound probe into the biliopancreatic ductal system became easier, even when sphincterotomy was not performed. Figure 7–7 shows a cholangiocarcinoma in the middle common bile duct. The bile duct is thickened by invading tumor and is clearly delineated with the adjacent organs. Using this technique, precise information regarding tumor stage may be obtained preoperatively. Ampullary lesions may also be imaged using this technique, as shown in Figure 7–8.

Figure 7–9 demonstrates an endosonograph obtained from within the main pancreatic duct in a patient with a mucin-producing pancreatic cancer. The endosonograph shows the small tumor and the dilated pancreatic duct with normal surrounding pancreatic parenchyma. However, because of the diameter of the duct—and because the ultrasound probe has no bending function—insertion of the probe to the tail of the pancreas is not always possible.

The most important indication for placing an ultrasound probe into the biliopancreatic ductal system is for tumor staging (e.g., determining the degree of tumor extension into the wall of the bile duct or adjacent organs or vascular structures). The standard echoendoscope and the ultrasonic probe have a complementary role in intracorporeal ultrasonic examinations. At the present time, the conventional echoendoscope is superior for detecting small lesions of the biliopancreatic system and diagnosing tumor extension into adjacent organs. However, continued advances in the area of ultrasound probe technology should provide instruments with enhanced diagnostic capabilities in the future.

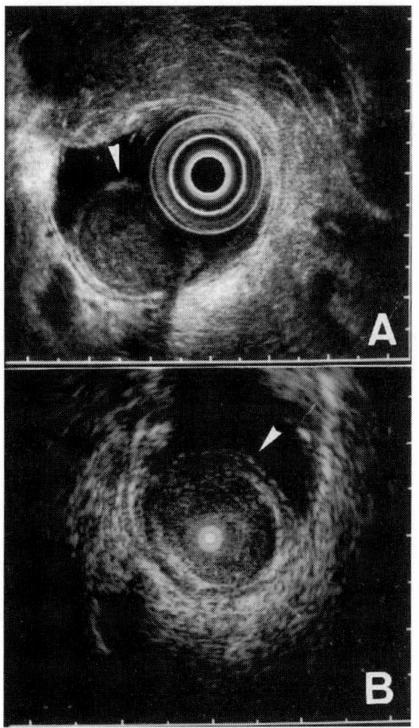


**FIGURE 7–8**

Endosonograph of an ampullary carcinoma (arrows) as demonstrated by endosonography on the papilla of Vater (**A**) and by an ultrasound probe cannulating the papilla of Vater (**B**).

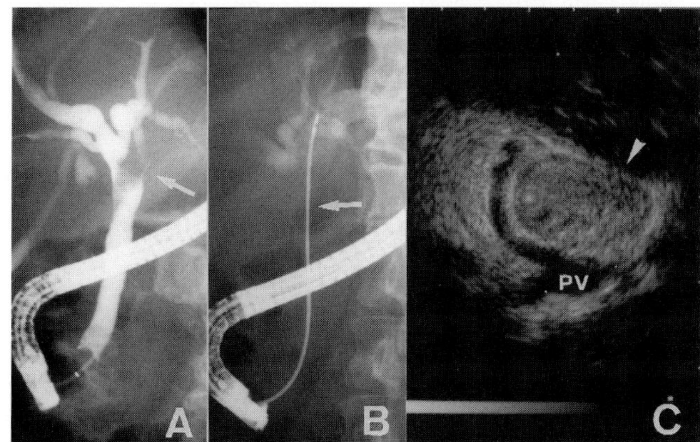


**FIGURE 7–7**

Cholangiocarcinoma growing into the common bile duct showing the tumor mass at the liver hilum as demonstrated by the transpapillary approach of the ultrasound probe. (**A**) ERCP shows the filling defect at the liver hilum (arrow). (**B**) Inserting the ultrasound probe (2.5 mm, 12 MHz) into the common bile duct (arrow). (**C**) Endosonograph of the tumor mass (arrow) in the common bile duct adjacent to the image of portal vein (PV).

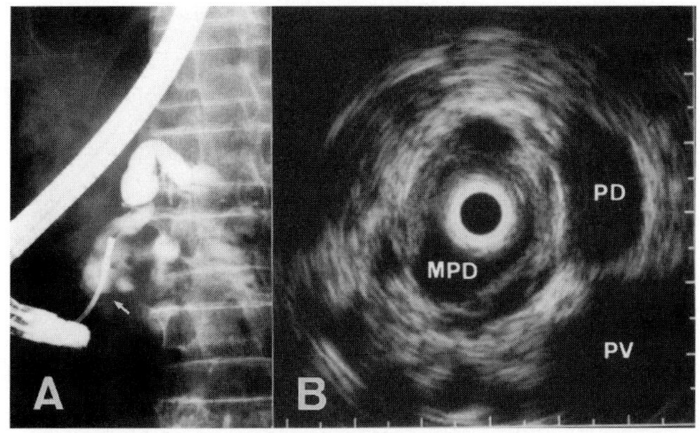


**FIGURE 7–9**

Intrapancreatic ductal endosonograph of mucin-producing pancreatic cancer. (**A**) Dilated pancreatic duct demonstrated by pancreatography. (**B**) Endosonograph demonstrating the cross section of a dilated pancreatic duct. The pancreatic parenchyma and adjacent blood vessels are shown. (MPD, main pancreatic duct; PD, pancreatic duct; PV, portal vein)

## Problems, Limitations, and Future Development of Ultrasound Probes

The ultrasound probe is still in the development stage. The biggest problem is that of durability. Use in the gastrointestinal tract via the accessory channel of standard endoscopes is not problematic. However, when used in the biliary or pancreatic ductal system, the probes have a reduced life expectancy. This is most likely due to the bending and torsion that takes place as the probes pass over the duodenoscope's elevator. Thus, probe design remains developmental, but newer, more durable designs are anticipated. Another problem is that of spontaneous rotation of the image and drift of the image during the ultrasonic scanning. These imaging problems are also attributed to the design of the probe shaft, and newer designs are under consideration.

The greatest limitation of the ultrasound probes, however, is the quality of the image relative to those obtained via the conventional echoendoscope. Compared with endosonographic images obtained by echoendoscopes, images obtained by ultrasound probes are inadequate, athough image quality is improving with each generation.

At present, ultrasound probes do not offer a substitute for conventional echoendoscopes in evaluating gastrointestinal tract or pancreaticobiliary lesions. Images of the entire pancreaticobiliary system are not possible by ultrasound probes because the depth of tissue penetration is limited. However, it is possible to obtain higher quality images of the esophagus and colon relative to images obtained using the conventional echoendoscopes. Furthermore, it is now possible to demonstrate the extent of lesions within the intra-biliopancreatic ductal system using ultrasound probes. After the current problems and limitations of the ultrasound probes are solved, these instruments will take their place among the array of conventional endoscopes and echoendoscopes in the well-equipped endoscopy suite.

## References

1. Silverstein FE, Martin RW, Kimmey MD. Experimental evaluation of an ultrasound probe: In vitro and in vivo canine studies. Gastroenterology 96:1058–1062, 1989.
2. Rösch TH, Classen M. A new ultrasonic probe for endosonographic imaging of the upper GI tract. Endoscopy 22:41–46, 1990.
3. Tio TL, Cheng J, Wijers OB, et al. Endosonographic TNM staging of extrahepatic bile duct cancer: Comparison with pathological staging. Gastroenterology 100:1351–1361, 1991.
4. Boyce HW Jr., Boyce GA. Endoscopic ultrasonography: Instruments and techniques. Gastrointest Endosc Clin North America 2:575–599, 1992.
5. Kimmey MB, Martin RW, Silverstein FE. Clinical application of linear ultrasound probes. Endoscopy 24(suppl 1):364–369, 1992.
6. Murata Y, Suzuki S, Ohta M, Mitsunaga A, Kazuhiko H, Yoshida K, Ide H. Small ultrasonic probes for determination of the depth of superficial esophageal cancer. Gastrointest Endosc 44:23–28, 1996.
7. Yanai H, Yoshida T, Harada T, Matsumoto Y, Nishiaki M, Shigemitsu T, Tada M, Okita K, Kawano T, Nagasaki S. Endoscopic ultrasonography of superficial esophageal cancers using a thin ultrasound probe system equipped with switchable radial and linear scanning modes. Gastrointest Endosc 44:578–582, 1996.
8. Hasegawa N, Niwa Y, Arisawa T, Hase S, Goto H, Hayakawa T. Preoperative staging of superficial esophageal carcinoma: Comparison of an ultrasound probe and standard endoscopic ultrasonography. Gastrointest Endosc 44:388–393, 1996.
9. Adrain AL, Cassiday MJ, Schiano TD, Liu J-B, Miller LS. High resolution endoluminal sonography (HRES) is a sensitive means of identifying Barrett's metaplasia. Am J Gastroenterol 91:1902A, 1996.
10. Yasuda K, Mukai H, Nakajima M. Clinical application of ultrasonic probes in the biliary and pancreatic duct. Endoscopy 24(suppl 1): 370–375, 1992.
11. Tamada K, Ueno N, Ichiyama M, Tomiyama T, Nishizono T, Wada S, Oohashi A, Tano S, Aizawa T, Ido K, Kimura K. Assessment of pancreatic parenchymal invasion by bile duct cancer using intraductal ultrasonography. Endoscopy 28:492–496, 1996.

SECTION

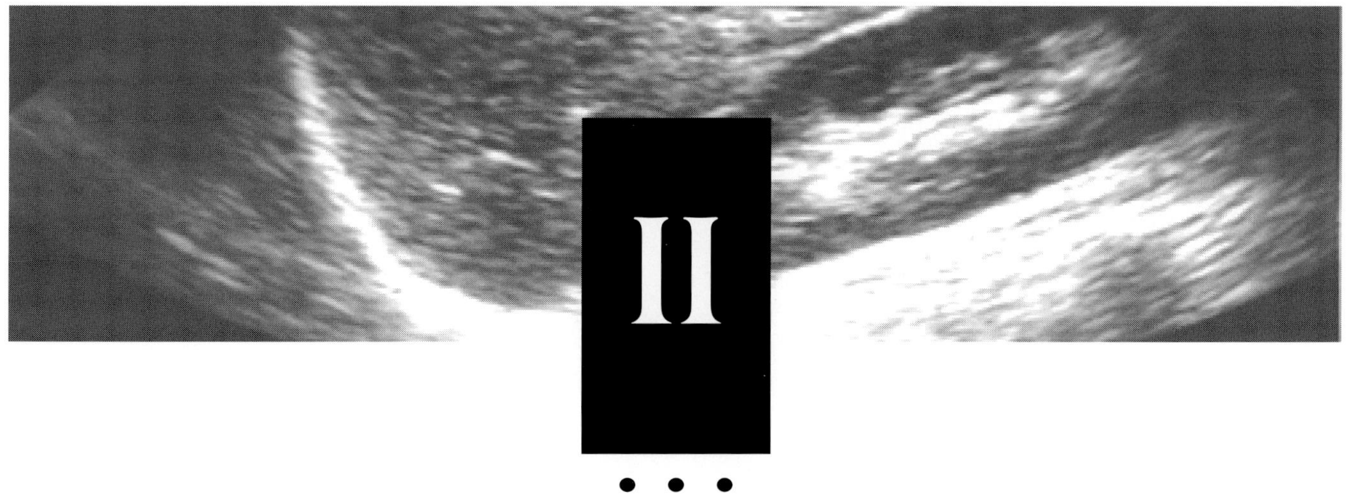

II

# Introduction to Endosonography: Getting Started

CHAPTER

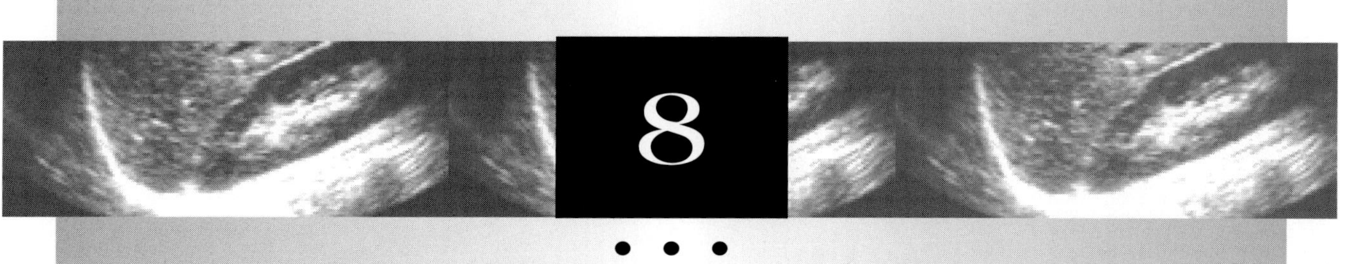

# 8

# The Gut Wall

Giancarlo Caletti
Paolo Bocus
Thomas Togliani
Enrico Roda

During the early developmental stages of endoscopic ultrasonography (EUS), investigators directed their attention toward obtaining better views of internal organs, especially those that were difficult to examine by conventional ultrasonography—the heart, the pancreas, the common bile duct, and so on. Subsequently, investigators focused on the application of EUS to the study of the gastrointestinal wall. The ability to delineate the architecture of the gastrointestinal tract wall has proven to be one of the major advantages of EUS.

Using EUS, the gastrointestinal wall appears as five ultrasonographic layers of different echogenicities. These layers are parallel to the mucosal surface in the image and are distinguished by their different echotexture and intensity. The first layer (innermost) is hyperechoic (bright or white), the second is hypoechoic (dark), the third is hyperechoic, the fourth is hypoechoic, and the fifth (outermost) is hyperechoic (Fig. 8–1).

Because the intestinal wall is comprised of five histologic layers (mucosa, muscularis mucosae, submucosa, muscularis propria, and serosa), it was originally thought that the sonographic layers corresponded directly to the histologic features of the wall. However, this simple hypothesis did not take into account the fact that an ultrasound image is made up of echoes produced by the interaction of the ultrasound wavefront at interfaces between the anatomic tissue layers and those created by the internal structure of the tissue layers.

An interface is an "infinitely" thin surface that constitutes the barrier between two media of different acoustic impedances (see Chapter 1). An incident pulse

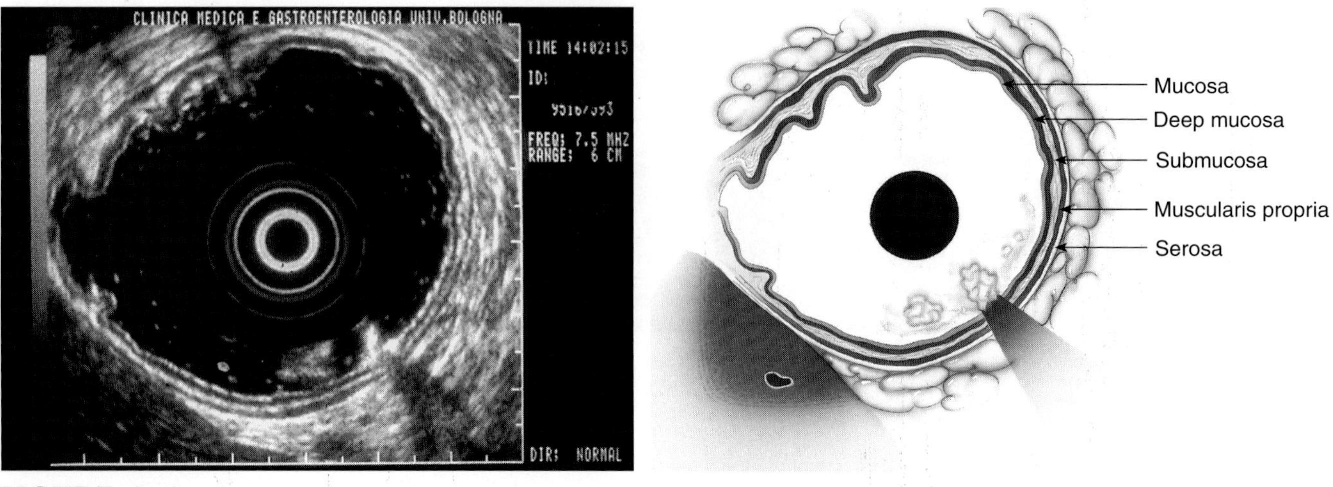


**FIGURE 8-1**

EUS 360° scanning of the normal gastric wall. The probe is positioned within the water-filled stomach. The five-layer structure is best visualized in an in vitro examination. A small amount of gastric debris is noted to cast a subtle acoustic shadow in the lower right portion of the figure.

directed toward an interface generates a reflected pulse (the echo) and a transmitted pulse. The intensity of the echo, and hence the ability to form an image at the interface, varies with the reflection coefficient of the interface—that is, the difference between the two acoustic impedances.

In biological media, the reflection coefficients are low so the transmission coefficients are high. Therefore, a single pulse can generate hundreds of echoes from the interfaces located on its course. Under certain circumstances, the reflection coefficient is very high, preventing the generation of an image of the structures located behind the interfaces, e.g., interfaces of soft tissue with bone, stone, or air.

Another important point is worth noting: The intensity of the reflected echoes at interfaces does not depend on the frequency used, but on the reflection coefficient. The thickness of an interface depends on the axial resolution of the equipment.

The sources of echoes in the tissues are due to the scattering phenomenon. Practically, a tissue that scatters ultrasound is one that exhibits acoustic inhomogeneity. When a pulse encounters a scatterer, a small fraction of the incident energy is re-emitted, not in a precise direction, but omnidirectionally. Consequently, only a very small part of the re-emitted energy can be received by the probe, thereby generating an echo of very low amplitude, called a back-scattered echo.

The scattering power of a small volume of a tissue depends on the volumic concentration of scatterers (e.g., biliary sludge) and on the ultrasonic frequency. The intensity of the back-scattered echoes rapidly increases as the ultrasonic frequency increases. The biological substances able to generate echoes are (1) macromolecular, with collagen in first place, then fibrin, elastin, and some lipids; (2) cellular, such as red blood cells, which generate the Doppler signal by scattering; (3) mineral, such as bone or lithiasis; and (4) gas.

Anatomically, the GI tract wall appears as a succession of concentric layers, distinct from one another; and the model proposed is based on two assumptions. First, the junction surface between two histologic layers is an acoustic interface, generating echoes of high intensities. Second, a histologic layer itself is supposed to be relatively homogeneous with regard to ultrasound, and echo-poor if compared with the two frontiers (junction–surface) limiting it. Consequently, the gastrointestinal tract wall should be conceived simply as a succession of hyperechogenic histologic discontinuities separated by the hypo- or nonechogenic histologic layers themselves.

All the sonographic layers distinguished by EUS have approximately the same thickness. This is problematic in relation to the hypothesis that the sonographic layers correspond to the histologic structure of the wall because the actual anatomic structures are *not* of equal thickness (1). The muscularis mucosae and the serosa are just a few microns thick, so it is unlikely that they themselves can produce ultrasonographically evident layers. The third ultrasonographic layer corresponds spatially to the submucosa, but it appears thicker by EUS than by actual histologic measurements. The fourth sonographic layer corresponds to the muscularis propria, but it is thinner at EUS than by actual measurements. Furthermore, the total thickness of the ultrasound image does not equal the total thickness of a histologic section of the wall (Fig. 8–2). It is clear, therefore, that no one-to-one relationship between the sonographic layers at EUS and the actual histologic features of the wall can exist.

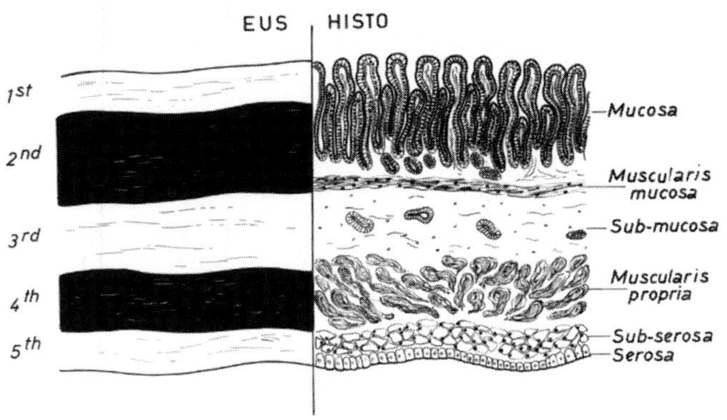


**FIGURE 8–2**

Relationship between EUS and anatomic layers of the normal gut wall. (1) Interface between stomach fluid and superficial mucosa; (2) lamina propria and muscularis mucosae; (3) submucosa and interface between submucosa and muscularis propria; (4) muscularis propria; (5) interface between serosa and surrounding tissue.

"Depth" or "thickness" in an ultrasound image is actually a measure of time, not of distance. Ultrasonographic thickness represents the time required for an ultrasound pulse emitted by a transducer to travel to and return from a reflective tissue interface rather than the distance traveled between transducer and tissue. Time *(t)* is related to distance *(d)* by the equation $d = vt$, where $v$ is the velocity of sound in the tissue being imaged. In soft tissues, this velocity is relatively constant at 1540 m/s. Thus, the only variable an endosonograph can measure is time—the time elapsed between the emission of an ultrasound pulse and the reception of its echo, as well as its conversion into lengths or distances as programmed for an average clarity of propagation of sound. Consequently, an infinitely thin interface appears on the image as an echogenic layer with an apparent thickness "*d*", where "*d*" appears to measure approximately 300–600 μ.

With the advent of newer endosonographic equipment, μ may be used to define the axial resolution of the equipment. The shorter the pulse, the better the axial resolution of the equipment. However, acoustic velocity is not equal in all tissues. It is probable that the velocity of ultrasound through the histologic layers varies according to differences in the acoustic impedance of the tissues that comprise the wall, thus suggesting the origin of different thicknesses. Unfortunately, the microscopic acoustic properties of tissues, such as velocity, reflective power of interfaces, and the scattering power of the individual tissue layers are not well known. Therefore, however sophisticated the techniques of measurement, they may be difficult to employ.

Two in vitro studies (2,3) have provided a more reasonable interpretation of the ultrasonic image of the gastrointestinal wall. Kimmey et al. (3), based on exacting correlation of ultrasound images with corresponding histologic sections, proposed an interpretation of ultrasound images of the gut wall that takes into account the tissue structure, its ultrasound characteristics, and the physics of ultrasound. It must be noted, however, that this interpretation is based on studies of resected tissue; thus it must be extrapolated to the interpretation of in vivo ultrasound images. Kimmey et al. hypothesized that the overall appearance of the ultrasound image is determined by a combination of the echoes from two sources: those created at interfaces between tissue layers with different acoustic impedances and those created by the internal structure of the tissue layers. According to Kimmey, if the more superficial tissue layer is echo-rich and the deeper layer is echo-poor, then the interface echo adds thickness to the superficial layer and subtracts thickness from the deeper layer. If, on the other hand, the more superficial layer is echo-poor and the deeper layer is echo-rich, the interface echo is not distinguishable from the deeper layer and therefore does not change the relative layer thickness.

Five major layers have been observed on ultrasound images of specimens of normal wall from the esophagus, stomach, colon, and rectum. The first hyperechoic layer corresponds to the superficial mucosa and the second hypoechoic layer to the deep mucosa. The third hyperechoic layer represents the submucosa plus the acoustic interface between the submucosa and the muscularis propria. The fourth hypoechoic layer corresponds to the muscularis propria minus the acoustic interface between the submucosa and the muscularis propria. The fifth layer corresponds to the serosa and subserosal fat. In vitro, the esophageal and colonic walls may separate into six layers if the transducer probe is at a distance from the mucosa—something that is impossible to obtain in vivo. In the laboratory, however, the fourth layer is separated by a thin hyperechoic layer within two hypoechoic layers. This thin echogenic line is produced by connective tissue between the inner circular and outer longitudinal components of the muscularis propria.

EUS imaging is achieved by applying the transducer directly to the wall, by scanning through water in the gastrointestinal lumen, or by scanning through a water-filled balloon surrounding the transducer. The best images of the gut wall are made when the transducer is not in direct contact with the mucosa and imaging is performed through luminal water. One reason for this is that the transducer can be placed at the proper distance from the wall so that the ultrasound beam is in optimal focus. Another possible reason for the better images is that no pressure is applied to the transducer, so compression cannot distort the image. However, it is not always possible to keep sufficient water in such areas of the gastrointestinal tract lumen as the esophagus, duodenum, and colon. In these areas, the transducer or its surrounding water-filled balloon must be placed in contact with the wall. The application of a balloon or transducer directly against the gastrointestinal wall can produce considerable compression unless it is carefully controlled.

Ødegaard et al. (4) have tested the hypothesis that the ultrasound appearance of the gastrointestinal wall is influenced by the amount of pressure applied when the transducer is in contact with the tissue. They examined the effect of increasing transducer pressure applied to fresh porcine gastrointestinal tissue on the resulting ultrasound images. Images were scrutinized for changes in wall thickness, tissue echogenicity, and the normal layered appearance. When the pressure against the wall increased, the images revealed changes in wall thickness, tissue echogenicity, and the number of layers. Wall echogenicity increased with increasing degrees of pressure and some layers were obliterated. The second ultrasound layer, or deep mucosa, appeared to be the most susceptible to compression. The stomach and rectum were more resistant to compression than the esophagus, duodenum, and colon. Images of the esophageal specimens showed a five-layer structure with pressure up to 10 kPa, but at 10 kPa a three-layer structure was observed because layer 2 was missing and layer 1 merged with layer 3. Ødegaard et al. concluded that endoscopic ultrasound imaging artifacts should be reduced by limiting the amount of pressure applied to the wall with the transducer (4). Thus, the correspondence between the histologic and the echographic aspect of the gastrointestinal wall is not obvious, and no automatic correspondence exists between the so-called "echographic" layers and the histologic layers.

## Appearance of Gut Wall In Vivo

The thickness of echographic layers of the gut wall is not static by EUS. Thickness can change in vivo according to the degree of distension of the gut and/or the functional state of the wall.

### Esophagus

It is usually difficult to visualize the several echographic layers of the esophageal wall, probably owing to difficulties in focusing the ultrasound beam on the wall when it is in direct contact with the transducer. The esophageal wall is 2–3 mm thick and, when brought into contact with the balloon surrounding the transducer, compresses easily. Thus it is very difficult to completely control the application pressure that can distort the EUS image (4). For these reasons only three layers are normally seen. The first hyperechoic layer corresponds to the balloon–mucosa–submucosa together with the submucosa–muscularis propria interface. The second hypoechoic layer corresponds to the muscularis propria, and the third hyperechoic layer represents the interface between the muscularis propria and the surrounding tissue (Fig. 8–3).

### Stomach and Duodenum

The typical five-layered sonographic pattern is recognized easily in the water-filled stomach (see Fig. 8–1). The gastric wall may be thinner in the fundus and body of the stomach, compared to the antrum. The muscularis propria (fourth hypoechoic layer) in the distal antrum and pyloric region may be especially evident.

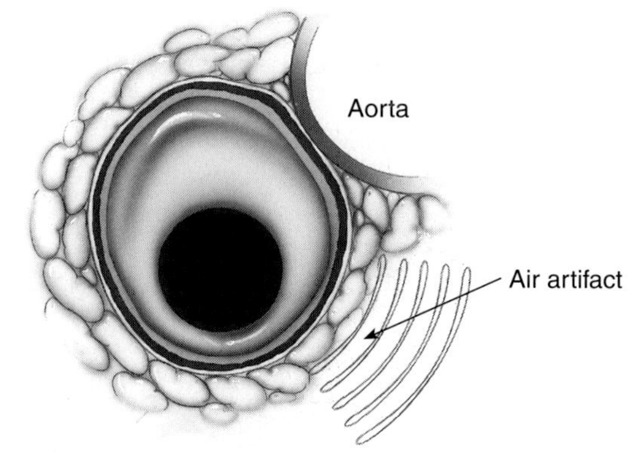


**FIGURE 8–3**

EUS 360° scanning of a normal esophagus. The balloon (B) is well filled by water. Only three layers are displayed (arrows).

It is very rare to distinguish five sonographic layers within the duodenal wall. The crescent-shaped folds show a homogeneous echo pattern, and only the muscular coat can be seen as a separate layer.

## Colon and Rectum

Five sonographic layers are usually well seen in the colon and rectum at EUS (Fig. 8–4). The thickness of the outer layers varies depending on how much periserosal fat is present. In the rectum, the fourth layer may be thicker as the muscularis propria is more developed in this segment of the gut, and it is divided in two layers in relation to the presence of two separate muscular coats (longitudinal and circular).

# Pathologic Alteration

The diagnosis of gastrointestinal diseases by EUS is based on changes in the typical sonographic layer pattern of the gut wall. Several questions about the clinical application of EUS arise in relation to this statement:

1. Does normal EUS sonographic appearance always mean that the wall is normal?
2. Does any change or modification of the normal sonographic pattern always indicate a pathologic condition of the wall?
3. Do the various disorders that involve the gut wall produce specific changes in the EUS images?
4. Is there a strict relationship between the extent of change in an EUS image and the actual extent of involvement of the wall by a disease process?
5. Is it possible to differentiate benign from malignant lesions?
6. What is the minimal size of a pathological lesion detectable by EUS?

The first question refers to the specificity and negative predictability of EUS. In our experience, EUS of the stomach has a specificity of 97% and a negative predictive value of 87%. Therefore, there can be a high degree of confidence that the wall is actually normal if the EUS image is normal. The second question refers to the sensitivity and positive predictive value of EUS when the wall is abnormal; these are 94% and 99%, respectively. Any deviation from the normal sonographic appearance of the wall almost always indicates a pathologic condition. EUS can detect changes that arise in one layer or are confined to one or more layers. This characteristic is often useful in diagnosis, especially in the case of lesions that arise within the wall such as a leiomyoma. Although there are no EUS images that are strictly diagnostic for a particular abnormality of the gut wall, the EUS appearance is fairly typical for certain lesions (e.g., leiomyoma, lymphoma, linitis plastica). In general, the extent of a lesion as defined by EUS corresponds to the actual anatomic extent of the abnormality. This accounts for the high degree of accuracy (in the range of 80–90%) of EUS in staging malignant lesions. EUS can also differentiate benign from malignant lesions, depending on the nature of the lesion. The minimum size of a pathologic lesion detectable by EUS remains uncertain.

The five-layer structure of the gut wall is obtained with the clinically available frequencies of 7.5 and 12 MHz. Higher frequencies, up to 20–25 MHz, have

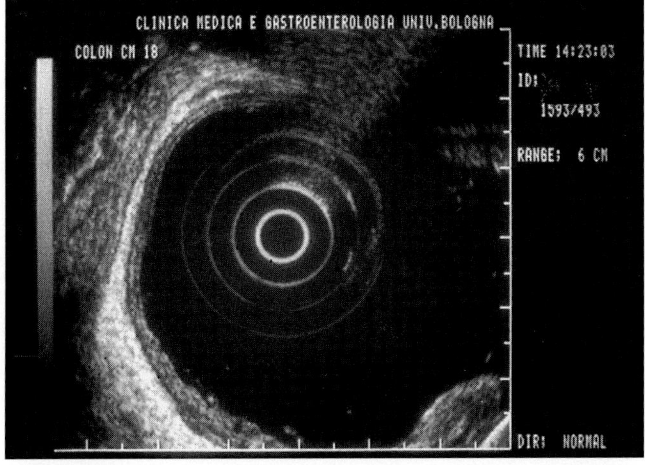


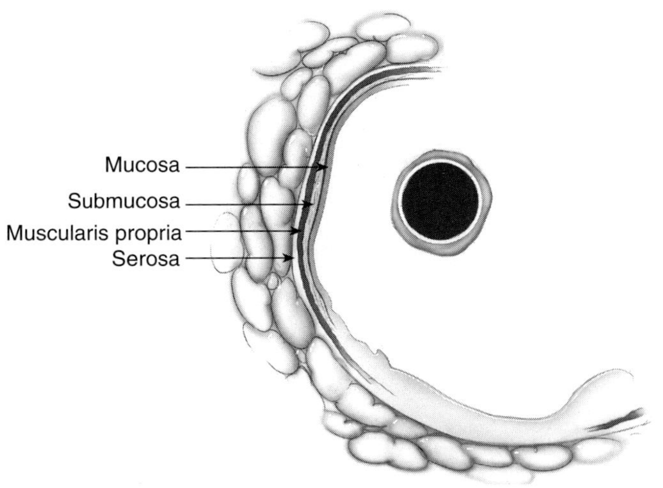


**FIGURE 8–4**

EUS 360° scanning of a normal colonic wall. The probe is positioned within the lumen of a water-filled colon. The five-layer structure is best visualized in an in vitro examination.

also been tested in order to obtain a more detailed view of the wall (5,6,7). The aim of these studies is to visualize the lamina propria and the muscularis mucosae in order to accurately stage early cancer. Seven, even nine, layers have sometimes been visualized. However, conflicting results have been obtained. But it is possible that in the future high-frequency endosonography will select patients for endoscopic treatment when Tis (tumor in situ) of the gut wall is exhibited.

## References

1. Bolondi L, Caletti GC, Casanova P, Villanacci V, Grigioni WF, Labò G. Problems and variations in the interpretations of the ultrasound features of the normal upper and lower GI tract wall. Scand J Gastroenterol 21(suppl 123):16–26, 1986.
2. Bolondi L, Casanova P, Santi V, Caletti GC, Barbara L, Labò G. The sonographic appearance of the normal gastric wall: An in vitro study. Ultrasound Med Biol 12:991–998, 1986.
3. Kimmey MB, Martin RW, Hagitt RC, Wang KY, Franklin DW, Silverstein FE. Histologic correlates of gastrointestinal ultrasound images. Gastroenterology 96:433–441, 1989.
4. Ødegaard S, Kimmey MB, Martin RW, Yee HC, Cheung AHS, Silverstein FE. The effects of applied pressure on the thickness, layers, and echogenicity of gastrointestinal wall ultrasound images. Gastrointest Endosc 38:351–356, 1992.
5. Wiersema MJ, Wiersema LM. High-resolution 25-megahertz ultrasonography of the gastrointestinal wall: Histologic correlates. Gastrointest Endosc 39:499–504, 1993.
6. Yanai H, Fujimura H, Suzumi M, et al. Delineation of the gastric muscularis mucosae and assessment of depth of invasion of early gastric cancer using a 20-megahertz endoscopic ultrasound probe. Gastrointest Endosc 39:505–512, 1993.
7. Murata Y, Suzuki S, Ohta M, et al. Small ultrasonic probes for determination of the depth of superficial esophageal cancer. Gastrointest Endosc 44:23–28, 1996.

# CHAPTER

# Normal EUS Anatomy

## THE ESOPHAGUS AND STOMACH

Charles J. Lightdale
Frank Van de Mierop

The forward oblique optics of the Olympus GF-UM20 echoendoscope do not provide an adequate endoscopic examination of the upper gastrointestinal tract, particularly the esophagus. Thus, when using this instrument, most endosonographic examinations should be preceded by a standard upper gastrointestinal tract examination using a gastroscope. However, the new GF-UM200 and GF-UM130 instruments provide a much improved video image that in most instances can provide a complete endoscopic examination. Alternatively, when imaging small esophageal or gastric lesions with high-resolution ultrasound probes, the endoscopic image becomes essential for targeting the lesion (1).

The endosonographic image should be oriented in a fashion similar to that of a CT scan, with anterior structures located at the top of the image and posterior structures at the bottom. Structures on the anatomic left appear on the right of the image and vice versa, as if facing a supine patient from the feet. This technique is most easily accomplished in the esophagus, which is essentially an axial organ, but can also be accomplished in the stomach (2–4).

### Esophagus

The esophagus is best examined using the water-filled balloon technique, being careful not to overdistend the balloon. In some instances, direct contact of the transducer to the mucosa or instillation of water into the lumen will improve imaging. The normal thickness of the esophageal wall when the lumen is distended with a 3-cm–diameter water-filled balloon is approximately 3 mm and is essentially uniform throughout (4,5).

Areas of interest are located by advancing the echoendoscope to distances from the incisor teeth corresponding to those measured on standard endoscopy. Some careful study within a localized area may be required to detect small lesions. For orientation, imaged anatomic structures are correlated with depth of insertion. Scanning of the esophagus usually begins at the gastroesophageal junction and continues with progressive retraction of the echoendoscope under ultrasound guidance.

For purposes of imaging, the esophagus may be divided into three parts: upper, middle, and lower. The upper portion of the esophagus extends from the oropharynx to the superior aspect of the aortic arch. The most useful landmarks visualized here include the vertebral column posteriorly and the tracheal air column anteriorly. The great vessels of the neck may be imaged in cross section as they emerge from the aortic arch, and the superior vena cava is readily observed (Fig. 9–1). The middle portion of the esophagus extends from the aortic arch to the subcarinal region, where the most useful landmarks are the aortic arch and the descending aorta posteriorly, and the trachea and carina anteriorly (Fig. 9–2). The area just distal to the aortic arch as it passes over the pulmonary artery, called the aorto-pulmonary window, can be scanned from this location. Opposite this area, the characteristic echoes from the right main bronchus are seen. The lower portion of the esophagus extends from the subcarinal region to the cardia; the descending aorta is posterior and the left atrium is anterior (Fig. 9–3). The intrahepatic portion of the inferior vena cava and hepatic veins are often evident from the cardia, and the inferior vena cava can be followed into the right atrium. The pericardium can usually be seen as a two-layer structure (5–7).

Six "stations" have been defined for endosonographic imaging of the esophagus (8). Station I, located in the cervical esophagus, is where the spine, trachea, left subclavian artery, and carotid artery may be observed. Station II, located in the proximal esophagus, is where images of the aortic arch, trachea, and spine may be obtained. Station III, located in the proximal esophagus, is where the trachea, spine, descending aorta, azygos vein, and superior vena cava may be imaged. Station IV, located in the mid esophagus, is where the left and right bronchus, spine, azygos vein, and descending aorta are best imaged. Station V, located in the near distal esophagus, is where the left atrium, spine, azygos vein, and left pulmonary vein are seen. Station VI, located in the most distal esophagus, is where the left ventricle, liver, inferior vena cava, hepatic veins, spine, aorta, and stomach are seen.

The azygos and hemiazygos veins are important anatomic landmarks. This is especially true for the larger azygos vein, as it passes from just above the diaphragm in a cephalad direction from posterior to anterior along the right side of the esophagus where it enters the superior vena cava at the level of the aortic arch. (Fig. 9–4) Lymph nodes along the entire length of the esophagus

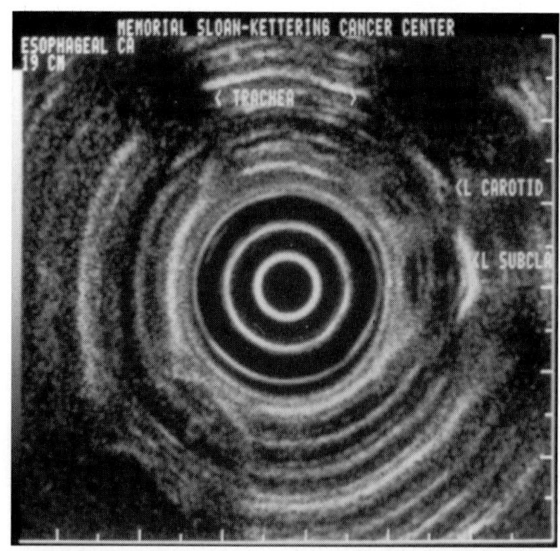


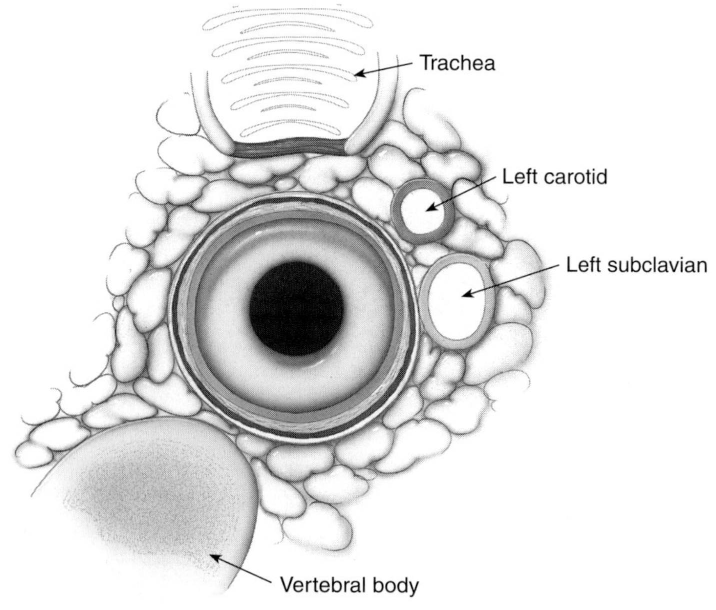


**FIGURE 9–1**

In the proximal esophagus, the anterior, air-filled trachea is seen at the top of the ultrasound image, and the posterior upper thoracic spine at the bottom (7 o'clock). The left carotid and left subclavian arteries emerging from the aortic arch are noted.

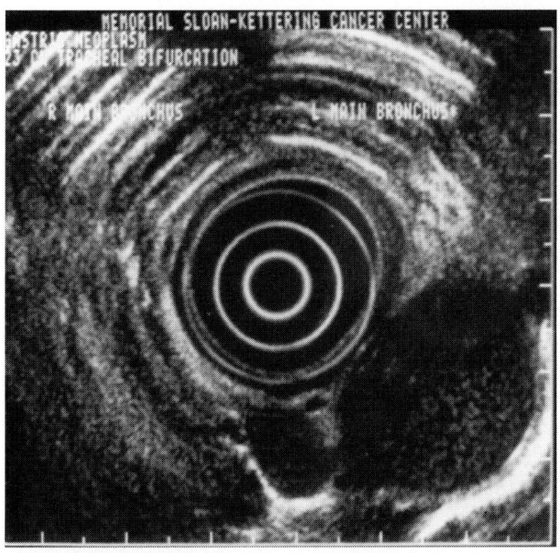


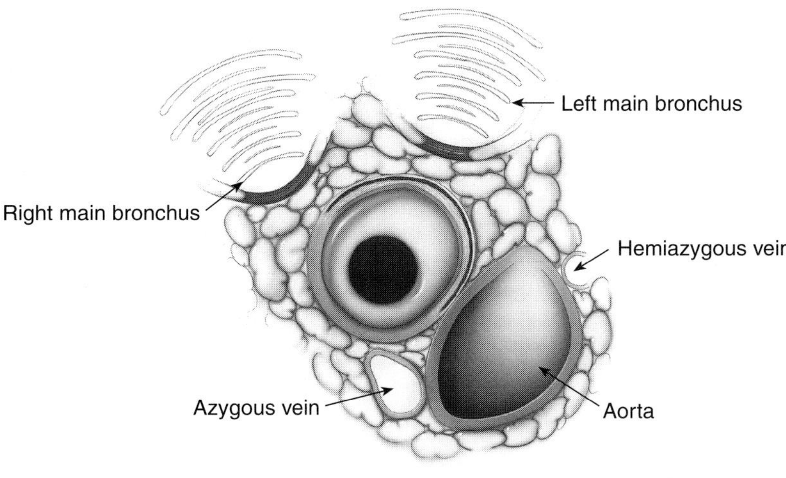


**FIGURE 9–2**

The image shown is obtained just below the carina. It demonstrates both the left and right mainstem bronchus. Note the elongation of the aorta in the 5-o'clock position demonstrating the arch of the aorta. The hypoechoic structures at either side of the aorta are the azygos (6 o'clock) and hemiazygos vein (3 o'clock).

may be imaged, including peritracheal, subcarinal, pericardial, and crural nodes.

The esophageal wall can usually be imaged as a five-layered structure. Often only three layers will be immediately evident because the wall is too close to the transducer for optimal acoustic focus. Inflating the balloon with de-aerated water will push the wall further from the transducer, but may concurrently compress the wall, causing poor definition of layers. Using the hand controls to angle the transducer can help to focus the beam on areas of interest. The amount of water in the balloon can be varied by alternately instilling and suctioning water. Balloon decompression is often needed when pulling the transducer back through the cardia into the esophagus and when passing the aortic arch. In the

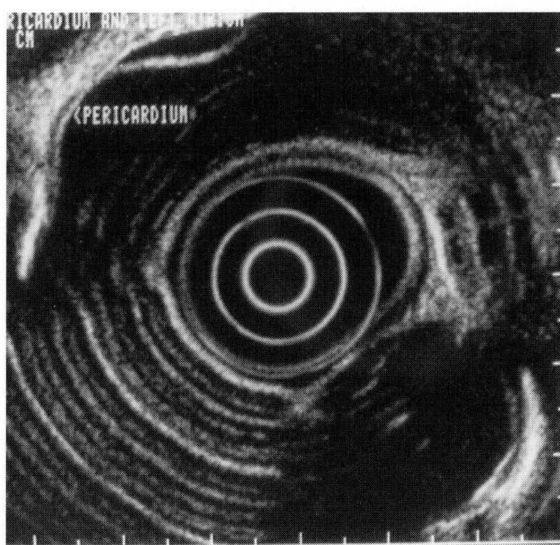


**FIGURE 9–3**

There is a close relationship between the esophagus and the left atrium anteriorly (at the top of the image), and the aorta posteriorly (at the bottom of the image at approximately 5 o'clock). The pericardium, imaged as two layers, can be seen adjacent to the left atrium.

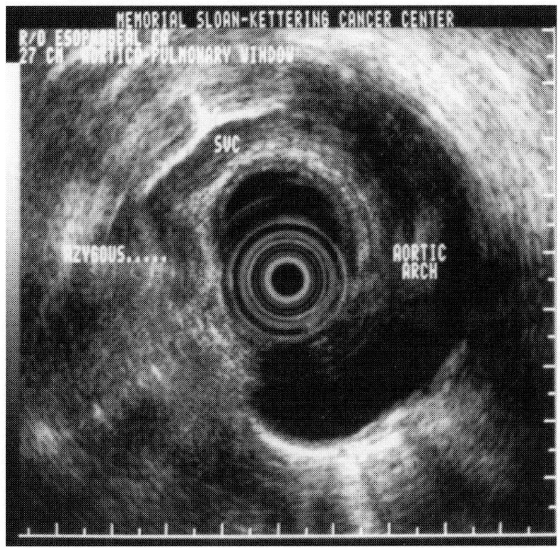


**FIGURE 9–4**

An endosonograph obtained in the mid-thoracic esophagus is shown. The azygos vein is observed emptying into the superior vena cava (SVC) at the level of the aortic arch.

**TABLE 9–1**

Gastric Wall Layers

| | Image Echogenicity | Correlation | Remark |
|---|---|---|---|
| I | Echo-rich | Border echo; lumen–wall | Closest to transducer. With high frequency (20 MHz) imaging of three layers possible, with delineation of muscularis mucosae |
| II | Echo-poor | Mucosa | |
| III | Echo-rich | Submucosa | |
| IV | Echo-poor | Muscularis propria | With high frequency (12–20 MHz), not one but three layers (thin echo-rich layer between two echo-poor layers) |
| V | Echo-rich | Border echo; fat/serosa/ subserosa | |

proximal esophagus, pressure on the trachea from the water-filled balloon may cause discomfort; if this occurs, the amount of water in the balloon should be decreased.

## Stomach

The gastric wall is best examined by filling the lumen with 300–600 mL of de-aerated water. With the water-filled lumen technique, the five layers of the gastric wall (3–4 mm thick) are usually very clearly delineated (Table 9–1). Optimally, the transducer is turned away from the wall as the focal length for the 7.5-MHz transducer is 2–2.5 cm for radial scanning. The prepyloric area and the gastric cardia are often difficult to completely fill with water, and the water-filled balloon method of examination must be used to image these areas. Air can be suctioned from the gastric lumen to collapse the stomach around the balloon. In addition, the position of the patient can be altered to facilitate water coating of the gastric wall (2,7). For examination of the gastric antrum, it may be necessary to place patients in a supine position while elevating the head of the bed. To visualize beyond the wall, the mucosa–transducer contact method or mucosa–balloon contact method is usually sufficient. The wall of the stomach gradually thickens toward the pylorus, the thickness increasing from approximately 4 to 8 mm. The pyloric sphincter is a thickened, echo-poor muscle layer contiguous with the fourth layer of the antrum.

The stomach is divided anatomically into the fundus, the body, and the antrum. The sonographic landmarks of the fundus are the aorta with the splenic vein and celiac axis posteriorly, the left hepatic lobe to the right, and the spleen to the left (Fig. 9–5). In slim patients, the left kidney and left adrenal gland can be seen as well. The celiac axis is an important landmark when imaging malignant lymph nodes for the staging of upper abdominal cancers.

Endosonographs of the body of the stomach will show the left hepatic lobe to the right and anteriorly, and the body and tail of the pancreas to the left and posteriorly (Figs. 9–6, 9–7). The splenic vein can be seen as a vessel demarcating the posterior border of the

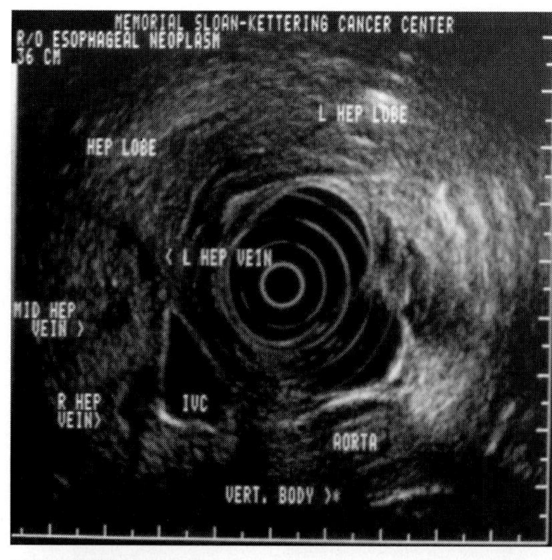


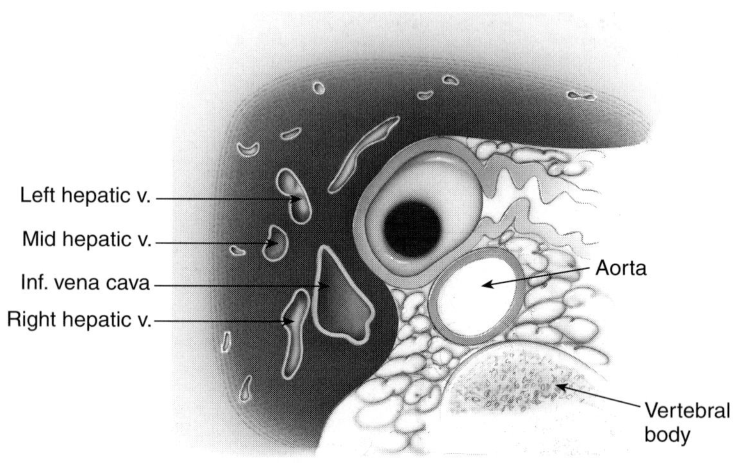


**FIGURE 9–5**

The gastric fundus is collapsed around the balloon by suction to demonstrate the surrounding structures. The left lobe of the liver is located anteriorly. The left, mid, and right hepatic veins are imaged draining into the inferior vena cava (IVC), which pulsates reflecting the right atrium. The aorta and vertebral body are located posteriorly.

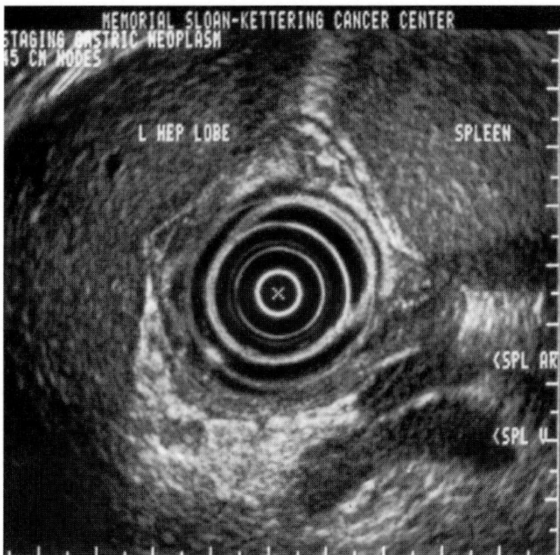


**FIGURE 9–6**

The splenic artery and vein are located posteriorly; the liver and spleen are located to the left and right.

pancreatic parenchyma. The splenic artery usually has a much more tortuous appearance, and is generally anterior to the vein. A double gastric wall image and two gastric lumens can be seen as the ultrasound beam passes through the angularis, imaging both the body and antrum simultaneously (4).

Endosonographs of the gastric antrum demonstrate the left lobe of the liver anteriorly and the pancreas, splenic vein, and portal vein posteriorly (Fig. 9–8). In the distal antrum, the gallbladder usually can be seen (Fig. 9–9).

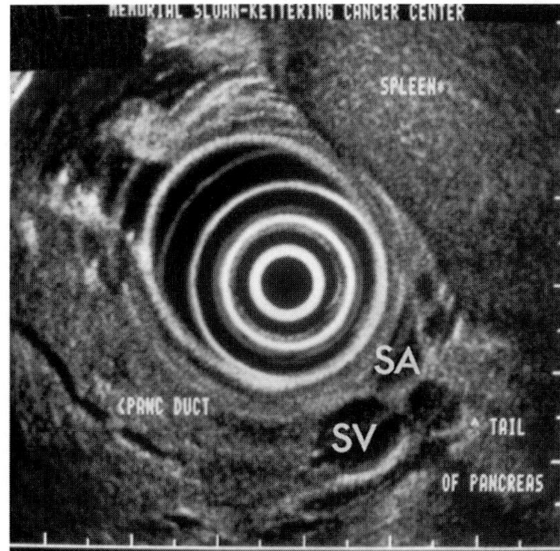


**FIGURE 9–7**

The tail of the pancreas is imaged through the posterior gastric wall with the pancreatic duct evident, as well as portions of the splenic artery (SA), splenic vein (SV), and spleen.

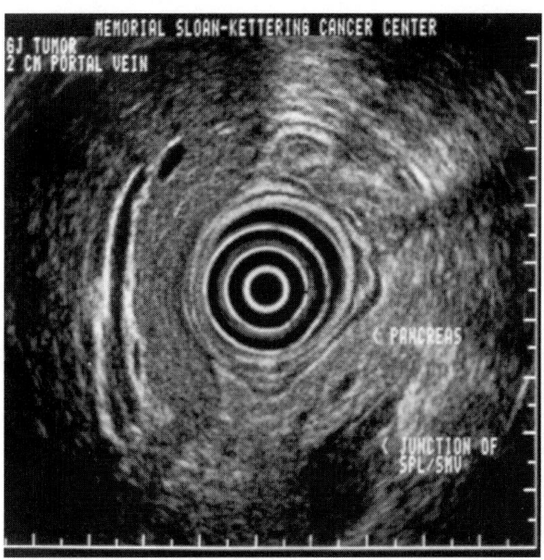


**FIGURE 9–8**

Portions of the pancreatic head and pancreatic body are observed posteriorly as imaged via the gastric antrum. At this level, the splenic vein (SPL) and superior mesenteric vein (SMV) join to form the portal vein. The left portal vein is demarcated by brightly echogenic vascular margins, characteristic of the intrahepatic portal venous system.

Lymph nodes can be imaged along both the lesser and greater curvature of the stomach. Lymph nodes tend to follow blood vessels, and must be distinguished from vascular structures by real-time imaging (7,9). Lymph nodes are discrete structures with internal echoes, compared to blood vessels, which show linear continuity and are essentially anechoic. The detection limit for regional lymph nodes is in the range of 3 mm. Blood vessels frequently show a hyperechoic distal wall enhancement not

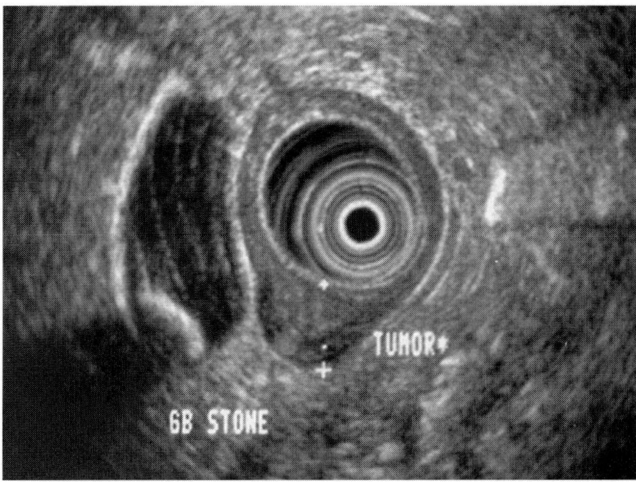


**FIGURE 9–9**

An endosonograph of the gallbladder containing a gallstone. The gallbladder is imaged from a position in the distal gastric antrum.

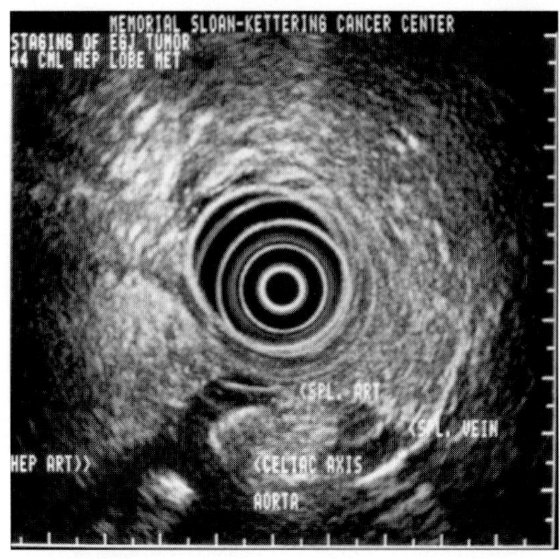


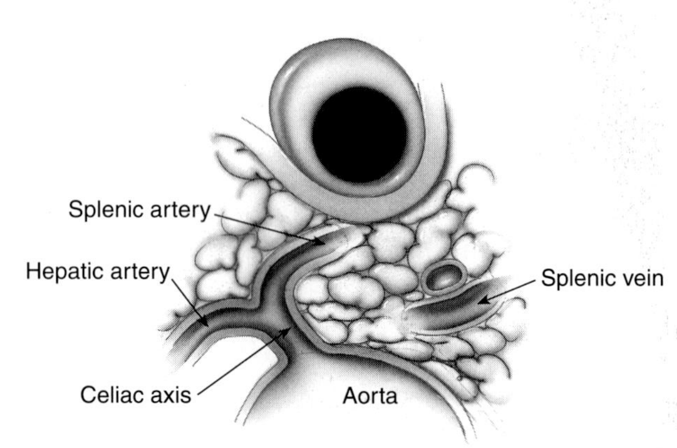


**FIGURE 9–10**

The celiac axis is located posteriorly. The top of the aorta, the origin of the hepatic and splenic arteries, and a small portion of the splenic vein are noted.

seen in normal lymph nodes, although pathologically homogeneous lymph nodes may also evidence this finding. Important areas of nodal drainage include those related to the celiac axis (Fig. 9–10), splenic artery, splenic hilum, hepatic artery, porta hepatis, and left gastric artery in the gastro-hepatic ligament between the liver and lesser curvature of the stomach.

Performed with care, endosonographic measurements of normal anatomy are accurate and interobserver variability is small. With good technique, training, and experience, misinterpretation of normal structures can be avoided. Pitfalls include tangential scanning of the GI tract wall, which can cause a thickened appearance. Extraluminal bowel loops can mimic tumors or lymph nodes; and the ventral pancreas, relatively echo-poor, may mimic a tumor, as can the caudate lobe of the liver. Artifacts that can occur during the procedure include a mirror image of the transducer (8).

## References

1. Chak A, Canto M, Stevens P, Lightdale CJ, Van de Mierop F, Cooper G, Pollack BJ, Sivak MV. Prospective evaluation of new ultrasound catheter systems: Comparison with ultrasound endoscopes. Gastrointest Endosc 43(4):A8, 1996.
2. Tio TL, Tytgat GNJ. Atlas of Transintestinal Ultrasonography. Mur-Kostverloren, Aalsmeer, The Netherlands, 1986.
3. Strohm WD, Classen M. Anatomical aspects in ultrasonic endoscopy. Scand J Gastroenterol 19(suppl 94):21–23, 1984.
4. Caletti GC, Bolondi L, Zani L, Labo G. Technique of endoscopic ultrasonography investigation: Esophagus, stomach, and duodenum. Scand J. Gastroenterol 21(suppl 123):1–5, 1986.
5. Thatcher BS, Sivak MV Jr, George C. Endoscopic ultrasonography: A preliminary report. Gastrointest Endosc 31:237–242, 1985.
6. Yasuda K, Kiyota K, Mukai K, Cho E. Anatomical aspects of endoscopic ultrasonography. In Kawai K (ed): Endoscopic Ultrasonography in Gastroenterology. New York: Igaku-Shoin, 1988.
7. Bótet JF, Lightdale CJ. Endoscopic sonography of the upper gastrointestinal tract. Am J Roent 156:63–68, 1991.
8. Catalano MF. Normal structures on endoscopic ultrasonography: Visualization measurement data and interobserver variation. Gastrointest Endosc Clin N Am 5(3):475–486, 1995.
9. Rösch T, Classen M. Normal anatomy on endosonographic examination. In: Gastroenterologic Endosconography. Stuttgart/New York: Thieme, 1992, pp. 13–35.
10. Yanai H, Fujimura H, Suzumi M, Matsuura S, Awaya N, Noguschi T, Karita M, Tada M, Okita K, Aibe T. Delineation of the gastric muscularis mucosae and assessment of depth of invasion of early gastric cancer using a 20 megahertz endoscopic ultrasound probe. Gastrointest Endosc 39:505–512, 1993.
11. Miller LS, Schiano TD. The use of high frequency endoscopic ultrasonography probes in the evaluation of achalasia. Gastrointest Endosc Clin N Am 5(3):635–47, 1995.
12. Grech P. Mirror-image artifact with endoscopic ultrasonography and reappraisal of the fluid–air interface. Gastrointest Endosc 39:700–703, 1993.

CHAPTER

# The TNM Classification for Staging Gastrointestinal Malignancies

Jacques Van Dam

Tumor staging is not a fixed science, but rather a dynamic process. As new information regarding the etiology of various types of cancers is acquired and as new methods of diagnosing and treating tumors develop, the classification and staging of cancer must also change. Consequently, the American Joint Committee on Cancer (AJCC) in cooperation with the International Union Against Cancer (UICC, Union Internationale Contre le Cancer) agreed in 1987 on a uniform classification system of malignancy, including gastrointestinal cancers. The new formulation of the TNM classification system was the result of a collaborative effort by a number of national TNM committees, including the American, British, Canadian, French, German, Italian, and Japanese (1). The AJCC was sponsored by the American Cancer Society, American College of Physicians, American College of Surgeons, College of American Pathologists, the National Cancer Institute, and others (2).

The AJCC/UICC classification is founded on the premise that cancers of similar sites of origin share similar properties of growth and extension. Specifically, the classification system relies upon the fact that the size of an untreated tumor (T) increases progressively until it involves regional lymph nodes (N) and finally metastasizes to distant sites (M). As the primary cancer (e.g., a gastrointestinal tumor) increases in size, there is a point at which local invasion occurs—a point detectable by newer, more sensitive diagnostic modalities such as endoscopic ultrasonography (EUS). Involvement of regional lymph nodes draining the area of the tumor may also be detectable by EUS. Metastatic disease is also demonstrable by EUS; for example, tumor involvement may be detected in celiac axis lymph nodes in association with primary esophageal carcinoma.

The history of tumor staging dates back to the 1920s with the League of Nations (3). The practice of dividing cancers into "stages" arose from the observation that those patients whose tumors were relatively localized had higher survival rates than those whose tumors had extended beyond the organ of origin. The staging of cancer is an accepted tradition as well as a necessity in understanding and communicating data regarding malignancies. Other reasons to stage cancer include the following:

1. To aid the clinician in planning therapy that provides the greatest potential benefit: specifically, to supply the statistical data needed to develop that plan.
2. To render some indication of prognosis, both for the clinician and the patient.
3. To assist in the evaluation of controlled trials of chemotherapy, radiation therapy, photodynamic therapy, surgical therapy, or combination therapy.
4. To facilitate the exchange of information between treatment centers.
5. To contribute to the continuing investigation of human cancers.

The principal purpose of the new, internationally agreed-upon cancer staging classification is, however, to provide a method of conveying clinical experience to others without ambiguity.

Staging of tumors at all anatomic locations is numbered from best (stage 0) to poorest prognosis (stage IV): Stage 0, carcinoma in situ; stage I, localized cancer; stage II, limited local or regional spread; stage III, extensive local or regional spread; stage IV, distant spread. The use of the "juxtaregional" lymph node classification has been abandoned in favor of classifying lymph nodes as either regional (N) or distant (M). The AJCC has eliminated the surgical staging classification (sTNM). The two major classifications in the new TNM system are the clinical (cTNM) and the pathologic (pTNM) classifications. The clinical classification is an expression of the anatomic extent of disease based on pretreatment clinical evaluation. It includes information obtained from patient history, physical examination, imaging techniques, endoscopic evaluation, biopsy specimens, and surgical exploration. The pathologic classification is based on the evidence acquired prior to therapy, supplemented or modified by the additional evidence adduced from pathologic examination of a resected specimen.

## Esophageal Carcinoma

The TNM classification for esophageal cancer has been completely revised. Prior to the reclassification for esophageal carcinoma in 1987, the extent of the tumor (T) was determined by its size and degree of obstruction: (T1) <5 cm or no obstruction; (T2) >5 cm, esophageal obstruction, or circumferential lesion; (T3) extension outside the esophagus. In the new TNM classification, tumor size, circumferential involvement, and degree of obstruction have been abandoned in favor of depth of invasion. The new classification reflects the improvement in imaging techniques such as EUS: (T0) no evidence of primary tumor; (Tis) carcinoma in situ; (T1) tumor invades lamina propria or submucosa; (T3) tumor invades adventitia; (T4) tumor invades adjacent structures (Table 10–1). The definition of regional lymph nodes has been modified and simplified. Regional lymph nodes for tumors of the cervical esophagus include cervical esophageal lymph nodes and the supraclavicular lymph nodes. Regional lymph nodes for tumors of the thoracic esophagus include the mediastinal and perigastric lymph nodes, but exclude the supraclavicular lymph nodes (Table 10–2). Involvement of more distant nodes, such as celiac axis lymph nodes is considered metastatic disease (M1).

Endosonography is highly accurate, and it is superior to computed tomographic scan (CT scan) for the preoperative staging of esophageal carcinoma (4–11). However, endosonography is not a substitute for CT scan, but rather a useful adjunct for the preoperative staging of esophageal cancer. There is a learning curve

**TABLE 10-1**

**AJCC/UICC Staging of Esophageal Cancer**

| | |
|---|---|
| ***Primary Tumor (T)*** | |
| TX | Primary tumor cannot be assessed |
| T0 | No evidence of primary tumor |
| Tis | Carcinoma in situ |
| T1 | Tumor invades lamina propria or submucosa |
| T2 | Tumor invades muscularis propria |
| T3 | Tumor invades adventitia |
| T4 | Tumor invades adjacent structures (1) |
| ***Regional Lymph Nodes (N)*** | |
| NX | Regional lymph nodes cannot be assessed |
| N0 | No regional lymph node metastasis |
| N1 | Regional lymph node metastasis (2) |
| ***Distant Metastasis (M)*** | |
| MX | Presence of distant metastasis cannot be assessed |
| M0 | No distant metastasis |
| M1 | Distant metastasis (3) |

(1) Cervical esophagus: Extends from the cricoid cartilage to the thoracic inlet (suprasternal notch) at approximately 18 cm from the incisors.
Thoracic esophagus: Extends from the thoracic inlet to the esophagogastric junction at approximately 40 cm from the incisors.
(i) upper thoracic—extends from the thoracic inlet to the tracheal bifurcation at approximately 24 cm from the incisors.
(ii) mid thoracic—extends to approximately 32 cm from the incisors.
(iii) lower thoracic—from approximately 32 cm from the incisors, includes the abdominal esophagus.
(2) Regional lymph nodes:
(i) cervical esophagus—the cervical nodes including the supraclavicular lymph nodes; all others distant.
(ii) thoracic esophagus—mediastinal and perigastric lymph nodes; all others distant, including supraclavicular and celiac lymph nodes.
(3) Most common sites include liver, lungs, pleura, kidneys, and celiac lymph nodes.

**TABLE 10-2**

AJCC/UICC Staging of Esophageal Cancer

| | Stage Grouping | | |
|---|---|---|---|
| Stage 0 | Tis | N0 | M0 |
| Stage I | T1 | N0 | M0 |
| Stage IIA | T2 | N0 | M0 |
| | T3 | N0 | M0 |
| Stage IIB | T1 | N1 | M0 |
| | T2 | N1 | M0 |
| Stage III | T3 | N1 | M0 |
| | T4 | Any N | M0 |
| Stage IV | Any T | Any N | M1 |

for the endosonographic staging of esophageal tumors, as noted by Rice et al. (12,13). The accuracy for preoperative T staging in their first 28 cases was 59%, but improved to 81% in the next 52 patients evaluated (12,13). Fockens et al. also demonstrated a learning curve for esophageal tumor staging using endoscopic ultrasonography. By assessing the preoperative T-stage accuracy in his first 100 cases (36 of whom underwent surgical exploration) and comparing it with his next 131 cases (35 of whom underwent surgical exploration), he concluded that acceptable accuracy rates could be achieved only after 100 examinations (14).

Endosonography is accurate in identifying the early stages of disease (including superficial esophageal carcinoma) and in detecting advanced, nonresectable esophageal carcinoma, considerable inter-observer variation notwithstanding (15–18). The most difficult assessment is for T2 tumors, for which the accuracy is poorest (11). Assessment of vascular involvement in patients with esophageal cancer has important implications for the approach to therapy. Relative to CT scan, endosonography provides a more sensitive and reliable determination of local vascular involvement (19). The differentiation of mucosal and submucosal disease in early esophageal cancer (T1) is problematic, however, and has led to overstaging in some cases. Endosonographic evaluation of patients with superficial esophageal carcinoma has demonstrated an overall accuracy of 72% for T staging (20).

The addition of high-resolution ultrasound probes for staging esophageal carcinoma has yielded mixed results (21–25). The ultrasound probes contain transducers with frequencies of up to (and sometimes more than) 15–20 MHz. These instruments may provide highly detailed images of superficial carcinomas but cannot image deeply into the tissue adjacent to the esophagus; thus they are generally incapable of assessing regional lymph node metastases (21). On average, 20-MHz probes penetrate no deeper than 2 cm (21). In addition, orientation when imaging from the stomach (to assess for celiac axis lymph adenopathy) may be problematic (22).

## Endosonographic Evaluation of Lymph Node Metastases (N Stage)

The endosonographic assessment of lymph node metastases has been shown to be more accurate than that provided by CT scan. However, the precise differentiation of malignant from benign lymph nodes remains problematic. Unlike CT scan—which can determine only lymph node size—endoscopic ultrasonography provides additional information, including lymph node shape, border characteristics, and central echogenicity (26). However, micrometastases currently detectable only by histologic evaluation may not produce endosonographically detectable changes, leading to understaging. Moreover, large inflammatory lymph nodes may be incorrectly classified as metastatic and hence overstaged. Attempts to classify lymph nodes by specific endosonographic features have improved the accuracy of lymph node classification, but they are cumbersome and subjective. Nor have they been widely studied (27,28).

In one study, Heintz et al. used computer-supported B-mode analysis (ProgramMicroscale, Digithurst; Nuremberg, Germany) to evaluate lymph node characteristics in vitro on resected specimens of patients with esophageal and gastric carcinoma (29). However, subjective evaluation or computer analysis did not reliably distinguish benign from malignant lymph nodes (29). Catalano et al. developed a system of analysis in which four endosonographic characteristics of lymph nodes (size, shape, border demarcation, and central echo pattern) were evaluated (27). Sensitivity and specificity were 89.1% and 91.7%, respectively, when such stringent criteria were used. The four criteria were demonstrated to be additive in their ability to predict lymph node metastases. When all four criteria were present, accuracy in predicting lymh node metastases was reportedly 100% (27). However, all four criteria were observed in regional lymph nodes in a minority of cases. A recently recognized association between depth of tumor penetration (T stage) and lymph node metastasis (N stage) may aid in reliably predicting lymph node metastases. In a recent review of the association between T stage and N stage for 103 patients with surgically resected specimens of esophageal carcinoma, lymph node involvement (%) increased with the depth of tumor penetration, as follows: Tis ($n$ = 4) N1 (0%); T1 ($n$ = 14) N1 (14.3%); T2 ($n$ = 18) N1 (33.3%); T3 ($n$ = 60) N1 (73.3%); T4 ($n$ = 7) N1 (85.7%) (30). Similarly, in their series of more than 400 cases, Dittler et al. reviewed the accuracy of endosonography for assessing lymph node metastases and noted that the incidence of lymph node metastases increased with advancing T stage: T1, 4%; T2, 52%; T3, 82%; T4, 91% (31). Therefore, if tumor involvement of lymph nodes increases with advancing T stage, it may be one of the most sensitive indicators of lymph node metastases (30,31).

The most accurate and effective approach to esophageal tumor staging is the combination of endosonography and CT scan. Using this approach, CT scan should be performed first to detect distant metastases (M stage). If no distant metastases are detected, endosonography should be performed to determine depth of tumor penetration and the presence of regional lymph adenopathy (T, N stage). The role of regional lymph node assessment by thoracoscopy is under investigation and preliminary results are promising (32). The relative safety and efficacy of this invasive technique are under intensive investigation. The relative merits of thoracoscopy vis à vis endoscopic ultrasound have not yet been determined, but the results of trials comparing the two techniques are anticipated. The addition of EUS-guided FNA has revolutionized the endoscopic assessment of regional lymph nodes for patients with esophageal cancer. However, more studies carefully assessing the safety and efficacy of the technique are required.

## Gastric Carcinoma

The TNM classification for gastric carcinoma has been substantially revised (2,33). Depth of tumor invasion is now the primary determinant of tumor classification (T), reflecting the improvements in imaging modalities such as EUS: (T0) no evidence of primary tumor; (Tis) carcinoma in situ, intra-epithelial tumor without invasion of the lamina propria; (T1) tumor invades lamina propria or submucosa; (T2) tumor invades the muscularis propria or the subserosa; (T3) tumor penetrates the serosa (visceral peritoneum) without invasion of adjacent structures; (T4) tumor invades adjacent structures (Tables 10–3 and 10–4). The definition of regional lymph nodes has been modified and the N3 category has been eliminated. N1 refers to metastases in regional lymph nodes consisting of perigastric lymph node(s) within 3 cm of the edge of the primary tumor. N2 refers to metastases either in perigastric lymph node(s) more than 3 cm from the edge of the primary tumor, or in lymph nodes along the left gastric, common hepatic, splenic, or celiac arteries.

Recent studies evaluating the use of EUS for the preoperative staging of gastric carcinoma have reported an overall accuracy of approximately 84% in determining depth of penetration of tumor (T) (34–36). Sensitivity of EUS for lymph node involvement was 81% and specificity 50% (35). Although certain echo patterns are considered characteristic for lymph node metastases, it is often difficult to differentiate granulomatous or inflammatory lymph nodes from those involved with tumor. Similarly, small lymph nodes with micrometastatic involvement cannot be distinguished from benign lymph nodes (35,36). Evaluation of EUS in the diagnosis of infiltrating cancers of the stomach is currently under way. Preliminary reports suggest that EUS may be both sensitive and specific in detecting and assessing gastric lymphoma (37). In addition, EUS may be useful in the diagnosis of linitis plastica, especially in cases in which biopsy results are negative (38).

**TABLE 10–3**

**AJCC/UICC Staging of Gastric Cancer**

| | |
|---|---|
| ***Primary Tumor (T)*** | |
| TX | Primary tumor cannot be assessed |
| T0 | No evidence of primary tumor |
| Tis | Carcinoma in situ: Intra-epithelial tumor without invasion of the lamina propria |
| T1 | Tumor invades lamina propria or submucosa |
| T2 | Tumor invades the muscularis propria or the subserosa |
| T3 | Tumor penetrates the serosa (visceral peritoneum) without invasion of adjacent structures (1) |
| T4 | Tumor invades adjacent structures (2) |
| ***Regional Lymph Nodes (N)*** | |
| NX | Regional lymph node(s) cannot be assessed |
| N0 | No regional lymph node metastasis |
| N1 | Metastasis in perigastric lymph node(s) within 3 cm of the edge of the primary tumor |
| N2 | Metastasis in perigastric lymph node(s) more than 3 cm from the edge of the primary tumor, or in lymph nodes along the left gastric, common hepatic, splenic, or celiac arteries (3) |
| ***Distant Metastasis (M)*** | |
| MX | Presence of distant metastasis cannot be assessed |
| M0 | No distant metastasis |
| M1 | Distant metastasis (4) |

(1) Tumor of muscularis propria without serosal penetration, but with spread to gastrohepatic or gastrocolic ligaments or to lesser or greater omentum is still considered T2.
(2) Adjacent structures are spleen, transverse colon, liver, diaphragm, pancreas, abdominal wall, adrenal gland, kidney, small intestine, and retroperitoneum.
(3) Regional lymph nodes include perigastric lymph nodes, not otherwise specified and those along the inferior (right) gastric, splenic, superior (left) gastric, including retropancreatic, hepatoduodenal, aortic, portal, retroperitoneal, and mesenteric.
(4) Most common metastatic sites include liver, lungs, supraclavicular lymph nodes, and widespread intraperitoneal sites.

**TABLE 10–4**

**AJCC/UICC Staging of Gastric Cancer**

| | *Stage Grouping* | | |
|---|---|---|---|
| Stage 0 | Tis | N0 | M0 |
| Stage IA | T1 | N0 | M0 |
| Stage IB | T1 | N1 | M0 |
| | T2 | N0 | M0 |
| Stage II | T1 | N2 | M0 |
| | T2 | N1 | M0 |
| | T3 | N0 | M0 |
| Stage IIIA | T2 | N2 | M0 |
| | T3 | N1 | M0 |
| | T4 | N0 | M0 |
| Stage IIIB | T3 | N2 | M0 |
| | T4 | N1 | M0 |
| Stage IV | T4 | N2 | M0 |
| | Any T | Any N | M1 |

## Ampullary Carcinoma

Primary cancers of the ampulla of Vater are not common, but are important owing to their strategic location. Prior to 1987, no specific anatomic staging for this cancer existed. The current classification for ampullary tumors is as follows: (T0) no evidence of primary tumor; (Tis) carcinoma in situ; (T1) tumor limited to the ampulla of Vater; (T2) tumor invades the duodenal wall; (T3) tumor invades 2 cm or less into the pancreas; (T4) tumor invades more than 2 cm into the pancreas and/or into adjacent organs (Tables 10–5 and 10–6). Regional lymph nodes are those adjacent to the head and body of the pancreas, anterior and pancreaticoduodenal, pyloric and proximal mesenteric lymph nodes, and common bile duct lymph nodes. The splenic lymph nodes and those at the tail of the pancreas are not considered regional lymph nodes, and tumor involvement of these lymph nodes is considered metastatic disease (M1). Tumors of the ampulla of Vater metastasize primarily by direct extension to adjacent structures.

Endoscopic ultrasonography is useful in detecting the presence and determining the extent of ampullary carcinoma (39–41). Reports evaluating the use of EUS in the preoperative staging of ampullary and pancreatic cancer have demonstrated a high degree of accuracy (41). In one study, the overall accuracy of EUS in determining the tumor stage (T) for ampullary carcinoma was 87%; however, the correct interpretation of lymph nodes remained problematic. The sensitivity of EUS for detecting metastatic lymph nodes in ampullary carcinoma was 80%, the specificity only 36%, and the positive predictive value 47% (41). The specificity was low owing to the difficulty in distinguishing nonmetastatic lymph node abnormalities from malignant involvement. In a larger study including 70 patients with pancreatic cancer and 32 patients with ampullary carcinoma, nonresectability was accurately assessed on the basis of vascular involvement (42). The overall accuracy for staging ampullary carcinoma was 84.4%. Thus, endoscopic ultrasonography remains the best method for the preoperative staging of this uncommon gastrointestinal cancer.

**TABLE 10-5**

AJCC/UICC Staging of Cancer of the Ampulla of Vater

| | |
|---|---|
| ***Primary Tumor (T)*** | |
| TX | Primary tumor cannot be assessed |
| T0 | No evidence of primary tumor |
| Tis | Carcinoma in situ |
| T1 | Tumor limited to the ampulla of Vater |
| T2 | Tumor invades duodenal wall |
| T3 | Tumor invades 2 cm or less into the pancreas |
| T4 | Tumor invades more than 2 cm into the pancreas and/or into other adjacent organs |
| ***Regional Lymph Nodes (N)*** | |
| NX | Regional lymph nodes cannot be assessed |
| N0 | No regional lymph node metastasis |
| N1 | Regional lymph node metastasis |
| ***Distant Metastasis (M)*** | |
| MX | Presence of distant metastasis cannot be assessed |
| M0 | No distant metastasis |
| M1 | Distant metastasis |

**TABLE 10-6**

Stage Grouping for Ampulla of Vater Cancer

| | | | |
|---|---|---|---|
| Stage 0 | Tis | N0 | M0 |
| Stage I | T1 | N0 | M0 |
| Stage II | T2 | N0 | M0 |
| | T3 | N0 | M0 |
| Stage III | T1 | N1 | M0 |
| | T2 | N1 | M0 |
| | T3 | N1 | M0 |
| Stage IV | T4 | Any N | M0 |
| | Any T | Any N | M1 |

## Colon and Rectal Carcinoma

There are numerous staging systems for colon and rectal cancer. Dukes, Kirklin, Astler–Coller, and TNM are some of the better known systems. The modified Astler–Coller–Dukes system (MAC) is the most commonly used staging system for colon cancer in the United States. The 1987 TNM classification for colon cancer has been modified to correspond directly with the Dukes classification (1,2). In 1990, the National Institutes of Health held a consensus conference on adjuvant therapy for patients with colon and rectal cancer (43). The primary goal of the conference was not to select a new staging system for colon and rectal cancer; however, the first "conclusion and recommendation" made by the committee was that "the TNM system can effectively describe risk groups for recurrence of colon and rectal cancer, and should be used in clinical trial research and clinical practice." Furthermore, in its 1991 report on the National Cancer Data Base, the American Cancer Society stated that in the future, data will be coded according to the TNM system (44).

The current classification for colon and rectal tumors is as follows: (T0) no evidence of primary tumor; (Tis) carcinoma in situ; (T1) tumor invades submucosa; (T2) tumor invades muscularis propria; (T3) tumor invades through the muscularis propria into the subserosa, or into nonperitonealized pericolic or perirectal tissues; (T4) tumor perforates the visceral peritoneum, or directly invades other organs or structures (Table 10–7). The classification for lymph nodes has also been modified and takes into account the number of lymph nodes involved: (N0) no regional lymph node metastases; (N1) metastasis in 1–3 pericolic or perirectal lymph nodes; (N2) metastases in 4 or more pericolic or perirectal lymph nodes; (N3) metastasis in

**TABLE 10-7**

AJCC/UICC Staging of Colon and Rectal Cancer

| | |
|---|---|
| ***Primary Tumor (T)*** | |
| TX | Primary tumor cannot be assessed |
| T0 | No evidence of primary tumor |
| Tis | Carcinoma in situ |
| T1 | Tumor invades submucosa |
| T2 | Tumor invades muscularis propria |
| T3 | Tumor invades through muscularis propria into the subserosa, or into nonperitonealized pericolic or perirectal tissues. |
| T4 | Tumor perforates the visceral peritoneum, or directly invades other organs or structures* |
| ***Regional Lymph Nodes (N)*** | |
| NX | Regional lymph nodes cannot be assessed |
| N0 | No regional lymph node metastasis |
| N1 | Metastasis in 1 to 3 pericolic or perirectal lymph nodes |
| N2 | Metastasis in 4 or more pericolic or perirectal lymph nodes |
| N3 | Metastasis in any lymph node along the course of a named vascular trunk |
| ***Distant Metastasis (M)*** | |
| MX | Presence of distant metastasis cannot be assessed |
| M0 | No distant metastasis |
| M1 | Distant metastasis |

* *Note:* Direct invasion of other organs or structures includes invasion of other segments of the colorectum by way of serosa (e.g., invasion of the sigmoid colon by a carcinoma of the cecum).

any lymph node along the course of a named vascular trunk (Table 10–8, Fig. 10–1). The current TNM staging of colon cancer may be directly correlated with the Dukes classification (Table 10–8).

Studies comparing EUS and CT scan for staging rectal cancers consistently found EUS more accurate than CT scan for determining the depth of cancer invasion; however, in many published reports, a rigid, nonoptical, endorectal ultrasound transducer was used (45–49). Additional reports comparing the GF-UM3 ultrasonographic fibergastroscope to CT scan for staging rectal cancers were in agreement with earlier reports demonstrating an overall higher accuracy for EUS (50). The advantage of using the GF-UM3 for rectal ultrasound is that both the 12- and 7.5-MHz frequencies are available for high-resolution imaging of rectal wall layers and imaging of deeper structures such as lymph nodes, respectively.

**TABLE 10-8**

AJCC/UICC Stage Grouping for Colon/Rectal Cancer

| | | | | Dukes |
|---|---|---|---|---|
| Stage 0 | Tis | N0 | M0 | |
| Stage I | T1 | N0 | M0 | A |
| | T2 | N0 | M0 | |
| Stage II | T3 | N0 | M0 | B |
| | T4 | N0 | M0 | |
| Stage III | Any T | N1 | M0 | C |
| | Any T | N2,N3 | M0 | |
| Stage IV | Any T | Any N | M1 | D |

*Note:* Dukes B is a composite of better (T3, N0, M0) and worse (T4, N0, M0) prognostic groups, as is Dukes C (Any T, N1, M0) and (Any T, N2, N3, M0).

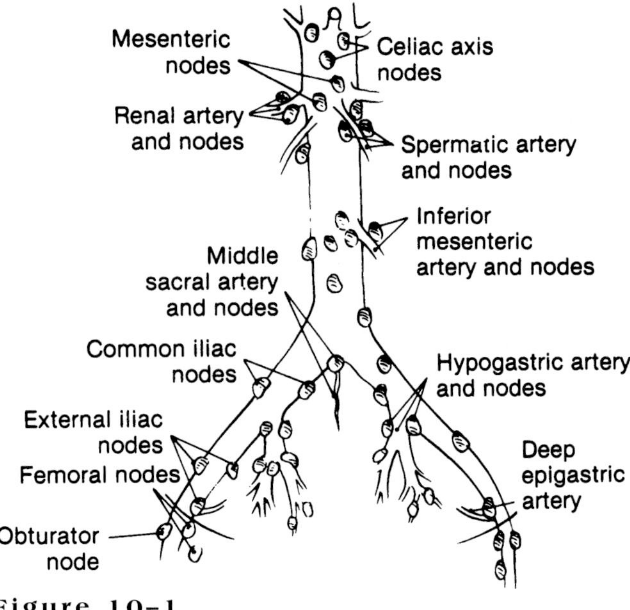


**Figure 10–1**

Lymph nodes along named vascular trunks. (Reproduced with permission from Manual for Staging of Cancer, 3rd ed. American Joint Committee on Cancer. Beahrs OH, Henson DE, Hutter RVP, Myers MH (eds). Philadelphia: JB Lippincott, 1988.)

With the advent of endoscopic mucosal resection (an endoscopic method for the removal of superficial lesions), EUS was evaluated to determine if it could reliably determine the stage of early colorectal tumor invasion (51). Sixty patients diagnosed with "early cancer" were prospectively analyzed. Forty lesions interpreted as mucosal by EUS were shown histologically to include 32 lesions in the mucosa and 8 in the submucosa or deeper. The overall accuracy was 77%. The authors concluded that EUS alone was not reliable for determining lesions resectable by endoscopic mucosal resection. However, similar studies utilizing high-frequency (20 MHz) ultrasound probes were shown to be more reliable for determining depth of early colorectal cancer penetration (52). In fact, high-frequency ultrasound probes had an accuracy of 88% and thus were deemed useful in directing therapeutic strategy. However, more studies evaluating EUS accuracy and interobserver variation are needed before firm conclusions may be drawn regarding the use of EUS for early colorectal cancer staging.

In conclusion, endoscopic ultrasonography has been shown to have an important impact on clinical decision making, especially in tumor staging (54–56). As additional options become available for the management of gastrointestinal tumors, more information will be required to determine how best to use our healthcare resources to benefit our patients. Endoscopic ultrasound is uniquely suited to provide such information in a relatively cost-effective and noninvasive manner.

## References


1. Sobin LH, Hermanek P, Hutter RVP. TNM classification of malignant tumors: A comparison between the new (1987) and the old editions. Cancer 61:2310–2314, 1988.
2. Manual for Staging of Cancer, 3rd ed. American Joint Committee on Cancer. Beahrs OH, Henson DE, Hutter RVP, Myers MH (eds). Philadelphia: J.B. Lippincott, 1988.
3. Rubin P. Concepts of cancer staging. In Calabresi P, Schein P, Rosenberg S (eds): Medical Oncology, Basic principles and Clinical Management of Cancer. New York: Macmillan, 1986, pp 157–177.
4. Bótet JF, Lightdale CJ, Zauber AG, Gerdes H, Urmacher C, Brennan MF. Preoperative staging of esophageal cancer: Comparison of endoscopic US and dynamic CT. Radiology 181:419, 1991.
5. Grimm H, Sollano J, Hamper K, Noar M, Soehendra N. Endoscopic ultrasound (EUS) of esophagogastric cancer: A new requirement for preoperative staging? [Abstract] Gastrointest Endosc 34:176, 1988.
6. Lightdale CJ, Bótet JF. Esophageal carcinoma. Pre-operative staging and evaluation of anastomotic recurrence. Gastrointest Endosc 36:S11, 1990.
7. Souquet JC, Napoleon B, Pujol B, Valette PJ, Chollet R, Lambert R. Endosonography-guided treatment of esophageal carcinoma. Endoscopy 24:(suppl 1)324, 1992.
8. Tio TL, Coene PPLO, Schouwink MH, Tytgat GNJ. Esophagogastric carcinoma: Preoperative TNM classification with endosonography. Radiology 173:411, 1989.
9. Tio TL, Cohen P, Coene PP, Udding J, Den Hartog Jager FCA, Tytgat GNJ. Endosonography and computed tomography of esophageal carcinoma: Preoperative classification compared to the new (1987) TNM system. Gastroenterology 96:1478, 1989.
10. Ziegler K, Sanft C, Semsch B, Friedrich M, Gregor M, Riecken EO. Endosonography is superior to computed tomography in staging tumors of the esophagus and cardia. [Abstract] Gastroenterology 94:517, 1988.
11. Souquet JC, Napoléon B, Pujol B, Keriven O, Ponchon T, Descos F, Lambert R. Endoscopic ultrasonography in the preoperative staging of esophageal cancer. Endoscopy 26:764, 1994.
12. Rice TW, Boyce GA, Sivak MV Jr. Esophageal ultrasound and the preoperative staging of carcinoma of the esophagus. J Thorac Cardiovasc Surg 101:536, 1991.
13. Rice TW. Esophageal ultrasound in the preoperative staging of esophageal carcinoma: The Cleveland Clinic experience. Presented at Endoscopic Ultrasonography: A Tutorial, March 21–22, 1991, Cleveland, Ohio.
14. Fockens P, Van den Brande JHM, van Dullemen HM, van Lanschot JJB, Tytgat GNJ. Endosonographic T-staging of esophageal carcinoma: A learning curve. Gastrointest Endosc 44:58–62, 1996.
15. Natsugoe S, Yoshinaka H, Morinaga T, Shimada M, Baba M, Fukumoto T, Stein HJ, Aikou T. Ultrasonographic detection of lymph-node metastases in superficial carcinoma of the esophagus. Endoscopy 28:674–679, 1996.
16. Tio TL, Den Hartog Jager FCA, Tytgat GNJ. The role of endoscopic ultrasonography in assessing local resectability of oesophagogastric malignancies. Scand J Gastroenterol 21(suppl 123):78, 1986.
17. Catalano MF, Sivak MV Jr, Bedford RA, Falk GW, van Stolk, R, Presa F, Van Dam J. Observer variation and reproducibility of endoscopic ultrasonography. Gastrointest Endosc 41:115, 1995.
18. Burtin P, Napoléon B, Palazzo L, Roseau G, Souquet J-C, Calès P. Interobserver agreement in endoscopic ultrasonography staging of esophageal cardia cancer. Gastrointest Endosc 43:20–24, 1996.
19. Ginsberg GG, Al-Kawas FH, Nguyen CC, Tio TL, Johnson MC, Fleischer DE, Zeman RK, Benjamin SB. Endoscopic ultrasound evaluation of vascular involvement in esophageal cancer: A comparison with computed tomography. [Abstract] Gastrointest Endosc 39:276, 1993.
20. Yoshikane H, Tsukamoto Y, Niwa Y, Goto H, Hase S, Shimodaira M, et al. Superficial esophageal carcinoma: Evaluation by endoscopic ultrasonography. Am J Gastroenterol 89:702, 1994.
21. McLoughlin RF, Cooperberg PL, Mathieson JR, Stordy SN, Halparin LS. High resolution endoluminal ultrasonography in the staging of esophageal carcinoma. J Ultrasound Med 14:725, 1995.
22. Fockens P, van Dullemen HM, Tytgat GNJ. Endosonography of stenotic esophageal carcinomas: Preliminary experience with an ultra-thin, balloon-fitted ultrasound probe in four patients. Gastrointest Endosc 40:226, 1994.
23. Murata Y, Suzuki S, Ohta M, Mitsunaga A, Hayashi K, Yoshida K, Ide H. Small ultrasonoic probes for determination of the depth of superficial esophageal cancer. Gastrointest Endosc 44:23–28, 1996.
24. Yanai H, Yoshida T, Harada T, Matsumoto Y, Nishiaki M, Shigemitsu T, Tada M, et al. Endoscopic ultrasonography of superficial esophageal cancers using a thin ultrasound probe system equipped with switchable radial and linear scanning modes. Gastrointest Endosc 44:578–582, 1996.
25. Hasegawa N, Yasuma N, Arisawa T, Hase S, Goto H, Hayakawa T. Preoperative staging of superficial esophageal carcinoma: Comparison of an ultrasound probe and standard endoscopic ultrasonography. Gastrointest Endosc 44:388–393, 1996.
26. Grimm H, Hamper K, Binmoeller KF, Soehendra N. Enlarged lymph nodes: Malignant or not? Endoscopy 24(suppl 1):320, 1992.
27. Catalano MF, Sivak MV Jr, Rice T, Gragg LA, Van Dam J. Endosonographic features predictive of lymph node metastasis. Gastrointest Endosc 40:442, 1994.
28. Vassallo P, Wernecke K, Roos N, Peters PE. Differentiation of benign from malignant superficial lymphadenopathy: The role of high-resolution US. Radiology 183:215, 1992.
29. Heintz A, Mildenberger P, Georg M, Braunstein S, Junginger Th. Endoscopic ultrasonography in the diagnosis of regional lymph nodes in esophageal and gastric cancer—Results of studies in vitro. Endoscopy 25:231, 1993.
30. Catalano MF, Sivak MV Jr, Rice TW, Bedford R, Van Dam J: Depth of tumor invasion of esophageal carcinoma (ECA) is predictive of lymph node metastasis. Role of endoscopic ultrasonography (EUS). [Abstract] Am J Gastroenterol 87(9):1245, 1992.
31. Dittler HJ, Rösch T, Lorenz R, Siewert JR, Classen M. Failure of endoscopic ultrasonography to differentiate malignant from benign lymph nodes in esophagogastric cancer. [Abstract] Gastrointest Endosc 38(2):240, 1992.
32. Krasna MJ, McLaughlin JS. Thoracoscopic lymph node staging for esophageal cancer. Ann Thorac Surg 56:671, 1993.
33. Kennedy BJ. The unified international gastric cancer staging classification system. Scand J Gastroenterol 22(suppl 133):11–13, 1987.
34. Tio TL, Coene PP, Schouwink MH, et al. Esophagogastric carcinoma: Preoperative TNM classification with endosonography. Radiology 173:411–417, 1989.
35. Tio TL, Schouwink MH, Cikot RJLM, et al. Preoperative TNM classification of gastric carcinoma by endosonography in comparison with the pathological TNM system: A prospective study of 72 cases. Hepato-gastroenterol 36:51–56, 1989.
36. Tio TL, Coene PPL, Luiken GJH, et al. Endosonography in the clinical staging of esophagogastric carcinoma. Gastrointest Endosc 36:S2–S10, 1990.
37. Caletti GC, Brocchi E, Gibilaro M, et al. Sensitivity specificity and predictive value of endoscopic ultrasonography (EUS) in the diagnosis and assessment of gastric lymphoma. Gastrointest Endosc 36:195A, 1990.
38. Andriulli A, Recchia S, De Angelis C, et al. Endoscopic ultrasonographic evaluation of patients with biopsy negative gastric linitis plastica. Gastrointest Endosc 36:611–615, 1990.
39. Tio TL, Tytgat GNJ. Endoscopic ultrasonography in staging local resectability of pancreatic and periampullary malignancy. Scand J Gastroenterol 21(suppl 123):135–142, 1986.
40. Yasuda K, Mukai H, Cho E, et al. The use of endoscopic ultrasonography in the diagnosis and staging of carcinoma of the papilla of Vater. Endoscopy 20:218–222, 1988.
41. Tio TL, Tytgat GNJ, Cikot RJLM, et al. Ampullopancreatic carcinoma: Preoperative TNM classification with endosonography. Radiology 175:455–461, 1990.
42. Tio TL, Sie LH, Kallimanis G, Luiken GJHM, Kimmings AN, Huibregste K, Tytgat GNJ. Staging of ampullary and pancreatic carcinoma: Comparison between endosonography and surgery. Gastrointest Endosc 44:706–713, 1996.
43. Steele GD, Augenlicht LH, Begg CB, et al. Adjuvant therapy for patients with colon and rectal cancer. JAMA 264:1444–1450, 1990.

44. Menck HR, Garfinkel L, Dodd GD. Preliminary report of the national cancer data base. CA—A Cancer J for Clin 41:7–18, 1991.
45. Rifkin MD, McGlynn ET, Marks G. Endorectal sonographic prospective staging of rectal cancer. Scand J Gastroenterol 21(suppl 123): 99–103, 1986.
46. Kramann B, Hildebrandt U. Computed tomography versus endosonography in the staging of rectal carcinoma: A comparative study. Int J Colorect Dis 1:216–218, 1986.
47. Beynon J, Mortensen NJMcC, Foy DMA, et al. Preoperative assessment of mesorectal lymph node involvement in rectal cancer. Br J Surg 76:276–279, 1989.
48. Rotte KH, Kluhs L, Kleinau H, et al. Computed tomography and endosonography in the preoperative staging of rectal carcinoma. Eur J Radiol 9:187–190, 1989.
49. Jochem RJ, Reading CC, Dozois RR, et al. Endorectal ultrasonographic staging of rectal carcinoma. Mayo Clin Proc 65:1571–1577, 1990.
50. Roubein LD, David C, DuBrow R, et al. Endoscopic ultrasonography in staging rectal cancer. Am J Gastroenterol 85:1391–1394, 1990.
51. Hizawa K, Suekane H, Aoyagi K, Matsumoto T, Nakamura S, Fujishima M. Use of endosonographic evaluation of colorectal tumor depth in determining the appropriateness of endoscopic mucosal resection. Am J Gastroenterol 91:768–771, 1996.
52. Saitoh Y, Obara T, Einami K, Nomura M, Taruishi M, Ayabe T, et al. Efficacy of high-frequency ultrasound probes for the preoperative staging of invasion depth in flat and depressed colorectal tumors. Gastrointest Endosc 44:34–39, 1996.
53. Roubein LD, Lynch P, Glober G, Sinicrope FA. Interobserver variability in endoscopic ultrasonography: A prospective evaluation. Gastrointest Endosc 44:573–577, 1996.
54. Jafri IH, Saltzman JR, Colby JM, Krims PE. Evaluation of the clinical impact of endoscopic ultrasonography in gastrointestinal disease. Gastrointest Endosc 44:367–370, 1996.
55. Nickl NJ, Bhutani MS, Catalano M, et al. Clinical implications of endoscopic ultrasound: The American Endosonography Club study. Gastrointest Endosc 44:371–377, 1996.
56. Chang KJ. Endoscopic ultrasonography: Moving towards permanence. Gastrointest Endosc 44:502–504, 1996.

CHAPTER

# Pitfalls in Endosonographic Imaging

Thomas Rösch
Meinhard Classen

Endoscopic ultrasonography (EUS) is a sensitive imaging method for staging a variety of gastrointestinal tumors, including esophageal, gastric, and pancreatic cancers. There are meticulous studies of EUS for imaging pancreatic duct anomalies (1) and detailing the endosonographic patterns of benign gastric ulcers and gastric carcinomas (2–4). Studies such as these suggest that microscopic changes may be detectable by EUS, a possibility that would extend endosonography to almost every field of gastroenterologic diagnosis. However, enthusiasm was tempered by skepticism as the limits of endosonographic imaging became evident. Ultrasonic images are imperfect because practical imaging systems have limited spatial, contrast, and temporal resolutions (5). The environment in which endoscopic ultrasound imaging operates is imposed by the physical and biologic properties of the imaged tissue. Imaging artifacts produced by the interaction between the ultrasound transducer and the target structure (tangential imaging, mirror-image artifact, etc.) are just some of the artifacts that can confound interpretation of endosonographic imaging (5,6). In addition, endosonographic interpretation is quite subjective, leading to substantial interobserver variation (7,8) and requiring a dedicated and prolonged period of instruction (9). The following sections offer practical advice based on our own experience together with the study and discussions of the results of other investigators.

## Pitfall: You Will See What You Expect to See

Many reports of the accuracy of EUS in detecting small lesions have not been based on blinded studies. This is problematic as the examiner's considerable bias in ultrasound imaging can lead to an overstatement of the role for EUS for certain indications (e.g., the differential diagnosis of esophageal, gastric, and pancreatic lesions). EUS is virtually never the primary method of investigation (with a few exceptions, such as the detection of pancreatic neuroendocrine tumors); rather, it is used to derive additional information about lesions that have already been diagnosed by other methods, mainly upper-gastrointestinal endoscopy. The experienced endosonographer is almost always able to create a tumor-like image somewhere in the pancreatic head or the gastric antrum. This is especially true when the endosonographer is expected to identify a tumor suspected from other imaging techniques such as x-ray, ERCP, etc. If, for example, biopsy specimens are equivocal for gastric lymphoma, a "slight thickening of the wall" in the region in question can almost always be seen at EUS even though the actual evidence of lymphoma is far from conclusive (Fig. 11–1).

## Pitfall: EUS Cannot Provide a Histologic Diagnosis

The high resolution of the images of the gastrointestinal wall and pancreas provided by EUS has encouraged the expectation that specific EUS criteria for malignant or benign changes must exist. The question of benign versus malignant is a common clinical problem with respect to many lesions such as the esophageal stricture, gastric ulcer, or pancreatic mass. This question cannot be answered by EUS, as has been demonstrated at least for gastric ulcers (2,10), pancreatic tumors (11,12), and regional lymph nodes in patients with esophageal carcinoma (13). On the contrary, EUS may add to the confusion inherent in these diagnostic problems. This is clearly the case in the differential diagnosis of esophageal stenosis. A prospective, blinded study is urgently needed before EUS can be recommended for the detection of carcinoma in Barrett's esophagus or achalasia (Fig. 11–2) when this diagnosis is not at least suspected at endoscopy or by CT scanning. In contrast to previous observations (14,15,16), EUS was found to be unreliable in the detection and staging of malignancy in patients with Barrett's esophagus and high-grade dysplasia using the dedicated echoendoscope (17). The use of high-resolution ultrasound probes may be more capable of detecting such superficial lesions in patients with Barrett's esophagus (18). Similarly, the distal esophageal wall thickening commonly observed in patients with achalasia must not be mistaken for tumor (pseudoachalasia). Patients with achalasia often have a tortuous esophagus, leading to tangential imaging and artifact production (6). As in the case of patients with Barrett's esophagus, the use of high-resolution ultrasound probes has been shown to be capable of imaging the intramural muscular layer

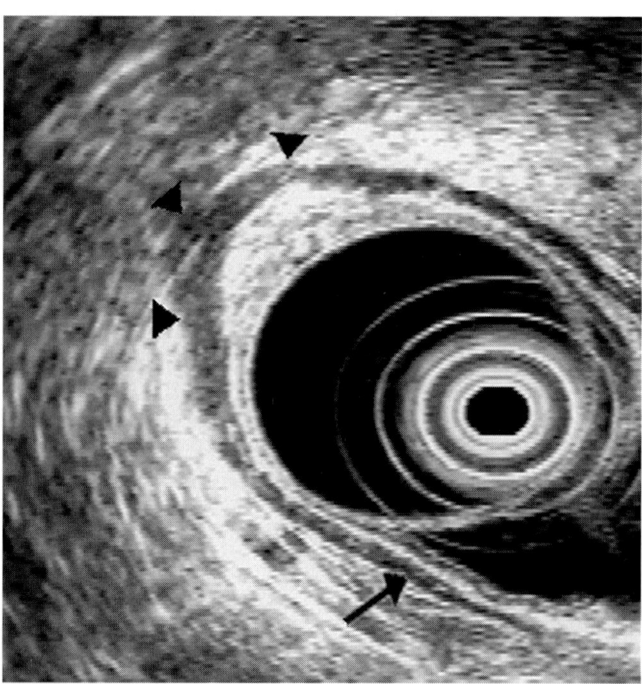

**FIGURE 11–1**

Oblique scanning of the gastric antrum leading to a significant broadening of the mucosa/submucosa (hyperechoic) and muscularis propia (hypoechoic) (arrowheads); the normal wall is demarcated by an arrow.

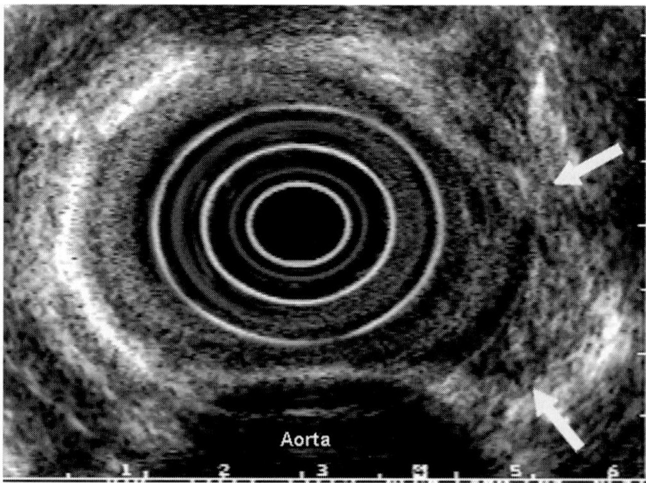


**FIGURE 11–2**

Oblique scanning of the cardia in a patient with achalasia leads to an eccentric "pseudo-tumorous" wall thickening (arrows); the remaining circumference exhibits diffuse thickening with the layer structure being hardly recognizable. This is due to a sphincter spasm and an insufficient focal distance between the transducer and wall.

thickening in patients with achalasia (19). Although high-resolution endoluminal sonography cannot be used to differentiate patients with achalasia from normal controls, it may be useful in the differential diagnosis of patients with esophageal motility disorders (19).

Although numerous studies confirm that EUS is highly accurate in the primary staging of esophageal, gastric, pancreatic, and rectal cancers (20–24), there are reservations about its accuracy for restaging these lesions. Malignant esophageal strictures limit the accuracy of esophageal cancer staging. They preclude passage of the dedicated echoendoscope, limiting the amount of tumor that can be studied endosonographically and increasing the risk of the procedure (25,26,27). Newer, high-resolution, nonendoscopic esophagoprobes may im-prove the ability to stage patients with high-grade malignant strictures as well as diminish the risk of esophageal perforation (28). It is likely that the fibrous and inflammatory changes that occur in response to radiotherapy and chemotherapy cannot be distinguished from residual malignancy by EUS. It may not be possible, therefore, for EUS to determine the actual response of a tumor to these therapeutic modalities (29,30).

## Pitfall: Producing Tumors by the "Oblique-Scanning Method"

Accurate discrimination of structures and determination of their size is possible only when the sector scan plane is nearly perpendicular to the surface of the imaged lesion. An oblique scanning plane broadens gastric, esophageal, and pancreatic lesions and blurs the layers and borders. With this incorrect technique, the EUS of a normal esophageal or gastric wall can be transformed to show localized thickening, even with loss of the normal layer structure, and the diagnosis of "tumor" is confirmed (Fig. 11–3). This pitfall is likely to occur in the gastric antrum with prominent but otherwise normal gastric folds, and in the esophagus immediately proximal to a stenosis. Oblique scanning may lead to overstaging of esophageal and gastric tumors by blurring the underlying (intact) wall layers. In pancreatic carcinoma, the relation of a tumor to a vessel (e.g., the portal vein in pancreatic head cancer) can be assessed correctly only if both structures are nearly perpendicular to the scanning plane. Many minor changes in the position of the transducer relative to the lesion are usually needed in order to determine whether the findings are due to artifact or actual tumor infiltration.

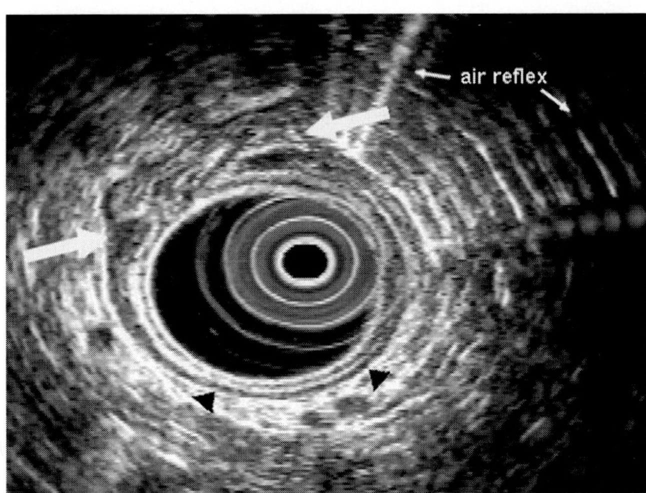


**FIGURE 11–3**

Oblique scanning through the angular fold leads to a diffuse broadening with a chaotic architecture of the layer pattern (arrows); the normal wall scanned perpendicularly is demarcated by arrowheads. Interfering gas (poor transducer and balloon contact with the wall) leads to air artifact.

## Pitfall: Measurement of Wall Thickness Is Not Exact

EUS diagnosis in certain disorders such as inflammatory bowel disease (31,32) or esophageal motility disorders (33–38) is based on measurements of wall thickness. Such measurements are subject to considerable interobserver variation, even when the same videotape is shown to different examiners. This is

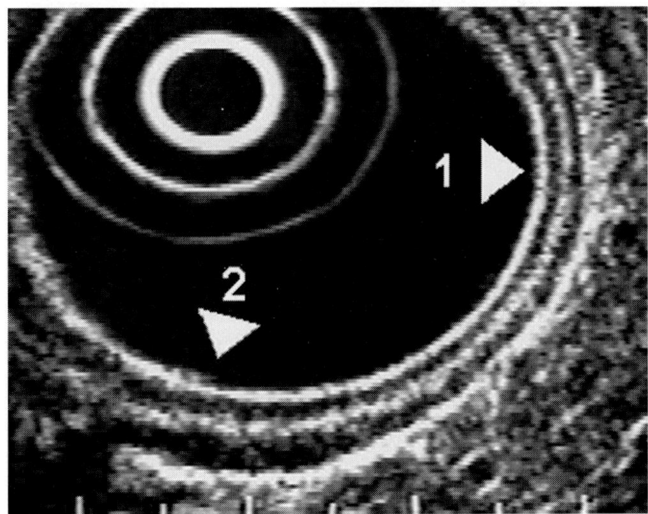


**FIGURE 11–4**

Thickness of wall layers is dependent on the angle of scanning (oblique versus perpendicular) and on the degree of balloon compression; for these reasons, the diameters of the layers vary greatly between positions 1 and 2.

because changes in the position of the ultrasound transducer relative to the wall produce changes in the size or thickness of the layers. Furthermore, variations in the degree of distension of the balloon with water when EUS is performed in the esophagus and duodenum result in changes in the apparent thickness of the wall layers (unpublished observations) (Fig. 11–4). Ødegaard and colleagues have shown in vitro that the amount of pressure applied to the gastrointestinal wall influences the endosonographic measurement of wall thickness (39). In the absence of standardized conditions, EUS measurements should be regarded as approximations and used with caution.

## Pitfall: Misinterpretation of Normal Structures

Knowledge of the EUS anatomy as well as various normal structures and lesions is mandatory to avoid misinterpretation of normal structures leading to clinically relevant false-positive diagnoses. In many cases the anatomic substrate of these structures is not precisely known. The most important pitfalls are the following:

- Para-aortic tissue in the area of the distal esophagus can be misinterpreted as tumor tissue surrounding or even enveloping the aorta, especially when there is a distal esophageal carcinoma (Fig. 11–5).
- The ventral anlage of the pancreas appears as a more hypoechoic triangular area in the lateral pancreatic head; in certain sections it may look rounded and hence be misinterpreted as a tumor. Repeated scanning will show that this area respects the borders of the pancreas and shows transition with the more echo-rich remaining pancreas. It can be found in one-third to two-thirds of all patients (40,41).
- The caudate lobe of the liver can be roundish and echo-poor on certain EUS sections and thus can be mixed up with a pancreatic tumor (Fig. 11–6).
- There are many small vascular structures around the duodenum, stomach, and esophagus whose exact nature is difficult or impossible to determine. Around the duodenum, such vascular structures may be misinterpreted as the pancreatic or common bile duct. Precise delineation of the pancreatic gland, according to the well-defined landmarks (large vessels), should be attempted before a small ductular structure is ascribed to these ducts.

Generally, endoscopic ultrasonography is a very precise imaging method that demonstrates structures and lesions at a size of 2–3 mm with an image resolution hitherto unknown. This, however, may lead to overinterpretations and overestimations. A critical approach is mandatory to correctly define the role of EUS in gastroenterologic diagnostics.

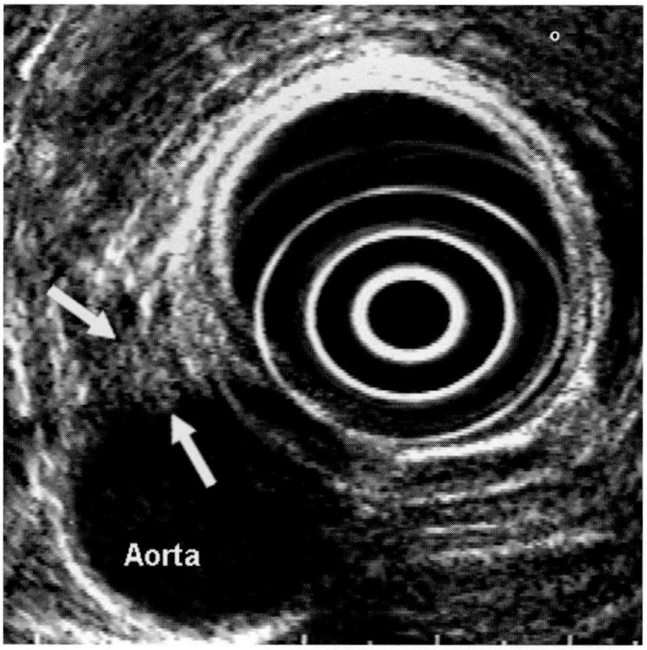

**FIGURE 11–5**

Triangle-like para-aortal tissue, as can often be seen from the distal esophagus in normal subjects.

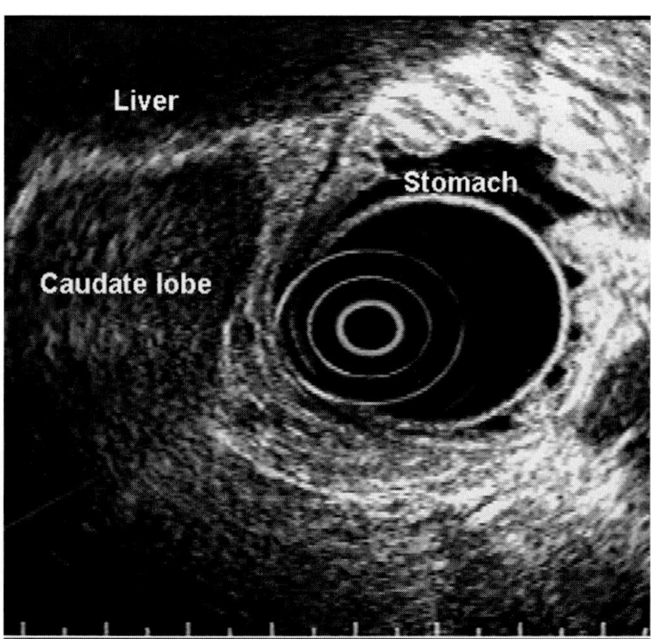


**FIGURE 11–6**

The caudate lobe can be misinterpreted as mass lesion.

## References


1. Mitake M, Nakazawa S, Naitoh Y, et al. Value of endoscopic ultrasonography in the detection of anomalous connections of the pancreatobiliary duct. Endoscopy 23:177–220, 1991.
2. Yasuda K, Nakajima M, Cho E, Kobayashi M, Kawai K. Benign versus malignant gastric ulcers: A role for endoscopic ultrasonography? In Dancygier H, Classen M (eds): 5th International Symposium on Endoscopic Ultrasonography. Munich: Demeter Verlag (Z Gastroenterol suppl.), 1989, pp 50–56.
3. Niwa Y, Nakazawa S, Yoshino J, et al. Qualifications of gastric ulcer healing by endoscopic ultrasonography. Gastrointest Endosc 36:116–122, 1990.
4. Takemoto T, Nakata K, Aibe T, Fukumoto Y. Endoscopic sonography of H2-blocker resistant peptic ulcer. In Dancygier H, Classen M (eds): 5th International Symposium on Endoscopic Ultrasonography. Munich: Demeter Verlag (Z Gastroenterol suppl.), 1989, pp 57–63.
5. Wells PNT, Harris RA, Halliwell M. The envelope that tissue imposes on achievable ultrasonic imaging. J Ultrasound Med 11:433–439, 1992.
6. Van Dam J. Endoscopic ultrasonography in achalasia. Endoscopy 26:792–793, 1994.
7. Catalano MF, Sivak MV Jr., Bedford RA, Falk GW, van Stolk R, Presa F, Van Dam J. Observer variation and reproducibility of endoscopic ultrasonography. Gastrointest Endosc 41:115–120, 1995.
8. Burtin P, Napoléon B, Palazzo L, Roseau G, Souquet J-C, Calès P. Interobserver agreement in endoscopic ultrasonography staging of esophageal and cardia cancer. Gastrointest Endosc 43:20–24, 1996.
9. Fockens P, Van den Brande JHM, van Dullemen HM, van Lanschot JJB, Tytgat GNJ. Endosongraphic T-staging of esophageal carcinoma: A learning curve. Gastrointest Endosc 44:58–62, 1996.
10. Rösch T, Lorenz R, von Wichert A, et al. Endoscopic ultrasonography is not useful in the differential diagnosis of gastric ulcer. Gastrointest Endosc 38:241(abstract), 1992.
11. Hildebrandt U. Transrectal endosonographic technique. In Dancygier H, Classen M (eds): 5th International Symposium on Endoscopic Ultrasonography. Munich: Demeter Verlag (Z Gastroenterol suppl.), 1989, pp 13–16.
12. Palazzo L, Roseau G, Gayet B, et al. Endoscopic ultrasonography in the diagnosis and staging of pancreatic adenocarcinoma. Results of a prospective study with comparison to ultrasonography and CT scan. Endoscopy 25:143–150, 1993.
13. Catalano MF, Sivak MV Jr., Rice TW, Gragg LA, Van Dam J. Endosonographic features predictive of lymph nodes metastasis. Gastrointest Endosc 40:442–446, 1994.
14. Srivastava A, Vanagunas A, Kamel P, et al. Endoscopic ultrasound in the evaluation of Barrett's esophagus. Gastrointest Endosc 37: 244b(abstract), 1991.
15. Dancygier H, Classen M. Endoscopic ultrasonography in esophageal diseases. Gastrointest Endosc 35:220–225, 1989.
16. Srivasta AK, Vanagunas A, Kamel P, Cooper R. Endoscopic ultrasound in the evaluation of Barrett's esophagus: A preliminary report. Am J Gastroenterol 89:2192–2195, 1994.
17. Falk GW, Catalano MF, Sivak MV Jr., Rice TW, Van Dam J. Endosonography in the evaluation of patients with Barrett's esophagus and high-grade dysplasia. Gastrointest Endosc 40:207–212, 1994.
18. Adrain AL, Cassidy MJ, Schiano TD, Liu J-B, Miller LS. High resolution endoluminal sonography (HRES) is a sensitive means of identifying Barrett's metaplasia. Am J Gastroenterol 91:1902A, 1996.
19. Miller LS, Liu J-B, Barbarevech CA, Baranowski RJ, Dhuria M, Schiano TD, Goldberg BB, Fisher RS. High-resolution endoluminal sonography in achalasia. Gastrointest Endosc 42:545–549, 1995.
20. Rösch T, Classen M. Gastroenterologic Endosonography. Stuttgart: Thieme, 1992.
21. Lightdale CJ. Endoscopic ultrasonography in the diagnosis, staging, and follow-up of esophageal and gastric cancer. Endoscopy 24:297–303, 1992.
22. Rösch T, Lorenz R, Braig C, et al. Endoscopic ultrasonography in diagnosis and staging of pancreatic and biliary tumors. Endoscopy 24:304–308, 1992.
23. Tio TL, Weijers OB, Hulsman F, et al. Endosonography of colorectal diseases. Endoscopy 24:309–314, 1992.
24. Rösch T, Lorenz R, Classen M. Endoscopic ultrasonography in the evaluation of colon and rectal disease. Gastrointest Endosc 36: S33–S39, 1990.
25. Catalano MF, Van Dam J, Sivak MV Jr. Malignant esophageal strictures: Staging accuracy of endoscopic ultrasonography. Gastrointest Endosc 535–539, 1995.
26. Roubein LD. Endoscopic ultrasonography and the malignant esophageal stricture: Implications and complications. Gastrointest Endosc 41:613–615, 1995.
27. Van Dam J, Rice TW, Catalano MF, Kirby T, Sivak MV, Jr. High grade malignant stricture is predictive of esophageal tumor stage: Risks of endosonographic evaluation. Cancer 71:2910–2917, 1993.
28. Binmoeller KF, Seifert H, Seitz U, Izbicki JR, Kida M, Soehendra N. Ultrasonic esophagoprobe for TNM staging of highly stenosing esopahgeal carcinoma. Gastrointest Endosc 41:547–552, 1995.
29. Dittler HJ, Rösch T, Fink U, et al. Endosonographic re-staging of carcinoma of the esophagus and cardia following radio- and chemotherapy. Gastrointest Endosc 38:241(abstract), 1992.
30. Hordijk ML, Kok TC, Wilson JHP, et al. Assessment of response of esophageal carcinoma to induction chemotherapy. Endoscopy 25: 1993. (in press).
31. Shimizu S, Tada M, Kawai K. Value of endoscopic ultrasonography in the assessment of inflammatory bowel diseases. Endoscopy 24:354–358, 1992.
32. Hildebrandt U, Kraus J, Ecker KW, et al. Endosonographic differentiation of mucosal and transmucosal non-specific inflammatory bowel disease. Endoscopy 24:359–363, 1992.
33. Devière J, Dunham F, Rickaert F, et al. Endoscopic ultrasonography in achalasia. Gastroenterology 96:1210–1213, 1989.
34. Devière J, Dunham F, Cremer M. Reply to letter by Ponsot et al. Gastroenterology 98:253, 1990.
35. Ponsot P, Chaussade S, Palazzo P, et al. Echoendoscopie et megaesophage: Frequence et particularites chez des malades ayant un epaississement de la musculeuse. Gastroenterol Clin Biol 13:240(abstract), 1989.
36. Ziegler K, Sanft C, Friedrich M, et al. Endosonographic appearance of the esophagus in achalasia. Endoscopy 22:1–4, 1990.
37. Van Dam J, Falk GW, Sivak MV Jr, Achkar E, Rice TW. Endosonographic evaluation of the patient with achalasia: Appearance of the esophagus using the echoendoscope. Endoscopy 27:185–190, 1995.
38. Ikeda M, Fujino MA, Nakamura T, et al. Dysphagia and thickening of the muscularis propria of the esophagus diagnosed by endoscopic ultrasonography. Gastroenterology 98:63(abstract), 1990.
39. Ødegaard S, Kimmey MB, Martin RW, et al. The effects of applied pressure on the thickness, layers, and echogenicity of gastrointestinal wall ultrasound images. Gastrointest Endosc 38:351–356, 1992.
40. Rösch T, Lorenz R, Birkenfeld G, et al. The normal pancreas in endoscopic ultrasound. Gastrointest Endosc 37:255(abstract), 1991.
41. Wiersema MJ, Hawes RH, Lehman GA, et al. Prospective evaluation of endoscopic ultrasonography and endoscopic retrograde cholangiopancreatography in patients with chronic abdominal pain of suspected pancreatic origin. Endoscopy 25:555–564, 1993.
42. Grech P. Mirror-image artifact with endoscopic ultrasonography and reappraisal of the fluid-air interface. Gastrointest Endosc 39:700–703, 1993.

SECTION

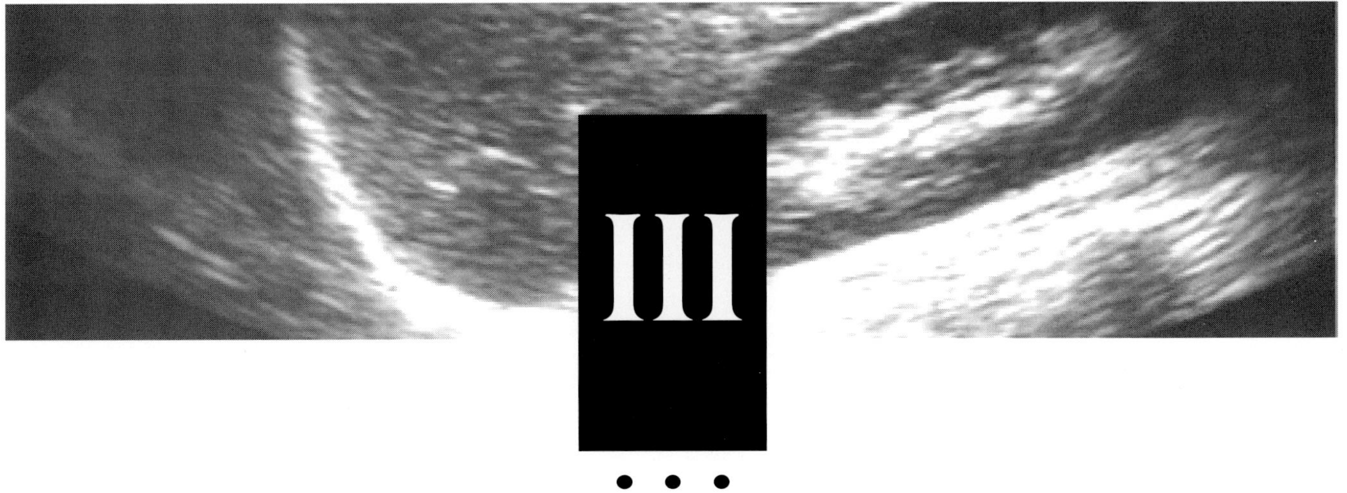

# III

# Endosonography of the Esophagus

CHAPTER

# Staging Esophageal Cancer
## THE CLEVELAND EXPERIENCE

Thomas W. Rice
Gregory Zuccaro, Jr.

Endoscopic ultrasonography (EUS) has been available at The Cleveland Clinic Foundation since 1987 for staging patients with esophageal cancer. EUS is uniquely suited to determine the depth of tumor invasion (T) of an esophageal malignancy, it is helpful in establishing the status of regional lymph nodes (N), and it may be used as a complementary imaging technique to assess the sites of distant metastases (M) that are in direct contact with the upper GI tract. We have used the clinical staging information acquired upon EUS as one of the major determinants of patient management, establishing operability and appropriateness of induction therapy. EUS has also been used in retreatment staging, assessing the response to induction therapy prior to planned surgical resection. In addition, we have utilized EUS in the surveillance of patients following resection of esophageal carcinomas and in patients with Barrett's esophagus.

## Pretreatment (Clinical) Staging of Esophageal Carcinoma

### Survival as a Function of Pretreatment Stage

The depth of tumor invasion (T) is the critical factor affecting survival in node-negative (N0) patients without evidence of distant metastases (M0) (1). Following surgical resection, patients with T*is* (intraepithelial) carcinomas and T1 intramucosal (limited to the lamina propria or muscularis mucosa) carcinomas have a similar five-year survival of 80–85% (2). For N0 patients, once the tumor breaches the muscularis mucosa, survival falls dramatically. Our data suggest that there is no survival difference between T1 submucosal (limited to the submucosa) carcinomas and T2 (limited to the muscularis propria) carcinomas, with a five-year survival of approximately 40–50% for each (1). When the tumor invades beyond the muscularis propria and into the periesophageal tissues (T3), survival falls even further (<25% at five years).

Stratification by T stage is not necessary if regional lymph node metastases (N1) have occurred. In our experience the survival of patients with T1N1M0, T2N1M0, and T3N1M0 carcinomas is similar. The survival rate for patients with N1 carcinomas is much worse than that of patients with T3N0M0 carcinomas (1). Although survival of patients with N1 disease is independent of T, an important relationship remains between T and N1. The esophagus is unique among gastrointestinal hollow viscus organs in that its lymphatics are found in the lamina propria and muscularis mucosa. In the stomach and the small and large intestines, lymphatics are not encountered by invading tumors until the submucosa. This superficial presence of lymphatics results in a small but significant 5% incidence of regional lymph node metastases (N1) in T1 intramucosal esophageal carcinomas (2). As the tumor invades deeper into the esophageal wall, the rate of regional lymph node metastases (N1) increases, with N1 disease found in approximately 25% of T1 submucosal tumors, 40–50% of T2 tumors, and 80% of T3 or T4 tumors. Since no lymphatics penetrate the basement membrane, regional lymph node metastases are not seen in Tis carcinomas.

Distant hematogenous metastatic disease (M1) further decreases survival. Our experience suggests that, although considered M1 disease by definition, celiac axis lymph node metastases (M1) in esophagogastric junction carcinomas do not reduce survival any more than do regional lymph node metastases (N1). It is thus our practice to treat this subset of M1 tumors in much the same way we manage tumors with regional lymph node metastases.

## The Role of Endoscopic Ultrasonography

Surgery is the most effective means of treating superficial esophageal carcinomas and carcinomas confined to the esophageal wall. Once the tumor has penetrated the muscularis propria or metastasized to regional lymph nodes, the likelihood of surgical cure at five years drops below 25% and no other effective standard therapy is available. Distant metastatic disease, except for celiac axis lymph node involvement, is incurable by any current therapy.

The information provided by endoscopic ultrasonography is unlikely to benefit those patients with underlying co-morbid illnesses that may exclude them from consideration for surgery. An EUS examination is part of the evaluation of all patients with newly diagnosed esophageal carcinoma who are considered operative candidates. Endoscopic ultrasonography is performed in such patients after distant metastatic disease has been excluded by CT scanning. The identification of both invasion beyond the esophageal wall (T3 or T4) and regional lymph node metastases (N1) is critical to patient outcome. Patients whose tumors are confined to the esophageal wall without regional lymph node metastases (T2N0M0 carcinomas or less) immediately undergo surgical resection. In the small subgroup of these patients whose pathologic staging demonstrates a more advanced carcinoma at resection, postoperative concurrent chemotherapy and radiation therapy are considered. It is our practice to offer patients with locally advanced carcinomas (T3N0M0 carcinomas or greater) multimodality therapy, since surgery alone is unlikely to be curative.

The pretreatment staging provided by EUS has proved essential in the evaluation of multimodality protocols administered at The Cleveland Clinic Foundation. When surgery is the first step in a multimodality regimen, the pathologic stage is directly comparable to the pretreatment stage. However, most multimodality regimens reserve surgery (and hence pathologic staging) until after an induction phase consisting of chemotherapy, radiation therapy, or both. In this case the pathologic stage may be very different from the pretreatment stage. Previous studies of induction therapy followed by surgery have been flawed not only by an inability to accurately determine the pretreatment stage of these patients but by the inability to accurately assess tumor response. Defining the appropriate patient population and stratification of these patients in a clinical trial are impossible without precise knowledge of depth of tumor invasion (T) or regional lymph node status (N). If pretreatment staging is inaccurate, the survival advantage attributed to treatment may reflect only an unequal distribution of better-prognosis patients.

In patients receiving multimodality therapy, pretreatment EUS identifies appropriate candidates and provides the reference point (pretreatment stage) that will be used to determine tumor response following induction therapy.

## Technique

We budget approximately 45 minutes for the complete EUS examination. For patients with high-grade malignant strictures, where neither the endoscope nor echoendoscope will pass, the required time is considerably shorter. Because the GF-UM20 echoendoscope provided an inadequate endoscopic inspection of the upper gastrointestinal tract, every EUS study was preceded by a standard EGD. However, with the introduction of the new videoscope, the initial endoscopic examination may be performed with the echoendoscope in most cases. The examination is extremely well tolerated with conscious sedation. We utilize high frequencies (12 MHz) to establish the T status of the primary tumor and lower frequencies (7.5 MHz) to establish the N status. We also use 7.5 MHz for transgastric scanning of distant sites (M) such as the celiac axis and the left lateral segment of the liver. Excessive balloon insufflation may lead to overdistension and the obliteration of the ultrasound layers of the esophageal wall, and hence overstaging of T. We currently prefer a gentle water insufflation technique combined with minimal balloon distension to prevent compression of the esophageal wall. In all patients with cervical and upper thoracic carcinomas, we perform bronchoscopy to exclude airway involvement. This examination is performed in the endoscopy suite immediately after the EUS examination.

## Clinical Experience

Our early experience with EUS staging of esophageal carcinoma demonstrated that there are both technical and interpretive learning periods (3). In this work, the accuracy of T determination was just 59%. A common error was overstaging, secondary to technical errors such as balloon overdistension and interpretive inexperience. With increased training, the accuracy of T determination has increased to 80% and is comparable to that of other centers (4).

In our initial experience, the accuracy of EUS in determination of regional lymph node status (N) was 70%; this has increased to 84% with improvement in our technical and interpretive skills (3,4,5). EUS is also accurate in staging cervical and abdominal lymph nodes in patients with superficial esophageal cancer (6–8). In a recent retrospective review of 100 consecutively staged patients, the EUS determination of N was 89% sensitive, 75% specific, and 84% accurate (5). The positive predictive value of EUS for N1 disease in this study was 86% and the negative predictive value was 79%. A patient was 24.4 times more likely to have N1 disease if EUS detected regional lymph nodes. The ultrasound evaluation of a visualized node should include assessment of size, shape, border characteristics, and internal echo pattern. In this study the single most sensitive parameter in detecting N1 disease was a hypoechoic internal echo pattern, followed by a sharp border, a round shape, and finally size greater than 10 mm. These features demonstrated an additive effect on accuracy of N1 prediction. When all four factors were present, the accuracy of N1 detection was 100%. Our recent experience with in vitro EUS examination of resected regional lymph node shows that size and the computer-assisted image analysis of echo pattern are the EUS characteristics with significant predictive value.

### *High-Grade Strictures*

Twenty-seven percent of patients who presented to The Cleveland Clinic Foundation for treatment of newly diagnosed esophageal carcinoma had high-grade strictures that would not permit passage of the echoendoscope. In our initial enthusiasm for EUS assessment of all patients, we routinely used wire-guided dilatation in these patients to facilitate EUS examination of the entire tumor, distal esophagus, and stomach. However, this procedure of dilatation and immediate complete EUS examination led to an unacceptably high perforation rate (25%), and has since been discontinued. EUS staging of just the proximal aspect of these tumors is inadequate. This partial staging by EUS in the area above the stricture has an accuracy of 33% at our institution. However, we have found that 91% of patients with high-grade malignant strictures that do not allow passage of the ultrasound endoscope have either stage III or IV disease at pathologic staging (9,10). The inability to pass the echoendoscope is perhaps the best predictor of advanced stage. We have established the presence of T4 disease in this setting with the use of miniature ultrasound probes (11). Our finding of an unacceptably high perforation rate for patients with high-grade malignant stenoses is not universal; others have reported lower perforation rates when same-day dilatation is performed for patients with malignant strictures (12). Others have also used high-resolution endoluminal ultrasonography for staging esophageal cancer (13,14).

## Retreatment Staging after Induction Therapy

Theoretically, determination of the stage following induction therapy (retreatment stage), if reliable, helps direct further treatment. Ideally, a complete response might justify cessation of therapy. A partial response or no response would mandate additional nonsurgical therapy or, alternatively, immediate resection. Disease progression might suggest the need for a purely palliative approach.

At present, retreatment staging is performed primarily to assess response. However, published response rates show wide variation—an observation that may be more a function of inconsistent and inaccurate staging than of variability in tumor response rates. The implications of a clinical response based on such imperfect tools as barium esophogram, computed tomography (CT), or esophagoscopy are unclear.

Preliminary reports using a new staging criterion for endoscopic ultrasonography to assess recurrence of esophageal cancer after combined chemoradiation therapy have been encouraging. Giovannini et al. have shown that complete endosonographic restoration of the esophageal wall (T0) after combined therapy predicted disease-free histology in 78% of cases (15). The ability to predict a complete response after combined therapy has important implications for therapy. However, additional study is required before definitive conclusions may be drawn regarding these results.

In our early experience with induction chemotherapy using EAP (etoposide, adriamycin, and cisplatin), EUS proved the most useful and accurate staging tool to determine post-chemotherapy response at the interim evaluation (16). However, this chemotherapeutic induction proved ineffective based both on EUS and on subsequent pathologic staging (17). Had the response rate been based upon symptom relief or endoscopy, this regimen would have been considered successful in 82% of the study patients.

Our most recent experience with highly effective chemotherapy and concurrent accelerated fractionated radiation therapy has been very different (18) (Figs. 12–1, 12–2). Whether using symptom relief, barium esophogram, endoscopy, CT, or EUS, we have been completely unable to predict, prior to surgery, which patients will have no residual, viable carcinoma. Persistent dysphagia may be a sign of residual tumor, but post-therapy fibrosis alone may also account for this. At endoscopy, the discovery of mucosally based residual tumor after induction chemoradiotherapy is extremely rare; most often, the exophytic tumor seen at initial endoscopy is replaced by scarring and visible ulceration. In theory, if residual tumor in these patients is truly submucosal, endoscopic ultrasound is ideally suited to assess response to chemoradiotherapy. However, our results with EUS restaging after induction therapy have been disappointing (19). After chemoradiotherapy, it is very difficult to distinguish inflammation, fibrosis, or necrotic tumor from viable tumor. We therefore erroneously identify hypoechoic mural thickening of the esophageal wall or penetration of periesophageal tissues as persistent tumor, when in fact these changes represent only residual inflammatory change or necrosis.

Assessment of N stage after chemoradiotherapy is likewise problematic (Fig. 12–3). The usual criteria used to assess lymph node status (size, shape, border characteristics, internal echo patterns) do not seem to apply. After induction therapy, nodes will often appear elliptical with indistinct borders, the typical hallmarks of benign, reactive nodes. However, at esophagectomy, residual cancer may be identified in nodes with this appearance; presumably, the endosonographic appear-

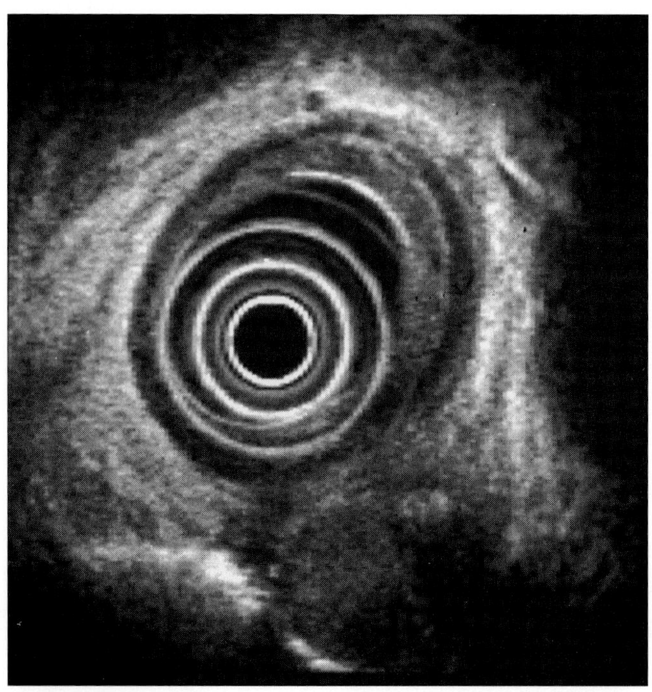

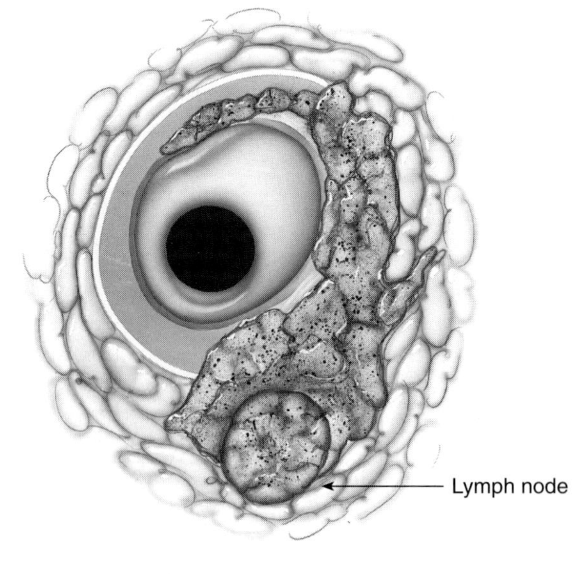


**FIGURE 12–1**

A T3N1 carcinoma prior to chemoradiotherapy. The tumor extends through the esophageal wall into the adventitia. A round, large lymph node with sharp borders and irregular internal echos is seen immediately adjacent to the primary tumor.

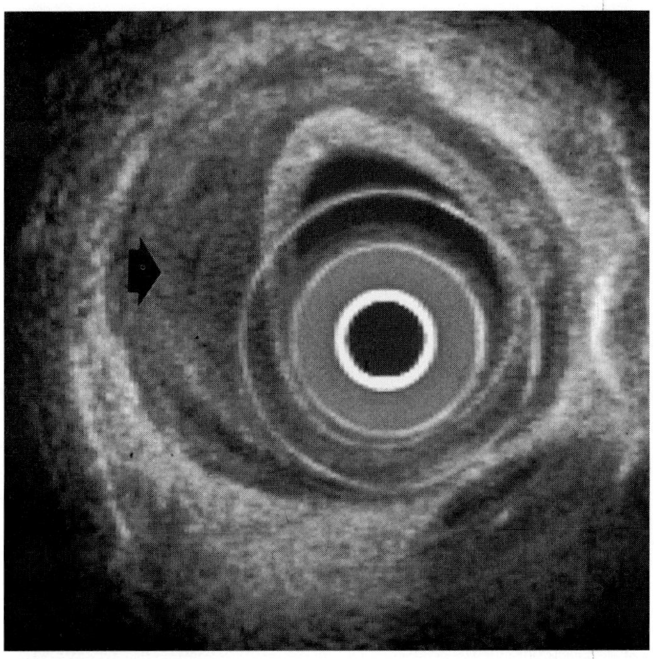

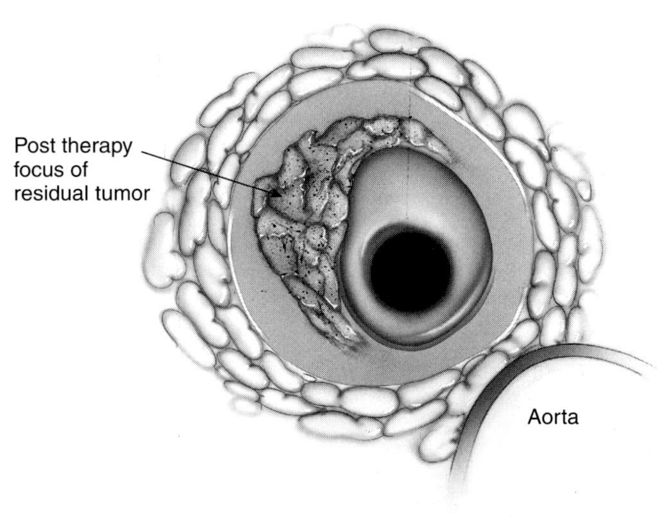


**FIGURE 12–2**

Endosonographic image of the same patient after chemoradiotherapy. Note that there is no apparent extension of tumor into the adventitia. Also, a nidus of hypoechoic residual tumor (arrow) is seen within the esophageal wall.

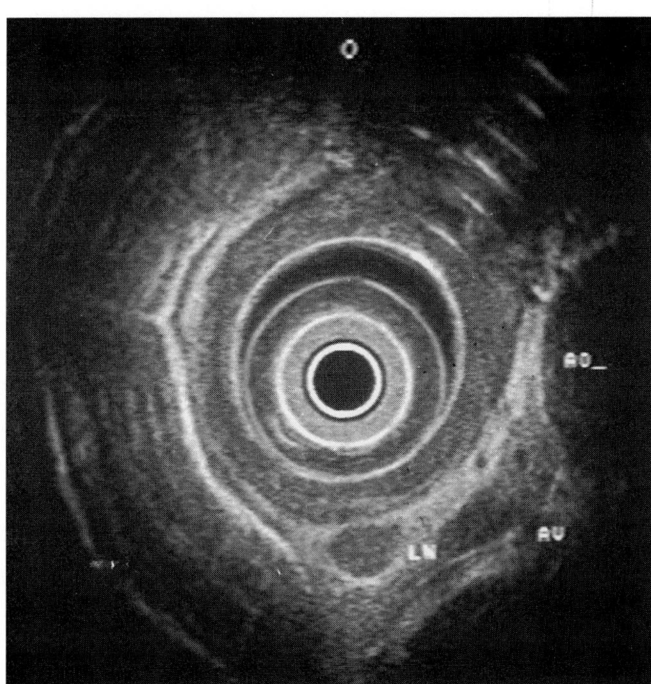


**FIGURE 12–3**

A lymph node visualized in the periesophageal tissues in a patient after chemoradiotherapy. The lymph node is irregular in shape, with indistinct borders. It fits some criteria for a reactive, rather than malignant lymph node. At pathologic staging, many nodes with this appearance are found to have residual cancer. The usual endosonographic criteria for evaluation of lymph nodes are unreliable after chemoradiotherapy.

ance of the nodes is altered by chemoradiotherapy, decreasing the reliability of the usual criteria for nodal assessment. Our poor results with interim EUS evaluation following induction therapy have been corroborated by other centers (20–22).

Although theoretically attractive, the inability to noninvasively differentiate viable carcinoma from inflammation, fibrosis, or necrotic carcinoma after effective induction chemoradiotherapy limits our ability to make treatment modifications based on EUS interim evaluations. Further research and new technologies may ultimately provide the refinements necessary for EUS to be useful in assessing induction response and determining the need for additional therapy. Although we continue to perform EUS at this juncture in our treatment protocols, the information gained is not used in clinical decision making.

## Surveillance

### Postoperative Surveillance

We have performed yearly EUS examinations of patients after resection of esophageal carcinoma (Figs. 12–4, 12–5). Submucosal thickening at the level of the anastomosis is a common and non-specific finding in the majority of patients and may be misinterpreted as an anastomotic recurrence. EUS examination of cervical

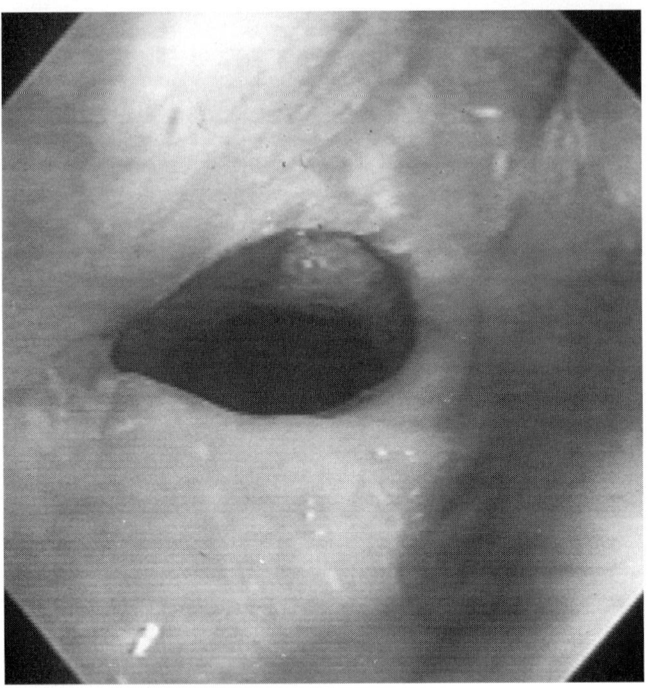

**FIGURE 12-4**

Esophagoscopy in a patient one year after successful esophagectomy.

esophagogastric anastomoses has been incomplete in many patients owing to the discomfort and intolerance of EUS examination in this location.

The use of EUS for detecting anastomotic recurrences was first reported by Lightdale et al. in a series of 40 patients with esophageal or gastric cancer (23). Twenty-four of 40 patients had local recurrence, and in 23 of the 24 it was detected by EUS. However, it was also detected by standard endoscopy and biopsy/cytology in 16 of 24 patients.

In a compilation of the early experiences at two institutions with surveillance EUS, 30 asymptomatic and 10 symptomatic patients were retrospectively reviewed (24). In the 30 asymptomatic patients, of the three recurrences two were endoscopically visible and were confirmed by biopsy within 2 months of detection. All three recurrences were detected at EUS; however, therapy was not altered by EUS detection. In addition, in one EUS study of an asymptomatic patient, anastomotic thickening was misinterpreted as a local recurrence; fortunately, no alteration of therapy resulted from this false-positive study. In the 10 symptomatic patients all four recurrences were detected by conventional esophagoscopy and biopsy. EUS confirmed these endoscopic findings.

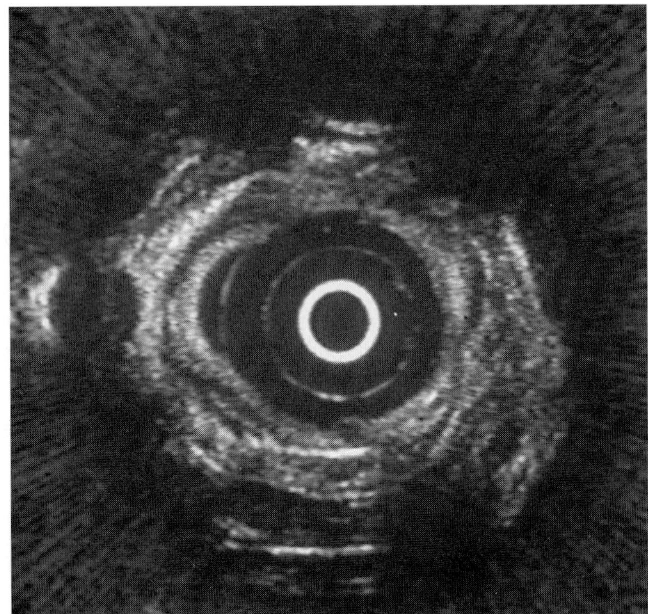

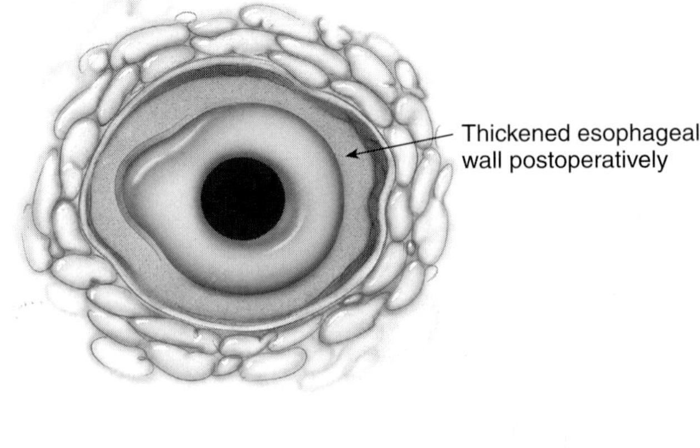


**FIGURE 12-5**

EUS of the esophageal wall at the level of the anastomosis. The submucosa is slightly thickened, which is simply postoperative change. There is no evidence of tumor recurrence.

In our experience, it is uncommon for EUS to uncover a recurrence not suspected by symptoms or documented by routine endoscopy and biopsy. EUS is not warranted in routine postoperative surveillance and should be reserved for the occasions when a local recurrence is suspected but cannot be documented by conventional endoscopic and radiographic examinations. In this instance EUS and EUS-guided needle aspiration of the perianastomotic tissue may prove beneficial.

## Surveillance for Patients with Barrett's Esophagus

We have used EUS to evaluate nine patients with high-grade dysplasia and no endoscopic evidence of invasive carcinoma in Barrett's esophagus prior to esophagectomy (25). EUS detected only one of three intramucosal carcinomas, but overstaged this early T1N0M0 (Stage I) carcinoma as a T2N1M0 (Stage IIB) carcinoma. At resection, there was no evidence of invasive carcinoma in six patients; in two of these, EUS predicted invasive T2N0M0 (Stage IIA) carcinomas. EUS did not provide the mucosal definition necessary to differentiate high-grade dysplasia from early intramucosal carcinoma. The artifacts associated with the EUS examinations of these patients caused many false-negative and false-positive studies. We do not use EUS in the surveillance of patients with Barrett's esophagus and reserve it for those patients undergoing resection of a Barrett's carcinoma.

## Summary

EUS can provide relevant information unobtainable by other means in the clinical staging of patients with esophageal carcinoma. Endosonographic staging criteria are continually being studied and refined (26). The information is essential in determining appropriate, stage-specific therapy. There is a learning curve in the performance and the interpretation of EUS examinations (27), and interobserver agreement is low for certain stages (28). Lymph node staging and the evaluation of high-grade malignant strictures present unique clinical problems. Positive correlations exist between advanced T and regional lymph node metastases (N1) and malignant strictures and advanced stage (III and IV). In the Cleveland Clinic Foundation experience, EUS has not been useful in retreatment staging following induction therapy, the routine surveillance of patients following resection of esophageal carcinomas, or the surveillance of patients with Barrett's esophagus.

## References

1. Killinger WA Jr, Rice TW, Adelstein DJ, Zuccaro G Jr, Medendorp SV, Kirby TJ, Goldblum JR. Stage II esophageal carcinoma: The significance of T and N. J Thorac Cardiovasc Surg 111:935–940, 1996.
2. Sabik JF, Rice TW, Goldblum JR, Koka A, Kirby TJ, Medendorp SV, Adelstein DJ. Superficial esophageal carcinoma. Ann Thorac Surg 60:896–902, 1995.
3. Rice TW, Boyce GA, Sivak MV. Esophageal ultrasound and the preoperative staging of carcinoma of the esophagus. J Thorac Cardiovasc Surg 101:536–544, 1991.
4. Rice TW, Sivak MJ Jr, Kirby TJ. Ultrasound staging of esophageal carcinoma. Can J Surg 34:399, 1991.
5. Catalano MF, Sivak MV Jr., Rice, TW, Gragg LA, Van Dam J. Endosonographic features predictive of lymph node metastasis. Gastrointest Endosc 40:442–446, 1994.
6. Natsugoe S, Yoshinaka H, Moringa T, Shimada M, Hokita S, Baba M, Takao S, Fukumoto T, Stein HJ, Aikou ST. Assessment of tumor invasion of the distal esophagus in carcinoma of the cardia using endoscopic ultrasonography. Endoscopy 28:750–755, 1996.
7. Yanai H, Yoshida T, Harada T, Matsumoto Y, Nishiaki M, Shigemitsu T, et al. Endoscopic ultrasonography of superficial esophageal cancers using a thin ultrasound probe system equipped with switchable radial and linear scanning modes. Gastrointest Endosc 44:578–582, 1996.
8. Hasegawa N, Niwa Y, Arisawa T, Hase S, Goto H, Hayakawa T. Preoperative staging of superficial esophageal carcinoma: Comparison of an ultrasound probe and standard endoscopic ultrasonography. Gastrointest Endosc 44:388–393, 1996.
9. Van Dam J, Rice TW, Catalano MF, Kirby TJ, Sivak MV Jr. High-grade malignant stricture is predictive of esophageal tumor stage. Cancer 71:2910–2917, 1993.
10. Catalano MF, Van Dam J, Sivak MV Jr. Malignant esophageal strictures: Staging accuracy of endoscopic ultrasonography. Gastrointest Endosc 41:535–539, 1995.
11. Zuccaro G Jr, Sivak MV Jr, Rice TW. Endoscopic ultrasound and the staging of esophageal and gastric cancer. Gastrointest Endosc Clin North America 2:625–636, 1992.
12. Kallimanis G, Gupta K, Kawas FH, et al. Endoscopic ultrasound for staging esophageal cancer with or without dilation is clinically important and safe. Gastrointest Endosc 41:540–546, 1995.
13. McLoughlin RF, Cooperberg PL, Mathieson JR, Stordy SN, Halparin LS. High resolution endoluminal ultrasonography in the staging of esophageal carcinoma. J Ultrasound Med 14:725–730, 1995.
14. Murata Y, Suzuki S, Ohta M, Mitsunaga A, Hayashi K, Yoshida K, Ide H. Small ultrasonic probes for determination of the depth of superficial esophageal cancer. Gastrointest Endosc 44:23–28, 1996.
15. Giovannini M, Seitz JF, Thomas P, Hannoun-Levy JM, Perrier H, Resbeut M, Delpero JR, Fuentes P. Endoscopic ultrasonography for assessment of the response to combined radiation therapy and chemotherapy in patients with esophageal cancer. Endoscopy 29:4–9, 1997.
16. Rice TW, Boyce GA, Sivak MV, Adelstein DJ, Kirby TJ. Esophageal carcinoma: Esophageal ultrasound assessment of preoperative chemotherapy. Ann Thorac Surg 53:972–977, 1992.
17. Adelstein DJ, Rice TW, Boyce GA, Sivak MV, Van Kirk MA, Kirby TJ, van Stolk RU, Bukowski RM. Adenocarcinoma of the esophagus and gastroesophageal junction: Clinical and pathologic assessment of response to induction chemotherapy. Am J Clin Oncol 17:14–18, 1994.
18. Adelstein DJ, Rice TW, Becker M, et al. Use of concurrent chemotherapy, accelerated fractionation radiation, and surgery for patients with esophageal carcinoma. Cancer 80:1011–1120, 1997.
19. Pimentel R, Zuccaro G, Adelstein DJ, Rice TW. Accuracy of endoscopic staging of esophageal carcinoma after successful induction chemoradiotherapy. Gastrointest Endosc 41:310, 1995.
20. Hordijk ML, Kok TC, Wilson JHP, Mulder AH. Assessment of response of esophageal carcinoma to induction chemotherapy. Endoscopy 25:592–596, 1993.

21. Dittler HJ, Fink U, Siewert GR. Response to chemotherapy in esophageal cancer. Endoscopy 26:769–771, 1994.
22. Roubein LD, DuBrow R, David C, et al. Endoscopic ultrasonography in the quantitative assessment of response to chemotherapy in patients with adenocarcinoma of the esophagus and esophagogastric junction. Endoscopy 25:587–591, 1993.
23. Lightdale CJ, Bótet JF, Kelsen DP, et al. Diagnosis of recurrent upper gastrointestinal cancer at the surgical anastomosis by endoscopic ultrasound. Gastrointest Endosc 35:407–412, 1989.
24. Catalano MF, Sivak MV Jr, Rice TW, Van Dam J. Postoperative screening for anastomotic recurrence of esophageal carcinoma by endoscopic ultrasonography. Gastrointest Endosc 42:540–544, 1995.
25. Falk GW, Catalano MF, Sivak MV Jr, Rice TW, Van Dam J. Endosonography in the evaluation of patients with Barrett's esophagus and high grade dysplasia. Gastrointest Endosc 40:207–212, 1994.
26. Brugge WR, Lee MJ, Carey RW, Mathisen DJ. Endoscopic ultrasound staging criteria for esophageal cancer. Gastrointest Endosc 45:147–152, 1997.
27 Fockens P, Van den Brande JHM, van Dullemen HM, van Lanschot JJB, Tytgat GNJ. Endosonographic T-staging of esophageal carcinoma: A learning curve. Gastrointest Endosc 44:58–62, 1996.
28. Burtin P, Napoléon B, Palazzo L, Roseau G, Souquet J-C, Calès P. Interobserver agreement in endoscopic ultrasonography staging of esophageal and cardia cancer. Gastrointest Endosc 43:20–24, 1996.

CHAPTER

# Staging Esophageal Cancer
## THE MUNICH EXPERIENCE

Thomas Rösch
Meinhard Classen

It is now generally accepted that staging of esophageal cancer is one of the main indications for upper gastrointestinal endoscopic ultrasonography (EUS) (1). Prior to surgery, EUS can predict the histopathologic stage of esophageal carcinoma according to the TNM system (2). The T-stage of esophageal carcinoma is determined by demonstrating tumor growth through the several layers of the wall (Figs. 13–1 to 13–6). The accuracy of EUS in the staging of esophageal cancer is reported as excellent in a number of studies that compare EUS with histopathology (5–9,11,13–24,29–31, 39,71) (Table 13–1). However, problems may be encountered when EUS is used to stage esophageal cancer in clinical practice.

## Do We Need EUS to Plan Therapy?

The management of patients with esophageal carcinoma is determined by the physician's attitude. The prognosis is generally poor, because most esophageal cancers are in an advanced stage at the time of diagnosis. If esophageal cancer is regarded by physicians as fatal, and if minimal, palliative measures are advocated as the only reasonable approach to management, EUS is of no clinical value. However, if a more aggressive approach, consisting of operation with or without pretreatment by chemotherapy and radiotherapy, is adopted, there is an

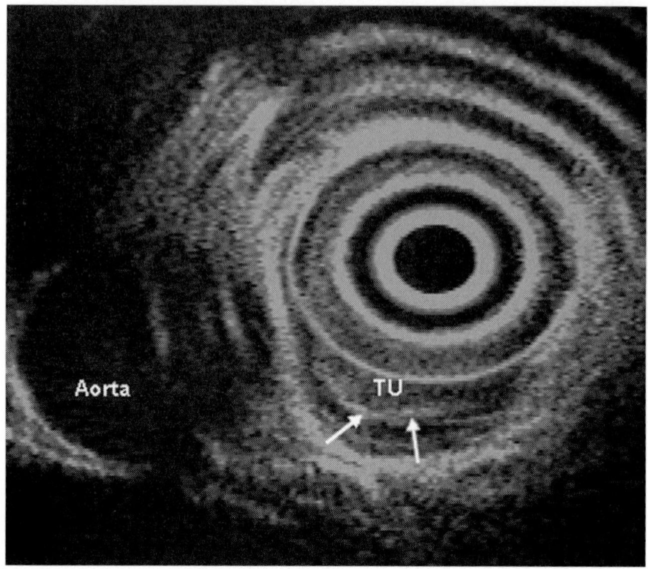


**FIGURE 13-1**

Stage T1 esophageal cancer (TU = tumor) observed as an echopoor thickening of the inner layers with the submucosa being preserved (arrows).

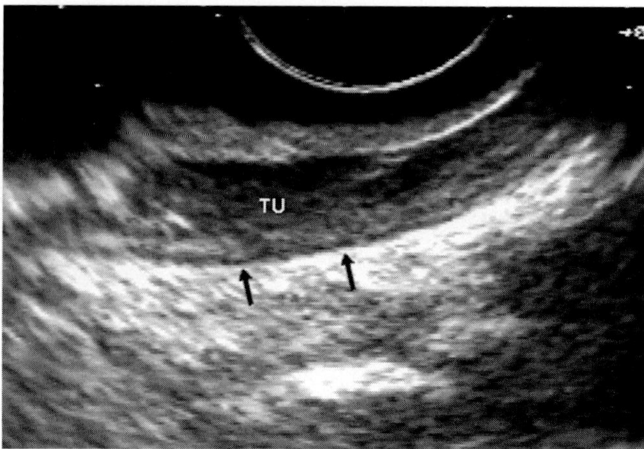


**FIGURE 13-3**

Stage T1 esophageal cancer (TU = tumor) observed as an echopoor focal wall thickening with the underlying submucosa and muscularis propria (arrows) remaining intact.

obvious need for meticulous preoperative tumor staging. Such an approach applies to stage-dependent treatment protocols, where early-stage cancers (i.e., those confined to the mucosa and therefore with low risk of lymph node metastases), may be treated by limited measures such as minimally invasive surgery, endoscopic resection ("strip biopsy") or photodynamic therapy. More advanced cancers (T3/4) may be pretreated with radio/chemotherapy in order to "downstage" these tumors (34). Meticulous local staging should only be performed in patients fit for major surgery and without evidence of distant metastases as excluded by ultrasonography and CT scan.

EUS, by virtue of its accuracy in tumor staging, provides accurate pretreatment assessment of a patient's prognosis. Previously, this has been possible only after surgery and a histopathologic examination of resection specimens. Tumor stage, according to the TNM tumor classification, correlates very closely with survival in patients with esophageal cancer (35). In patients with esophageal cancer, it has been shown that the pre-

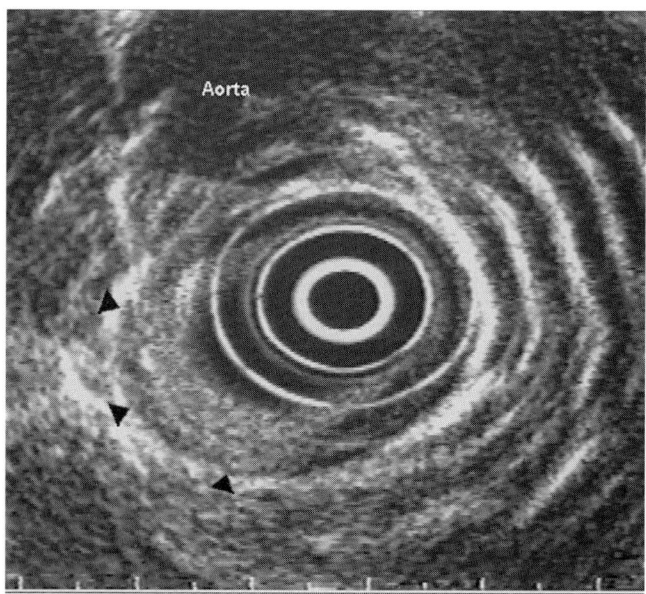


**FIGURE 13-2**

Esophageal cancer observed as focal, echopoor wall thickening with loss of the layer structure, but smooth outer margins (arrowheads).

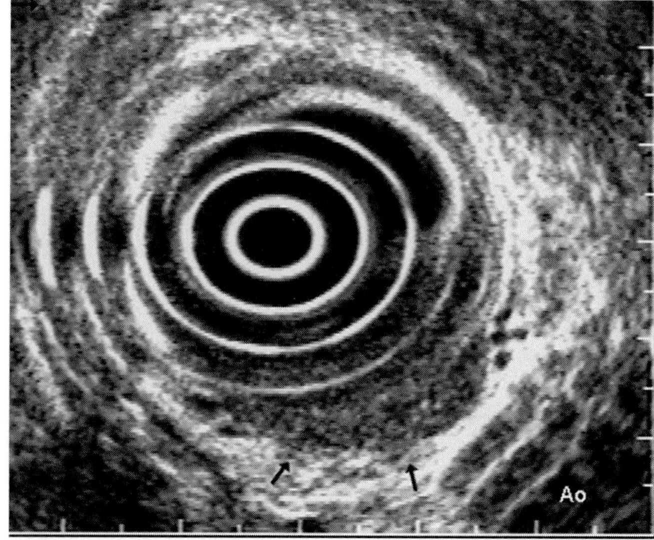


**FIGURE 13-4**

Stage T3 esophageal cancer with eccentric echopoor wall thickening and irregular outer margins (arrows).

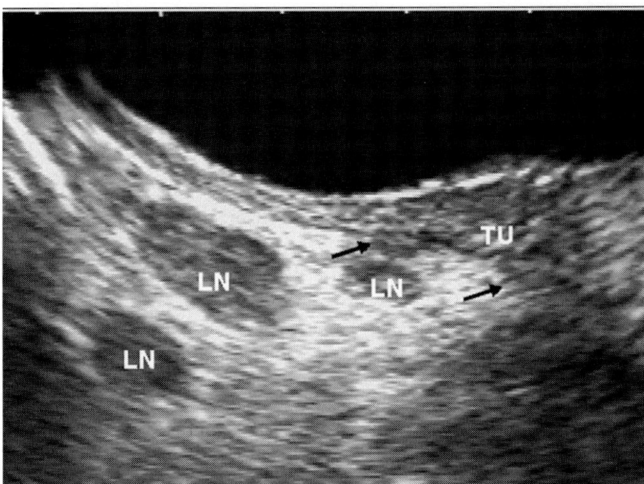


**FIGURE 13-5**

Stage T3 esophageal cancer with irregular outer margins (arrows) of the tumorous wall thickening and peritumorous lymph nodes (LN).

operative T and N stages, as determined on the EUS, have excellent correlation with survival following surgery (36) or following alternative treatment modalities such as radiotherapy or laser treatment (8).

EUS helps in determining whether a tumor is locally resectable or whether palliative measures should be primarily applied. EUS was shown to predict resectability of esophageal carcinoma preoperatively with reasonable accuracy, but difficulties may arise in esophageal squamous cell cancer owing to microscopic submucosal tumor spread beyond the macroscopic tumor margins (6,14,37). Palliative therapy of esophageal cancer is no longer limited to surgical therapies, but by endoscopic modalities as well. Furthermore, it is known that only patients with an expected radical resection (R0-resection) benefit from surgery. EUS may improve and shorten the diagnostic process of decision making be-tween surgery or palliation for patients with esophageal carcinoma or patients with gastric cardia cancer involving the distal esophagus (38). Because no other imaging method provides information on tumor stage with an accuracy that approaches that of EUS, this procedure has become the essential examination when surgical or other forms of therapy are being considered within stage-dependent treatment options.

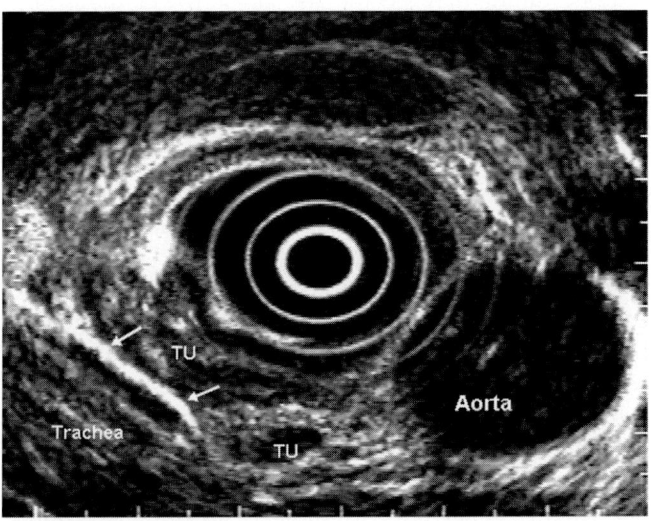


**FIGURE 13-6**

Stage T4 esophageal cancer (TU = tumor) observed as a massive echopoor and inhomogeneous wall thickening, infiltrating into the trachea (arrows).

**TABLE 13-1**

Accuracy of EUS in Staging Esophageal Cancer in the Literature

| First Author | *n* | T-staging | N-staging |
|---|---|---|---|
| Murata (71) | 173 | 88% | 88% |
| Dittler (5) | 167 | 86% | 90% |
| Tio (7) | 102 | 89% | 81% |
| Souquet (8) | 82 | 77% | 72% |
| Grimm (9) | 67 | 86% | 90% |
| Heintz (11) | 63 | 74% | 84% |
| Vilgrain (39) | 51 | 85% | 75% |
| Bótet (13) | 50 | 92% | 88% |
| Fok (29) | 45 | 89% | — |
| Rösch (14) | 44 | 82% | 70% |
| Nattermann (15) | 44 | 80% | 55% |
| Hordijk (16) | 41 | 76% | — |
| Ziegler (17) | 37 | 89% | 69% |
| Nobre-Leitao (18) | 36 | 80% | 79% |
| Peters (30) | 34 | 76% | 82% |
| Sugimachi (19) | 33 | 90% | — |
| Kalantzis (20) | 28 | 82% | 72% |
| Rice (21) | 22 | 59% | 69% |
| Napolitano (31) | 21 | 71% | 80% |
| Schüder (22) | 21 | 86% | 81% |
| Date (23) | 20 | 85% | — |
| Takemoto (24) | 18 | 72% | 79% |

## Can EUS Replace CT Scan?

Various studies have compared EUS with computed tomography scanning (CT scan) in the preoperative staging of esophageal carcinoma. With regard to accurate detection of tumor penetration (T-stage) and recognition of lymph node metastases (N-stage), EUS is superior to CT scan (Table 13–2). However, one report has shown a less impressive superiority of EUS over CT scan in the prediction of tumor extent when all patients (including those with an impassable tumor stenosis) are taken together (39). It is probably not fair to evaluate CT scan according to parameters that may not be suitable for this method (e.g., differentiation between stages T2 and T3). If other criteria such as the assessment of resectability are adopted (which must clearly

TABLE 13-2

Accuracy of EUS versus CT in the Different T and N Stages of Esophageal Carcinoma*

| Stage | *n* | EUS | CT |
|---|---|---|---|
| T1/2 | 69 | 65% | 29% |
| T3 | 143 | 92% | 71% |
| T4 | 80 | 91% | 49% |
| N0 | 66 | 63% | 77% |
| N1 | 158 | 89% | 47% |

*Pooled data from ref. 3,12,13,15,17,25.

TABLE 13-3

Percent of Nontraversable Tumor Stenoses in Patients with Esophageal Cancer in the Literature*

| First Author | *n* | Non-traversible Stenoses |
|---|---|---|
| Ziegler (17) | 37 | 19% |
| Tio (3) | 74 | 24% |
| Bótet (13) | 50 | 26% |
| Dittler (5) | 167 | 26% |
| Van Dam (42) | 79 | 26% |
| Grimm (10) | 49 | 26% |
| Rösch (14) | 44 | 32% |
| Heyder (72) | 35 | 36% |
| Murata (71) | 269 | 36% |
| Hordijk (8) | 41 | 37% |
| Heintz (12) | 40 | 45% |
| Vilgrain (39) | 51 | 50% |
| Dancygier (37) | 32 | 63% |

*Includes only studies to which this parameter refers.

be defined since these vary from institution to institution), CT scan may yield better results. For advanced tumors, CT scan appears more reliable.

CT scanning with the most up-to-date equipment and meticulous examination technique should be applied in clinical studies to avoid underestimating the accuracy of EUS. More recent studies also show significantly better results for CT scan (14,40,41). Evaluation by CT scan is necessary in patients with esophageal carcinoma to search for distant metastases in the liver and lungs. In patients with nontraversable tumor stenoses, CT scan is useful in the search for distant lymph node metastases (N2) around the celiac axis. For these reasons, CT scans of the chest and upper abdomen is advisable for esophageal carcinoma patients who are fit for surgery. If no distant metastases are present, EUS is performed.

## EUS in Nontraversable Tumor Stenoses

Based on a review of the literature, the rate of passage of the EUS instrument beyond the distal margin of esophageal cancers varies considerably, presumably owing to differences in patient selection (Table 13–3). When esophageal dilation is performed solely for the purpose of passage of the EUS instrument, the risk of perforation may be considerable, especially when, after bouginage, the echoendoscope is inserted blindly into the esophagus (42,43,44,45) in the same session. However, other studies cast doubt on this finding (46, 47). Should endosonographic staging of these tumors be required, careful step-wise dilation in several sessions and performance of EUS on a separate day are recommended (48).

Accurate EUS staging of esophageal carcinomas associated with marked stenosis of the lumen is possible in a variable percentage of cases. Lightdale et al. (49) failed to pass the EUS instrument through the stenoses in 26% of cases although the results of EUS staging were incorrect in only 8% for the T-stage and 12% for the N-stage. Tio et al. (3) reported an accuracy rate of 89% for the T-stage and 80% for the N-stage, although it was possible to pass the EUS instrument completely beyond the lesion in only 74% of the cases. Dittler et al. (6) found that for 97 patients in whom it was possible to pass the echoendoscope through the tumor, the determination of the T-stage was correct in 86% of cases. For 38 impassable tumors, the accuracy was 72%. In Vilgrain et al. (39), the accuracy for T and N staging (73% and 50% respectively) was considerably improved if the impassable tumors (50%) were eliminated from consideration. Then, EUS correctly predicted T-stage in 85% of cancers and lymph node involvement in 84%.

A possible solution to the problem of the markedly stenotic tumor may be the use of narrower ultrasound probes. A 7-mm blind echoprobe recently developed that can be introduced over a guide wire, possibly also following previous bouginage, was described to be safe and efficient in a limited number of patients (50). Small ultrasound probes ("miniprobes"), which can be introduced through the accessory channel of a conventional endoscope (51), were also shown to be reasonably accurate, although results in the literature vary (2,8,52–54,55, 56–58,69–71). In one report, the ultrasound probe was compared to the standard echoendoscope and found to be more accurate for detecting and staging "superficial" esophageal carcinoma (56). However, it is difficult to achieve a satisfactory water interface between the probe and the tissue. In addition, the depth of penetration of the ultrasound beam is frequently insufficient for accurate staging of advanced tumors. With further technical improvements the ultrasound probe might become an alternative, especially since the endoscope evaluation (with biopsy capability) and endosonographic evaluation can be combined in a single procedure.

## Overstaging by Means of EUS

Overstaging of esophageal carcinoma is encountered in up to 20% of cases and seems to occur mainly with T2 lesions. This has been attributed to peritumorous inflammatory and/or fibrous changes, but there are no detailed comparisons of histology and EUS images. Such overstaging seems to occur predominantly in early cancers (8). Whether such a histologic analysis would provide valuable information and reduce overstaging is speculative. However, the differentiation between stages T2 and T3 has considerable importance with respect to prognosis and choice therapy, especially for cancers in the proximal esophagus.

## Recognition of Metastatic Lymph Nodes

The recognition of metastatic lymph nodes at EUS is a long-standing topic of discussion. There is debate as to whether size alone (e.g., if greater than 1 cm in diameter) or additional features, such as echopattern and border features, should be considered in deciding the nature of a lymph node detected by EUS. Lymph nodes as small as 2–3 mm can be detected by EUS, but EUS studies of lymph nodes have some methodological problems. For example, it is difficult to correlate EUS findings with resected specimens in a node-by-node comparison. An in vitro study by Tio and Tytgat (59) showed evidence that hypoechoic, sharply demarcated lymph nodes are probably malignant, but this finding has been disputed (2). A more recent study using computer analysis of the gray scale of lymph nodes in a resection specimen did not find significant differences between malignant and benign nodes (60).

The probability that malignant lymph nodes are present (N1) increases with advancing T-stage. It is necessary to perform a radical lymphadenectomy in order to be certain that the N-stage is actually N0. Specific data in relation to lymph nodes (e.g., the number removed during surgery) are absent in many reports. The concomitant T-stage is probably the best parameter to assess the dignity of endosonographically visualized lymph nodes (61). EUS-guided fine needle aspiration (EUS FNA) of lymph nodes is one method to better define their nature; initial results have been encouraging (62–63). However, sampling error can occur when the needle traverses the primary tumor. EUS FNA is even more important in distant lymph nodes (e.g., those around the celiac axis [stage M1]) because, if positive for malignant disease, these metastatic lymph nodes alter the treatment from curative to palliative or preoperative neoadjuvant therapy.

## Follow-up

EUS used for follow-up in patients with esophageal (and gastric) cancer was shown to be highly sensitive and reasonably specific in one 1989 study (64). However, these results have not been duplicated by others. In our experience, granulation or fibrous tissue can sometimes mimic recurrence so that therapeutic decisions such as re-operation should not be based on EUS findings alone.

The issue of whether EUS is useful for tumor restaging after radiotherapy and/or chemotherapy of esophageal cancer has not yet been fully resolved. EUS correctly predicted the lack of response to chemotherapy (65) and showed a reduction in wall thickness and of number and size of lymph nodes in patients who did not undergo operations (66). Other studies of patients operated on after radio/chemotherapy were somewhat variable but most showed that EUS did not reliably predict the T-stage following treatment (67,68,63,69). Clearly, further work and possibly better EUS criteria are needed.

## Conclusions

EUS is the most reliable imaging method for local tumor staging of esophageal carcinoma. It is therefore recommended that EUS be performed in every patient with esophageal carcinoma found to be fit for surgery and without evidence of distant metastases. EUS provides significant information for planning therapy. Marked degrees of tumor stenosis and overstaging remain problematic, but these should be resolved at least in part by improvements in the understanding of peritumorous changes and by the development of new technology such as the ultrasound probe. The ultimate effect of EUS on the outcome is, at present, difficult to assess (70) because no treatment (surgery, chemotherapy, radiotherapy—alone and in various combinations) has been shown to be clearly superior to others, especially in advanced stages. As stage-dependent treatment protocols become the preferred therapy for patients with esophageal carcinoma, EUS will have an even more important role in improving patient outcome.

## References

1. Armengol-Miro JR, Benjamin S, Binmoeller K, et al. Clinical applications of endoscopic ultrasonography in gastroenterology—state of the art 1993. Results of a consensus conference, Orlando, Florida, 19 January 1993. Endoscopy 25:358–366, 1993.
2. Rösch T, Classen M. Gastroenterologic Endosonography. Stuttgart–New York: Thieme, 1992.
3. Tio TL, Cohen P, Coene PP, et al. Endosonography and computed tomography of esophageal carcinoma. Gastroenterology 96:1478–1486, 1989.
4. Tio TL, Cohen P, Coene PP, et al. Preoperative TNM classification of esophageal carcinoma by endosonography and computed

tomography: A comparison with the new (1987) TNM classification. Gastroenterology 96:512 (abstract), 1989.

5. Dittler HJ, Siewert JR. Role of endoscopic ultrasonography in esophageal carcinoma. Endoscopy 25:156–161, 1993.
6. Dittler HJ, Bollschweiler E, Siewert JR. Was leistat die Endosonographie im präoperativen Staging das Ösophaguskarzinoms? Dtsch Med Wschr 116:561–566, 1991.
7. Tio TL, Coene PP, den Hartog Jager FCA, et al. Preoperative TNM classification of esophageal carcinoma by endosonography. Hepato-Gastroenterol 37:376–381, 1990.
8. Souquet JC, Napoleon B, Pujol B, et al. Endosonography-guided treatment of esophageal carcinoma. Endoscopy 24:324–328, 1992.
9. Grimm H, Binmoeller K, Hamper K, et al. Endosonography for pre-operative locoregional staging of esophageal and gastric cancer. Endoscopy 25:224–230, 1993.
10. Grimm H, Hamper K, Maas R, Soehendra N. Präoperatives Staging von Ösophagus- und Magenkarzinom mit der Endosonographie. Vergleich mit der Computertomographie. In Henning H, Soehendra N (eds). Fortschritte der gastroenterologischen Endoskopie. 20th ed. Munich: Demeter Verlag, 1990, pp 74–79.
11. Heintz A, Wahl W, Mildenberger P, et al. Endosonographie biem Ösophaguscarcinom. Ergebnisse einer klinischen Untersuchung und einer In-vitro-Analyse. Chirung 63:629–633, 1992.
12. Heintz A, Höhne U, Schweden F, et al. Endosonographie versus Computertomographie bei der präoperativen Stadienbeurteilung von Oesophaguskarzinomen. Z Gastroenterol 29:49–52, 1991.
13. Bótet JF, Lightdale CJ, Zauber AG, et al. Preoperative staging of esophageal cancer: Comparison of endoscopic US and dynamic CT. Radiology 181:419–425, 1991.
14. Rösch T, Lorenz R, Zenker K, et al. Local staging and assessment of resectability in carcinoma of esophagus, stomach and duodenum by endoscopic ultrasonography. Gastrointest Endosc 38: 460–467, 1992.
15. Nattermann C, Dancygier H. Endoskopischer Ultraschall im präoperativen TN-staging des Ösophaguskarzinoms. Eine vergleichende Studie zwischen Endosonographie und Computertomographie. Ultraschall Med 14:100–105, 1993.
16. Hordijk ML, Zander H, van Blankenstein M, et al. Influence of tumor stenosis on the accuracy of endosonography in preoperative T staging of esophageal cancer. Endoscopy 25:171–175, 1993.
17. Ziegler K, Sanft C, Zeitz M, et al. Evaluation of endosonography in TN staging of esophageal cancer. Gut 32:16–20,1991.
18. Nobre-Leito C, Santos AA, Miodes Correira J, et al. Esophageal carcinoma: Preoperative staging with endosonography. Endoscopy 24(suppl. I):379 (abstract), 1992.
19. Sugimachi K, Ohno S, Fujishima H, et al. Endoscopic ultrasonographic detection of carcinomatous invasion and of lymph nodes in the thoracic esophagus. Surgery 107:366–371, 1990.
20. Kalantiz N, Kallimanis G, Laoudi F, et al. Endoscopic ultrasonography and computed tomography in preoperative (TNM) classification of esophageal carcinoma. Endoscopy 24:653 (abstract), 1992.
21. Rice TW, Boyce GA, Sivak MV. Esophageal ultrasound and the preoperative staging of carcinoma of the esophagus. J Thorac Cardiovasc Surg 101:536–544, 1991.
22. Schüder G, Koch B, Seitz G, et al. Endosonographisches Staging beim Oesophaguskarcinom—Ein prospektiver Vergleich mit herkömmlichen bildgebenden Verfahren. Z Gastroenterol 28:534 (abstract), 1990.
23. Date H, Miyashita M, Sasajima K, et al. Assessment of adventitial involvement of esophageal carcinoma by endoscopic ultrasonography. Surg Endosc 4:195–197, 1990.
24. Takemoto T, Itoh T, Fukumoto Y, Aibe T, Okita K. Endoscopic ultrasonography in preoperative staging of esophageal cancer. In Dancygier H, Classen M (eds). 5th International Symposium on Endoscopic Ultrasonography. Munich: Demeter Verlag (Z Gastroenterol suppl.):34–38, 1989.
25. Grimm H, Maydeo A, Hamper K, et al. Results of endoscopic ultrasound and computed tomography in preoperative staging of esophageal cancer: A prospective controlled study. Gastrointest Endosc 37:279 (abstract), 1991.
26. Dittler HJ, Bollschweiler E, Siewert JR. Was leistet die Endosonographie im präoperativen Staging des Ösophaguskarzinoms? Dtsch Med Wschr 116:561–566, 1991.
27. Souquet JC, Valette PJ, Pujol B, et al. Accuracy of endosonography for the diagnosis of superficial cancers of the gastro-intestinal tract. Endoscopy 20:92 (abstract), 1988.
28. Dancygier H, Classen M. Endoscopic ultrasonography in esophageal diseases. Gastrointest Endosc 35:220–225, 1989.
29. Fok M, Cheng SW, Wong J. Endosonography in patient selection for surgical treatment of esophageal carcinoma. World J Surg 16: 1098–1103, 1992.
30. Peters JH, Hoeft SF, Heimbucher J, et al. Selection of patients for curative or palliative resection of esophageal cancer based on preoperative endoscopic ultrasonography. Arch Surg 129:534–539, 1994.
31. Napolitano V, Allaria A, Amato G, et al. Accuracy of endoscopic ultrasonography in the preoperative staging of esophageal cancer. Endoscopy 26:823 (abstract), 1994.
32. Fockens P, Van den Brande JHM, van Dullemen HM, van Lanschot JJB, Tytgat GNJ. Endosonographic T-staging of esophageal carcinoma: A learning curve. Gastrointest Endosc 44:58–62, 1996.
33. Brugge WR, Lee MJ, Carey RW, Mathisen DJ. Endoscopic ultrasound staging criteria for esophageal cancer. Gastrointest Endosc 45:147–152, 1997.
34. Siewert JR, Dittler HJ. Esophageal carcinoma: Impact of staging on treatment. Endoscopy 25:28–32, 1993.
35. Siewert, Roder JD, Fink U. Fortschritte in der chirurgischen Behandlung des Plattenepithelkarzinoms der Speiseröhre. Internist 31:131–142, 1990.
36. Hiele M, Lerut A, Schurmans P, et al. Endoscopic ultrasound accurately predicts outcome in patients undergoing surgery for esophageal or esophagogastric carcinoma. Gastrointest Endosc 38: A286 (abstract), 1992.
37. Tio TL, Tytgat GNJ. Evaluation of resectability of gastrointestinal tumors. In Kawai K (ed). Endoscopic ultrasonography in gastroenterology. Tokyo–New York: Igaku Shoin, 1988, pp 106–118.
38. Natsugoe S, Yoshinaka H, Moringa T, Shimada M, Hokita S, Baba M, Takao S, Fukumoto T, Stein HJ, Aikou ST. Assessment of tumor invasion of the distal esophagus in carcinoma of the cardia using endoscopic ultrasonography. Endoscopy 28:750–755, 1996.
39. Vilgrain V, Mompoint D, Palazzo L, et al. Staging of esophageal carcinoma: Comparison of results with endoscopic sonography and CT. AJR 155:277–281, 1990.
40. Lehr L, Rupp N, Siewert JR. Assessment of resectability of esophageal cancer by computed tomography and magnetic resonance imaging. Surgery 103:344–350, 1988.
41. Halvorsen RA Jr, Thompson WM. Computed tomographic staging of gastrointestinal tract malignancies. Part I: Esophagus and stomach. Invest Radiol 22:2–16, 1987.
42. Van Dam J, Rice TW, Catalano MF, et al. High-grade malignant strictures predicative of esophageal tumor stage. Risks of endosonographic evaluation. Cancer 71:2910–2917, 1993.
43. Rösch T, Dittler HJ, Fockens P, et al. Major complications of endoscopic ultrasonography: Results of a survey of 42,105 cases. Gastrointest Endosc 39:A341 (abstract), 1993.
44. Catalano MF, Van Dam J, Sivak MV Jr. Malignant esophageal strictures: Staging accuracy of endoscopic ultrasonography. Gastrointest Endosc 41:535–539, 1995.
45. Roubein LD. Endoscopic ultrasonography and the malignant esophageal stricture: Implications and complications. Gastrointest Endosc 41:613–615, 1995.
46. Kallimanis G, Gupta K, Kawas FH, et al. Endoscopic ultrasound for staging esophageal cancer with or without dilation is clinically important and safe. Gastrointest Endosc 41:540–546, 1995.
47. Ikenberry S, Gren F, Savider T, et al. Savary dilation of esophageal cancer prior to endoscopic ultrasound examination. Gastrointest Endosc 41:350 (abstract), 1995.
48. Armengol-Miro JR, Benjamin S, Binmoeller K, et al. Clinical applications of endoscopic ultrasonography in gastroenterology—State of the art. 25:358–366, 1993.
49. Lightdale CJ, Bótet JF, Zauber A, et al. Endoscopic ultrasonography compared to computerized tomography for pre-operative staging of esophageal cancer. Gastrointest Endosc 36:191 (abstract), 1990.
50. Binmoeller KF, Seifert H, Seitz U, Izbicki JR, Kida M, Soehendra N. Ultrasonic esophagoprobe for TNM staging of highly stenosing esophageal carcinoma. Gastrointest Endosc 41:547–552, 1995.

51. Rösch T, Classen M. A new ultrasound probe for endosonographic imaging of the upper GI tract. Endoscopy 22:41–46, 1990.
52. Rösch T, Dittler HJ, Classen M. First clinical application of an ultrasonic probe for endoluminal ultrasound in esophago-gastric tumors: Comparison with conventional endosonography. Gastrointest Endosc 36:216 (abstract), 1990.
53. Mizuno S, Ikeda E, Mizuma Y, et al. Clinical evaluation of an ultrasonic probe in the diagnosis of esophageal and gastric diseases. Endoscopy 24:654 (abstract), 1992.
54. Nesje LB, Oldegaard S, Matre K, et al. Evaluation of esophageal stenotic lesions using a 20 MHz linear transendoscopic ultrasound system. Endoscopy 24:655 (abstract), 1992.
55. McLoughlin RF, Cooperberg PL, Mathieson JR, Stordy SN, Halparin LS. High resolution endoluminal ultrasonography in the staging of esophageal carcinoma. J Ultrasound Med 14:725–730, 1995.
56. Hasegawa N, Niwa Y, Arisawa T, Hase S, Goto H, Hayakawa T. Preoperative staging of superficial esophageal carcinoma: Comparison of an ultrasound probe and standard endoscopic ultrasonography. Gastrointest Endosc 44:388–393, 1996.
57. Murata Y, Suzuki S, Ohta M, Mitsunaga A, Hayashi K, Yoshida K, Ide H. Small ultrasonic probes for determination of the depth of superficial esophageal cancer. Gastrointest Endosc 44:23–28, 1996.
58. Yanai H, Yoshida T, Harada T, Matsumoto Y, Nishiaki M, Shigemitsu T, et al. Endoscopic ultrasonography of superficial esophageal cancers using a thin ultrasound probe system equipped with switchable radial and linear scanning modes. Gastrointest Endosc 44:578–582, 1996.
59. Tio TL, Tytgat GNJ. Endoscopic ultrasonography in analyzing peri-intestinal lymph node abnormality. Preliminary results of studies in vitro and in vivo. Scand J Gastroenterol 20(suppl. 123):158–163, 1986.
60. Heintz A, Mildenberger P, Georg M, et al. Endoscopic ultrasonography in the diagnosis of regional lymph nodes in esophageal and gastric cancer—results of an in vitro study. Endoscopy 25: 231–235, 1993.
61. Dittler HJ, Rösch T, Lorenz R, et al. Failure of endoscopic ultrasonography to differentiate malignant from benign lymph nodes in esaphago-gastric cancer. Gastrointest Endosc 38:240 (abstract), 1992.
62. Giovannini M, Seitz JF, Monger G, et al. Fine-needle aspiration biopsy guided by endoscopic ultrasonography. Results in 141 patients. Endoscopy 27:171–172, 1995.
63. Isenberg G, Chak A, Canto M, et al. Endoscopic ultrasound in restaging of esophageal cancer alter adjacent chemoradiation. Gastrointest Endosc 43:418 (abstract), 1996.
64. Lightdale CJ, Bótet JF, Kelsen DP, et al. Diagnosis of recurrent upper gastrointestinal cancer at the surgical anastomosis by endoscopic ultrasound. Gastrointest Endosc 35:407–412, 1989.
65. Roubein LD, DuBrow R, David C, et al. Endoscopic ultrasonography, in the quantitative assessment of response to chemotherapy in patients with adenocarcinoma of the esophagus and esophagogastric junction. Endoscopy 25:587–591, 1993.
66. Tio TL, Blank LECM, den Hartog Jager FCA, et al. Endosonography in the clinical TNM staging and follow-up after combined radiotherapy of inoperable esophageal carcinoma. Gastrointest Endosc 37:242 (abstract), 1991.
67. Dittler HJ, Rösch T, Fink U, et al. Endosonographic re-staging of carcinoma of the esophagus and cardia following radio- and chemotherapy. Gastrointest Endosc 38:241 (abstract), 1992.
68. Hordijk ML, Kok TC, Wilson JHP, et al. Assessment of response of esophageal carcinoma to induction chemotherapy. Endoscopy 25:592–596, 1993.
69. Faigel DO, Ginsberg GG, Kadish SL, et al. Effect of neoadjuvant therapy on cancer staging by endoscopic ultrasonography. Gastrointest Endosc 43:415 (abstract), 1996.
70. Rösch T. Endoscopic ultrasonography—more questions than answers? Endoscopy 25:600–602, 1993.
71. Murata Y, Suzuki S, Hashimoto H. Endoscopic ultrasonography of the upper gastrointestinal tract. Surg Endosc 2:180–183, 1988.
72. Heyder N, Lux G. Malignant lesions of the upper gastrointestinal tract. Scand J Gastroenterol 21(suppl. 123):47–51, 1986.
73. Rösch T, Lorenz R, Dancygier H, et al. Endosonographic diagnosis of submucosal upper GI tract tumors. Scand J Gastroenterol 27:1–8, 1992.

CHAPTER

# Postoperative Recurrence of Esophageal Cancer

Charles J. Lightdale
Frank Van de Mierop

Locally recurrent upper gastrointestinal cancer is a common problem after surgical resection. Gignoux et al. (1) reported 67% of recurrent esophageal cancer to have a local component, and 32% of recurrences to be limited to local recurrence only. Gunderson and Sosin (2) reported that, in their series, 87% of patients with recurrent gastric cancer had a local component, and in 53% this was the sole site of recurrence.

Symptoms due to locally recurrent upper gastrointestinal cancer, however, are essentially indistinguishable from those due to postoperative dysmotility, inflammation, or fibrous stricture (3). The diagnosis of anastomotic recurrence is often difficult—particularly when recurrent cancer is submucosal or extramucosal—and endoscopy with biopsy is not diagnostic. Endoscopic ultrasonography is useful for detecting regional lymph node recurrence (4). The diagnosis of lymph node involvement by tumor, which had been dependent on subjective image analysis (4), is now complemented by endoscopic ultrasound-guided fine needle aspiration (FNA) for cytologic confirmation (5). CT scan lacks efficacy in detecting tumor recurrence and is limited by varying anastomotic morphology and artifacts generated by movement and by retained metallic clips and staples (6–8). Exploratory surgery is diagnostic in most cases of recurrent malignancy, but has a high morbidity and is rarely reported to be curative (9–13). However, an accurate diagnosis of recurrent anastomotic cancer provides critical prognostic guidance for appropriate patient management, and earlier diagnosis has the potential to improve treatment results.

## Recurrent Esophagel Cancer: A Study

Endoscopic ultrasonography was used to examine the upper gastrointestinal tract in 40 symptomatic patients suspected of having recurrent upper gastrointestinal cancer following surgical resection (14) (Table 14–1). After esophagectomy, there was a gastroesophageal anastomosis in 20 patients, a gastrojejunostomy after distal gastrectomy in 16 patients, and an esophagojejunostomy after total gastrectomy in 4 patients. Of the 40 patients, 24 were documented to have recurrent anastomotic cancer by histopathology. In 16 patients, diagnosis was made at initial endoscopy and biopsy (15 patients) or cytology (1 patient); and in 2 patients, on repeat endoscopy and biopsy. Six patients were diagnosed at surgery which was performed for persistent symptoms in spite of negative endoscopic examination. CT scans were consistent with recurrence in 7 of the 24 patients (metastases to liver, lung, and peritoneum), but none was diagnostic of anastomotic recurrence.

Using endoscopic ultrasonography, locally recurrent cancer was correctly identified by nodular, irregular, hypoechoic thickening of the anastomosis in 23 of the 24 patients (Figs. 14–1 through 14–3). There was one false-negative result. Absence of anastomotic recurrence was correctly diagnosed in 13 of 16 patients with 3 false positives. In diagnosing locally recurrent cancer, EUS had a sensitivity of 95%, specificity of 80%, positive predictive accuracy of 88%, and negative predictive accuracy of 92% (14).

Others have reported successful use of EUS for anastomotic recurrence, but have also noted difficulty in differentiating recurrence from inflammatory changes in some patients (15). A gastric remnant recurrence may have the appearance of an infiltrating linitis plastica. In their study, Catalano et al. reported their experience in symptomatic and asymptomatic anastomotic recurrence after esophageal resection (16). They correctly diagnosed 6 out of 6 local anastomotic recurrences in the symptomatic patients. In the asymptomatic patients, documented recurrences were predominantly extramucosal. Results of both studies (14,16) in symptomatic patients are depicted in Table 14–2.

**TABLE 14–1**

**Endosonographic Evaluation of Symptomatic Patients Suggesting Recurrent Upper Gastrointestinal Cancer in the Region of the Surgical Anastomosis**

| | Pathology | |
|---|---|---|
| **EUS** | ***Positive*** | ***Negative*** |
| positive | 23 | 3 |
| negative | 1 | 13 |

(Sensitivity = 23/24 = 95%; PV (+) = 23/26 = 88%; Specificity = 13/16 = 80%; PV (-) = 13/14 = 92%)

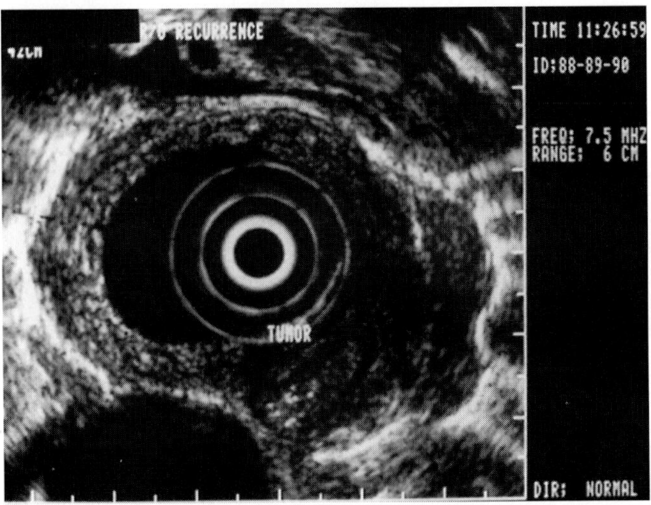


**FIGURE 14–1**

Endosonograph of recurrent gastroesophageal cancer at the esophagogastric anastomosis. The image demonstrates the nodular, hypoechoic tumor extending deeply in a posterior direction to the left lateral wall of the descending aorta (6 o'clock).

## Technique

Gastrojejunostomy anastomoses are best examined with a combination of the water-filled–balloon and water-filled–lumen techniques. Esophagogastrostomy or esoph-

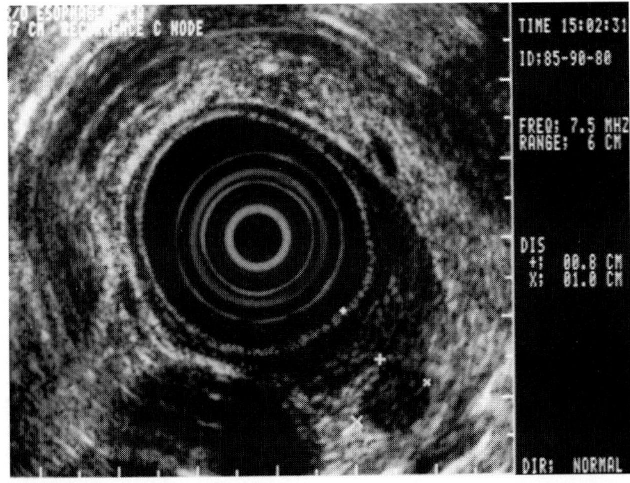


**FIGURE 14–2**

Recurrence of esophageal cancer at the gastroesophageal anastomosis is seen as a hypoechoic disruption measuring 0.8 cm in thickness and located from 2 o'clock to 6 o'clock on the endosonograph. Outside the recurrence in the wall of the anastomosis there is a discrete, hypoechoic, round, sharply demarcated 1.0-cm–diameter lymph node infiltrated by cancer.

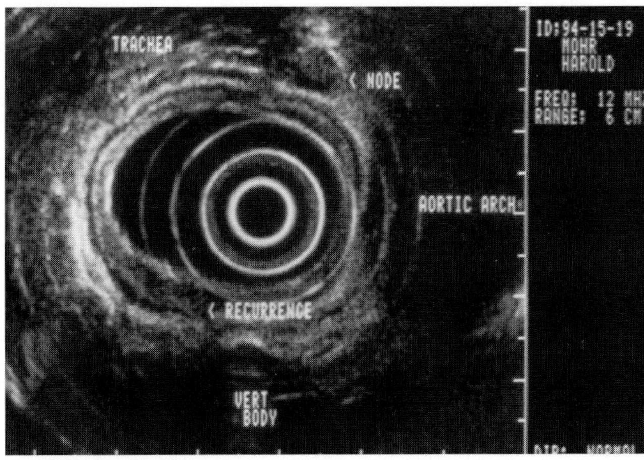


**FIGURE 14–3**

Recurrent adenocarcinoma of the esophagus associated with Barrett's epithelium is seen as a hypoechoic interruption of the esophagogastric anastomosis from 6 o'clock to 7 o'clock at the level of the aortic arch. A 6-mm paratracheal lymph node metastasis is evident at 1 o'clock.

agojejunostomy are best examined primarily by the water-filled–balloon method; although injecting small amounts of water into the lumen sometimes helps image the anastomosis in more detail and avoids trapped-air artifacts. In addition to local anastomotic recurrences, lymph nodes should be assessed for abnormalities. Careful *real-time* analysis is necessary when imaging the anastomosis because overlapped folds (due either to surgical technique or to pulling back when the balloon is filled) may mimic abnormalities. If the anastomosis cannot be passed with the UM-20, one may use newly available catheter probes that can be passed over a guidewire (17) or under direct vision across a strictured anastomosis (18–21). These new probes have the advantage of being thinner; however, some also use higher frequencies (12 and 20 MHz), which may or may not be advantageous. Most stapled anastomoses show a single hyperechoic or three-layer image with a central hypoechoic layer. The anastomotic area is usually smooth and less than 6 mm in thickness.

Radiation and chemotherapy may result in fibrous wall thickening which may mimic recurrent cancer. The effect of radiotherapy seems to be time-limited. Because of such inflammatory changes, EUS T-staging within 3 months of radiation seems to be of limited value. At longer periods after therapy the wall thickening decreases, and it becomes easier to differentiate between the layers (22). Whether adjuvant treatments will cause decreased EUS specificity in the evaluation of anastomotic recurrences remains to be evaluated.

For diagnosing distant metastases in patients after surgery, CT scan remains a useful test; however, it is not useful for the diagnosis of anastomotic recurrence where EUS appears to be highly sensitive. Specificity of EUS for diagnosis of anastomotic recurrence is good, but should be improved with the use of EUS-guided deep needle biopsy (23).

**TABLE 14–2**

Results of the Endosonographic Evaluation of 50 Symptomatic Patients with Suspected Anastomotic Recurrence

| | Pathology | |
|---|---|---|
| EUS | *Positive* | *Negative* |
| positive | 29 | 3 |
| negative | 1 | 17 |

(Sensitivity = 96%; specificity = 85%; positive predictive value = 90%; negative predictive value = 94%)

## References

1. Gignoux M, Roussel A, Paillot B, Gillet M, et al. The value of preoperative radiotherapy in esophageal cancer: Results of a study of the E.O.R.T.C. World J Surg 11:426–432, 1987.
2. Gunderson LL, Sosin H. Adenocarcinoma of the stomach: Areas of failure in re-operation series (second or symptomatic look). Int J Radiat Oncol Biol Phys 8:1–11, 1982.
3. Allum WH, Hockey MS, Fielding JWL. Gastric remnant recurrence—Detection and implications for the management of gastric cancer. Clin Oncol 10:333–339, 1984.
4. Catalano MF, Sivak MV Jr, Rice TW, Gragg LA, Van Dam J. Endosonographic features predictive of lymph node metastasis. Gastrointest Endosc 40:442–446, 1994.
5. Wiersema MJ, Chak ML. Real-time endoscopic ultrasound guided FNA of a mediastinal lymph node. Gastrointest Endosc 39:429–431, 1993.
6. Mauro MA, Lee JKT, Heiken JP, Balfe DM. Radiologic staging of gastrointestinal neoplasms. Surg Clin North Am 64:67–88, 1984.
7. Halvorsen RA, Thompson WM. Computed tomographic evaluation of esophageal carcinoma. Semin Oncol 11:113–128, 1984.
8. Mullin D, Shirkhoda A. Computed tomography after gastrectomy in primary gastric carcinoma. J Comput Assist Tomogr 9:30–33, 1985.
9. Kasai M, Mori S, Watanabe T. Follow-up results after resection of thoracic esophageal carcinoma. World J Surg 2:543–550, 1978.
10. Thompson FB, Robins RE. Local recurrence following subtotal resection for gastric carcinoma. Surg Gynecol Obst 95:341–344, 1952.
11. Wangensteen OH, Lewis FJ, Arhelger SW, Muller JJ, Maclean LD. An interim report upon the "second look" procedure for cancer of the stomach, colon and rectum and for "limited peritoneal carcinosis." Surg Gynecol Obst 99:257–267, 1954.
12. Ellis H, Jayasekara G. Is second look surgery justified in suspected recurrence of cancer of the stomach? Br J Surg 62:226–230, 1975.
13. Skinner DB. En bloc resection for neoplasms of the esophagus and cardia. J Thorac Cardiovasc Surg 85:59–69, 1983.
14. Lightdale CJ, Bótet JF, Kelsen DP, Turnbull AD, Brennan MF. Diagnosis of recurrent upper gastrointestinal cancer at the surgical anastomosis by endoscopic ultrasound. Gastrointest Endosc 35:407–412, 1989.
15. Dancygier H, Classen M. Endoscopic ultrasonography in esophageal diseases. Gastrointest Endosc 35:220–225, 1989.
16. Catalano MF, Sivak MV, Rice TW, Van Dam J. Postoperative screening for anastomotic recurrence of esophageal carcinoma by EUS. Gastrointest Endosc 42(6):540–544, 1995.
17. Fockens P, Van Dullemen HM, Tytgat GNJ. Endosonography of stenotic esophageal carcinoma: Preliminary experience with an ultra-thin balloon-fitted ultrasound probe in 4 patients. Gastrointest Endosc 40:226–228, 1994.
18. Chak A, Canto M, Stevens P, Lightdale CJ, Van de Mierop F, Cooper G, Pollack BJ, Sivak MV. Prospective evaluation of new

ultrasound catheter system: Comparison with ultrasound endoscopes. Gastrointest Endosc 43(4):A8, 1996.

19. Murata Y, Suzuki S, Ohta M, Mitsunaga A, Kazuhiko H, Yoshida K, Ide H. Small ultrasonic probes for determination of the depth of superficial esophageal cancer. Grastrointest Endosc 44:23–28, 1996.
20. Yanai H, Yoshida T, Harada T, Matsumoto Y, Nishiaki M, Shigemitsu T, Tada M, Okita K, Kawano T, Nagasaki S. Endoscopic ultrasonography of superficial esophageal cancers using a thin ultrasound probe system equipped with switchable radial and linear scanning modes. Gastrointest Endosc 44:578–582, 1996.
21. Hasegawa N, Niwa Y, Arisawa T, Hase S, Goto H, Hayakawa T. Preoperative staging of superficial esophageal carcinoma: Comparison of an ultrasound probe and standard endoscopic ultrasonography. Gastrointest Endosc 44:388–393, 1996.
22. Hordijk ML. Restaging after radiotherapy and chemotherapy: Value of endoscopic ultrasonography. Gastrointest Endosc Clin N Am 5(3):601–608, 1995.
23. Wiersema MJ, Wiersema LM, Khusro Q, Cramer HM, Liang-Che T. Combined endosonography and fine-needle aspiration cytology in the evaluation of gastrointestinal lesions. Gastrointest Endosc 40:199–206, 1994.

# SECTION

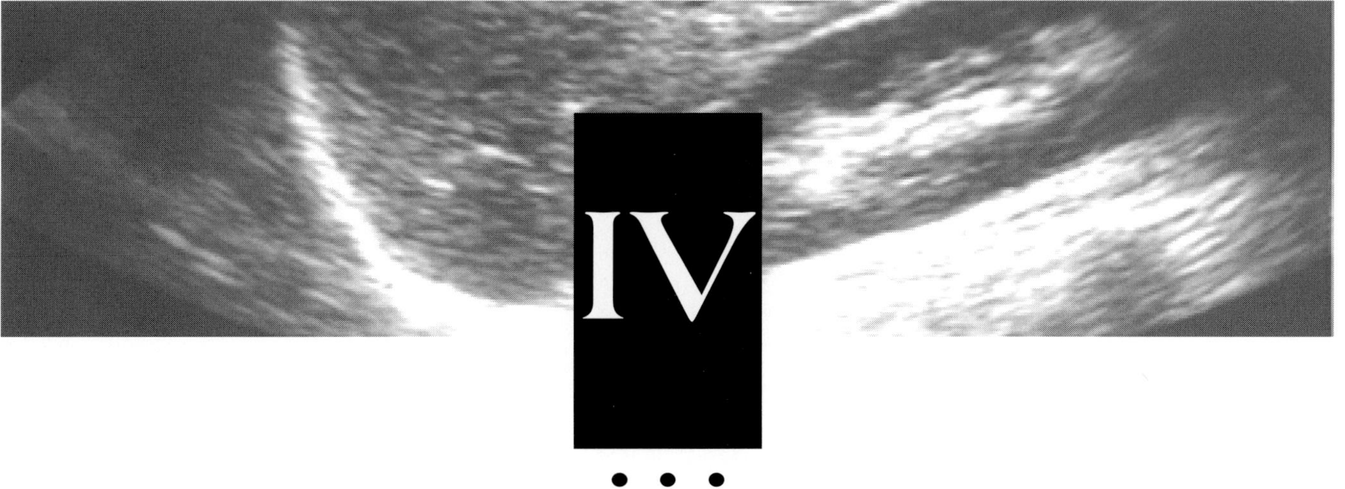


# Gastric Endosonography

CHAPTER

# 15

# Subepithelial Lesions

Rosalind U. van Stolk

Subepithelial lesions are often referred to as submucosal lesions. But with the advent of endoscopic ultrasonography—and with it the ability to accurately delineate the layers of the gastrointestinal tract, including the submucosa—we now know that many, if not most, "submucosal" lesions do not emanate from the submucosa. Thus, they are more accurately named subepithelial lesions. Subepithelial lesions involving the gastrointestinal tract come to clinical attention much less frequently than mucosal lesions. Their rate of occurrence is difficult to assess because most are asymptomatic. Hence they tend to be found incidentally during evaluation for other reasons—at barium contrast radiography, endoscopy, surgery, or autopsy (1). The most common lesion of the upper gastrointestinal tract presenting as a subepithelial lesion is the leiomyoma. On autopsy, leiomyoma is reported in up to 5% of specimens of the esophagus (2), and in the stomach of 50% of patients over age 50 (3). This prevalence, emphasizes the fact that most leiomyomas never come to clinical attention. Larger lesions may ulcerate, however, thus presenting with bleeding or pain.

Subepithelial lesions usually are diagnosed by gastrointestinal contrast radiography or endoscopy. Single-contrast barium studies may suggest a subepithelial lesion as evidenced by a smooth defect in the barium column (Fig. 15–1). Double-contrast techniques may reveal a double contour outlining a smooth filling defect (4). Endoscopy reveals a protrusion into the lumen covered by normal-appearing mucosa (Fig. 15–2A). Abdominal ultrasound may provide information about abnormalities of organs adjacent to the gastrointestinal tract, but its resolution is not sufficient to evaluate the gastrointestinal tract wall itself. Thin cuts taken during computed tomography may show thickening of the gastrointestinal tract wall or low-attenuation lesions projecting into the gastrointestinal tract lumen (5). However, the limitations of CT scanning in the assessment of the gastrointestinal wall are well described. In brief, small lesions are easily missed (6).

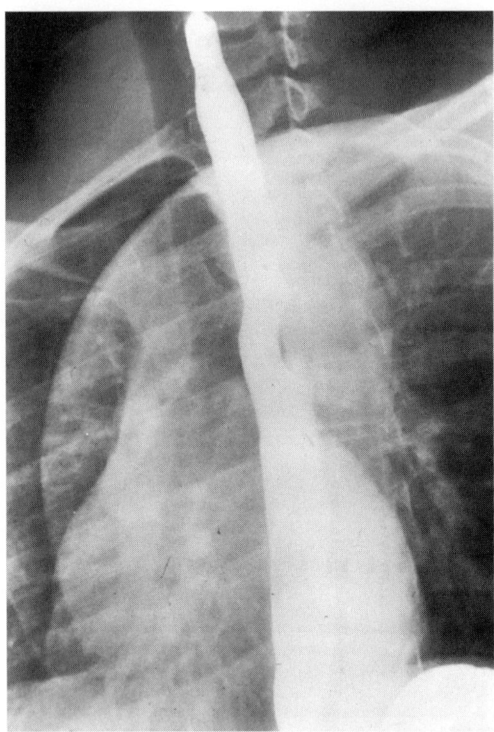

**FIGURE 15-1**

Barium-contrast radiograph demonstrating the smooth contour of an esophageal lesion. (Courtesy J. Van Dam)

Currently, most subepithelial lesions are diagnosed endoscopically. However, endoscopy shows only the mucosal aspect of the lesion and can evaluate neither the depth nor the extent of the lesion (7,8). In addition, endoscopy often cannot differentiate between true lesions involving the submucosa, lesions involving the other layers of the gastrointestinal tract wall, and adjacent extrinsic lesions. Endoscopic biopsies are rarely diagnostic because they sample small pieces limited to the superficial layers of the gastrointestinal tract wall (9).

Endoscopic ultrasound is a uniquely useful adjunct in the diagnosis of subepithelial lesions. The placement of high-frequency transducers immediately adjacent to the gastrointestinal tract wall affords high-resolution imaging of the wall configuration itself and that of adjacent extraluminal structures as well (10,11,12). Scanning at 20 MHz using endoscopic ultrasound probes provides the highest-resolution images of the gastrointestinal tract wall. Using the 12-MHz–transducer echoendoscope provides high-resolution images of the gastrointestinal tract wall, and the 7.5-MHz setting allows visualization of organs and lesions extrinsic to the gastrointestinal tract wall (13). The size and location of subepithelial tumors can be clearly elucidated. In the majority of cases, the clinical management of patients is changed as a result of the information obtained by EUS (14). Several reviews have addressed the characteristic endosonographic appearance of subepithelial lesions (15–19) (Table 15–1).

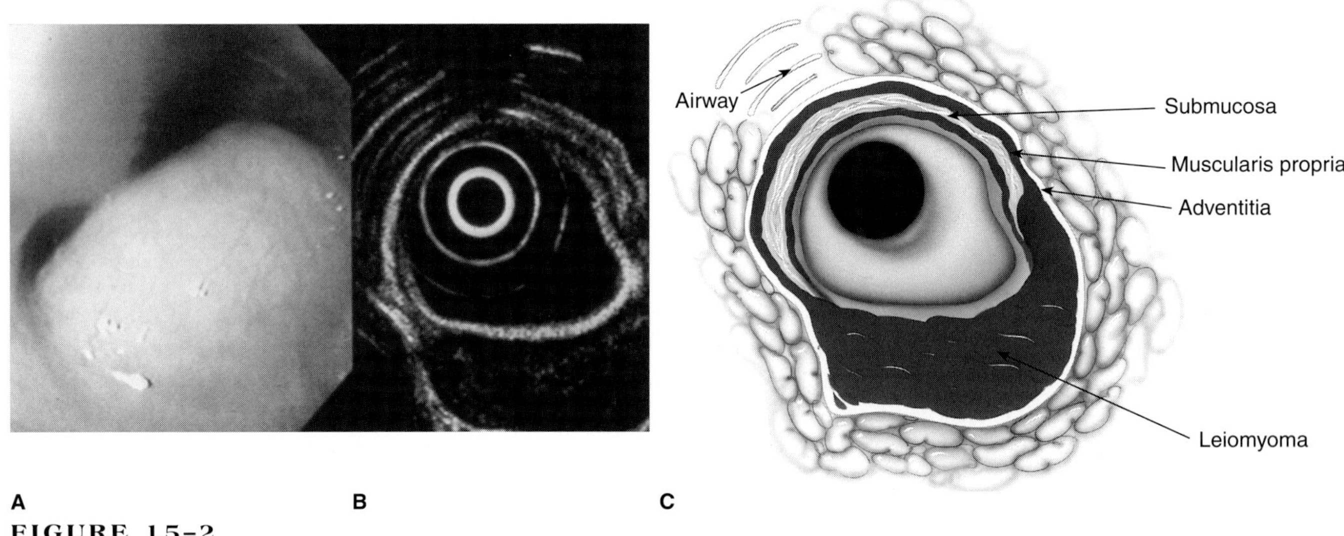


**FIGURE 15-2**

(**A**) Endoscopic photograph of an esophageal leiomyoma. The lesion is covered by endoscopically and histologically normal esophageal mucosa. The mass lesion projects into the lumen of the esophagus and may produce symptoms of dysphagia. (*See color insert for color plate.*) (**B**) Endoscopic ultrasound of the leiomyoma pictured in (A). The endosonograph shows the typical hypoechoic lesion contiguous with the muscularis propria layer (fourth, hypoechoic layer) of the gastrointestinal tract wall. (**C**) Artist's rendering of the endosonograph. (Courtesy J. Van Dam)

**TABLE 15-1**

**Published Series of EUS in Evaluating Subepithelial Lesions**

| Author | *n* | Site | *n*/Site | Most Common Lesion | *n* | % |
|---|---|---|---|---|---|---|
| Yasuda (1990) | 308 | Esophagus | 128 | Varix | 82 | 64 |
| | | Stomach | 174 | Leiomyoma * | 60 | 34 |
| | | | | Cyst | 28 | 16 |
| | | | | Aberrant Pancreas | 24 | 14 |
| | | Duodenum | 6 | Leiomyoma | | |
| Boyce (1991) | 91 | Esophagus | 28 | Leiomyoma ** | 15 | 54 |
| | | Stomach | 55 | Leiomyoma | 18 | 33 |
| | | | | Varix | 10 | 18 |
| | | Duodenum | 8 | Lipoma | 2 | |
| Tio (1990) | 42 | Esophagus | 12 | Leiomyoma | 7 | |
| | | Stomach | 28 | Leiomyoma | 15 | |
| | | | | Leiomyosarcoma | 18 | |
| | | Duodenum | 2 | Leiomyoma | 2 | |
| Rösch (1992) | 37 | Esophagus | 14 | Leiomyoma | 7 | |
| | | Stomach | 20 | Leiomyoma | 5 | |
| | | Duodenum | 3 | | | |
| Caletti (1989) | 25 | Stomach only | 25 | Leiomyoma | 10 | |
| | | | | Normal | | |
| | | | | Adjacent organ | 6 | |
| | | | | Pancreatic cyst | 2 | |

* Angiographic or pathologic confirmation.
** Varices excluded.

Endoscopic ultrasound is especially useful when an extraluminal structure compresses the lumen of the gastrointestinal tract, mimicking a subepithelial lesion. One such structure is the splenic artery (or splenic artery aneurysm), which EUS has been reported to readily identify (20). Moto et al. reported the utility of EUS in 19 patients in whom extraluminal compression by an adjacent structure was the cause of an apparent subepithelial lesion (11). In 16 of the 19 patients, the extraluminal compression was due to an adjacent normal structure or organ (splenic artery 7, spleen 5, normal pancreas 2, gallbladder 1, and colon 1). In 3 instances, the extraluminal compression was caused by an extraluminal tumor (hepatic 2, omental 1). Endoscopic ultrasonography was 100% accurate in differentiating the extraluminal etiology of the mass from a potential subepithelial or intramural source. In addition, EUS was found to be superior to standard abdominal ultrasonography or CT scan in this regard.

## Diagnosis of Subepithelial Lesions by Endosonography

In the largest series of subepithelial lesions evaluated by endoscopic ultrasound, Yasuda et al. examined more than 300 lesions (15). Sixty-eight percent of the lesions described were subepithelial tumors, 75% of which were located in the stomach. The majority of other lesions were esophageal or gastric varices (29%), while a small number (3%) were ultimately diagnosed as gastric lymphoma. Histologic material was obtained in 131 out of 158 gastric lesions (83%). The most common subepithelial tumor was the leiomyoma, accounting for 46% of the lesions detected. Gastric wall cysts and ectopic pancreatic tissue were the next most common lesions, representing 21% and 18% of the gastric lesions, respectively. Leiomyosarcomas and lipomas accounted for 5–6% of the group. Carcinoid tumors (2), an eosinophilic granuloma (1) and a granular cell myoblastoma (1) completed the series for which pathologic tissue was available (Table 15–2).

In the next-largest reported series of supepithelial lesions (91 lesions), leiomyomas were again the most common lesion, representing 53% of esophageal lesions and 40% of nonvariceal gastric lesions (16). In comparison to Yasuda's series, a smaller number were cysts or pancreatic tissue (6%), but varices represented a similar large percentage (18%). Endoscopic ultrasound was able to accurately diagnose four cases of gastric adenocarcinoma (linitus plastica) which presented as a submucosal gastric lesion. Two leiomyosarcomas were found in the stomach and lipomas were found in three cases—one in the stomach and two in the duodenum. Other lesions represented less than 2% of all the cases. Endoscopic ultrasound correctly predicted the histologic layer from which the lesion originated in 32 of 33 cases in the esophagus or stomach (Table 15–3).

Similar series of subepithelial lesions were reported by Tio, Rösch, Caletti, and Catalano; these series contained respectively 42, 37, 25, and 122 cases of subepithelial tumors evaluated by endoscopic ultrasound (17–19,13). A variety of lesions similar to those reported in the above series was seen, and the characteristic endosonographic appearance of the most common lesions was confirmed.

**TABLE 15-2**

**Gastric Submucosal Tumors Examined by EUS with Histologic Confirmation**

| | |
|---|---|
| Leiomyoma | 60 |
| Leiomyosarcoma | 8 |
| Cyst | 28 |
| Aberrant pancreas | 24 |
| Lipoma | 7 |
| Carcinoids | 2 |
| Eosinophilic granuloma | 1 |
| Granular cell myoblastoma | 1 |
| Total | 131 |

Reprinted with permission from Yasuda K. Gastrointestinal Endoscopy 36: S17–S20, 1990.

TABLE 15-3

EUS Prediction of Histologic Layer or Extrinsic Organ Involved

| Esophagus Diagnosis | Pathologic confirmation ($N$ = 11) | Stomach Diagnosis | Pathologic confirmation ($N$ = 22) |
|---|---|---|---|
| Leiomyoma | 5/5 | Leiomyoma | 9/9 |
| | | Leiomyosarcoma | 2/2 |
| Bronchogenic carcinoma | 3/3 | Carcinoma (linitus plastica) | 4/4 |
| Metastatic breast carcinoma | 1/1 | | |
| Lymphoma | 1/1 | | |
| Fibrovascular polyp | 1/2* | Varix | 7/7** |

* One case interpreted as leiomyoma
** 4-Pathologic; 3-Angiographic confirmation
Adapted with permission from Boyce G, et al. Gastrointestinal Endoscopy 37:449, 1991.

## Comparison between Endoscopic Ultrasound and Other Imaging Modalities

The benefit of endoscopic ultrasound in the diagnosis of subepithelial lesions was reported in a study of 42 cases (17). Tio et al. compared endoscopic ultrasound with CT scanning in patients in whom upper gastrointestinal subepithelial tumors were suspected on the basis of endoscopy or barium contrast radiographs. Histologic material was available for 24 patients, who underwent surgical resection either because of the size of the lesion or bleeding (12 cases) or because of suspected malignancy (12 cases). The remaining 18 cases were small lesions. These were followed by endoscopic ultrasound and computed tomography to confirm their benign nature. In the first group (benign lesions with histologic confirmation) the accuracy of endoscopic ultrasound was 83%.

When compared to endoscopy, barium studies or CT scanning, endoscopic ultrasound has been reported to more accurately assess the size and location of subepithelial lesions (16,17). In most instances, pathologic diagnosis is unobtainable by diagnostic endosonography; however, the correct diagnosis may often be inferred from the endosonographic configuration, which reveals the lesion to be solid, cystic, or vascular. Endosonography also establishes the precise location of the lesion within the gastrointestinal wall. The narrow differential diagnosis of subepithelial lesions afforded by the addition of endoscopic ultrasound enhances the ability to provide appropriate management decisions. It also permits continued observation (surveillance) of patients with suspected benign lesions and the choice of operative management for a smaller number of patients with suspected malignant lesions.

## Endoscopic Characteristics of Specific Lesions

The characteristics of specific subepithelial lesions examined by endoscopic ultrasound (Table 15–4) have been described in all five published series and in numerous single reports. The need for confirmatory histopathologic assessment varies with the nature of the lesion as imaged by endosonography (21).

### Leiomyoma

Leiomyomas involving the gastrointestinal wall are benign smooth muscle tumors usually arising from the muscularis propria. Rarely, they may arise from the muscularis mucosae and, when emanating from this superficial muscle layer, may often be endoscopically resected (22). Leiomyomas are usually solitary, well-circumscribed, and submucosal. As indicated by autopsy studies, they may be quite common in the esophagus and stomach, but they may be detected throughout the length of the gastrointestinal tract. Most lesions are <2 cm and asymptomatic. Patients with lesions >2 cm may present with

TABLE 15-4

Endoscopic Ultrasonographic Features of Submucosal Lesions

| Diagnosis | EUS Findings Reported |
|---|---|
| Leiomyoma | Hypoechoic; contiguous with muscularis propria; smooth outer margin |
| Leiomyosarcoma | Hypoechoic, contiguous with muscularis proria; large lesions may have irregular outer margin; adenopathy; small lesions identical to leiomyoma |
| Lipoma | Hyperechoic; submucosal |
| Bronchogenic carcinoma<br>Breast carcinoma metastatic | Hypoechoic; disrupts submucosa and muscularis propria; irregular outer margin |
| Granular cell tumors | Hypoechoic; submucosa; smooth margin |
| Linitus plastica | Hypoechoic, disrupts submucosa and muscularis propria; adjacent adenopathy |
| Varices | Anechoic; submucosal; serpentine |
| Aberrant pancreas | Submucosal; ductular structure may be present |
| Pancreatic pseuodcyst | Anechoic; smooth margin; compresses adjacent wall |
| Carcinoid | Submucosal; hypoechoic |
| Splenic remnant | Submucosal; multiple vascular structures within lesion |
| Fibrovascular polyp | Submucosal; mixed echogenicity |
| Lymphoma | Hypoechoic, disrupts submucosa and muscularis propria; adenopathy (?) |
| Gastric cyst | Anechoic; smooth border; submucosal |

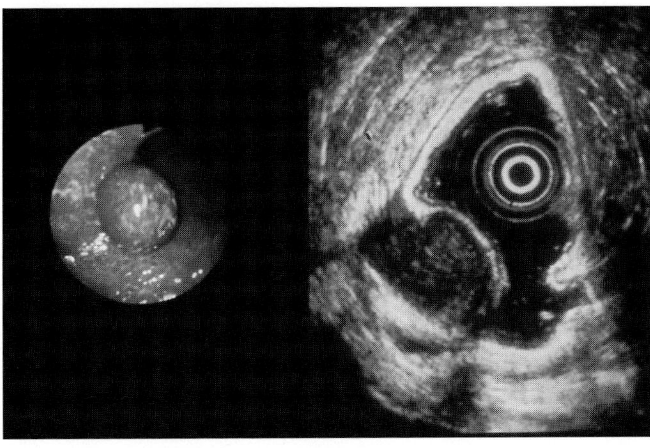

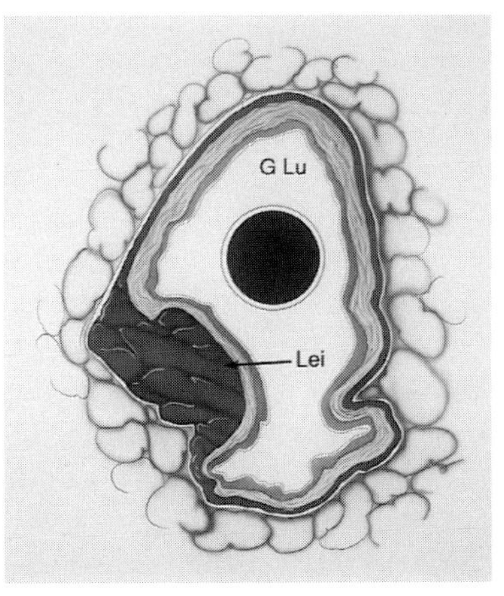


A B C

**FIGURE 15-3**

(**A**) Endoscopic photograph of a gastric leiomyoma. The lesion is covered by endoscopically and histologically normal gastric mucosa. The mass lesion projects into the lumen of the stomach and may produce symptoms of bleeding if ulcerated. (*See color insert for color plate.*) (**B**) Endoscopic ultrasound of the leiomyoma pictured in (A). The endosonograph shows the typical appearance of a hypoechoic lesion contiguous with the muscularis propria layer (fourth, hypoechoic layer) of the gastrointestinal tract wall. (**C**) Artist's rendering of the endosonograph.

bleeding or anemia. Endoscopically, larger lesions may have a central umbilication or may ulcerate centrally. Histologically, they appear as circular palisades of smooth muscle cells with prominent nuclei (23).

Endosonographically, a leiomyoma appears as an echo-poor mass contiguous with the fourth hypoechoic layer (Figs. 15–2, 15–3). This layer has previously been confirmed to represent the muscularis propria (24). The lesion is usually well rounded and well demarcated with a smooth outer border. Characteristically, esophageal leiomyomas are rounder and have a consistent hypoechoic appearance (Fig. 15–2B).

The location of the lesion may be either intraluminal or extraluminal, or it may be a combination; however, the ultrasound appearance of a well-circumscribed echo-poor lesion and its relationship to the fourth hypoechoic layer allows a correct presumptive diagnosis (Fig. 15–4). In the Yasuda and Boyce series, endoscopic ultrasound correctly diagnosed leiomyoma in more than 95% of cases (15,16).

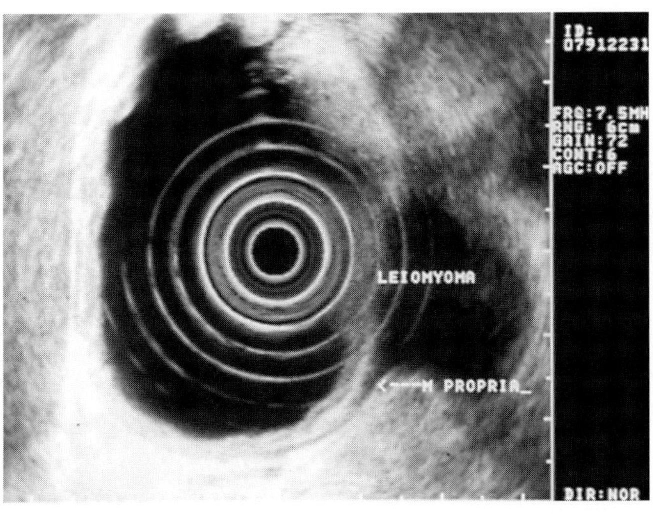


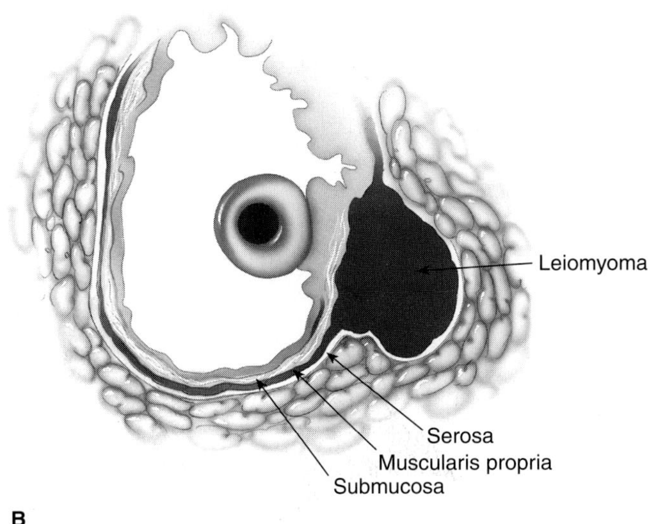


A B

**FIGURE 15-4**

(**A**) Endosonograph of an extragastric leiomyoma arising from the muscularis propria of the stomach. The upper GI barium-contrast radiograph and upper GI endoscopy were normal. The lesion does not protrude into the lumen of the stomach, but rather into the peritoneum. The lesion was resected laparoscopically. (Courtesy J. Van Dam) (**B**) Artist's rendering of the endosonograph.

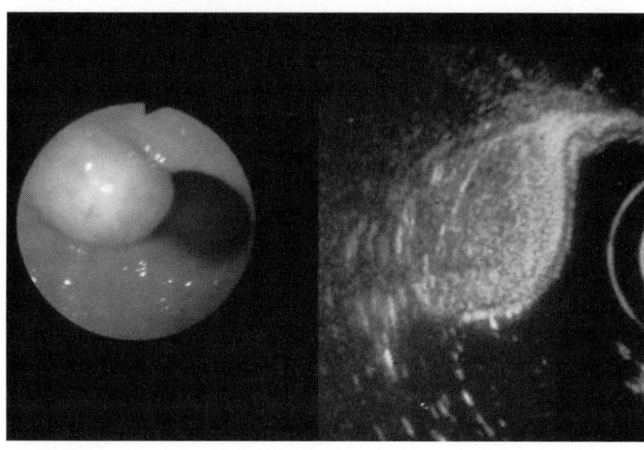

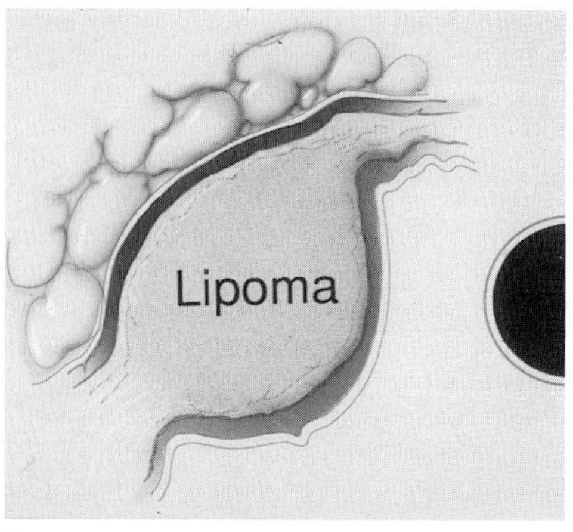


A B C

**FIGURE 15–5**

(**A**) Endoscopic photograph of a gastric lipoma. The lesion is covered by endoscopically and histologically normal gastric mucosa. The mass lesion projects into the lumen of the stomach and may produce symptoms of bleeding if ulcerated. (*See color insert for color plate.*) (**B**) Endoscopic ultrasound of the lesion pictured in (**A**). The endosonograph shows the typical appearance of a hyperechoic lesion contiguous with the submucosal layer (third, hyperechoic layer) of the gastrointestinal tract wall. (**C**) Artist's rendering of the endosonograph.

## Lipoma

Lipomas are benign tumors composed of fatty tissue. They may involve the gastrointestinal tract throughout its length. Most are solitary and submucosal. Histopathologic assessment of lipomas reveals a circumscribed collection of adipose tissue with a collagen capsule (25). At endosonography, lipomas appear as more diffuse lesions filled with bright echoes (Figs. 15–5, 15–6). They appear to arise from the echo-rich layer just superficial to the muscularis propria which corresponds to the submucosa. Thus, lipomas may be accurately described as "submucosal" lesions. Endosonographic evaluation of gastric lipomas is essential before a decision can be made regarding endoscopic resection (26).

## Varices

Varices are enlarged, tortuous vessels found primarily in patients with portal hypertension. They appear in the gastrointestinal tract at porto–systemic venous confluences. Esophageal varices—the most common form of

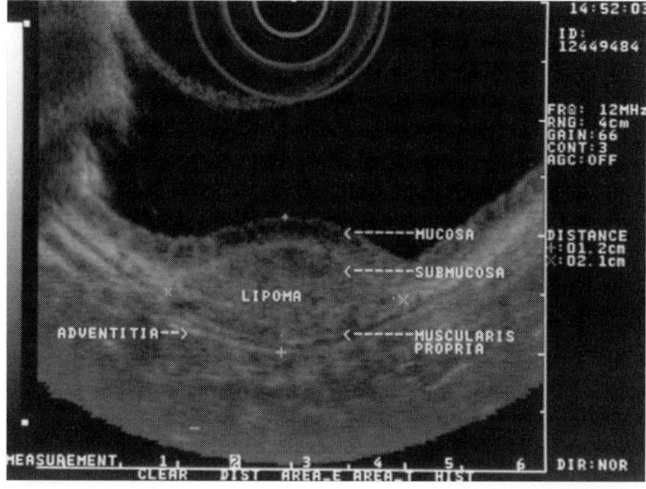


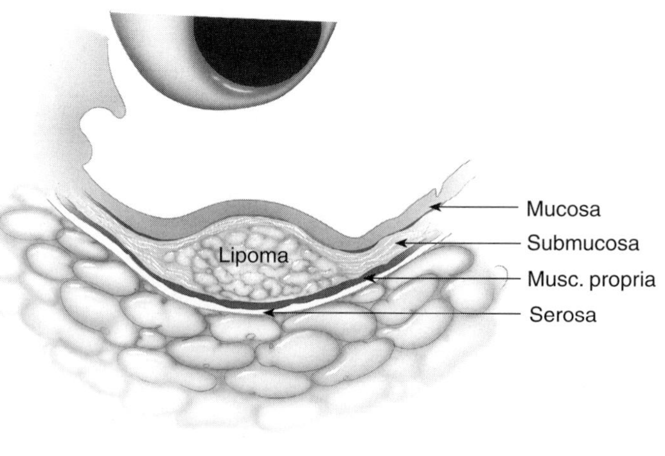


A B

**FIGURE 15–6**

(**A**) Endosonograph of a small gastric lipoma (1.2 × 2.1 cm). The lesion was detected endoscopically as a subepithelial lesion in the gastric antrum. The endosonograph shows the typical appearance of a hyperechoic lesion contiguous with the submucosal layer (third, hyperechoic layer) of the gastrointestinal tract wall. (Courtesy J. Van Dam) (**B**) Artist's rendering of the endosonograph.

varices—can usually be diagnosed correctly by endoscopy because of their characteristic configuration and bluish hue. Gastric varices may be more difficult to detect owing to the confounding appearance of the gastric rugae and the thicker glandular mucosal layer (Fig. 15–7A).

Endosonographically, gastric varices appear as echo-free serpentine structures with smooth margins (Fig. 15–7B). The fact that varices are easily compressed by the ultrasound balloon, aids in the correct diagnosis. Endoscopic ultrasound has also been instrumental in elucidating the nature of large vessels extrinsic to the gastrointestinal wall. The real-time performance of endoscopic ultrasound allows the operator to scan over and along a hypoechoic lesion, verifying the linear appearance that distinguishes vessels from cysts. When large gastric folds are seen at endoscopy, endoscopic ultrasound may be an invaluable indicator of the vascular nature of the lesion, thereby avoiding inappropriate and potentially hazardous large-particle biopsies for diagnosis.

## Cysts

Cysts may appear in the submucosal layer of the gastrointestinal tract or involve closely adjacent organs such as the pancreas, adrenal gland, or spleen. Yasuda et al. described gastric cysts as echo-free rounded lesions within the submucosal layer (Fig. 15–8) (15). The lesions cannot be compressed as readily as varices and are sharply demarcated.

Van Dam et al. first described the utility of endoscopic ultrasound to detect upper gastrointestinal foregut cysts and to sample such cysts endoscopically using needle aspiration (27). Foregut cysts are a diverse group of anomalies that form during embryonic development. In adults, foregut cysts usually are asymptomatic and are discovered incidentally during radiographic or endoscopic examination. Chest CT scan often fails to provide an accurate preoperative diagnosis of mediastinal cysts, because of its relative inability to distinguish solid from cystic lesions when compared with ultrasound. Other

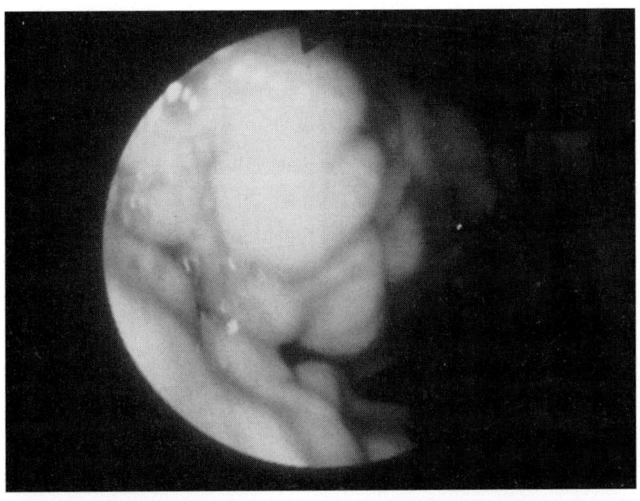

A

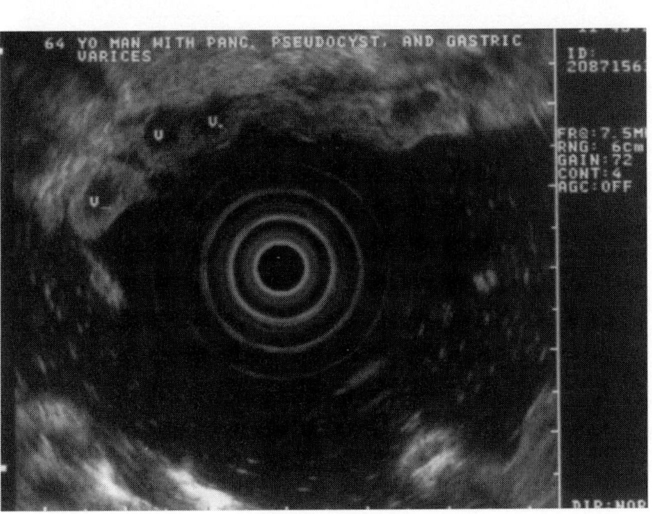


B

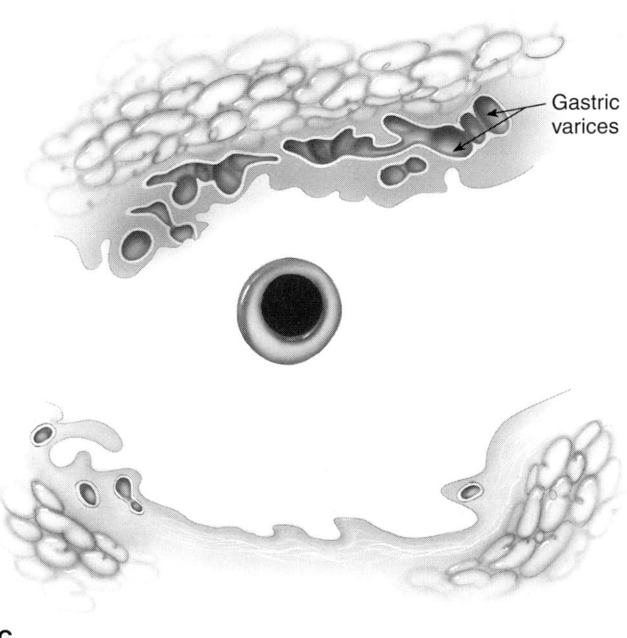


C

**FIGURE 15–7**

The patient is a 66-year-old man with pancreatitis, no endoscopic evidence of esophageal varices, a pancreatic pseudocyst, and presumed splenic vein involvement. (**A**) Endoscopic photograph of gastric varices. The lesion is covered by endoscopically and histologically normal gastric mucosa. The serpentine lesion projects into the lumen of the stomach and may produce symptoms of profound bleeding similar to that of esophageal varices. (*See color insert for color plate.*) (**B**) Endosonograph of the lesion pictured in (**A**). The endosonograph shows the typical appearance of a hypoechoic vascular lesion within the gastrointestinal tract wall. (**C**) Artist's rendering of the endosonograph.

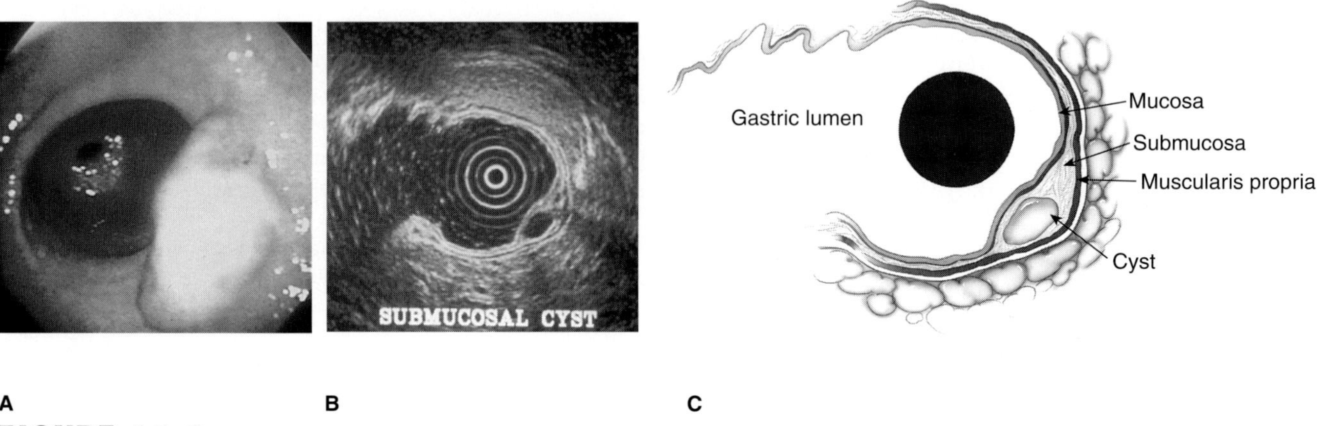


A B C

**FIGURE 15–8**

Gastric cyst. (**A**) The endoscopic photograph on the left shows a gastric subepithelial lesion at the junction of the gastric antrum and body. The lesion is covered by endoscopically and histologically normal gastric mucosa. (*See color insert for color plate.*) (**B**) Endosonograph of the lesion shown in (A). Note the anechoic composition of the lesion. Its endosonographic density is similar to that of the fluid-filled gastric lumen. It is located precisely within the submucosal layer (third, hyperechoic layer) of the gastrointestinal tract wall. (Courtesy J. Van Dam) (**C**) Artist's rendering of the endosonograph.

published reports have confirmed the ability of endoscopic ultrasonography to accurately detect and diagnose esophageal duplication cysts (28–30).

Gastric cysts are a rare clinical entity and usually asymptomatic. Endosonography has been used to detect and diagnose gastric duplication cysts (31). In addition, endosonography has been used to detect rare gastric bronchogenic cysts and gastric cysts containing papillary tumors that abdominal ultrasound and abdominal CT scan failed to detect (32, 33). Endosonography has been shown to be essential prior to attempting endoscopic drainage of gastric duplication cysts (Fig. 15–9) (34).

## Aberrant Pancreas

Pancreatic rests are lesions of ectopic pancreatic tissue. Primarily found in the distal stomach, often along the greater curvature of the antrum, these lesions are usually small. On endoscopy, they may exhibit a characteristic central dimple. Ectopic pancreatic tissue is not as characteristic endosonographically as the previously described lesions. It may appear either as a hypoechoic or mixed echogenic lesion within the gut wall. Its position may vary from mucosal to serosal. A ductal structure may be present, this is seen as a distinct, echo-poor structure within the lesion (Fig. 15–10).

## Rare Lesions

Uncommon lesions reported in the endosonographic literature include granular cell tumor, fibrovascular polyp, spontaneous esophageal hematoma, duodenal carcinoid tumor, esophageal hemangioma, mediastinal granulomas, pancreatic pseudocyst, neurolemmoma, histiocytoma, fibroma, splenic implant, primary liposarcoma of the stomach, and Brunner's gland nodule (Figs. 15–11, 15–12) (12, 15, 16, 18, 35–39, 40, 41). The appearance of the various lesions at endoscopic ultrasound have been described, but the number of lesions is too small to determine if the appearance described is characteristic. Similarly, extrinsic malignant tumors infiltrating the gut wall and presenting as submucosal lesions have also been described. These include bronchogenic carcinoma, breast carcinoma, and mediastinal neural tumors (16) (see Table 15–4). In some instances, endoscopic ultrasound has assisted or directed endoscopic therapy either by the snare resection technique (40) or by the endoscopic, band ligation-assisted technique (41).

# Differential of Benign and Malignant Submucosal Tumors

The most common subepithelial lesion in the upper gastrointestinal tract, the leiomyoma, exhibits characteristic features at endosonography. However, studies confirm that the endoscopic ultrasound appearance of these benign lesions overlaps with that of malignant leiomyosarcoma or leiomyoblastoma. Malignant smooth muscle tumors involving the gastrointestinal wall tend to be larger lesions, having inhomogeneous internal echoes and an irregular outer border (Fig. 15–13). But unless the mass is clearly seen to disrupt the outer margin of the muscularis propria layer, thus indicating invasion, the differentiation between benignity and malignancy cannot be made with certainty (17).

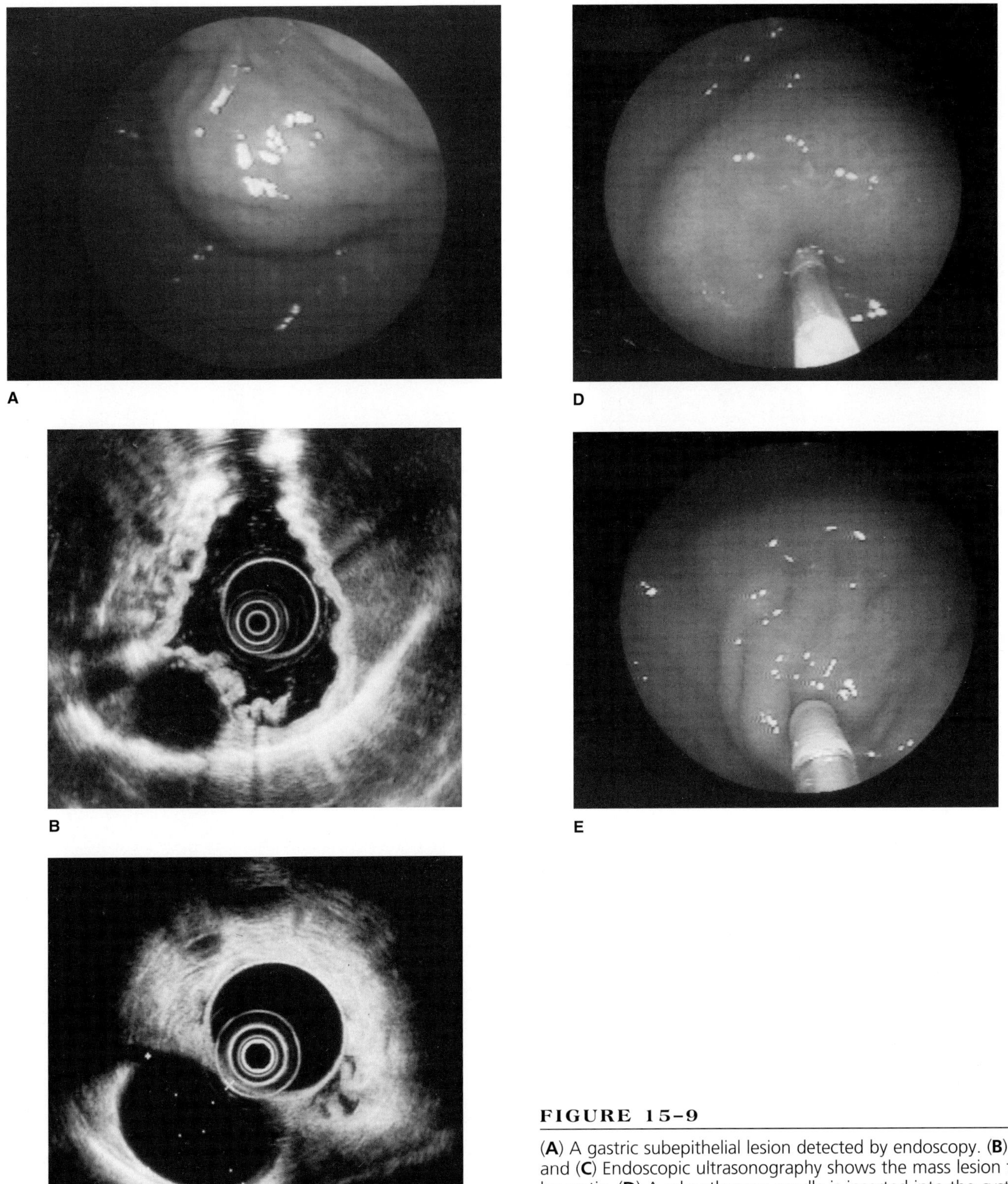



**FIGURE 15-9**

(**A**) A gastric subepithelial lesion detected by endoscopy. (**B**) and (**C**) Endoscopic ultrasonography shows the mass lesion to be cystic. (**D**) A sclerotherapy needle is inserted into the cyst endoscopically. (**E**) The cyst is drained. (Reprinted with permission from Ferrari AP, Van Dam J, Carr-Locke DL. Endoscopy 27:270, 1995.) (*See color insert for color plates **A**, **D**, and **E**.*)

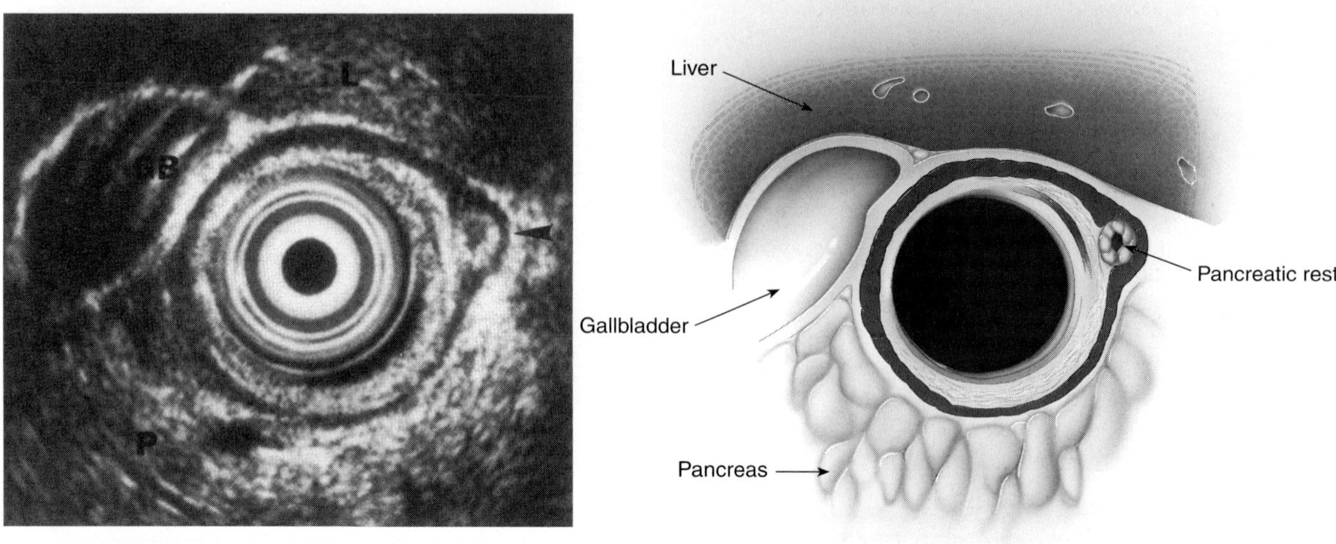


**FIGURE 15-10**

Endosonograph of a pancreatic rest. A small lesion with a central ductal structure located within the submucosal layer (third, hyperechoic layer) of the gastrointestinal tract wall (arrow). (GB) gallbladder; (P) pancreas; (L) liver. (Courtesy G. Boyce)

Rösch et al. reported on the endoscopic ultrasound characteristics of 26 smooth muscle tumors presenting as subepithelial tumors, and conducted a thorough review of the literature (18). He tabulated criteria described for the lesions in an effort to clarify and differentiate points between leiomyoma and leiomyosarcoma. Although symptoms were more common with malignant lesions, they were also present in almost 40% of benign lesions. Rösch confirmed that size and configuration alone are not reliable differentiating factors, since 12–33% of the leiomyomas exceeded 3 cm and occasionally had areas of central necrosis. However, because small smooth muscle tumors are very rarely malignant, a policy of close followup using endoscopic ultrasound, especially for patients with an elevated risk of surgery, may be justified. Growth of the lesion, a change in the echogenic pattern, or necrosis would allow the clinician to refer a small subgroup of patients for excisional surgery.

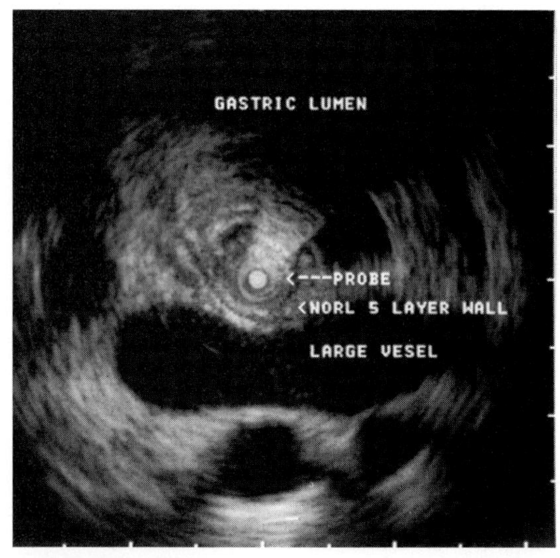


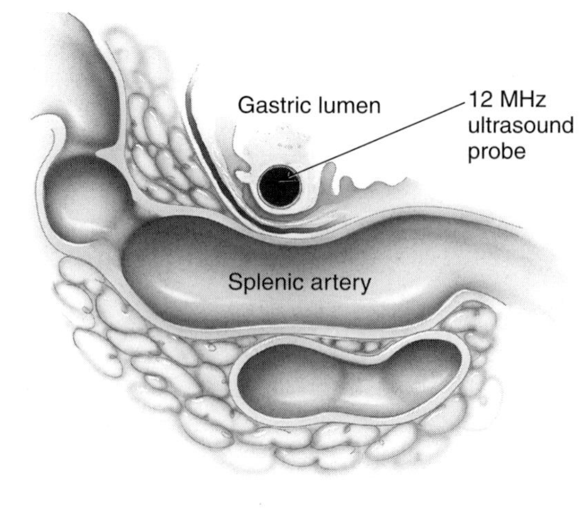


**FIGURE 15-11**

Endosonograph of an enlarged splenic artery presenting as a gastric subepithelial mass lesion in an individual undergoing endoscopy for peptic-type symptoms. The determination of vascularity was made using a 12-MHz endoscopic ultrasound probe passed through the accessory channel of the gastroscope. Confirmation of the lesion as being the splenic vein was made using a standard radial echoendoscope. (Courtesy J. Van Dam)

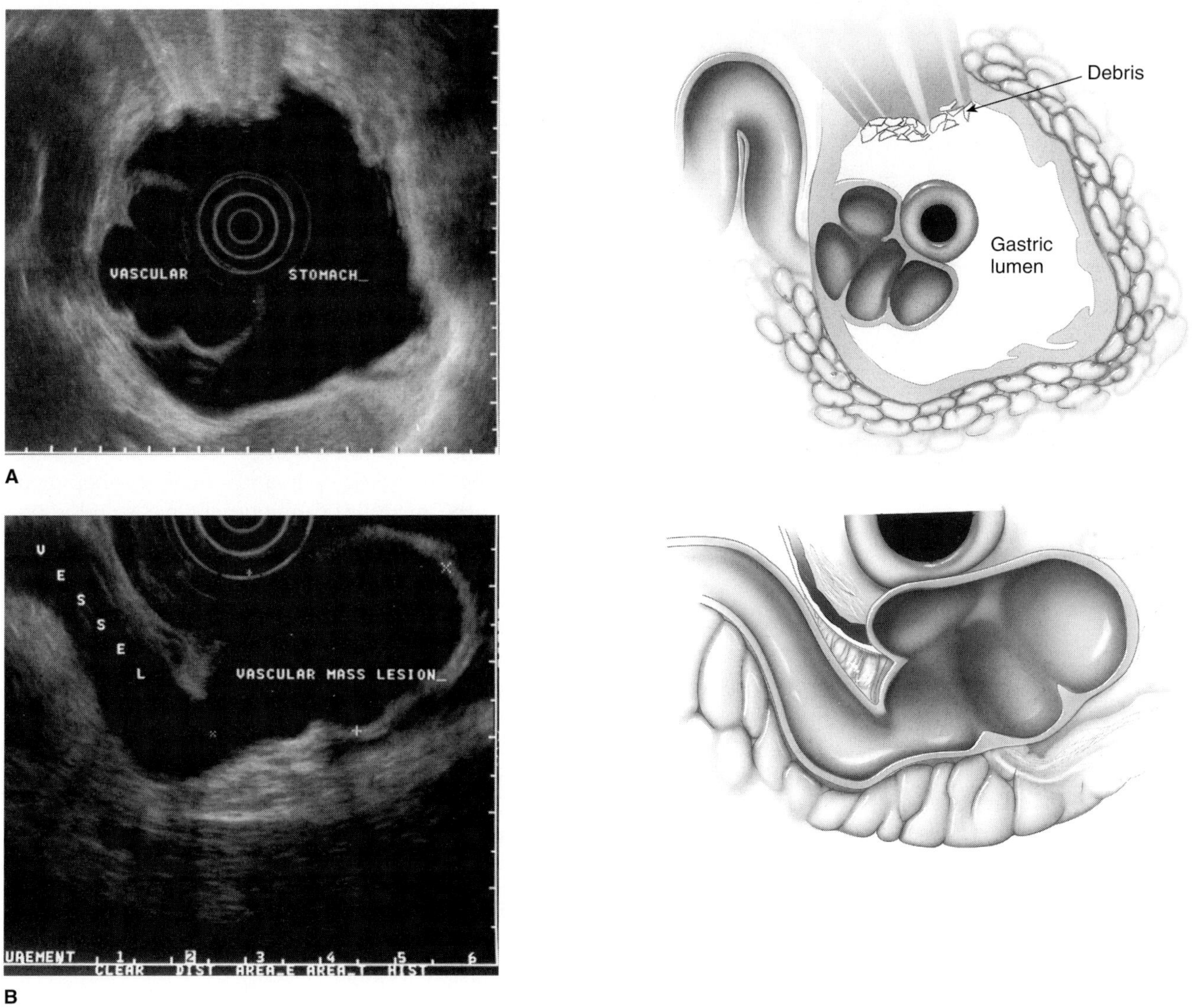


**FIGURE 15-12**

(**A**) Endosonograph of a single gastric varix presenting as a gastric subepithelial mass lesion in an individual undergoing endoscopy for peptic-type symptoms. The lesion is quite large and serpentine. (**B**) In another view, the lesion can be seen emanating from a branch of the portal vein adjacent to the gastric fundus. (Courtesy J. Van Dam)

## Rectal Submucosal Lesions

Submucosal lesions in the rectum are rare. Rectal varices have been described, as well as rare neurologic tumors. Carcinoid tumors may occur in the rectum and represent approximately 20% of all gastrointestinal carcinoid lesions (42). Rectal carcinoids usually arise from the submucosal layer and often have a smooth surface; therefore, they are usually described endoscopically as being submucosal lesions. Small lesions may well be amenable to endoscopic removal. Matsumoto et al. described the endosonographic features of five patients with small rectal carcinoid lesions. Endoscopic ultrasound accurately defined the masses as restricted to the submucosal layer and allowed the correct choice of endoscopic polypectomy or local excision for these lesions rather than radical surgery (43).

## Special Techniques for the Histologic Assessment of Subepithelial Lesions

Despite its advantages, endoscopic ultrasound does not provide a histologic diagnosis of subepithelial lesions. Standard endoscopic biopsy techniques are disappointing in the diagnosis of these lesions. Jumbo biopsies have been utilized but often fail to reach tissue beneath the submucosa (9). Recently, there have been several

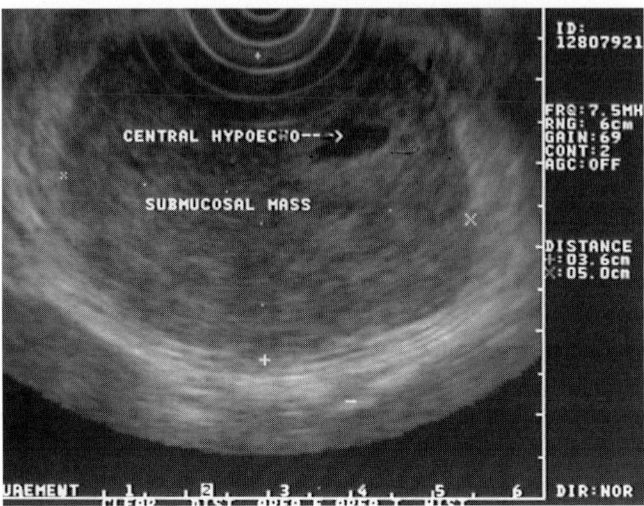


**FIGURE 15–13**

Gastric spindle cell tumor consistent with gastrointestinal stromal tumor. Note the internal echoes and the area devoid of echoes within the substance of the lesion. Pathologic assessment detected numerous mitoses per high-power field. (Courtesy J. Van Dam)

reports of special techniques used in conjunction with endoscopic ultrasound to obtain histologic material for the diagnosis of such lesions.

Small shallow lesions may be seen at endoscopy but may be difficult to pinpoint at endoscopic ultrasound. Tanaka et al. have described a method of injecting saline into the submucosal layer adjacent to a lesion (44). The endosonographic appearance of submucosal saline allows accurate placement of the ultrasound probe and clear imaging of the boundary between the saline and the lesion. A corollary use of submucosal saline injection, called strip-biopsy, has been described by Japanese investigators (45). The injection raises a small mucosal or submucosal lesion off the muscular wall and permits safe snare polypectomy with a fast pure-cut cautery. This technique provides a whole pathologic specimen of small lesions for diagnosis.

Wiersema et al. have described fine-needle aspiration cytology under endoscopic ultrasound guidance. In their series a cytologic diagnosis was made in 17 out of 20 patients with extrinsic or submucosal masses suspected to be malignant. All of these lesions had prior negative conventional biopsies or brush cytology (46). Other reports have confirmed the clinical utility of EUS-guided fine needle aspiration to determine the malignant status of subepithelial lesions (47).

Caletti et al. described the use of a unique flexible needle passed through the endoscope biopsy channel. The needle has a guillotine tip similar to a true-cut forceps. This group reported on biopsy specimens from 21 patients with gastric submucosal tumors. Adequate tissue was obtained in 18 cases (85%) and no major complications occurred (48). Other investigators are evaluating similar techniques for obtaining core biopsy material under EUS guidance (49). The advantage of obtaining a core biopsy over that of aspiration cytology is to obtain a quantity of material sufficient for histologic evaluation.

## Summary

Subepithelial lesions involving the gastrointestinal tract are difficult to diagnose definitively by conventional imaging with gastrointestinal radiography, abdominal ultrasound, or computed tomographic scanning. Endoscopic views are limited and standard biopsy techniques have a low yield.

Endoscopic ultrasound is a major addition to our imaging armamentarium for these lesions. An improved assessment of the size, depth, and extent of subepithelial lesions can be made. The unique ability of endoscopic ultrasound to visualize the layers of the gastrointestinal tract wall allows assessment of the specific layer of the wall from which the lesion arises.

A very characteristic endosonographic appearance has been described for submucosal smooth muscle tumors, cysts, varices, and lipomas. Additionally, accurate information regarding extrinsic lesions compressing the gastrointestinal tract is possible. Finally, special new techniques for obtaining histologic or cytologic material from submucosal lesions have been reported in which endoscopic ultrasound is the guiding imaging technique.

### References

1. David GR: Neoplasms of the stomach. In Sleisinger MG (ed): Gastrointestinal Disease. Philadelphia: W.B. Saunders, 1989, pp 766–767.
2. Postlewait RW. Benign tumors and cysts of the esophagus. Surg Clin North Am 63:925, 1983.
3. Morson BC, Dawson IMP. Nonepithelial tumors. In: Gastrointestinal Pathology. Oxford: Blackwell Scientific Publications, 1979, pp 187–199.
4. Phillips JC, Lindsay JW, Kendall JA. Gastric leiomyosarcoma: Roentgenologic and clinical findings. Am J Dig Dis 15:239–246, 1975.
5. Megibow AJ, Balthazar EJ, Hulnick DH, et al. CT evaluation of gastrointestinal leiomyomas and leiomyosarcomas. AJR 144: 727–731, 1985.
6. Pillazi G, Weinzeb J, Vernace F, et al. CT of gastric masses: Image pattern and a note on potential pitfalls. Gastrointest Radiol 8: 11–17, 1983.
7. Faivre J, Bory R, Moulinier B. Benign tumors of esophagus: Value of endoscopy. Endoscopy 10:264–268, 1978.
8. Papazian A, Gineston JL, Capron JP, Quenum C. Leiomyoblastoma of the stomach: Endoscopic treatment. Endoscopy 16:157–169, 1984.
9. Kaneko E, Kumagai J, Honda N, et al. Evaluation of the new giant biopsy forceps in the diagnosis of mucosal and submucosal gastric lesions. Endoscopy 15:322–326, 1983.
10. Kawai K. In: Endoscopic Ultrasonography in Gastroenterology. New York: Igaku-Shoin, 1988.
11. Moto Y, Ohta H, Satomura Y, Watanabe H, Yamakawa O, Yamaguchi Y, Mouri I, Sawabu N. Endoscopic ultrasonography in the diagnosis of extraluminal compressions mimicking gastric submucosal tumors. Endoscopy 26:239–242, 1994.

12. Inai M, Sakai M, Kajiyama T, Imada-Shirakata Y, Kin G, Inoue K, Ueda S, Okuma M. Endosonographic characterization of duodenal elevated lesions. Gastrointest Endosc 44:714–719, 1996.
13. Catalano MF, Geenen JE, Schmalz MJ, Johnson GK, Hogan WJ. Evaluation of submucosal lesions of the upper gastrointestinal tract by endoscopic ultrasound (EUS). Gastrointest Endosc 41:361A, 1995.
14. Geller AJ, Nguyen CC, Axelrad AM, Fleischer DE, Al-Kawas FH, Lewis JH. The impact of endoscopic ultrasonography (EUS) on the management of patients with gastric lesions diagnosed by other methods. Gastrointest Endosc 41:321A, 1995.
15. Yasuda K, Cho E, Nakajima M, Kawai K. Diagnosis of submucosal lesions of the upper gastrointestinal tract by endoscopic ultrasonography. Gastrointest Endosc 36:S17–S20, 1990.
16. Boyce GA, Sivak MV, Rösch T, et al. Evaluation of submucosal upper gastrointestinal tract lesions by endoscopic ultrasound. Gastrointest Endosc 37:449–454, 1991.
17. Tio TL, Tytgat GNJ, den Hartog Jager FCA. Endoscopic ultrasonography for the evaluation of smooth muscle tumors in the upper gastrointestinal tract: An experience with 42 cases. Gastrointest Endosc 36:342–350, 1990.
18. Rösch T, Loren R, Dancygier H, et al. Endosonographic diagnosis of submucosal upper gastrointestinal tract tumors. Scand J Gastroenterol 27:1–8, 1992.
19. Caletti G, Zani L, Bolondi L, et al. Endoscopic ultrasonography in the diagnosis of gastric submucosal tumor. Gastrointest Endosc 35:413–418, 1989.
20. Bashir RM, Gupta PK. Endoscopic ultrasonographic diagnosis of a splenic artery aneurysm. Pract Gastroenterol 19:24B–24D, 1995.
21. Catalano, MF. Endoscopic ultrasonography in the diagnosis of submucosal tumors: Need for biopsy. Endoscopy 26:788–791, 1994.
22. Kajiyama T, Sakai M, Torii A, et al. Endoscopic aspiration lumpectomy of esophageal leiomyoma derived from the musculari mucosae. Amer J Gastroenterol 90:417–422, 1995.
23. Ranchod M, Kempson R. Smooth muscle tumors of the gastrointestinal tract and retroperitoneum. A pathologic analysis of 100 cases. Cancer 39:255, 1977.
24. Bolondi L, Casanova P, Santi V, et al. The sonographic appearance of the normal gastric wall: An in vitro study. Ultrasound Med Biol 12:991–998, 1986.
25. Fenoglio-Preiser C, Pascal R, Perzin K. Tumors of the Intestines. Washington, D.C.: Armed Forces Institutes of Pathology, 1990.
26. Nakamura S, Iida M, Suekane H, et al. Endoscopic removal of gastric lipoma: Diagnostic value of endoscopic ultrasonography. Amer J Gastroenterol 86:619–621, 1991.
27. Van Dam J, Rice TW, Sivak MV Jr. Endoscopic ultrasonography and endoscopically guided needle aspiration for the diagnosis of upper gastrointestinal tract foregut cysts. Amer J Gastroenterol 87:762–765, 1992.
28. Geller A, Wang KK, DiMagno EP. Diagnosis of foregut duplication cysts by endoscopic ultrasonography. Gastroenterology 109: 838–842, 1995.
29. Bhutani MS, Hoffman BJ, Reed C. Endosonographic diagnosis of an esophageal duplication cyst. Endoscopy 28:396–397, 1996.
30. Faigel DO, Burke A, Ginsberg GG, Stotland BR, Kadish SL, Kochman ML. The role of endoscopic ultrasound in the evaluation and management of foregut duplications. Gastrointest Endosc 45:99–103, 1997.
31. Van Dam J, Zuccaro G Jr., Sivak MV Jr. Endosonographic diagnosis of a submucosal gastric cyst. J Ultrasound Med 11:61–63, 1992.
32. Tanaka M, Akahoshi K, Chijiiwa Y, Sasaki I, Nawata J. Diagnostic value of endoscopic ultrasonography in an unusual case of gastric cyst. Amer J Gastroenterol 90:662–663, 1995.
33. Carpenter S, Bansal R, Scheiman JM. Endosonography of an abdominal bronchogenic cyst. Gastrointest Endosc 44:197–199, 1996.
34. Ferrari AP, Van Dam J, Carr-Locke DL. Endoscopic needle aspiration of a gastric duplication cyst. Endoscopy 27:270–272, 1995.
35. Lawrence SP, Larsen BR, Stacy CC, McNally PR. Echoendosonographic and histologic correlation of a fibrovascular polyp of the esophagus. Gastrointest Endosc 40:81–84, 1994.
36. Mion F, Bernard G, Valette P-J, Lambert R. Spontaneous esophageal hematoma: Diagnostic contribution of echoendoscopy. Gastrointest Endosc 40:503–505, 1994.
37. Yoshikane H, Suzuki T, Yoshioka N, et al. Duodenal carcinoid tumor: Endosonographic imaging and endoscopic resection. Amer J Gastroenterol 90:642–644, 1995.
38. Yoshikane H, Suzuki T, Yoshioka N, Ogawa Y, Ochi T, Hasegawa N. Hemangioma of the esophagus: Endosonographic imaging and endoscopic resection. Endoscopy 27:267–269, 1995.
39. Savides TJ, Gress FG, Wheat LJ, Ikenberry S, Hawes RH. Dysphagia due to mediastinal granulomas: Diagnosis with endoscopic ultrasonography. Gastroenterology 109:366–373, 1995.
40. Yamamoto K. Primary liposarcoma of the stomach resected endoscopically. Endoscopy 27:711, 1996.
41. Chang KJ, Yoshinaka R, Nguyen P. Endoscopic ultrasound-assisted band ligation: A new technique for resection of submucosal tumors. Gastrointest Endosc 44:720–722, 1996.
42. Morgan JG, Marks C, Hearn D. Carcinoid tumors of the gastrointestinal tract. Ann Surg 180:720–727, 1974.
43. Matsumoto T, Iida M, Suekane H, et al. Endoscopic ultrasonography in rectal carcinoid tumors: Contribution to selection of therapy. Gastrointest Endosc 37:539–542, 1991.
44. Tanaka M, Bandou T, Watanabe A, Sasaki H. A new technique in endoscopic ultrasonography of the upper gastrointestinal tract. Endoscopy 22:221–225, 1990.
45. Tada M, Shimada M, Murakami F, et al. Development of the strip-off biopsy (in Japanese). Gastroenterol Endosc 26:833–839, 1984.
46. Wiersema MJ, Hawes RH, Tao LC, et al. Endoscopic ultrasonography as an adjunct to fine needle aspiration cytology of the upper and lower gastrointestinal tract. Gastrointest Endosc 38: 35–39, 1992.
47. Dy E, Ciaccia D, Bekal P, Thomas A, Gress F. Diagnosis of gastric and esophageal submucosal lesions by EUS-guided fine needle aspiration. Amer J Gastroenterol 91:2012A, 1996.
48. Caletti GC, Brocchi E, Ferrari A, et al. Guillotine needle biopsy as a supplement to endosonography in the diagnosis of gastric submucosal tumors. Endoscopy 23:251–254, 1991.
49. Harada N, Kouzu T, Arima M, Isono K. Endoscopic ultrasound-guided histologic needle biopsy: Preliminary results using a newly developed endoscopic ultrasound transducer. Gastrointest Endosc 44:327–330, 1996.

CHAPTER

# Needle Biopsy of Subepithelial Lesions

Giancarlo Caletti
Paolo Bocus
Thomas Togliani
Enrico Roda

The diagnosis of submucosal tumors (SMT) of the gastrointestinal tract has always been difficult. A variety of differing submucosal lesions produce the same endoscopic appearance, including benign or malignant pathologic tumors within the wall itself and contiguous normal or pathologic organs and structures that compress the gut wall. Biopsy specimens obtained at endoscopy by standard methods are usually inadequate for diagnosis because of the superficial nature and small size of the samples. The technique of obtaining multiple biopsies at a single site is usually not diagnostic for similar reasons. More aggressive techniques for obtaining larger specimens from deep within submucosal lesions may be unsafe and are of no value in cases of extrinsic compression (1).

Endoscopic ultrasonography (EUS) displays the structure of the gut wall and neighboring organs. The gastrointestinal wall appears ultrasonographically as layers of different echogenicities. These correspond closely to the anatomic architecture (2–5). EUS diagnosis is based on alterations that occur in this layered structure. EUS can differentiate SMT from extrinsic compression, and it provides precise information about the site, size, and nature (solid or liquid) of these lesions. The margins of the lesion are better defined by EUS than by any other imaging modality. A histologic diagnosis may be suggested by identification of the layer of origin within the wall and other acoustic characteristics (6,7).

The EUS appearance of a leiomyoma is that of a hypoechoic mass arising in the fourth hypoechoic layer which, for practical purposes, represents the muscularis propria (6,7) (Fig. 16–1). However, attempts to differentiate leiomyosarcoma from leiomyoma on the basis of size, shape, and sonographic appearance have been disappointing.

Yasuda et al. (6,8) state that a well-demarcated lesion located within the fourth hypoechoic layer with the same echodensity as this layer is likely to be a leiomyoma or a leiomyosarcoma. Unfortunately, the EUS appearance of these two tumors is the same, and the absence of distinguishing features makes differential diagnosis impossible (6,8). Aibe and Takemoto (9) report that malignant SMTs destroy the sonographic layers of the wall, while the normal pattern remains intact in benign SMT. Nakazawa et al. (10) maintain that irregularly shaped sonolucent areas within these tumors correspond to liquefaction necrosis and are thus indicative of leiomyosarcoma. Tio et al. (11) assert that leiomyosarcoma (or leiomyoblastoma) appears at EUS as a nonhomogeneous hypoechoic mass, relatively large, with sharply demarcated boundaries or irregular margins; occasionally, this mass has a central ulcer or fistulous tract. Although large tumor size and the demonstration of necrosis or fistulization suggest malignancy, the only reliable signs of malignancy relate to the biologic behavior of the tumor (i.e., frank infiltration of surrounding organs and structures or remote metastasis). However, all authorities on this subject, in the absence of a histologic diagnosis, recommend a careful follow-up or occasionally surgical resection (Fig. 16–2).

A number of different devices have been developed to obtain biopsy and cytology specimens.

## Fine Needle Aspiration Biopsy (FNAB)

Needle biopsy (a form of aspiration cytology) has increasingly been used to obtain tissue at bronchoscopy, and "skinny needle" (22-gauge) biopsies are now routinely used by invasive radiologists to obtain tissue specimens from sites hitherto inaccessible (12–17). Moreover, the availability of flexible needles for injecting esophageal varices raises the possibility that needle aspiration cytology could be applied to gastrointestinal lesions visualized endoscopically. This technique may allow samples to be obtained from lesions lying deep to necrotic debris or to normal mucosa, and hence hard to diagnose by conventional means.

Aspiration samples are taken using a transbronchial aspiration needle (21-gauge/13 mm long) or a sclerotherapy needle (23-gauge/4 mm long), both retractable at the distal end. At the proximal end a 10-mL disposable syringe is attached. After visualizing the proposed target, the needle is passed through the endoscope with its needle tip retracted. The needle is then protruded beyond the protective sheath and inserted into the suspect lesion. Suction is applied at the proximal end while the needle is plunged in and out of the lesion. After easing off the suction, the needle is retracted and the entire unit is withdrawn. The aspirated material is then expressed onto clean glass slides, air-dried, and stained with May–Grünwald–Giemsa stain to be examined by an experienced cytologist.

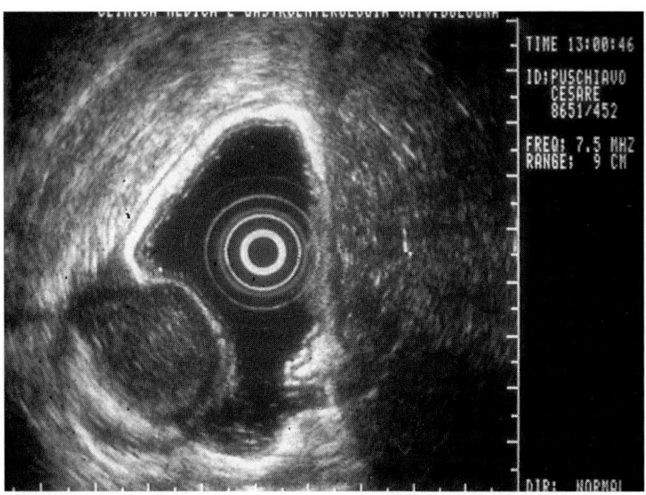


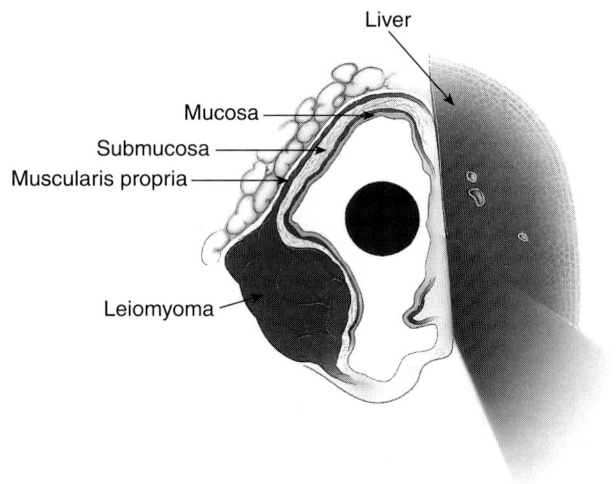


**FIGURE 16–1**

Gastric leiomyoma. EUS shows a solid hypoechoic mass originating from the fourth hypoechoic layer deep to the first three layers, which are normal.

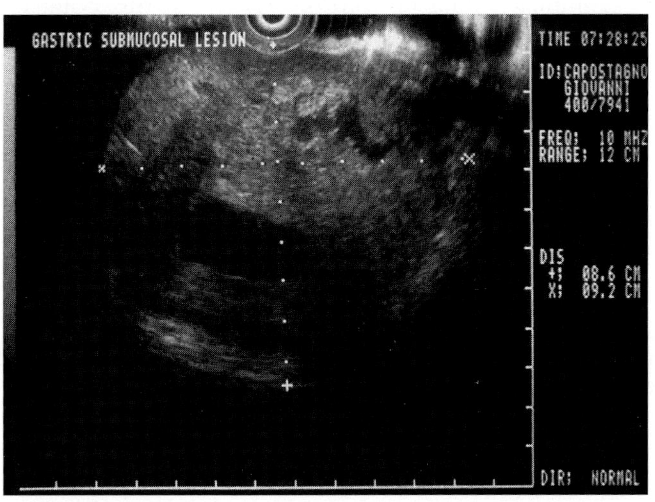


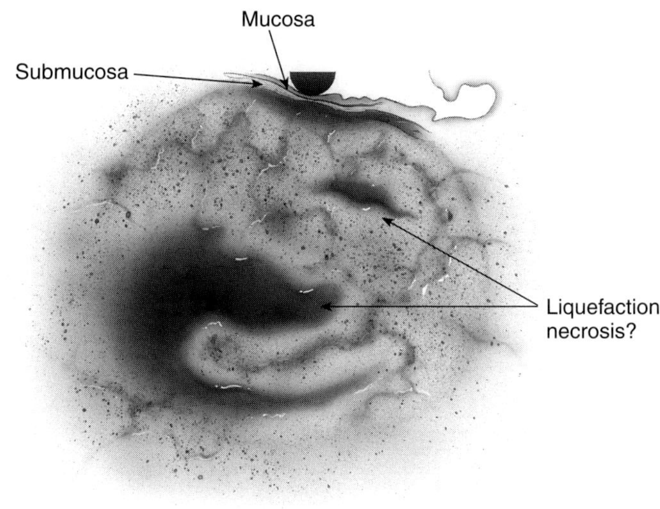


**FIGURE 16–2**

EUS shows a solid hypoechoic gastric mass originating from the fourth layer deep to the first three layers, which are normal. The irregularly shaped sonolucent areas within the tumor correspond to liquefaction necrosis, which is indicative of leiomyosarcoma. A large benign smooth muscle tumor was found at surgery.

In the case of concomitant brush cytology or forceps biopsy, samples must be obtained in the following order: needle aspiration, brush cytology, and forceps biopsy.

Several studies have advocated endoscopic aspiration cytology to add to the diagnostic accuracy of upper GI endoscopic biopsies and brush cytology. Zargar et al. (18) in a series of 318 lesions sampled, report 14 patients with submucosal malignancies and 5 with benign submucosal lesions. The diagnostic accuracy of aspiration cytology was significantly higher than that of biopsy or brush cytology in submucosal, infiltrative, and ulceronecrotic malignancies (92.9% versus 7.1% and 14.3% respectively; $p < 0.001$). The higher yield of needle aspiration in these lesions was due to its ability to allow adequate cytological sampling from the deeper layers. Kochhar et al. (19) describe interesting results of transproctoscopic fine needle aspiration cytology in the diagnosis of rectal lesions. Fifty-one consecutive patients referred with a presumptive diagnosis of rectal mass were subjected to proctoscopic examination when fine needle aspiration cytology, brush cytology, and biopsy samples were taken. Of the 30 patients for whom malignancy of the rectum was confirmed and in whom all three sampling techniques were applied, the biopsy was positive in 27 (90%), brush cytology in 25 (83.3%), and fine needle aspiration cytology in 29 (96.6%). A combination of fine needle aspiration cytology with brush cytology had a positive yield in 96.6% while that of fine needle aspiration cytology with biopsy had a yield of 100%. Fine needle aspiration cytology was most helpful in infiltrative tumors. All 10 patients with tumor in the pouch of Douglas or rectovescical pouch were correctly diagnosed at fine needle aspiration cytology, as was the case for submucosal rectal carcinoma. There were no false-positive results and no complications with this latter technique.

Fine needle aspiration cytology does, however, have certain limitations. First, the role of this technique in benign lesions lies primarily in excluding malignancy. Second, a negative aspirate does not necessarily rule out the possibility of a malignancy. Third, fine needle aspiration cytology cannot be used for typing benign lesions.

## EUS and FNAB

To improve the accuracy of diagnosing submucosal lesions, Wiersema et al. (20) combined endoscopic ultrasonography with fine needle aspiration cytology. Seventeen of 20 consecutive patients with gastrointestinal lesions suspicious for malignancy and/or not amenable to standard biopsy technique had diagnostic results with the combination of endoscopic ultrasonography and fine needle aspiration cytology. Endoscopic ultrasonography appeared to be helpful in determining the feasibility of fine needle aspiration as well as directing the biopsy approach. The intraluminal imaging method allowed definition of the regional anatomy surrounding the mass and the assessment of malignant features.

Van Dam et al. (21) reported a case of a mediastinal foregut cyst in which the diagnosis was made with EUS and confirmed with endoscopically guided needle aspiration. Endoscopy in a 63-year-old woman revealed an extraluminal right-sided mass 19–21 cm from the incisor teeth. The overlying esophageal mucosa appeared endoscopically normal. At EUS the lesion appeared homogeneously hypoechoic, with an echogenicity similar to that of the water-filled ballon (i.e., cystic). The cyst measured 2.0 × 2.5 cm in its largest dimension and had a notably thin wall. To assess the nature of the lesion further, and to ensure benignity, partial cyst aspiration was performed using a standard sclerotherapy needle under direct endoscopic visualization. Aspiration yielded 3 mL of turbid, yellow fluid. No complication was reported. Needle aspiration of foregut cysts may thus be both diagnostic and therapeutic, if sufficient volume of cystic fluid is removed to reduce symptoms. These authors successfully documented needle drainage of bronchogenic cysts and now recommend this approach together with close observation, to avoid thoracotomy.

## Guillotine Needle Biopsy

A newly devised biopsy needle—the "guillotine needle" (Flexi-Temno®, Bauer Company, Pieve di Cento; Bologna, Italy)—recently has been presented by us (22,23). It can be used to obtain adequate tissue samples for final histologic confirmation from solid submucosal lesions previously detected at endoscopic ultrasonography. This new biopsy needle is a unique flexible needle for endoscopes with a standard biopsy channel. Its tip is a guillotine device that allows the endoscopist to obtain submucosal samples 8 mm in length and 1.1–2.1 mm in section diameter. The guillotine is controlled by means of a handle similar to that of a biopsy forceps. The flexible part comes in several lengths for various applications and it is protected by a Teflon sheath (Fig. 16–3). When facing the submucosal tumor, the sheath is retracted, the guillotine device is opened, and the needle is completely pierced into the tumor. At this point the guillotine device is closed and the needle gently withdrawn.

The guillotine needle biopsy was performed in 47 patients (15 with esophageal SMTs and 32 with gastric SMT). One to four punctures (mean 3) were necessary to obtain one adequate sample. In the esophageal SMT group the guillotine biopsy diagnosed 15 leiomyomas (three surgically confirmed) (Fig. 16–4). In the gastric SMT group the guillotine biopsy could not obtain a sample in three surgically confirmed leiomyomas: two <2 cm located on the prepyloric lesser curve, and one >4 cm located on the greater curve of the body. In the remaining 29 patients the guillotine biopsy diagnosed 1 leiomyoblastoma, 5 lipomas (Figs. 16–5, 16–6), and 21 leiomyomas, while it detected two unsuspected leiomyosarcomas (EUS-diagnosed leiomyomas). One was <4 cm and one >4 cm (Fig. 16–7). No major complication was encountered during this study.

Biopsy diagnosis was confirmed at surgery in 16 patients: 1 lipoma, 1 leiomyoblastoma, 2 leiomyosarcomas, and 12 leiomyomas. Four lipomas and 9 leiomyomas, all asymptomatic and <4 cm size, in which EUS and bioptic diagnosis were coincident, are being followed at 12-month intervals with endoscopic ultrasonography and guillotine needle biopsy.

The guillotine needle biopsy has also been easily performed in infiltrative gastric disorders (6 lymphomas, 5 linitis plastica, 3 Menetrier's disease), the duodenum [1 leiomyoblastoma (Fig. 16–8), 1 ampullary cancer], and rectum [1 submucosal cancer recurrence (Fig. 16–9)].

The guillotine needle biopsy allows a definitive diagnosis; thus malignancies can be detected when endoscopic ultrasonography findings are not significant. In this way patients with small asymptomatic solid sub-

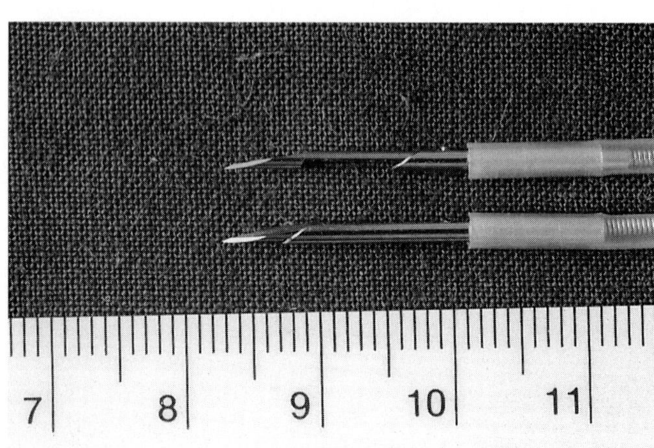


**FIGURE 16–3**

The newly devised biopsy needle, the Flexi-Temno®.

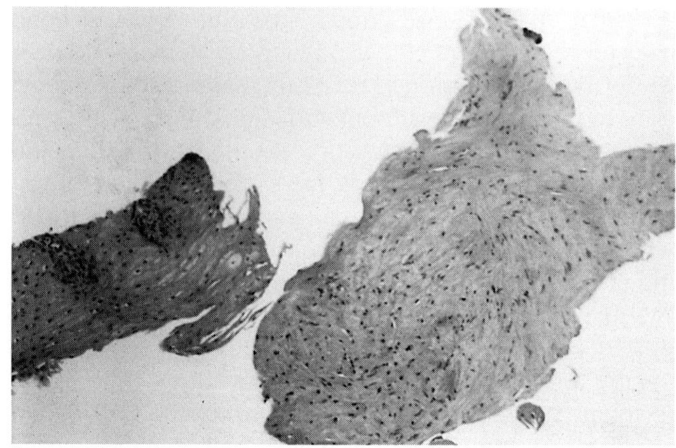

**FIGURE 16–4**

Guillotine needle sample of an esophageal leiomyoma. (hematoxylin–eosin, ×100) (*See color insert for color plate.*)

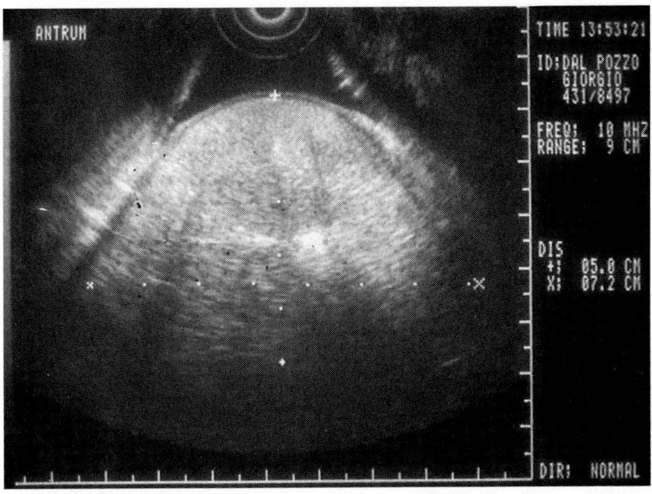


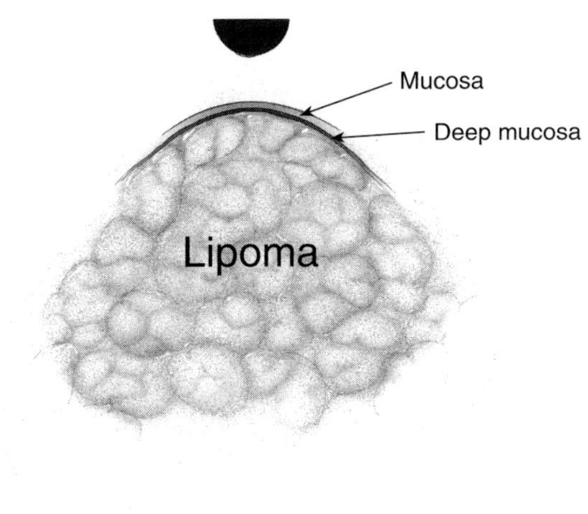


**FIGURE 16–5**

Gastric lipoma. EUS shows a large solid hyperechoic mass originating from the third hyperechoic layer deep to the first two layers, which are normal.

mucosal tumors can be regularly followed up, first with EUS and then with guillotine needle biopsy, and operated on when a malignancy is revealed.

## EUS-Guided FNAB

The combination of endosonography and endoscopic FNAB or guillotine needle biopsy is limited by the fact that EUS and biopsy are separate procedures and that the selection of the biopsy site depends on demonstration of an endoluminal abnormality. In fact, conventional mechanical radial scanning echoendoscopes do not allow one to visualize the entry of the biopsy needle into the lesion. The study of Tio et al. (24) is the only one in which a radial scanning echoendoscope is used in conjunction with FNA to detect pancreatic adenocarcinoma in a patient with submucosal gastric abnormalities.

The introduction of convex linear array echoendoscopes equipped with a biopsy channel has made FNAB under direct endosonographic guidance possible. This is because the scanning plane is parallel to the long axis of the endoscope, so that the biopsy needle can be visualized along its full length during its insertion into the target lesion.

Vilmann et al. (25) reported the successful use of EUS-guided FNA to diagnose a pancreatic cystadenoma

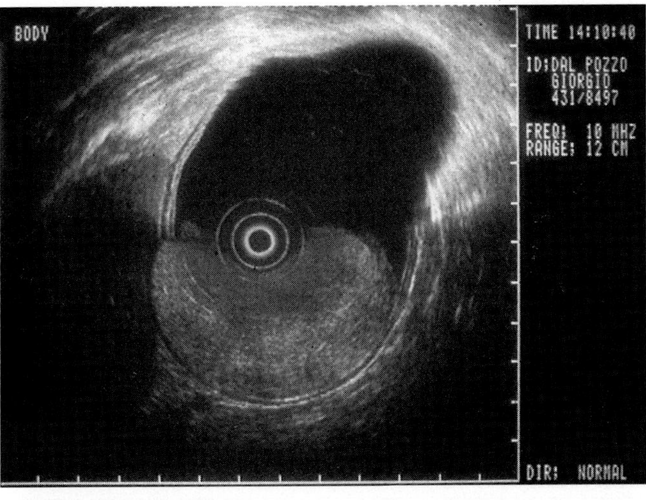


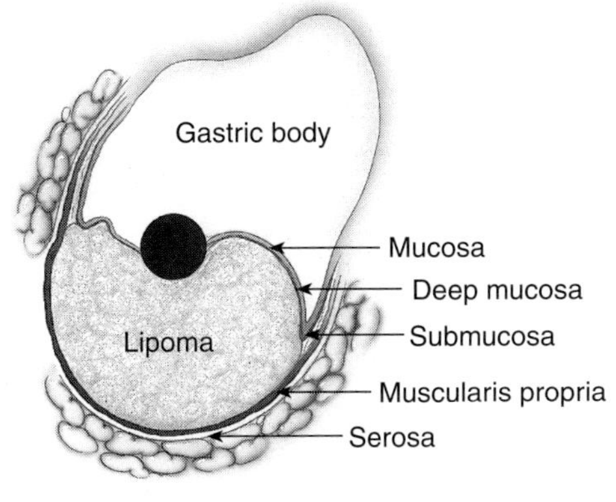


**FIGURE 16–6**

Another EUS view of the gastric lipoma shown in Figure 16–5. The fourth hypoechoic layer is clearly depicted and is normal.

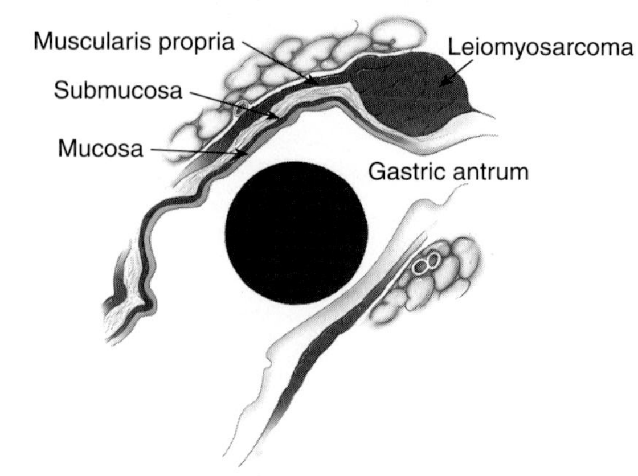


**FIGURE 16-7**

EUS shows a solid hypoechoic mass originating from the fourth hypoechoic layer deep to the first three layers, which are normal. The EUS pattern is characteristic for a leiomyoma. The guillotine needle biopsy demonstrated a leiomyosarcoma.

in a patient in whom ERCP was normal while US with needle aspiration biopsy and CT interpreted the lesion as chronic pancreatitis. Grimm et al. (26) used the EUS-guided technique to drain a pancreatic pseudocyst in a patient that did not have endoscopic evidence of extramural bulging. Wiersema et al. (27), using EUS-guided FNAB in a patient with lung cancer, detected malignancy in a paraesophageal lymph node not readily accessible by mediastinoscopy, transbronchial biopsy, or percutaneous FNAB. These authors also reported promising results with the same methods (28) in the diagnostic evaluation of patients with mediastinal lymph nodes, pancreatic masses, extrapancreatic abdominal masses, and infiltrative luminal lesions with a sensitivity of 100%, 82%, 100%, and 100%, respectively. Vilmann et al. (29,30) made a substantial contribution to the field of EUS-guided FNAB, by helping to develop a suitable needle sufficiently long and stable and by describing this biopsy technique well. They reported a predictive value of positive cytologic diagnosis of 100%, and a predictive value of negative cytologic diagnosis of 83%. Other preliminary case series published on EUS-guided FNAB (31–33) confirm that this new method can be safely applied in the evaluation of both extraluminal and submucosal lesions of the gastrointestinal tract with a high degree of diagnostic accuracy (87%) and that it may have a significant impact on the staging and management of patients with gastrointestinal and pulmonary malignancies. Giovannini et al. (34), in the diagnosis of malignancy, reported a sensitivity and specificity of 77% and 100%, respectively. The results were better for mediastinal masses (sensitivity

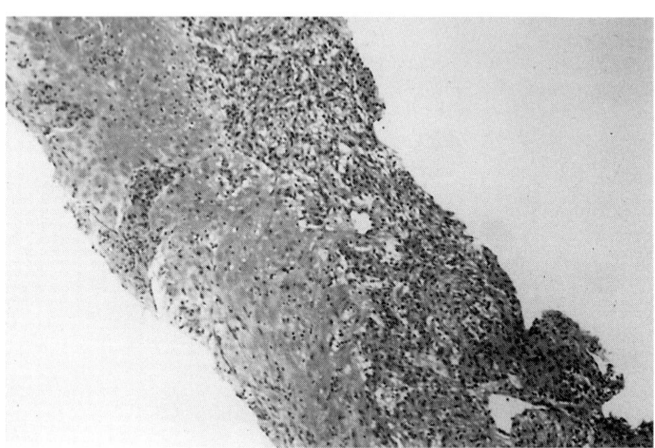

**FIGURE 16-8**

Guillotine needle sample of a duodenal leiomyoblastoma. (hematoxylin–eosin, ×100) (*See color insert for color plate.*)

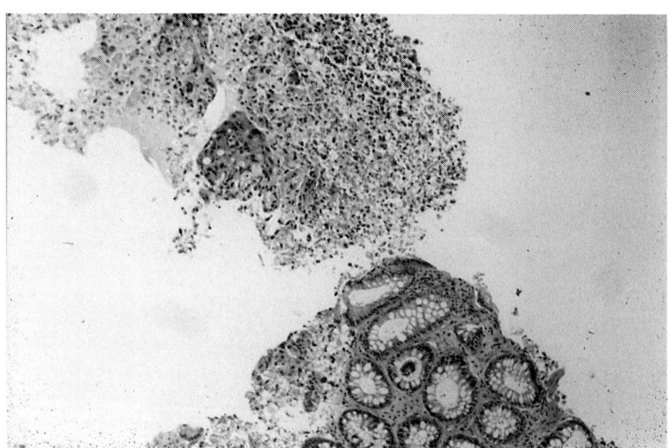

**FIGURE 16-9**

Guillotine needle sample of a submucosal cancer recurrence of the rectum. (hematoxylin–eosin, ×100) (*See color insert for color plate.*)

88%), mediastinal lymph nodes (81%), and celiac lymph nodes (80%) than for pancreatic tumors (75%) and submucosal tumors (60%):

In all published series no complications were encountered.

## References


1. Bjork JT. Nonepithelial neoplasms of the stomach. Gastrointest Endosc 23:162–163, 1981.
2. Aibe T, Fuji T, Okita K, Takemoto T. A fundamental study of normal layer structure of the gastrointestinal wall visualized by endoscopic ultrasonography. Scand J Gastroenterol 21(suppl 123):1–5, 1986.
3. Bolondi L, Caletti GC, Casanova P, Villanacci V, Grigioni W, Labò G. Problems and variations in the interpretation of the ultrasound feature of the normal upper and lower GI tract wall. Scand J Gastroenterol 21(suppl 123):16–26, 1986.
4. Bolondi L, Casanova P, Grigioni W, Caletti GC, Barbara L, Labò G. The sonographic appearance of the normal gastric wall: An in vitro study. Ultrasound Med Biol 12:991–995, 1986.
5. Kimmey MB, Martin RW, Hagitt RC, Wang KY, Franklin DW, Silverstein FE. Histologic correlates of gastrointestinal ultrasound images. Gastroenterology 96:433–441, 1989.
6. Yasuda K, Nakajima M, Yoshida S, Kiyota K, Kawai K. The diagnosis of submucosal tumors of the stomach by endoscopic ultrasonography. Gastrointest Endosc 35:10–15, 1989.
7. Caletti GC, Zani L, Bolondi L, Brocchi E, Rollo V, Barbara L. Endoscopic ultrasonography in the diagnosis of gastric submucosal tumor. Gastrointest Endosc 35:413–418, 1989.
8. Yasuda K, Cho E, Nakajima M, Kawai K. Diagnosis of submucosal lesions of the upper gastrointestinal tract by endoscopic ultrasonography. Gastrointest Endosc 36:S17–S20, 1990.
9. Aibe T, Takemoto T. Benign lesions of gastrointestinal tract. In Kawai K (ed): Endoscopic Ultrasonography in Gastroenterology. Tokyo: Igaku-Shoin, 1988, pp 44–55.
10. Nakazawa S, Yoshino J, Nakamura T, Yamanaka T, Hase S, Kojima Y, Ohasi S, Niwa Y. Endoscopic ultrasonography of gastric myogenic tumor. A comparative study between histology and ultrasonography. J Ultrasound Med 8:353–359, 1989.
11. Tio TL, Tytgat GNJ, Den Hartog Jager FCA. Endoscopic ultrasonography for the evaluation of smooth muscle tumors in the upper gastrointestinal tract: An experience with 42 cases. Gastrointest Endosc 36:342–350, 1990.
12. Iishi H, Yammamoto R, Tatsuta M, Okuda S. Evaluation of fine-needle aspiration biopsy under direct vision gastrofiberoscopy in diagnosis of diffusely infiltrative carcinoma of the stomach. Cancer 57:1365–1369, 1986.
13. Lundgreen R. A flexible thin needle for transbronchial aspiration biopsy through the flexible fiberoptic bronchoscope. Endoscopy 12:180–182, 1980.
14. Oho K, Kato H, Ogawa I, Hiyashi N, Hayata Y. A new needle for transfiberoptic bronchoscopic use. Chest 76:492, 1979.
15. Nguyen GK. Fine-needle aspiration biopsy cytology of hepatic tumors in adults. Pathol Ann 21:321–349, 1986.
16. Nguyen CK. Percutaneous fine-needle aspiration cytology of the pancreas. Pathol Ann 20:221–238, 1985.
17. Dickey JE, Haaga JR, Stellato TA, Schultz CL, Hau T. Evaluation of computed tomography guided percutaneous biopsy of the pancreas. Surg Gynecol Obstet 163:497–503, 1986.
18. Zargar SA, Khuroo MS, Mahajan R, Jan GM, Dewani K, Koul V. Endoscopic fine needle aspiration cytology in the diagnosis of gastro-oesophageal and colorectal malignancies. Gut 32:745–748, 1991.
19. Kochhar R, Rajwanshi A, Dev Wig J, Gupta NM, Kesiezie V, Bhasin DK, Malik AK, Gupta SK, Metha SK. Fine needle aspiration cytology of rectal masses. Gut 31:334–336, 1990.
20. Wiersema MJ, Hawes RH, Tao LC, Wiersema LM, Kopecky KK, Rex DK, Kumar S, Lehman GA. Endoscopic ultrasonography as an adjunct to fine needle aspiration cytology of the upper and lower gastrointestinal tract. Gastrointest Endosc 38:35–39, 1992.
21. Van Dam J, Rice TW, Sivak MV. Endoscopic ultrasonography and endoscopically guided needle aspiration for the diagnosis of upper gastrointestinal tract foregut cysts. Am J Gastroenterol 87:762–765, 1992.
22. Caletti GC, Gullini S, Brocchi E, Boccia S, Gibilaro M, Cantarini D, Ferrari A, Carfagna L, Barbara L. Endoscopic ultrasonography (EUS) with the guillotine needle biopsy in the diagnosis of gastric submucosal tumors (GMST). Gastrointest Endosc 36:222, 1990.
23. Caletti GC, Brocchi E, Ferrari A, Bonora G, Santini D, Mazzoleni G, Barbara L. Guillotine needle biopsy as a supplement to endosonography in the diagnosis of gastric submucosal tumors Endoscopy 23:251–254, 1991.
24. Tio TL, Sie LD, Tytgat GNJ. Endosonography and cytology in diagnosing and staging pancreatic body and tail carcinoma. Dig Dis Sci 38:59–64, 1993.
25. Vilmann P, Jacobsen GK, Henriksen FW, Hancke S. Endoscopic ultrasonography with guided fine needle aspiration biopsy in pancreatic disease. Gastrointest Endosc 38:172–173, 1992.
26. Grimm H, Binmoeller KF, Soehendra N. Endosonography-guided drainage of a pancreatic pseudocyst. Gastrointest Endosc 38: 170–171, 1992.
27. Wiersema MJ, Kochman ML, Chak A, Cramer HM, Kesler KA. Real-time endoscopic ultrasound-guided fine-needle aspiration of a mediastinal lymph node. Gastrointest Endosc 39:429–431, 1993.
28. Wiersema MJ, Kochman ML, Cramer HM, Tao LC, Wiersema LM. Endosonography-guided real-time fine-needle aspiration biopsy. Gastrointest Endosc 40:700–707, 1994.
29. Vilmann P, Hancke S, Henriksen FW, Jacobsen GK. Endosonographically-guided fine needle aspiration biopsy of malignant lesions in the upper gastrointestinal tract. Endoscopy 25: 523–527, 1993.
30. Vilmann P, Hancke S, Henriksen FW, Jacobsen GK. Endoscopic ultrasonography-guided fine-needle aspiration biopsy of lesions in the upper gastrointestinal tract. Gastrointest Endosc 41: 230–235, 1995.
31. Wegener M, Adamek RJ, Wedman B, Pfaffenbach B. Endosonographically guided fine-needle aspiration puncture of paraesophagogastric mass lesion: Preliminary results. Endoscopy 26:586–591, 1994.
32. Binmoeller KF, Seifert H, Soehendra N. Endoscopic ultrasonography-guided fine-needle aspiration biopsy of lymph nodes. Endoscopy 26:780–783, 1994.
33. Chang KJ, Katz KD, Durbin TE, Erickson RA, Butler JA, Lin F, Wuerker RB. Endoscopic ultrasound-guided fine-needle aspiration. Gastrointest Endosc 40:694–699, 1994.
34. Giovannini M, Seitz JF, Monges G, Perrier H, Rabbia I. Fine-needle aspiration cytology guided by endoscopic ultrasonography: Results in 141 patients. Endoscopy 27:171–177, 1995.

CHAPTER

# Gastric Lymphoma, Infiltrative Disorders, and Large Gastric Folds

Giancarlo Caletti
Paolo Bocus
Thomas Togliani
Enrico Roda

## Gastric Lymphoma

The gastrointestinal tract is the most common site of primary extranodal lymphoma, and about half of all gastrointestinal lymphomas are located in the stomach. Primary gastric lymphoma accounts for 2–8% of all gastric malignancies. The possible therapeutic approaches are different in patients with gastric malignant lymphoma as compared with gastric cancer, as gastric lymphoma has a better prognosis than gastric carcinoma owing to the sensitivity of the former to radiation therapy (RT) or chemotherapy (CT). It has also been pointed out by Shiu et al. (1) that a considerably better prognosis has been obtained when the true diagnosis was known preoperatively and the surgical treatment planned accordingly. It is therefore important to establish a correct preoperative differential diagnosis between gastric lymphoma and cancer.

Such a diagnosis is generally considered difficult. Fork et al. (2) report that endoscopy, including examination of biopsies, established a correct diagnosis in just 44% of his cases. Schutze et al. (3) report that the sensitivity of endoscopy was higher (85%), but the specificity of endoscopic biopsy was suboptimal, with only 60% of specimens having a positive outcome for lymphoma. In fact, in our experience with gastric cancers and primary lymphomas, endoscopic biopsies were correct in 93% of cancers and in 84% of lymphomas (4). In order to ameliorate the difficulties in endoscopic diagnosis of early primary gastric lymphoma, Suekane et al. (5) recently suggested performing endoscopic mucosal resection when forceps biopsy is negative and the endoscopic findings strongly indicate lymphoma. The prognosis of these patients depends mainly on two variables: depth of tumor invasion and lymph node metastasis (6). A strong correlation is also recognized among tumor size, depth of invasion, stage of the disease, and prognosis (7). Moreover, prognosis after surgery in these diseases depends on the radicality of surgery. A sufficient distance from tumor to margins of resection is a prerequisite for radical surgery, as residual tumor at surgical margins does reduce survival time (8,9). For all these reasons a correct preoperative staging is required.

## Linitis Plastica

The term "linitis plastica" refers to a scirrhous form of carcinoma that spreads predominantly in the submucosa, eliciting a marked desmoplastic response in the gastric wall. These lesions are almost always thought to involve the distal half of the stomach, arising near the pylorus and gradually extending upward from the antrum into the body and fundus. In advanced cases, the stomach may be diffusely infiltrated by tumor.

This diffuse type of gastric cancer has a great tendency to spread over the peritoneum and to engulf the remaining gastrointestinal tract. Consequently, the majority of patients with this tumor are initially seen with advanced disease. Under these conditions, surgery for these patients is usually palliative.

Palliative surgery, even total gastrectomy, has to be restricted to those patients who have tumors limited to the stomach or regional lymph nodes, in which case only 20% of patients would benefit from resection. Patients who have liver, peritoneal, or serosal involvement, or extension of the tumor locally (into the pancreas or diaphragm) will not benefit from a total gastrectomy. One alternative would be chemotherapy with or without radiation therapy (10).

Although endoscopy combined with biopsies and brushings has a reported overall sensitivity of 95–98% in detecting gastric cancer, it is a less reliable technique for diagnosing scirrhous tumors. The endoscopist often has difficulty recognizing these lesions because the overlying mucosa appears normal. False-negative findings from endoscopic biopsies or brushings may occur not only because these scirrhous tumors are located predominantly in the submucosa, but also because the tumor cells are often separated by large areas of fibrosis. Thus, excessive reliance on negative endoscopic findings can lead to a significant delay in the diagnosis and treatment of these tumors (11).

For all these reasons, an early diagnosis is important and correct staging is required before a therapeutic decision is made.

Unfortunately CT scan may reveal only thickening of the stomach wall with poor definition of the plane between the stomach and the adjacent organs, and infiltration of the perigastric fat. Endoscopic ultrasonography seems ideal for this purpose.

## Large Gastric Folds

The evaluation of the patient found to have greatly enlarged rugal folds presents many problems to the gastroenterologist, the surgeon, and the pathologist. Several different disease processes must be considered, and these diseases are difficult to separate by means of endoscopic appearance, radiology, and even biopsy. The prototype disease in this category, Menetrier's disease, is known by some 37 different names, perhaps reflecting an imprecise understanding of what the limits of this disease or related diseases are (12). If sufficient clinical and pathologic information is available, most patients presenting with enlarged gastric folds can be diagnosed with reasonable precision. Except for those cases in which the rugae are enlarged by a neoplastic infiltrate, the expansion of the folds is due to an expansion of one or more of three basic components: the submucosa, the surface foveolar epithelium, or the glandular component (parietal cells). The eponym Menetrier's disease remains the most commonly used name for this disease process; of the 36 other synonyms used, the descriptive term hyperplastic gastropathy has gained a measure of acceptance. In its purest form, the disease exhibits the following four features. First, the folds of the body and fundus are enlarged; these can be readily observed radiographically, endoscopically, and in gross specimens. Second, there is low gastric secretion after stimulation. Third, there is low serum albumin, reflecting serum protein loss through the mucosa. Finally, there are histologic findings of glandular atrophy and foveolar hyperplasia. These findings can be related to the low acid output and protein loss, respectively. With such increased mucosal thickness, standard biopsy techniques are unlikely to yield a specimen in which all of the features of Menetrier's disease can be appreciated. On occasion, prominent foveolar hyperplasia can be seen and may provide confirmation of the diagnosis in a highly typical clinical setting. A useful technique in evaluating patients with large folds is the macroparticle biopsy, which is taken with a polypectomy diathermy snare. While there is potential for perforation, this type of procedure is worth considering because it makes a surgical full-thickness biopsy unnecessary. With this type of biopsy, typical features of Menetrier's disease can be seen; and, if properly sampled, a normal-appearing biopsy can be used as strong evidence against the other diseases that can cause giant folds. While there is a significant risk for developing gastric carcinoma in Menetrier's disease, the exact magnitude of this risk is uncertain because of the difficulties in clearly defining the disease. Localized expansions of the gastric folds may occasionally produce a polyploid appearance in the absence of neoplasia, and histologic confirmation is necessary before diagnosing adenoma or carcinoma.

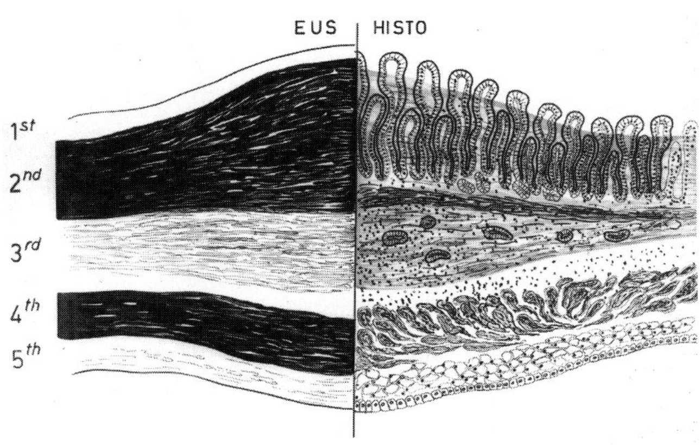


**FIGURE 17-2**

Schematic drawing showing the relationships between EUS and anatomic layers of the gastric wall T1 lymphoma.

## Endoscopic Ultrasonography (EUS) in Gastric Lymphoma and Infiltrative Disorders

EUS is able to investigate the intestinal wall which is made up of five ultrasonographic layers of different echogenicities (13) (Fig. 17–1). Thus the diagnosis of gastrointestinal diseases by EUS has been possible on the basis of changes in the layer structure of the gastrointestinal wall.

Neoplasms are detected at EUS as a disruption in the continuity of the normal ultrasonographic layer pattern or by diffuse layer thickening. Infiltrating gastric neoplasms produce diffuse thickening of all ultrasound layers without causing layer disruption. A change in the echogenicity of the ultrasound layers is another sign of tissue pathology. Neoplasms usually have an intermediate echogenicity: less echogenic than the central layer but more echogenic than the second and the fourth layers (13).

Lymphomatous involvement of the gastric wall proceeds mainly by longitudinal (or horizontal) growth within the wall, while the growth of carcinoma is predominantly vertical, with early invasion of the deep wall. Mucosal involvement in lymphoma is often less extensive than the infiltration of the underlying layers. Extended infiltration of the second and third layers with localized mucosal ulcerations is pathognomonic of lymphoma. In the early stages of gastric lymphoma, EUS discloses abnormal thickening of the second or the second and the third layers of the wall, with preservation of these layers as distinctive structures (Figs. 17–2 through 17–5). In advanced cases, thickening is diffuse with a typical hypoechoic pattern and the individual sonographic layers are no longer distinguishable (Figs. 17–6 through 17–9). These pathologic alterations are found not only within and around the lesions observed at endoscopy, but also in areas where the mucosa appears at endoscopy to be normal (14,15).

In infiltrative carcinoma, the involvement of the gastric wall is always transmural and more echogenic than in gastric lymphoma, and the implication of extramural

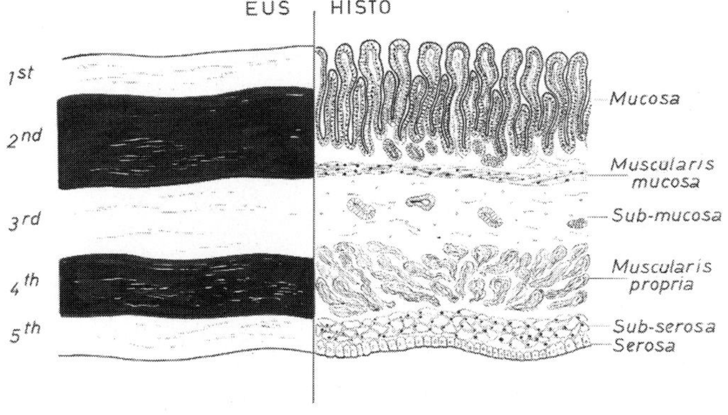


**FIGURE 17-1**

Schematic drawing showing the relationships between EUS and anatomic layers of the normal gastric wall: (1) Interface between stomach fluid and superficial mucosa, (2) lamina propria and muscularis mucosae, (3) submucosa and interface between submucosa and muscularis propria, (4) muscularis propria, (5) interface between serosa and surrounding tissues.

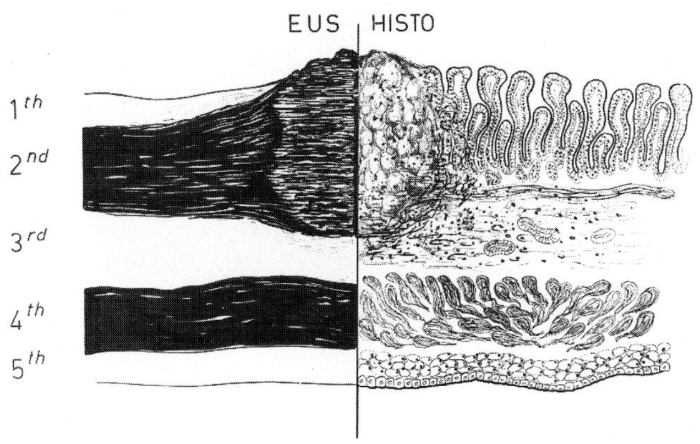


**FIGURE 17-3**

Schematic drawing showing the relationships between EUS and anatomic layers of the normal gastric wall in T1 cancer.

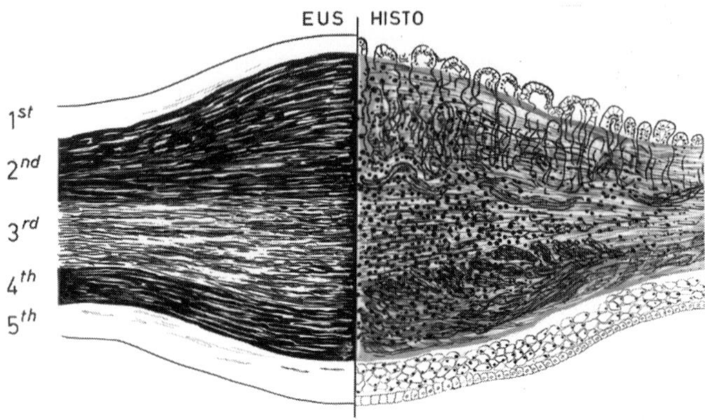


**FIGURE 17-4**

Schematic drawing showing the relationships between EUS and anatomic layers of the normal gastric wall in T2 lymphoma.

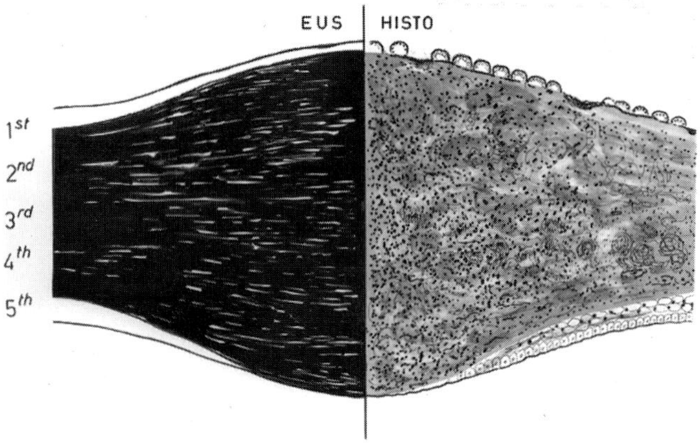


**FIGURE 17-6**

Schematic drawing showing the relationships between EUS and anatomic layers of the normal gastric wall in T3 lymphoma.

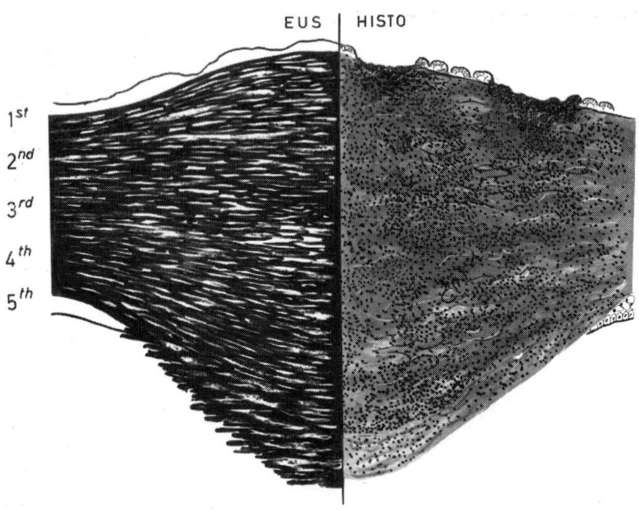


**FIGURE 17-8**

Schematic drawing showing the relationships between EUS and anatomic layers of the normal gastric wall in T4 lymphoma.

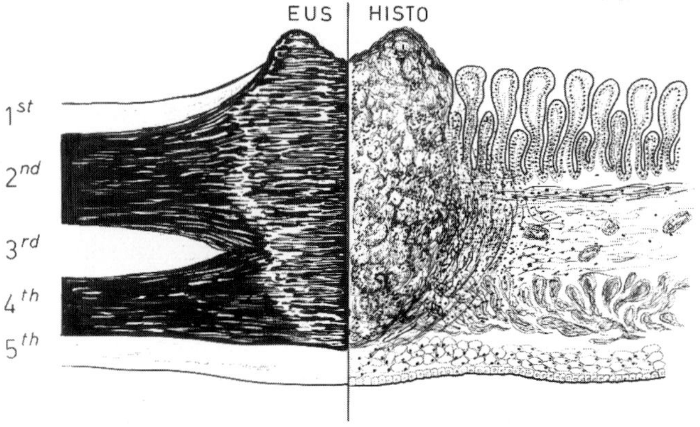


**FIGURE 17-5**

Schematic drawing showing the relationships between EUS and anatomic layers of the normal gastric wall in T2 cancer.

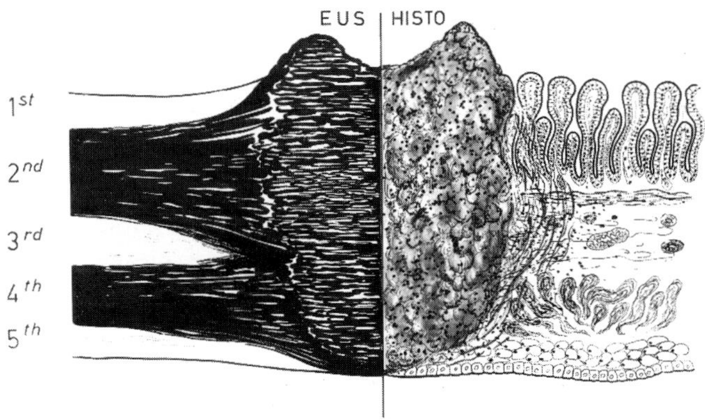


**FIGURE 17-7**

Schematic drawing showing the relationships between EUS and anatomic layers of the normal gastric wall in T3 cancer.

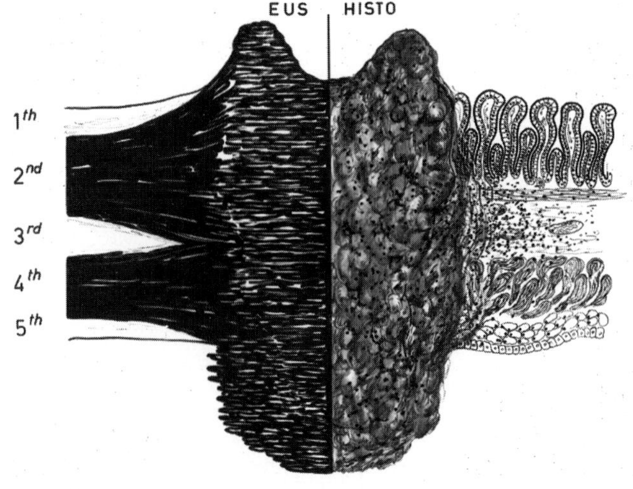


**FIGURE 17-9**

Schematic drawing showing the relationships between EUS and anatomic layers of the normal gastric wall in T4 cancer.

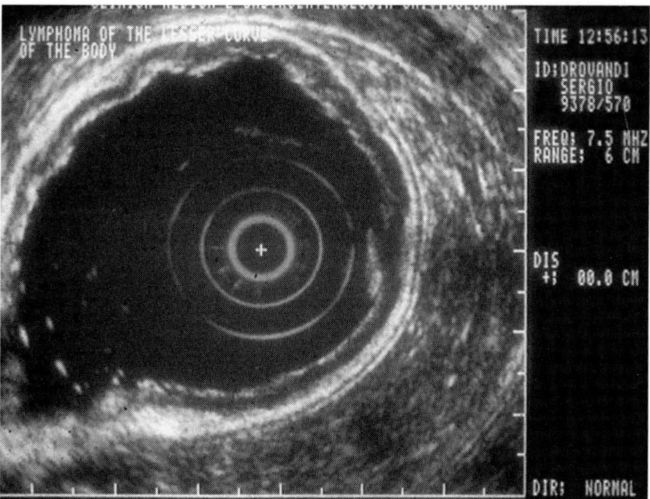


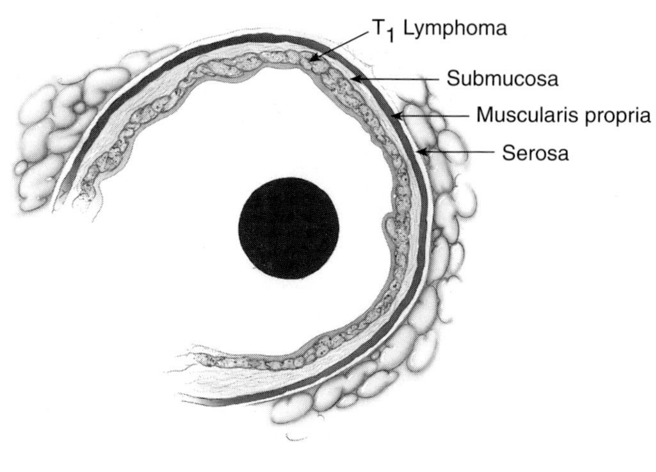


**FIGURE 17-10**

EUS of a T1 lymphoma. Hypoechoic tumor located in the mucosa.

structure and perigastric lymph nodes detectable by EUS is much more common (14).

Several EUS studies of gastric cancer and lymphoma have demonstrated specific ultrasonographic features that allow correct diagnosis and staging in the majority of patients. EUS is considered to be a useful tool for preoperative staging of these diseases (16–23).

EUS appears to be a very useful tool for preoperative staging of gastric lymphoma (4,24). As shown in Figures 17–10 through 17–13, EUS shows not only tumor depth and local spread, but also the passage from a pathologic to a normal wall (see Fig. 17–2). Moreover, EUS is able to display the relationship of the tumor to neighboring organs and early lymph node metastasis.

Numerous published reports described the preliminary experience with EUS in the diagnosis of primary gastric cancer and lymphoma (14–16). Subsequently, the sensitivity, specificity, and predictive value of EUS were reported (4).

In a recent report, EUS was performed in 82 primary gastric lymphomas (25). EUS made a correct diagnosis of lymphoma in 76 of the 82 patients with a sensitivity of 93%. Positive predictability was 91%, specificity 98%, and negative predictability 98%. Diagnostic accuracy was 97%. In the evaluation of lymphoma depth of invasion, EUS was correct in 87% of cases. EUS displayed metastatic perigastric lymph nodes in 15 of 27 patients with a sensitivity of 56%. Positive predictability was 100%, speci-

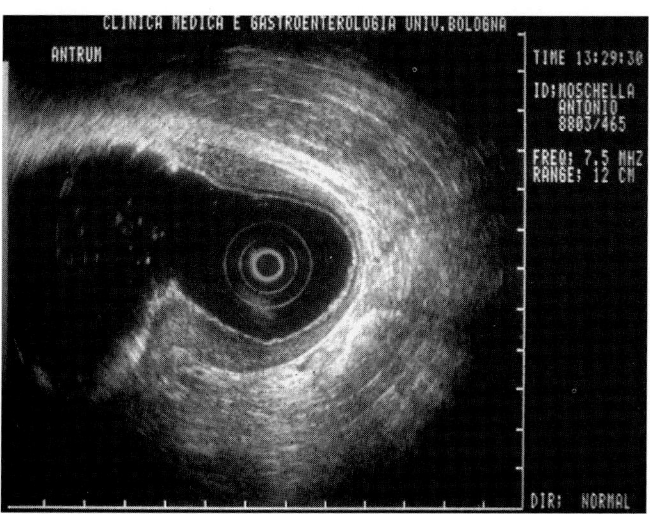


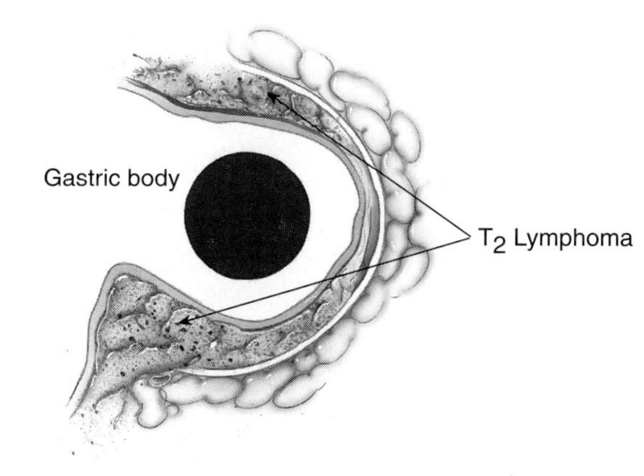


**FIGURE 17-11**

EUS of a T2 lymphoma. Hypoechoic tumor located in the mucosa and submucosa extending locally into the muscularis propria.

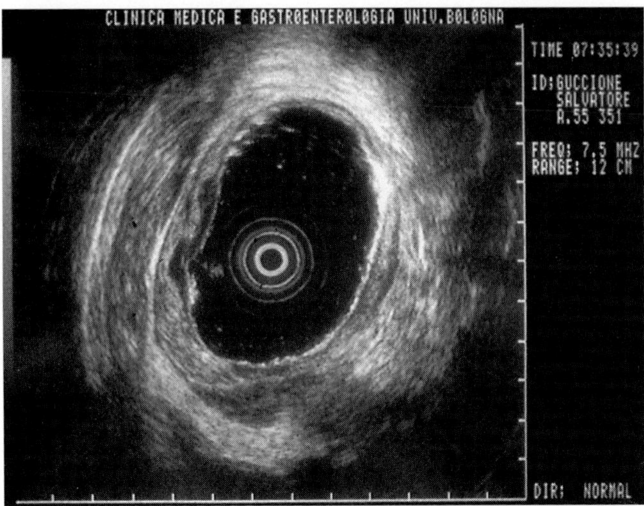


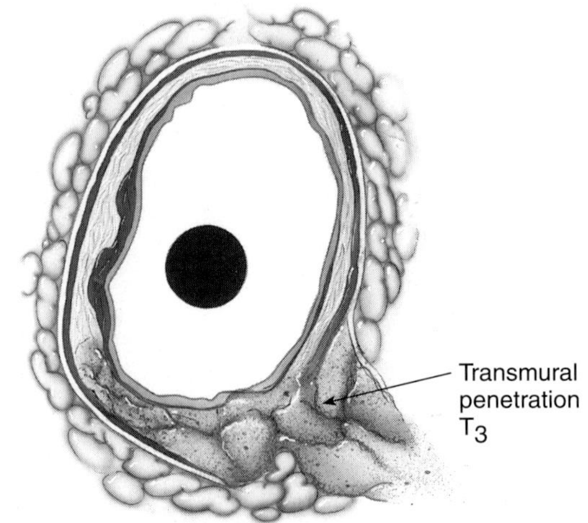


**FIGURE 17–12**

EUS of a T3 lymphoma. Transmural hypoechoic tumor with penetration into the serosa.

ficity 100%, and negative predictability 82%. Diagnostic accuracy was 85%.

The EUS differential diagnosis among lymphoma, linitis plastica, and Menetrier's disease is difficult. All three lesions have more or less the same echo pattern, displayed as an extended thickening of the second and third layers with preservation of layers as distinctive structures. However, it is possible to find small differences. In linitis, the layer thickening is hypoechoic as in lymphoma, but much more longitudinally extended and sometimes involves circularly all the gastric wall (Fig. 17–14). Menetrier's disease is displayed as a more localized thickening which is hyperechoic rather than hypoechoic (Fig. 17–15).

Large-particle biopsy has to be considered when the EUS diagnosis of these diseases is uncertain.

Suekane et al. (26) reported that EUS findings correlated well with the endoscopic, macroscopic, and histologic findings in 15 patients with primary gastric lymphoma. They also suggested that EUS may provide important information for the distinction between the MALT-type and other types of lymphoma. If their results are confirmed, EUS may prove helpful in guiding the choice of therapy in patients with gastric lymphoma. With respect to EUS staging of very early lymphoma (MALT), however, our data have been disappointing—probably because these lesions are localized to the mucosa and current EUS instruments cannot discrimi-

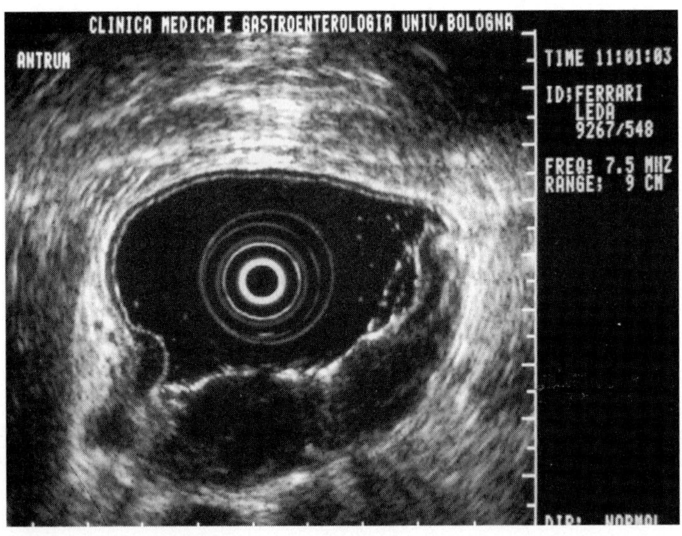


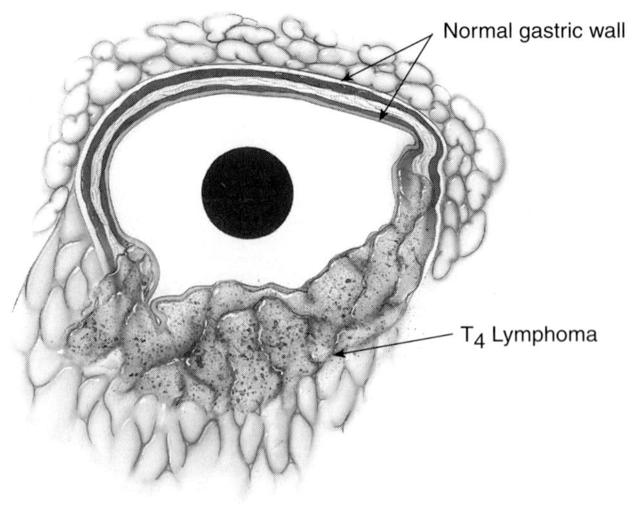


**FIGURE 17–13**

EUS of a T4 lymphoma. Transmural hypoechoic tumor with penetration into adjacent structures.

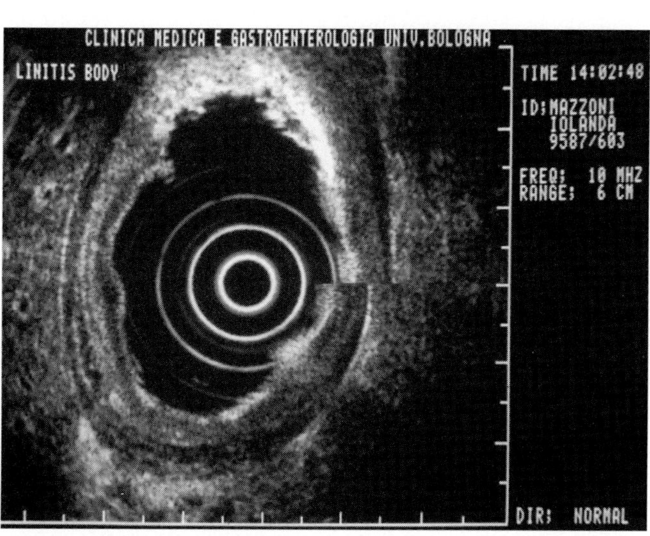


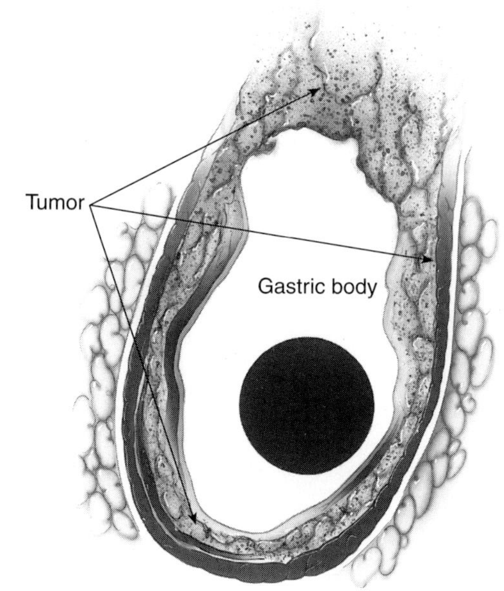


**FIGURE 17-14**

EUS in linitis plastica. There is an extended thickening of the second and third layers with preservation of layers as distinctive structures. The thickening is hypoechoic as in lymphoma and involves the gastric wall circumferentially.

nate this layer alone. Moreover, it is not completely clear how Suekane et al. (26) are able to differentiate MALT from non-MALT lymphomas relying solely on EUS imaging; this differentiation is normally made on histologic bases.

EUS can be of significant assistance in deciding whether a gastric lymphoma can be resected or not. Another question is whether or not EUS can help to spare some patients from a total gastrectomy by correctly defining tumor-free margins. Palazzo et al. (27) and Schüder et al. (28) report different conclusions on this point. Palazzo reports that EUS underestimated tumor surface extension in 37.5% of cases, concluding that EUS is incapable of accurately determining the extent of gastric resection. On the other hand, Schüder, in a smaller series, found the information provided by EUS to be accurate enough to guide surgical resection. In comparison with a historical control group, they

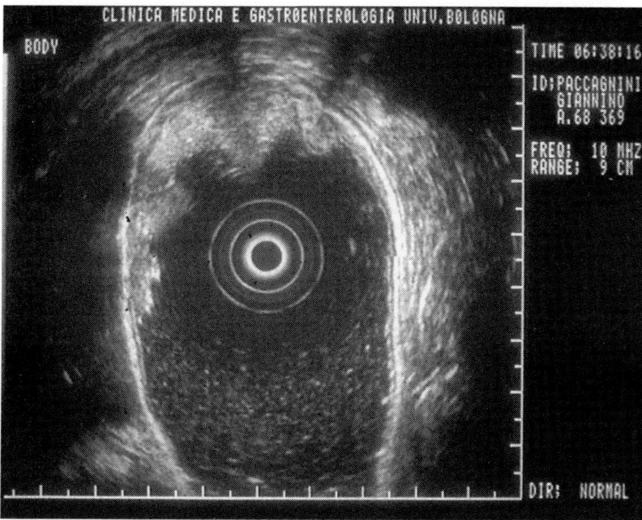


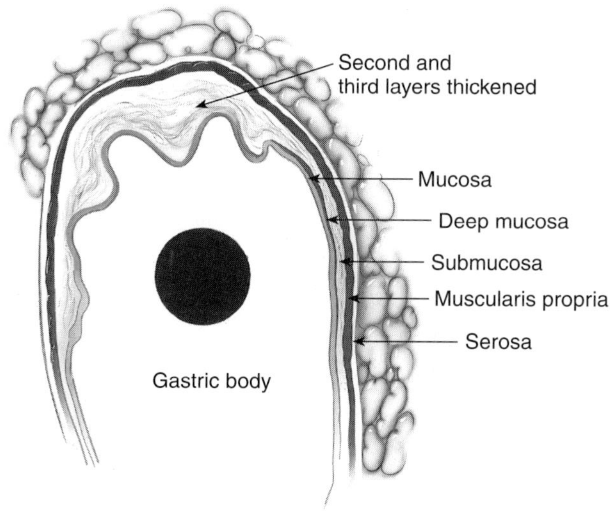


**FIGURE 17-15**

EUS in Menetrier's disease. There is an extended thickening of the second and third layers with preservation of the layers as distinctive structures. The thickening is more localized and is hyperechoic rather than hypoechoic.

reported that the rate of total gastrectomy decreased (from 65% to 10%) in the period during which EUS was used for lymphoma staging while the percentage of RO resection increased from 72% to 100% at the same time. As in every dispute, the truth probably lies in the middle. For the moment we can recommend following Schüder's suggestion to perform several retrograde needle biopsies of the wall in order to detect microtumoral invasion even where the wall seems normal at EUS. Finally, although prospective studies are few, EUS appears to be a sensitive method for assessing the response to radiation and chemotherapy for patients with primary gastric lymphoma (29). However, the possibility of EUS T-overstaging must be kept in mind because it is impossible to differentiate reactive fibrosis from tumor growth (30).

## Endoscopic Ultrasonography in Large Gastric Folds (LGF)

EUS is very useful in assessing patients with LGF. By allowing a detailed visualization of the different layers of the gastric wall, it can accurately show which layers are thickened and whether the layer structure is preserved. For a final diagnosis, however, EUS should always be combined with endoscopic (conventional-forceps or large-particle) biopsy after the exclusion of intramural vessels as a cause of gastric wall thickening.

Mendis et al. (31) examined the utility of EUS in 28 patients with endoscopically or radiographically diagnosed LGF most of whose endoscopic biopsies were inconclusive for malignancy. EUS demonstrated gastric varices in four patients in whom biopsy specimens were not taken. In three patients biopsy results were negative for malignancy. Owing to ultrasonographic findings of wall thickening involving layers 3 and 4, however, these patients underwent laparotomy, which revealed primary gastric carcinoma. In the remaining patients, large-forceps endoscopic biopsy revealed acute or chronic inflammation in sixteen (67%), malignancy in four (16%), and Menetrier's disease in one (4%). Malignancy did not develop in any of the patients with gastric wall thickening limited to layer 2 and negative biopsy results during a mean follow-up period of 35 months. Mendis concluded that when EUS abnormalities involve only the mucosal layer, endoscopic biopsies are diagnostic. Abnormalities involving the muscularis propria in the absence of ulceration strongly suggest malignancy and should be further investigated if endoscopic biopsy findings are negative. Moreover, potentially dangerous biopsies of gastric varices can be avoided.

Songur et al. (32), analyzing the EUS features in 35 patients with giant gastric folds, described some findings that could be useful in characterizing each type of lesion. According to these authors, when the second layer alone is thickened, Menetrier's disease may be one of the possible pathologic entities; and when the third layer alone is abnormally enlarged, anisakiasis might be suspected. Most of the patients with scirrhous carcinoma showed an abnormally enlarged third and fourth layer. The second and third layer may be thickened in healthy subjects with simple hyperrugosity, but also in patients with gastric lymphoma. The fourth layer was significantly thickened only in malignant conditions. The authors concluded that EUS can visualize the structure of giant gastric folds and may facilitate the differentiation of benign from malignant etiologies.

Maunoury et al. (33) reported that endosonographic aspects may be useful in distinguishing Menetrier's disease from lymphocytic gastritis, although biopsies are necessary for final confirmation of diagnosis because some overlapping endosonographic aspects may persist. Okada et al. (34) described two patients having gastritis cystica profunda presenting as giant gastric folds in which the diagnosis was made based on findings from EUS and mucosectomy.

Finally, LGFs may also result from infectious or inflammatory disorders. *Helicobacter pylori* gastritis is a common cause of gastric wall thickening. Avunduk et al. (35) demonstrated that EUS allows intrinsic localization of gastric wall thickening in patients with LGFs and *H. pylori* infection, and documents the resolution of this wall thickening upon eradication of *H. pylori* and resolution of gastritis.

### References

1. Shiu MH, Karas M, Nisce L, Lee BJ, Filippa DA, Lieberman PH. Management of primary gastric lymphoma. Ann Surg 195:196–202, 1982.
2. Fork FTh, Haglund U, Hogstrom H, Wehlin L. Primary gastric lymphoma v. gastric cancer. An endoscopic and radiographic study of differential diagnostic possibilities. Endoscopy 17:5–7, 1985.
3. Schutze WP, Halpern NB. Gastric Lymphoma. Surg Gynecol Obstet 172:33–38, 1991.
4. Caletti GC, Ferrari A, Brocchi E, Barbara L. Accuracy of endoscopic ultrasonography in the diagnosis and staging of gastric cancer and lymphoma. Surgery 113:14–27, 1993.
5. Suekane H, Iida M, Kuwano Y, Kohrogi N, Yao T, Iwashita A, Fujishima M. Diagnosis of primary early gastric lymphoma. Usefulness of endoscopic mucosal resection for histologic evaluation. Cancer 71:1207–1213, 1993.
6. Maruyama K. The most important prognostic factors for gastric cancer patients. A study using univariate and multivariate analyses. Scand J Gastroenterol 22(suppl 133):63–68, 1987.
7. Sato T, Sakai Y, Ishiguro S, Furukawa H. Radiologic manifestations of early gastric lymphoma. AJR 146:513–517, 1986.
8. Hornig D, Hermanek P, Gall FP. The significance of the extent of proximal margins of clearance in gastric cancer surgery. Scand J Gastroenterol 22(suppl 133):69–71, 1987.
9. Kirchner R, Henke W, Wittekind C, Farthmann EH. The surgeon's estimation of radicality and results of pathologic examination at margins of resection in gastric cancer surgery. Scand J Gastroenterol 22(suppl 133):72–75, 1987.
10. Aranha GV, Georgen R. Gastric linitis plastica is not a surgical disease. Surgery 106:758–763, 1989.

11. Levine MS, Kong V, Rubesin SE, Laufer I, Herlinger H. Scirrhous carcinoma of the stomach: Radiologic and endoscopic diagnosis. Radiology 175:151–154, 1990.
12. Appelman HD. Localized and extensive expansions of the gastric mucosa: Mucosal polyps and giant folds. In Appelman HD (eds.): Pathology of the Esophagus, Stomach, and Duodenum. Contemporary Issues in Surgical Pathology, 4th Ed. New York: Churchill Livingstone, 1984, p 79.
13. Kimmey MB, Martin RW, Hagitt RC, Wang KY, Franklin DW, Silverstein FE. Histologic correlates of gastrointestinal ultrasound images. Gastroenterology 96:433–441, 1989.
14. Bolondi L, Casanova P, Caletti GC, Grigioni W, Zani L, Barbara. Primary gastric lymphoma versus gastric carcinoma: Endoscopic US evaluation. Radiology 165:821–826, 1987.
15. Caletti GC, Zani L, Bolondi L, Guizzardi G, Brocchi E, Barbara L. Impact of endoscopic ultrasonography on diagnosis and treatment of primary gastric lymphoma. Surgery 103:315–320, 1988.
16. Caletti GC, Bolondi L, Brocchi E, Casanova P, Zani L, Gaiani S, Testa S, Guizzardi G, Labò G. Staging of gastric cancer by means of endoscopic ultrasonography. Gastroenterology 84:1366, 1983.
17. Tio TL, Den Hartog Jager FCA, Tytgat GNJ. The role of endoscopic ultrasonography in assessing local resectability of oesophagogastric malignancies. Scand J Gastroenterol 21(suppl 123): 78–86, 1986.
18. Aibe T, Ito T, Ioscida T, Noguchi T, Ohtani T, Fuji T, Takemoto T. Endoscopic ultrasonography of lymph nodes surrounding the upper GI tract. Scand J Gastroenterol 21(suppl 123):164–169, 1986.
19. Tio TL, Den Hartog Jager FCA, Tytgat GNJ. Endoscopic ultrasonography of non-Hodgkin lymphoma of the stomach. Gastroenterology 91:401–408, 1986.
20. Heyder N. Endoscopic ultrasonography of tumours of the oesophagus and the stomach. Surg Endosc 1:17–23, 1987.
21. Tio TL, Schouwink MH, Cikot RJLM, Tytgat GN. Preoperative TNM classification of gastric carcinoma by endosonography in comparison with the pathological TNM system: A prospective study of 72 cases. Hepato-Gastroenterol 36:51–56, 1989.
22. Tio TL, Coene PLO, Schouwink MH, Tytgat GNJ. Esophagogastric carcinoma: Preoperative TNM classification with endosonography. Radiology 173:411–417, 1989.
23. Tio TL, Coene PPLO, Luiken GJHM, Tytgat GNJ. Endosonography in the clinical staging of esophagogastric carcinoma. Gastrointest Endosc 36:S2–S10, 1990.
24. Tacke W, Kruis W, Zehnter E, Ziegenhagen D, Velasco S, Diehl V. Endosonographic findings in the upper gastrointestinal tract in staging of malignant nodal and extranodal lymphomas. Z Gastroenterol 32(8):431–435, 1994.
25. Caletti GC, Ferrari A. Endoscopic ultrasonography. Endoscopy 28:156–173, 1996.
26. Suekane H, Iida M, Yao T, Matsumoto T, Masuda Y, Fujishima M. Endoscopic ultrasonography in primary gastric lymphoma: Correlation with endoscopic and histologic findings. Gastrointest Endosc 39:139–145, 1993.
27. Palazzo L, Roseau G, Ruskone-Fourmestraux A, Rougier Ph, Chaussade S, Rambaud JC, Couturier D, Paolaggi A. Endoscopic ultrasonography in the local staging of primary gastric lymphoma. Endoscopy 25:502–508, 1993.
28. Schüder G, Hildebrandt U, Ecker KW, Seitz G, Feifel G. Role of endosonography in the surgical management of non-Hodgkin's lymphoma of the stomach. Endoscopy 25:509–512, 1993.
29. Van Dam J. The role of endoscopic ultrasonography in monitoring treatment: response to chemotherapy in lymphoma. Endoscopy 26:772–773, 1994.
30. Hordijk ML. Restaging after radiotherapy and chemotherapy: Value of endoscopic ultrasonography. Gastrointest Endosc Clin NA 5(3): 601–608, 1995.
31. Mendis RE, Gerdes H, Lightdale CJ, Bótet JF. Large gastric folds: A diagnostic approach using endoscopic ultrasonography. Gastrointest Endosc 40:437–441, 1994.
32. Songur Y, Okai T, Watanabe H, Motoo Y, Sawabu N. Endosonographic evaluation of giant gastric folds. Gastrointest Endosc 41: 468–474, 1995.
33. Maunoury V, Klein O, Houcke ML, Colombel JF. Endoscopic ultrasonography in the diagnosis of hypertrophic gastropathy (Letter). Gastroenterology 106:820, 1994.
34. Okada M, Iizuka Y, Oh K, Murayama H, Maekawa T. Gastritis cystica profunda presenting as giant gastric mucosal folds: The role of endoscopic ultrasonography and mucosectomy in the diagnostic work-up. Gastrointest Endosc 40(5):640–644, 1994.
35. Avunduk C, Navab F, Hampf F, Coughlin B. Prevalence of *Helicobacter pylori* infection in patients with large gastric folds: Evaluation and follow-up with endoscopic ultrasound before and after antimicrobial therapy. Am J Gastroenterol 90:1969–1973, 1995.

CHAPTER

# Staging Gastric Cancer
## THE NEW YORK EXPERIENCE

Charles J. Lightdale
Frank Van de Mierop

Gastric cancer is a highly lethal disease which, in Western countries, usually presents at an advanced stage in symptomatic patients (1). Despite advances in diagnosis and therapy, most patients with gastric cancer die of their disease (2–6). The average five-year survival for patients with gastric cancer is 17% (7). The mainstay of treatment is surgery, and survival after surgery remains highly dependent on stage, defined as the anatomic extent of disease at the time of operation, and preoperatively assessed resectability (8,9). In Japan, where gastric cancer is a major health problem, screening asymptomatic individuals has resulted in the diagnosis of patients with earlier stages of cancer and has improved survival after resection (5,6,10).

Of recent concern in the United States is the documented rising incidence of adenocarcinoma of the distal esophagus, esophagogastric junction, and gastric cardia in the setting of slight declines in the incidence of squamous cell carcinoma of the esophagus and adenocarcinoma of the distal stomach (11,12). Many of these adenocarcinomas of the distal esophagus, esophagogastric junction, and cardia are associated with the development of Barrett's metaplastic epithelium in the distal esophagus (11,12) Endoscopic ultrasonography can provide the surgeon with additional information on the extent of esophageal infiltration in patients with carcinoma of the gastric cardia (13).

## Diagnosis

The diagnosis of gastric cancer is based on upper gastrointestinal endoscopy and biopsy, which may be performed as a primary procedure or following barium contrast x-ray examination. Endoscopic ultrasonography (EUS) has its greatest impact as a staging procedure after histologic diagnosis rather than as a diagnostic test (14,15). The inability to reliably distinguish between neoplastic tissue and inflammation and fibrosis is a current limitation of EUS. For example, the differential diagnosis of benign versus malignant ulcer often cannot be made by EUS, despite initial enthusiasm (16,17). The exception to the rule that EUS is useful for staging but not diagnosis occurs in some patients with linitis plastica–type infiltrating gastric cancer who present with thickened enlarged gastric folds which must be differentiated from benign disease. In some of these patients, the disease is nearly all submucosal and repeated attempts at endoscopic biopsy do not reveal the diagnosis (18). By showing diffuse hypoechoic infiltration of the submucosa and muscularis propria, endoscopic ultrasound can suggest the presence of malignancy in these patients, even in the presence of normal endoscopic biopsies (18–23). Large gastric folds may also be found in relation to infection with *Helicobacter pylori* or in cases of Menetrier's disease, in which case evaluation by endoscopic ultrasonography may be of clinical benefit (20,21). Endoscopic ultrasound directed needle biopsies, large forceps biopsies, or snare biopsies (+/– saline injection) may add further accuracy in such cases (22). The presence of ascites or malignant-appearing perigastric nodes on EUS may also suggest malignancy (19).

## Staging

The American Joint Committee on Cancer (AJCC) published its most recent recommendations for staging cancer of the stomach in a revised staging classification (8). These classifications are based on the TNM staging system, which defines the anatomic extent of the disease:

- T indicates the depth of primary tumor invasion of these carcinomas, which originate in the mucosa and invade progressively deeper layers of the gastrointestinal tract wall as they advance.
- N indicates the spread of cancer to specified regional lymph nodes. In gastric cancer, lymph node metastases within 3 cm of the edge of the primary tumor are considered N1; lymph node metastases more than 3 cm from the tumor edge or those along major arterial trunks (e.g., the celiac, common hepatic, splenic, or left gastric arteries) are classified as N2.
- M indicates distant metastases to lymph nodes outside specified regional nodes, or to organs such as liver, lung, and adrenal glands not involved by direct extension from the primary cancer.

In the AJCC staging classification, it is important to note that clinical, surgical, and pathologic stages are based on the same TNM anatomic criteria. Symptoms or laboratory tests have no role in the classifications. T stage is based solely on the depth of invasion of the primary tumor. The length of the tumor, the extent of involved circumference, or degree of lumenal compromise are not factors in staging.

The Borrmann classification for gastric cancer is based on visual inspection of the mucosal surface of the resection specimen. Pertaining to gastric cancers invading into the muscularis propria, it is a descriptive classification (24), it has been largely abandoned except in the Japanese literature.

For early gastric cancer limited to the mucosa and submucosa, the Japanese Gastroenterological Endoscopy Society (25) made a new visual or endoscopic classification: Type I, a protruded tumor; type II, a superficial tumor (with subtypes a/elevated, b/flat, c/depressed); type III, an excavated tumor. On EUS, Japanese investigators (26) have proposed a subclassification of the T1-stage in the TNM staging. They divide T1 into a T1m (limited to the mucosa, layers 1–2) and a T1sm (within submucosa, <layer 3) (26).

## Clinical Staging

Modern imaging methods comprise the backbone of efforts to clinically stage the anatomic extent of gastric cancer. However, a thorough evaluation begins with a physical examination with particular attention to sites of possible metastases, especially the supraclavicular lymph nodes, the liver, and the lungs. Blood tests can provide a clue to possible liver metastases, and chest x-ray will help identify pulmonary and mediastinal extension; but in recent years, far more reliance has been placed on computerized tomography (CT). Multiple contradictory reports have been published in the literature regarding the efficacy of CT for staging (27–30). However, it seems clear that the ability to correctly stage the depth of tumor invasion (T) based on wall thickness and contour is open to frequent error, particularly in early stage disease. For example, it is not possible to tell T1 from T2 disease, and in advanced cancer involvement of adjacent organs or structures

(T4) is often problematic. The determination of lymph node metastasis is based solely on the size of the imaged node, and results have also been disappointing. On the other hand, CT has shown good accuracy in the detection of metastases to distant organs such as the lungs and liver (31). Magnetic resonance imaging (MRI) is still in an early phase of development, but as yet has shown no improvement over CT scan in staging gastric cancer (27–30).

## Endoscopic Ultrasonography

The largest experience in staging gastric cancer with EUS has been with the Olympus GF-UM3, GF-UM20, and more recently the GF-UM130, which have switchable frequencies of 7.5 MHz and 12 MHz or 20 MHz (14–16,32,33). The forward oblique optics allow easy visual examination of the stomach, which is best performed by filling the gastric lumen with water and/or placing a water-filled balloon over the transducer. Filling the lumen with water allows excellent definition of the gastric wall structure, but it is frequently difficult to cover the wall of the cardia and prepyloric areas with water; hence the water-filled balloon method is particularly helpful in these areas. It may be necessary to change the patient's position to prone or right oblique to submerge the desired area.

The great strength of EUS lies in its ability to image the wall of the gastrointestinal tract in greater detail than any other current method. The interaction of the gut wall with high-frequency ultrasound is complex; but, in general, five wall layers of alternating hyperechoic and hypoechoic bands are routinely imaged (34). The histologic correlates of the five layers involve the overlap of boundary echoes; but for clinical purposes, a simplified yet effective scheme equates the first two layers with the superficial and deep mucosa, the third layer with the submucosa, the fourth with the muscularis propria, and the fifth with the subserosal fat and serosa (see Chapter 9: Normal EUS Anatomy). Cancer of the stomach is usually imaged as a hypoechoic disruption of the wall layers. The compatibility of the AJCC staging classification for T in gastric cancer with EUS is good, but some difficulties remain. Using the balloon method in the cardia and the antrum, the first two wall layers are often too close to the transducer to be in focus; however, filling the balloon with additional water may cause compression of these layers with a resultant three-layer image. This problem can often be overcome by changing the position of the patient to effect water covering of the area under endoscopic control. Another difficult area is distinguishing between some T2 and T3 gastric cancers. The serosa of the stomach is very thin or nonexistent in some areas; even the pathologist handling a resected specimen may have difficulty separating a cancer that extends through the muscularis propria into the subserosa (T2) from one that penetrates the serosa (T3). Examples of surgical pathology–confirmed T1, T2, T3, and T4 cancers of the stomach imaged by EUS are shown in Figures 18–1 through 18–4. Lymph nodes along both lesser and greater curvatures of the stomach can be imaged. Lymph nodes tend to be arranged along blood vessels, and must be distinguished from vascular structures by real-time imaging (Fig. 18–5, 18–6). Lymph nodes are discrete structures with internal echoes, as opposed to blood vessels which show linear continuity and are essentially anechoic. Blood vessels frequently show a hypoechoic distal wall enhancement not seen in normal lymph nodes, although pathologically homogeneous lymph nodes may also

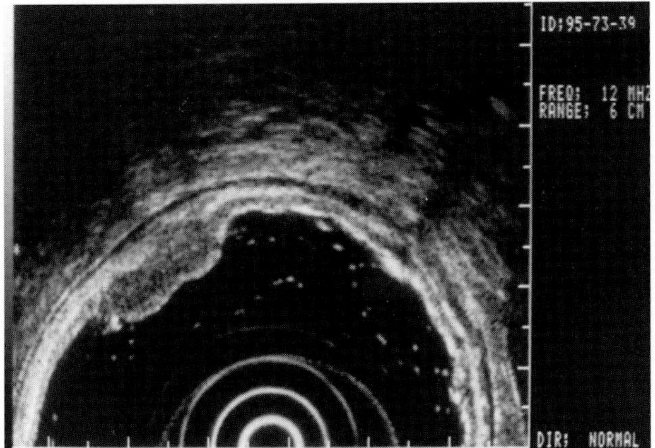


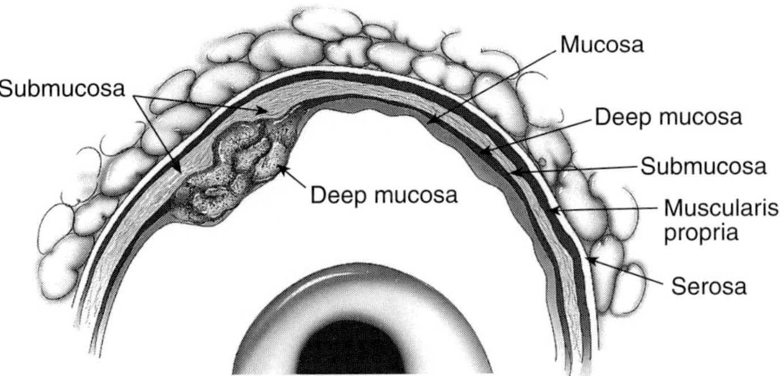


**FIGURE 18–1**

T1 gastric cancer limited to the first three layers of the wall of the gastric fundus.

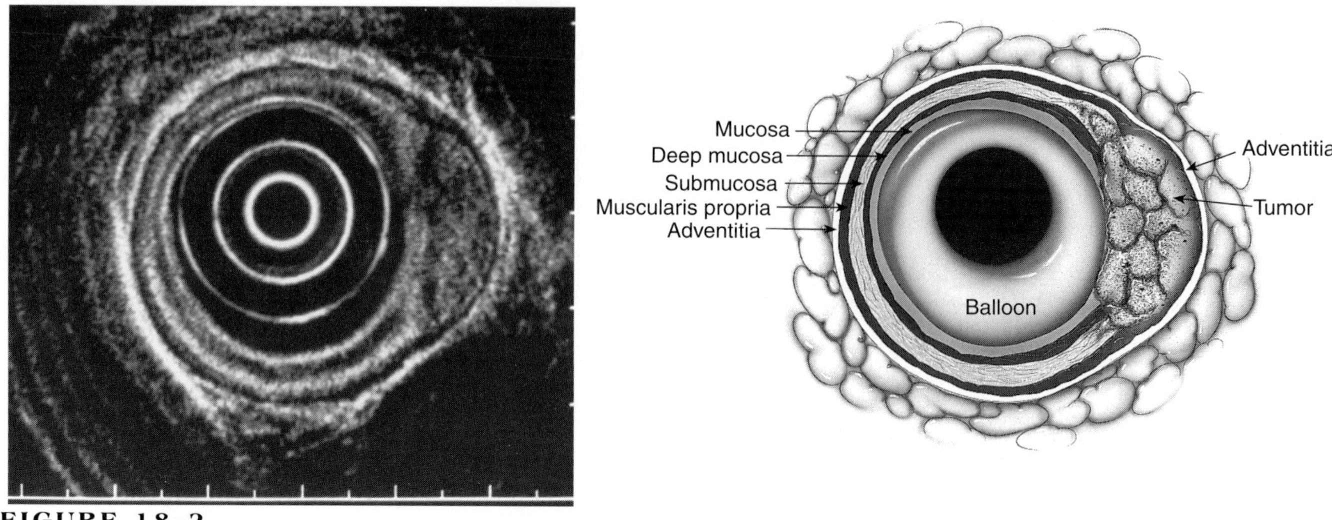


**FIGURE 18–2**

T2 cancer of the esophagogastric junction at 3 o'clock invading into but not through the fourth layer.

manifest this finding. Important areas of nodal drainage for cancer staging are the celiac axis, splenic artery, splenic hilum, hepatic artery, porta hepatis, and left gastric artery in the gastrohepatic ligament between the liver and the lesser curvature of the stomach. For ease of interpretation, EUS images should be oriented in the same fashion as CT scan—anterior structures at the top, posterior at the bottom, left structures at the right, and right at the left—as if facing a supine patient from the feet. This is usually easily accomplished by applying slight torque to the insertion tube with the GF-UM3, and is done electronically from the keyboard control panel of the GF-UM20 and GF-UM30.

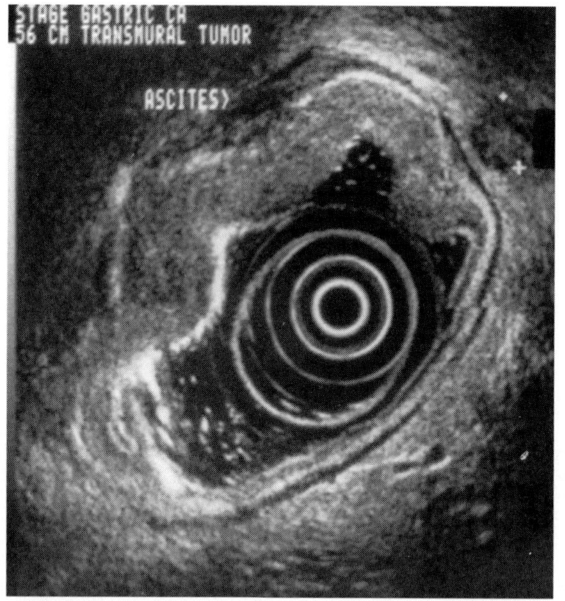


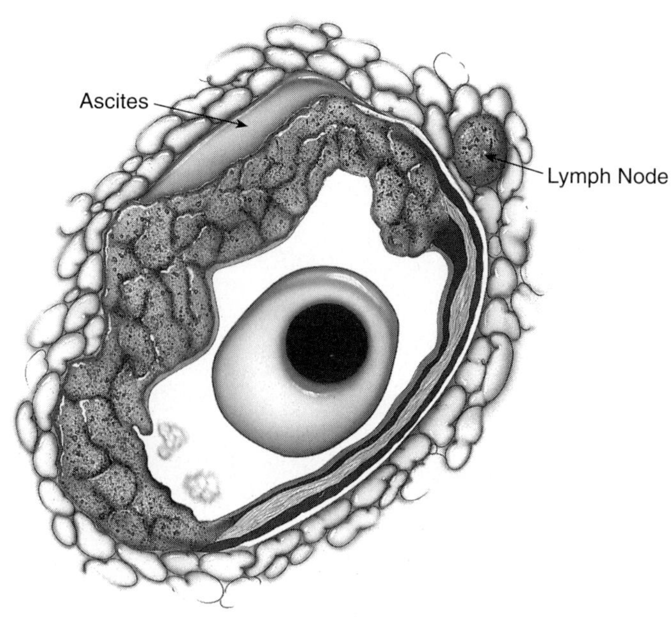


**FIGURE 18–3**

T3 gastric cancer of the lesser curvature of the stomach invading through all five wall layers. A thin anechoic area outside the cancer represents a small amount of ascitic fluid.

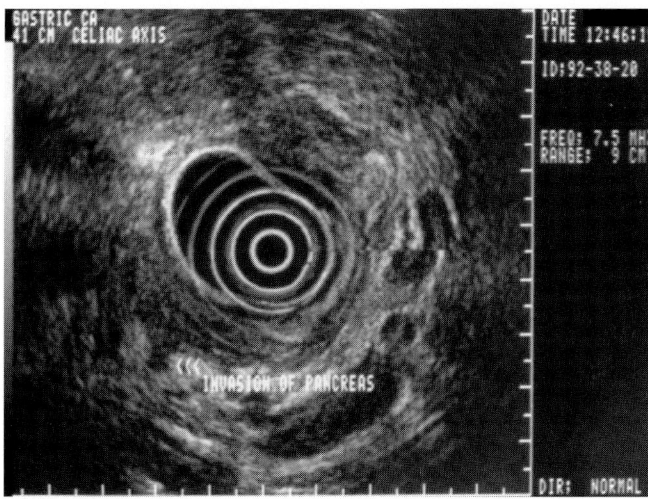


**FIGURE 18-4**

T4 gastric cancer. A tongue-like projection of hypoechoic tumor extends posteriorly from the stomach wall into the pancreas above the splenic vein.

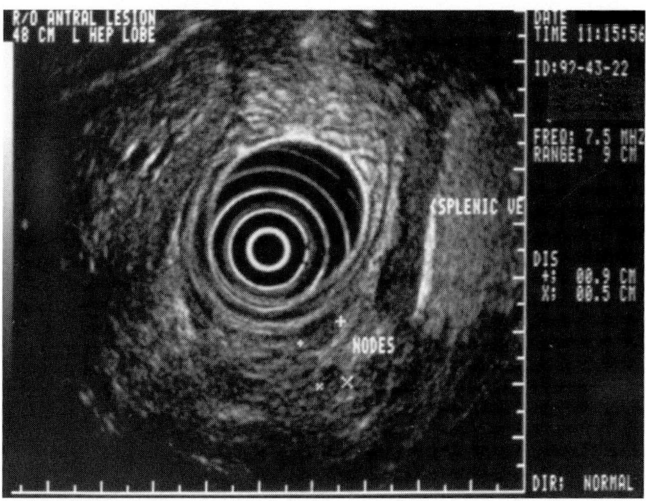


**FIGURE 18-6**

N2 regional lymph node metastases 0.5 cm and 0.9 cm in diameter in the area of the celiac axis, near the splenic vein and more than 3.0 cm from the edge of the primary cancer in the gastric antrum.

## Preoperative Staging with EUS

The available data demonstrate convincingly that EUS is highly accurate in determining the depth of primary cancer invasion or T stage. High-frequency EUS is limited in staging for distant metastases by its short depth of field, and therefore initial staging should be performed with a body imaging method such as CT. However, the accumulating literature shows a much higher staging accuracy for EUS compared to CT for staging depth of tumor penetration (T) and regional lymph node metastases (N). In a recent review, the accuracy of EUS for T was 78% and for N 70% in data from 22 centers reporting 2,263 patients (26,35). In all studies where comparisons have been made, EUS is more sensitive than CT for staging T and N, but not effective for staging M (26,31).

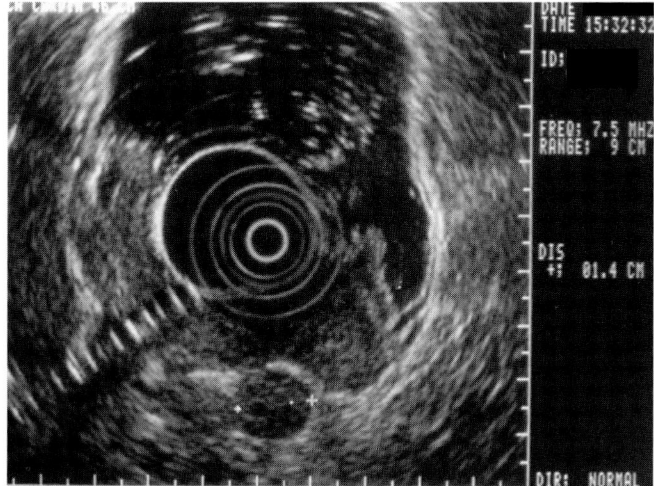


**FIGURE 18-5**

Large ulcerated cancer of the gastric cardia has broken through the entire wall structure (T3). In addition, an N1 regional lymph node metastasis is seen as a sharply demarcated, round structure, 1.4 cm in diameter, with a hypoechoic echo pattern similar to that of the adjacent primary cancer.

When analyzing patient survival ratio for gastric cancer surgery, it appears that only complete tumor removal is associated with a satisfactory prognosis. As such the R (resection) classification preoperatively is important ($R_0$, resectable; $R_1$, unresectable). EUS is highly accurate in predicting this resectability for gastric carcinoma, with almost identical predicted (by EUS) and actual rates of $R_0$ resections (9,31). Linear and radial scanning appear to be equally effective in staging for gastric cancer (26).

## Limitations of Endoscopic Ultrasonography

EUS is less than perfect in the local/regional staging of gastric cancer for several reasons. Understaging occurs because micrometastases cannot be imaged, whether in deeper wall layers or in lymph nodes. Overstaging is more common in gastric cancer, especially in the T1 and T2 stages (26,35). Many gastric cancers are ulcerated, and inflammation and fibrosis may involve deeper wall layers than the malignancy itself—hence the overstaging (14,36). Large reactive lymph nodes may also be difficult to distinguish from metastatic nodes. A further problem is the inability to distinguish by EUS the subserosal fat from the actual serosa or visceral peritoneum, which may tent away from the gastric wall, particularly at the curvatures of the stomach. Thus, in a patient with apparent disruption of the fifth layer on EUS, pathology may reveal complete penetration of the muscularis propria by cancer with infiltration of the subserosa. A patient with such pT2 disease is usually identified as uT3. The presence of ascites may help in a more accurate EUS diagnosis in such situations. These difficulties probably explain why the accuracy of EUS for T2 stage gastric cancer is lower than that for other T stages (26,35). In one report, accuracy for T2 staging was 71% compared to 86% for T1 and 89% for T3 lesions (26).

In staging nodal disease, the differentiation of benign from malignant nodes remains problematic. When evaluating lymph nodes at EUS, five descriptors are used: size, border, echo texture, echo intensity, and shape. We found the size of imaged lymph nodes to be an unreliable criterion of malignancy. Malignant nodes as small as 3 mm can be imaged with EUS. Nodes larger than 10 mm, however, are very suggestive for malignancy. As also emphasized by Tio et al. (14), we have found that malignant nodes tend to be rounded, sharply defined, and hypoechoic in echo intensity (Figs. 18–5, 18–6) compared to benign nodes, which tend to be elongated, hazier, and more echogenic. Determination of nodal malignancy by these criteria remains rather subjective, and requires improvement. Echo texture rather than echo intensity is thought by some authors to be more suggestive for malignancy (37). Heterogeneous echo texture (instead of homogeneous) seems more suggestive for malignancy. Subjective or computer-analysis (via gray-scale analysis) of the echo intensity of lymph nodes does not appear to aid in differentiation (37). If the criteria of large size (>10 mm), heterogeneous echo texture, and distinct border are used for gastric cancer staging, sensitivity for malignant lymph nodes is 85% and specificity between 45% and 85% (37). Sesame oil has been used for better detection of metastatic lymph nodes (38). EUS-guided FNA may be helpful in differentiating benign from malignant lymph nodes (39). Thus, differenting benign from malignant nodes is difficult; moreover, it appears that some lymph nodes are not imaged at all—especially the more distant lymph node metastases and prepyloric and pericardia lymph nodes (26).

EUS is not an appropriate method to detect distant metastases from gastric cancer. Due to its limited depth of penetration, high-frequency EUS can be used to scan the left liver lobe but only a portion of the right lobe; nor is it useful in evaluating pulmonary metastates and distant peritoneal metastates. In our experience in staging gastric cancer, the greatest accuracy for overall stage was achieved using CT for M and EUS for T and N (32).

## Endoscopic Ultrasonography for Early Gastric Carcinoma

Use of the GF-UM20 or GF-UM130 to evaluate early gastric cancer has been amplified by the introduction of miniprobes (40–45) whose small diameter (2.5 mm) allows passage through the accessory channel of a standard endoscope (41,45). Utilizing radial scanning transducers at 12 MHz and 20 MHz, ultrasound miniprobes can be used in patients with stenotic lesions that cannot be traversed with conventional dedicated echoendoscopes. Under direct endoscopic vision, small, early gastric cancers can be detected more easily (44,45). Staging early gastric cancer for possible endoscopic treatment is becoming increasingly important. The overall accuracy rate for staging early gastric cancer with miniprobes is in the range of 80% (44). But because of the higher frequency and limited depth of penetration, miniprobes are not as useful for imaging advanced lesions (beyond the muscularis propria) or large lesions. The accuracy of determining malignant involvement of lymph nodes using ultrasound probes is less than that for conventional endoscopic ultrasonography, and remains a major limitation for staging gastric cancer.

Use of miniprobes with high frequencies also leads to a more detailed imaging of the gastric wall. A seven-layer image can be obtained with the 20 MHz probes, differentiating the muscularis propria layer into a circular and longitudinal muscular layer. From Japanese centers, where experience is extensive with early gastric cancer (limited to the mucosa and submucosa), some authors believe they can differentiate the muscularis mucosae using high-frequency ultrasound miniprobes (20 MHz) (40). The muscularis mucosae was presumably visualized as a hypoechoic layer between layer 2 and 3.

Using higher frequencies has led several Japanese authors to subdivide the T1 stage of gastric cancer into T1m (mucosa) and T1sm (submucosa) (40,46). Shimizu et al. also believe that the disruption patterns of the third layer can predict infiltration or depth of EGC (46). The importance of these detailed examinations of the gastric wall is to accurately define the depth of invasion of an EGC, because the positivity of lymph nodes rises from 1% to 18% in EGC that go beyond the muscularis mucosae (43).

## Results

We prospectively studied results of EUS staging for T and N in 50 patients with gastric cancer, then compared our results to CT scan using the standard of surgical pathology (32). For T staging, EUS was accurate in 92% of cases, and for N staging, 78% (Figs. 18–7, 18–8). In

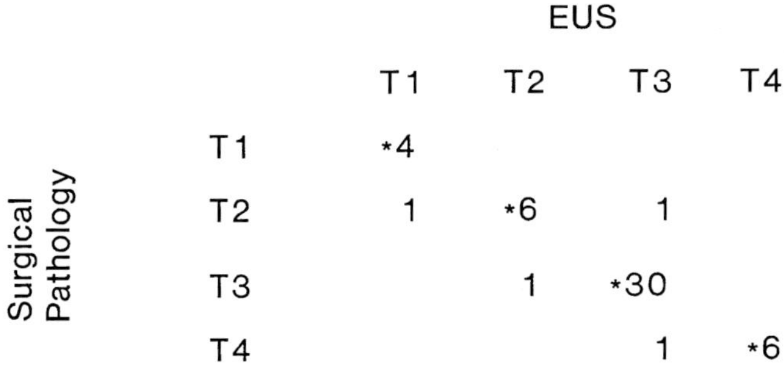


**FIGURE 18–7**

EUS staging for depth of invasion of primary gastric cancer (T) compared to surgical pathology.

all cases, modern CT scanning were used with 2-second scan time and dynamic technique, with intravenous and oral contrast in an effort to obtain the greatest accuracy. CT scan was performed after EUS and reviewed independently to avoid bias. EUS was significantly more accurate than dynamic CT scan in staging T and N in patients with gastric cancer (Fig. 18–9). Whether spiral CT will improve CT scan results has yet to be tested.

We were able to follow 43 patients with gastric cancer staged with EUS after attempted curative resection (47). After a median of 13 months postoperatively, we saw no recurrence in patients with T1 disease ($n$ = 3) and only 10% of those with stage T2 ($n$ = 10) experienced recurrence. On the other hand, during the same period, 58% with stage T3 ($n$ = 26) and 75% with T4 disease ($n$ = 4) experienced recurrence. At a median follow-up of 25 months, there was still no recurrence among the T1 patients, while one additional patient with stage T2 recurred (20%). Nineteen patients with EUS stage T4 recurred (Fig. 18–10). Thus, at a median of 25 months, 2 of 13 patients (15%) with EUS stage T1-2 had recurred, while 23 of 30 (77%) with EUS stage T3-4 had recurred ($p$ < .001).

| Surgical Pathology | EUS N0 | EUS N1 | EUS N2 |
|---|---|---|---|
| N0 | *10 | | 1 |
| N1 | 7 | *15 | |
| N2 | 1 | 2 | *14 |

*concordance = 39/50 = 78%

**FIGURE 18–8**

EUS staging for regional lymph node metastases from gastric cancer (N) compared to surgical pathology. There was a statistically significant tendency to understage nodal metastases ($p$ < .016).

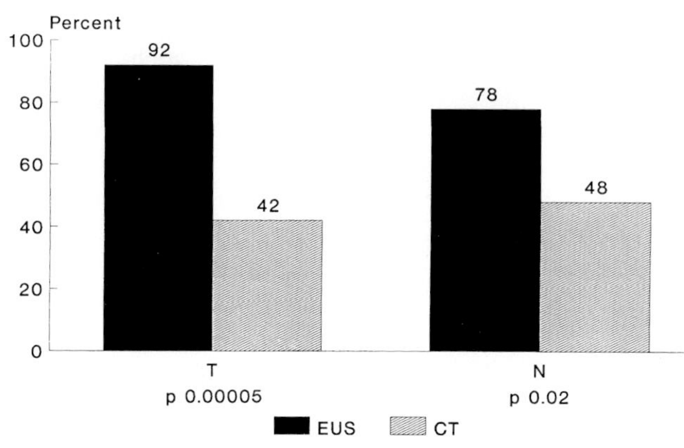


**FIGURE 18–9**

Results of EUS staging in 50 patients with gastric cancer. EUS was significantly better than dynamic CT scan in staging for depth of primary tumor invasion (T) and regional lymph node metastases (N), using the standard of surgical pathology. From Bótet et al, Radiology, 1991.[32]

## Conclusions

Our results contributed to the accumulating data demonstrating that endoscopic ultrasound adds significantly to the local/regional staging accuracy in gastric cancer, and

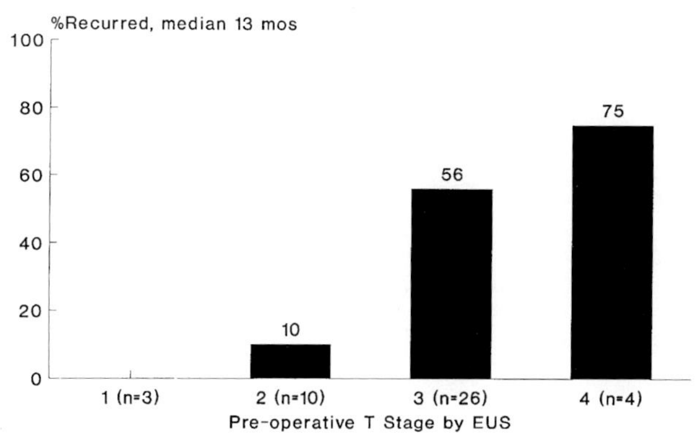


**FIGURE 18–10**

Percent recurrence by preoperative EUS T-stage. Recurrence of gastric carcinoma according to endoscopic ultrasound T-stage at 13 and 25 months median follow-up. In patients with EUS stage T3 and T4 recurrence was significantly more likely than in patients with EUS stage T1 and T2 at a median of 13 months ($p$ = .03) and at a median of 25 months ($p$ = .0002). From Smith et al, J Clin Oncol, 1993.[47]

suggest that EUS is more accurate than CT scan for this purpose. Potential clinical applications include patient selection for operative versus nonoperative management, such as endoscopic therapy in early cancer, and for radical versus palliative operations in advanced disease.

Our follow-up study showed that endoscopic ultrasound can be used to predict the risk of recurrence in patients with gastric carcinoma after resection with curative intent. Patients shown to have T1 and T2 lesions are best treated by surgery alone. Patients with T3 and T4 disease are significantly more likely to recur after surgery and should be considered for management programs that involve more than surgical resection (47). This prediction of poor outcome can be made preoperatively; thus, in an effort to improve the prognosis of patients with EUS T3-4 gastric cancer, an experimental program of treatment is being offered to many patients—one that includes preoperative systemic chemotherapy.

## References


1. Rohde H, Geilbensleben B, Bauer P, et al. Has there been any improvement in staging of gastric cancer? Cancer 64:2465–2481, 1989.
2. Breaux JR, Bringaze W, Chappuis C, et al. Adenocarcinoma of the stomach: A review of 35 years and 1,710 cases. World J Surg 14:580–586, 1990.
3. Cady B, Ramsden DA, Choe DS. Treatment of gastric cancer. Surg Clin North Am 56:599–605, 1976.
4. Shiu MH, Perotti, Brennan MF. Adenocarcinoma of the stomach: A multivariate analysis of clinical, pathologic and treatment factors. Hepato-gastroenterol 36:7–12, 1989.
5. Maruyama K, Okabayshi K, Kinoshita T. Progress in gastric cancer surgery in Japan and its limits of radicality. World J Surg. 11: 418–425, 1987.
6. Noguchi Y, Imadra T, Matsumoto A, et al. Radical surgery for gastric cancer: A review of the Japanese data. Cancer 64:2053–2062, 1989.
7. Boring CC, Squires TS, Tong T, Montgomery S. Cancer statistics 1994. CA Cancer J Clin 44:7–26, 1994.
8. Beahrs OH, Henson DE, Hutter RVP, et al. Manual for Staging of Cancer. Philadelphia: JB Lippincott, 1988, pp 69–74.
9. Dittler HJ, Siewert JR. Role of endoscopic ultrasonography in gastric carcinoma. Endoscopy 25:162–166, 1993.
10. Songür Y, Okai T, Watanabe H, Fujii T, Motoo Y, Sawabu N. Preoperative diagnosis of mucinous gastric adenocarcinoma by endoscopic ultrasonography. Am J Gastroenterol 91:1586–1590, 1996.
11. Blot WJ, Devesa SS, Kneller RW, Frsaumeni JF Jr. Rising incidence of adenocarcinoma of the esophagus and gastric cardia. JAMA 265:1287–1289, 1991.
12. Pera M, Cameron AJ, Trastek VF, Carpenter HA, Zinsmeister AR. Increasing incidence of adenocarcinoma of the esophagus and esophagogastric junction. Gastroenterology 104:510–513, 1993.
13. Natsugoe S, Yoshinaka H, Moringa T, Shimada M, Hokita S, Baba M, Takao S, Fukumoto T, Stein HJ, Aikou T. Assessment of tumor invasion of the distal esophagus in carcinoma of the cardia using endoscopic ultrasonography. Endoscopy 28:750–755, 1996.
14. Tio TL, Schouwink MH, Cikot RJLM, Tytgat GNJ. Preoperative TNM classification of gastric carcinoma by endosonography in comparison with the pathological TNM system: A prospective study of 72 cases. Hepato-gastroenterol 36:51–56, 1989.
15. Abe S, Lightdale CJ, Brennan MF. The Japanese experience with endoscopic ultrasonography in the staging of gastric cancer. Gastrointest Endosc 39:586–591, 1993.
16. Yasuda K, Nakajima M, Cho E, et al. Benign versus malignant gastric ulcers: A role for endoscopic ultrasonography? In Classen M, Dancygier H (eds.): 5th International Symposium on Endoscopic Ultrasonography. Demeter, Munich (Z Gastroenterol suppl) 1989; 50–58.
17. Polensky A, Ziegler K, Sauft C. Endosonographische Befunde benigner und maligner Lasionen der Magenwand. Dtsch Med Wschr 113:1263–1270, 1988.
18. Andriulli A, Recchia S, DeAngelis C, et al. Endoscopic ultrasonographic evaluation of patients with biopsy negative gastric linitis plastica. Gastrointest Endosc 36:611–615, 1990.
19. Mendes R, Gerdes H, Bótet JF, Lightdale CJ. Large gastric folds: A diagnostic approach using endoscopic ultrasonography. Gastrointest Endosc 40:437–441, 1994.
20. Avunduk C, Navab F, Hampf F, Coughlin B. Prevalence of *Helicobacter pylori* infection in patients with large gastric folds: Evaluation and follow-up with endoscopic ultrasound before and after antimicrobial therapy. Am J Gastroenterol 90:1969–1973, 1995.
21. Songür Y, Okai T, Watanabe H, Motoo Y, Sawabu N. Endosonographic evaluation of giant gastric folds. Gastrointest Endosc 41:468–474, 1995.
22. Wiersema MJ, Gatzimos K, Nisi R, Wiersema LM. Staging of non-Hodgkin's gastric lymphoma with endosonography-guided fine-needle aspiration biopsy and flow cytometry. Gastrointest Endosc 44:734–736, 1996.
23. Jacob Ph, Pujol B, Napoleon B, Keriven-Souquet O, Souquet JC. Accuracy of endoscopic ultrasonography (EUS) in the staging of gastric MALT lymphoma. Endoscopy 28:S38A, 1996.
24. Borrmann R. Geschwulste des Magens. Handbuch der Speziellen Pathologischen Anatomie and Histologie (Herausgegeben von Henke, F.U. and Lubarsch, O.) Vol. 4, Berlin, Springer, 1926.
25. Japan Research Society for gastric cancers. The general rules for the gastric cancer study in surgery and pathology. Part I. Clinical classification. Jpn J Surg 11(2):127–139, 1981.
26. Rösch T. Endosonographic staging of gastric cancer: A review of literature results. Gastroentest Endosc Clin NA 5(3):549–557, 1995.
27. Scatarige JC, Disantis DJ: CT of the stomach and duodenum. Radiol Clin North Am 27:687–706, 1989.
28. Cook AO, Levine BA, Sirinek KR: Evaluation of gastric adenocarcinoma: Abdominal computed tomography does not replace celiotomy. Arch Surg 121:603–606, 1986.
29. Sussman SK, Halvorsen RA, Illescas FF, et al: Gastric adenocarcinoma: CT versus staging. Radiology 167:335–340, 1988.
30. Halvorsen RA, Thompson WM. Computed tomographic staging of gastrointestinal tract malignancies. Part I. Esophagus and stomach. Invest Radiol 22:2–16, 1987.
31. Greenberg J, Durkin M, Van Drunen M, Aranka GV. Computed tomography or endoscopic ultrasonsography in preoperative staging of gastric and esophageal tumors. Surgery 116:696–702, 1994.
32. Bótet JF, Lightdale CJ, Zauber AG, et al. Endoscopic ultrasonography in the pre-operative staging of gastric cancer: A comparative study with dynamic CT. Radiology 181:426–432, 1991.
33. Rösch T, Lorenz R, Zenker K, et al. Local staging and assessment of resectability in carcinoma of the esophagus, stomach, and duodenum by endoscopic ultrasonography. Gastrointest Endosc 38: 460–467, 1992.
34. Kimmey MB, Martin RW, Haggitt RC, et al. Histologic correlates of gastrointestinal ultrasound images. Gastroenterology 96:433–441, 1989.
35. Rösch T, Classen M. Gastroenterologic Endosonography. Stuttgart: Thieme, 1992, pp 71–80.
36. Fein J, Gerdes H, Karpeh M, Lauers G, Bótet JF, Kelsen D, Brennan MF, Lightdale CJ. Overstaging of ulcerated gastric cancers by endoscopic ultrasonography (abstract). Gastrointest Endosc 39:274, 1993.
37. Heintz A, Mildenberger P, Georg H, Braunstein S, Jurginger Th. Endoscopic ultrasonography in the diagnosis of regional lymph nodes in esophageal and gastric cancer. Results of studies in vitro. Endoscopy 25:231–235, 1993.
38. Aibe T, Fujimara H, Yanai H. Endosonographic diagnosis of metastatic lymph nodes in gastric carcinoma. Endoscopy 24: 315–319, 1992.
39. Hoffman BJ, Hawes RH. Endoscopic ultrasonography-guided puncture of the lymph nodes: First experience and clinical consequences. Gastrointest Endosc Clin NA 5(3):587–593, 1995.

40. Yanai M, Fujimiza H, Suzumi M, Matsuura S, Awaya N, Noguchi T, Karita M, Tada M, Okita K, Aibe T. Delineation of the gastric muscularis mucosae and assessment of depth of invasion of early gastric cancer using a 20 megahertz endoscopic ultrasound probe. Gastrointest Endosc 39:505–512, 1993.
41. Yasuda K. Development and clinical use of ultrasonic probes. Endoscopy 26;816–817, 1994.
42. Akahoshi K, Chijiwa Y, Tanaha M, Hasada N, Nawata H. Endosonography probe-guided endoscopic mucosal resection of gastric neoplasms. Gastrointest Endosc 42:248–252, 1995.
43. Yasuda K, Nakajima M, Kanai K. Endoscopic diagnosis and treatment of early gastric cancer using endoscopic ultrasonography. Gastrointest Endosc Clin North Am 2:495–507, 1992.
44. Chak A, Canto M, Stevens P, Lightdale CJ, Van de Mierop F, Cooper G, Pollack BJ, Sivak MV. Prospective evaluation of new ultrasound catheter system: Comparison with ultrasound endoscopes. Gastrointest Endosc 43(4):A8, 1996.
45. Yanai H, Tada M, Karita M, Okita K. Diagnostic utility of 20-megahertz linear endoscopic ultrasonography in early gastric cancer. Gastrointest Endosc 44:29–33, 1996.
46. Shimizu S, Tada M, Kanai K: Endoscopic ultrasonography in early gastric cancer. Endoscopy 26:767–768, 1994.
47. Smith JW, Brennan MF, Bótet JF, Gerdes H, Lightdale CJ. Preoperative endoscopic ultrasound can predict the risk of recurrence after operation for gastric carcinoma. J Clin Oncol 11: 2380–2385, 1993.

CHAPTER

# Staging Gastric Cancer

## THE MUNICH EXPERIENCE

Thomas Rösch
Meinhard Classen

The diagnosis of gastric cancer is made primarily by endoscopy and biopsy. The main purpose of endoscopic ultrasonography (EUS) is preoperative staging according to the TNM system (1987) (1). Local and regional tumor spread can be demonstrated within the different echo layers of the gastric wall, and adjacent lymph nodes may be classified as benign or malignant by reference to size and/or echo pattern (1) (Figs. 19–1 through 19–5).

## Accuracy of EUS in Assessing Local Tumor Invasion (T-Stage)

During recent years, a variety of studies have evaluated gastric cancer staging. The accuracy of EUS for staging gastric cancer is minimally less than EUS staging of esophageal cancer, but still in a high range (3–6,8–26,28) (Table 19–1). In two Japanese studies of 67 (14) and 147 (5) patients, early gastric cancer was differentiated from advanced cancer in 90% of cases. Almost all information about tumor staging comes from studies using echoendoscopes with 360° scanning perpendicular to the shaft axis. A recent study suggests that linear-type echoendoscopes (scanning plane parallel to the axis of the insertion tube) yield accuracy rates comparable to the conventional 360° instruments in the staging of gastric cancer and other malignancies (29). This is despite the limited overview provided by linear-type echoendoscopes. However, determining the depth of tumor infiltration is possible using linear-type echoendoscopes. The delineation of the circumferential tumor extent is more difficult on EUS and may require a 360° sector scanner. Using such

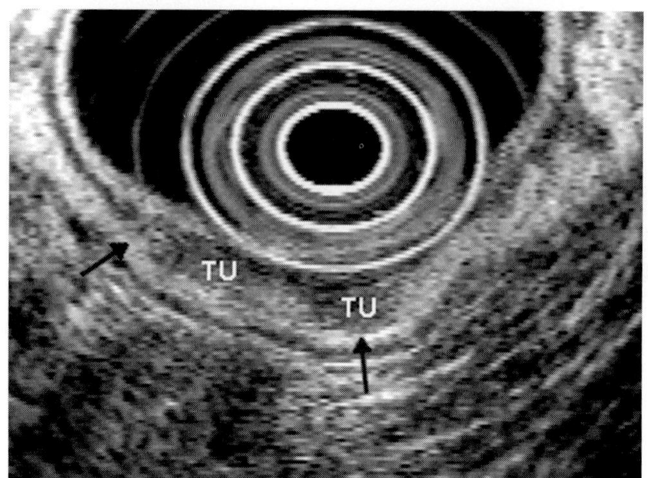


**FIGURE 19-1**

Early gastric cancer (TU), visible as echo-poor thickening of the inner layer; the underlying submucosa (arrows) is intact. (radial echoendoscope)

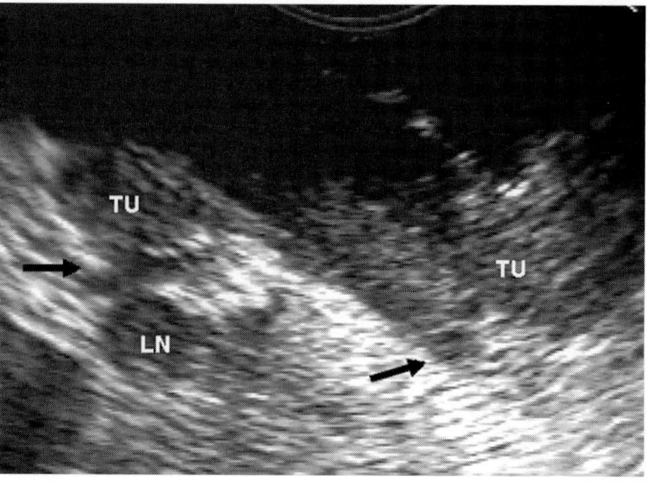


**FIGURE 19-3**

Gastric carcinoma in stage T3 (TU) with an echo-poor wall thickening and irregular outer borders (arrows) and a paratumorous lymph node metastasis (LN), indicating stage N1. (linear echoendoscope)

an instrument, resection lines of gastric cancers could well be predicted, with the notable exception of ulcerated gastric cancers (30). Ulcerated carcinomas also give rise to overstaging due to peritumorous inflammatory changes which can occur in up to 40% of cases (31) (see also below). In comparative studies, the accuracy of EUS for the T stage exceeds that of computed tomography (CT) by a factor of 15–60% depending on the stage of the tumor (Table 19–2).

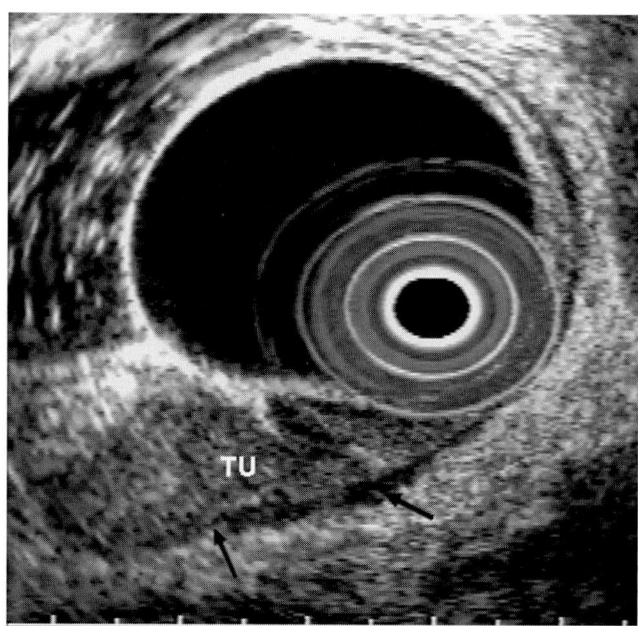


**FIGURE 19-2**

Gastric carcinoma in stage T2 (TU); the echo-poor wall thickening with the loss of the first three layers reaches the muscularis propria (arrows) but does not pass through it. (radial echoendoscope)

## Differential Diagnosis of Gastric Ulceration by Endoscopic Ultrasonography

Meticulously performed studies from Japan (5,32) have shown that benign ulcers exhibit changes at EUS which are very difficult to distinguish from those of ulcerative malignancy. Earlier studies suggested that EUS was accurate in differentiating between benign and malignant ulcers (33). A more recent study, however, showed EUS to be only 67% accurate in differentiating malignant from benign (chronic) ulcers; five of seven benign ulcers were

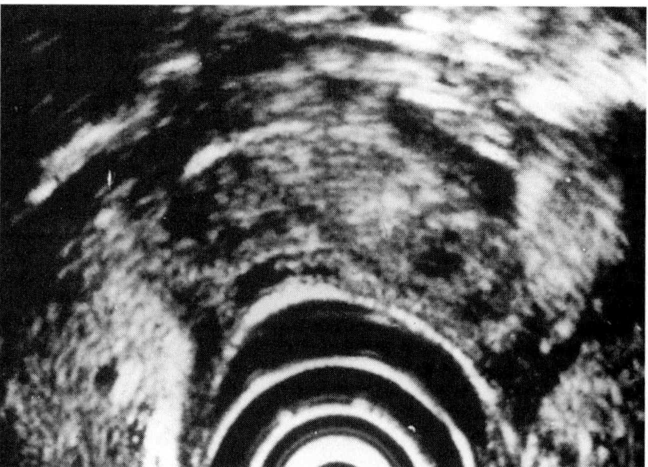

**FIGURE 19-4**

Large gastric carcinoma in stage T4 (TU) infiltrating into the pancreas. (radial echoendoscope)

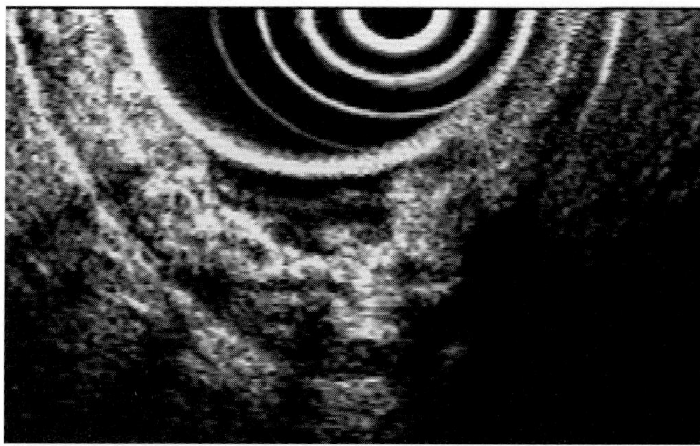

**FIGURE 19-5**

Gastric linitis plastica, seen on EUS as wall thickening; the layer structure is barely being visible, but the outer margin remains intact. (radial echoendoscope)

misinterpreted as malignant (34). Therefore, the differentiation of benign from malignant gastric ulcer is not a good indication for EUS. It has been suggested that EUS showing diffuse wall changes which are much more extended than the actual ulcer size determined on endoscopy may be indicative of malignancy and hence prompt further aggressive diagnostic steps; but this is not based on prospective data. In summary, EUS cannot reliably exclude malignancy in gastric ulcers. In ulcerated cancers, the actual extent of the tumor infiltration may be overestimated due to peritumorous inflammatory changes (2,31).

**TABLE 19-1**

Accuracy of EUS Compared to Histopathology in the Preoperative Staging of Gastric Cancer

| First Author | *n* | T Stage | N Stage |
|---|---|---|---|
| Yasuda (23) | 500 | 79% | — |
| Kida (24) | 321 | 82% | — |
| Dittler (3) | 254 | 83% | 66% |
| Ohashi (4) | 174 | 67% | — |
| Yoshikawa (28) | 166 | 72% | — |
| Yasuda (5) | 147 | 78% | — |
| Grimm (6) | 147 | 78% | 87% |
| Murata (8) | 146 | 79% | — |
| Ito (9) | 141 | 74% | — |
| Saito (10) | 110 | 81% | — |
| Zeigler (11) | 108 | 86% | 74% |
| Kimura (25) | 100 | 85% | — |
| De Angelis (26) | 86 | 80% | 75% |
| Akahoshi (12) | 74 | 81% | 50% |
| Tio (13) | 72 | 84% | 68% |
| Aibe (14) | 67 | 73% | 69% |
| Froment (15) | 53 | 79% | 70% |
| Bótet (16) | 50 | 92% | 78% |
| Nattermann (17) | 50 | 82% | 78% |
| Caletti (18) | 42 | 91% | 69% |
| Rösch (19) | 41 | 71% | 75% |
| Yoshimi (20) | 40 | — | 73% |
| Cerizzi (21) | 27 | 90% | 55% |
| Heintz (22) | 19 | 79% | 72% |

**TABLE 19-2**

Comparison of EUS and CT in the Preoperative Staging of Gastric Carcinoma

| | | T Staging | | N Staging | |
|---|---|---|---|---|---|
| First Author | *n* | *EUS* | *CT* | *EUS* | *CT* |
| Grimm (7) | 117* | 85%* | 15%* | 87% | 25% |
| Zeigler (11) | 108 | 86% | 43% | 74% | 51% |
| Bótet (16) | 50 | 92% | 42% | 78% | 48% |
| Nattermann (17) | 50 | 82% | 25% | 78% | 48% |

*Only stage T4 is used for comparison; comparative data for T staging are not available for other stages. N staging is compared in all 117 patients.

## Diagnosis of Gastric Linitis Plastica

Gastric linitis plastica represents an unusual form of gastric cancer. EUS may be useful in differentiating gastric linitis plastica from other causes of gastric wall thickening (35–39), gastric cysts (40,41), and perhaps gastric lymphoma (42,43). Patients with gastric linitis plastica may be difficult to diagnose on endoscopy and biopsy owing to diffuse, intramural tumor spread. In such cases, EUS demonstrates an echo-poor and inhomogeneous wall thickening with loss both of the uniform five-layered structure and of expandability on instillation of water. Such images are highly suggestive of gastric malignancy, even when histology is negative (44–47). Such findings should prompt the clinician to seek additional histology, using more aggressive techniques such as large-particle biopsy. Whether negative histology obtained on repeated occasions of unequivocal EUS findings of gastric linitis plastica should form the basis of treatment decisions is still a matter for debate. A high rate of false positives (up to 30%) in benign gastric wall thickening may exacerbate this controversy (46,47).

## Recognition of Malignant Lymph Nodes

The general comments concerning the detection of malignant lymph nodes in esophageal cancer apply to lymph nodes associated with gastric carcinoma (see Chapter 13: Esophageal Carcinoma). Whether the echo pattern of a given lymph node yields reliable information about the status of the node remains doubtful (2). Whether EUS-guided fine needle aspiration of lymph nodes (48) is accurate and clinically helpful remains to be determined. The accuracy of the EUS diagnosis of the metastatic lymph nodes associated with gastric cancer is somewhat lower than for lymph nodes involved by esophageal cancer (see Table 19–1). This may also relate to the greater difficulty of the meticulous scanning of the larger perigastric area and to difficulty in scanning more distant nodes (i.e., stage N2) because of the limited penetration of the EUS (7,19).

## Problems in Endosonographic Tumor Staging

Stenosis of the gastric lumen is seldom a problem for endosonography in gastric cancer, with the exception of rare antral tumors. Overstaging the depth of penetration of the cancer occurs in approximately 10–20% of the T2 and is especially frequent in ulcerated gastric cancers (31). Overstaging may result if the tumor is scanned from an oblique direction, as the resulting artifactual blurring of the deeper layers appears to suggest malignancy. There are some difficult locations for EUS scanning, including the lesser curvature of the antrum or the subcardial fundus region. Visualization of tumors in these areas may pose problems especially in early and discrete lesions. Generally, examiners take the absence of endosonographic wall changes in the area of an endoscopically localized early gastric cancer as evidence of T1. This is particularly the case in the flat or slightly excavated forms of these early tumors. Differentiation between mucosal and submucosal infiltration in early gastric cancer is also difficult and results are worse than for all gastric cancers (5,14). Accuracy rates of EUS in correctly diagnosing mucosal and submucosal tumor spread range from 72% to 80% (mucosal) and from 62% to 82% (submucosal) (5,10,14,24,25,49). Using high-frequency miniprobes (20 MHz), staging results in differentiating mucosal from submucosal invasion could not be substantially improved (accuracy 67%) (50,51). When the use of high US frequency permitted visualization of the muscularis mucosae, staging accuracy was slightly better (50). In another study, probe scanning of early gastric cancer was accurate in six of seven patients with three additional failures to visualize the lesion (52).

## Implications of EUS Findings for Tumor Therapy

Generally, gastrectomy is considered the treatment of choice for stage T1–T3 and even T4 lesions. Therefore, precise staging by EUS does not influence the choice of therapy in most patients with this cancer. However, endosonographic staging might be useful for advanced carcinomas (T3, T4, and N2) if preoperative treatment with chemotherapy is used in an effort to ‘downstage’ the tumor. The accuracy of EUS in relation to advanced stages is reported to be as high as 90% and more (2). However, it has yet to be shown that this accuracy is maintained when these advanced cancers are restaged after such therapeutic measures. The presence of fibrous and inflammatory changes may compromise the ability to accurately determine the stage of the remaining tumor. EUS can also be used to predict resectability of gastric carcinoma and was shown to be 80–90% accurate in this respect (19,53).

There is increasing interest in endoscopic therapy of early gastric cancer. Only tumors with infiltration into the mucosa (as opposed to involvement of the submucosa) are suitable since these lesions are associated with a very low rate of lymph node metastases. EUS might be valuable in the identification of suitable candidates for this type of treatment (54). Use of EUS to select suitable patients, however, needs improvement in terms of image resolution to reliably differentiate between mucosal and submucosal inflammation. This indication could also require an improved differential diagnosis of lymph node metastases.

## Conclusion

EUS is very accurate in staging the local spread of gastric cancer according to the TNM classification system. It has no place in the primary diagnosis of gastric cancers or the differentiation of benign and malignant gastric ulcers. The clinical value of EUS and its implications for therapy of gastric cancer might become more evident with increasing use of endoscopic or other forms of minimally invasive therapy for early gastric carcinoma as well as with other stage-dependent treatment protocols.

### References


1. Sobin LH, Hermanek P, Hutter RP. TNM classification of malignant tumors. Cancer 61:2310–2314, 1988.
2. Rösch T, Classen M. Gastroenterologic Endosonography. Stuttgart: Thieme, 1992.
3. Dittler HJ, Siewert JR. Role of endoscopic ultrasonography in gastric carcinoma. Endoscopy 25:162–166, 1993.
4. Ohashi S, Nakazawa S, Yoshino J. Endoscopic ultrasonography in the assessment of invasive gastric cancer. Scand J Gastroenterol 24:1039–1048, 1989.
5. Yasuda K, Nakajima M, Cho E, Kobayashi M, Kawai K. Benign versus malignant gastric ulcers: A role for endoscopic ultrasonography? In Dancygier H, Classen M (eds): 5th International Symposium on Endoscopic Ultrasonography. Munich: Demeter Verlag (Z Gastroenterol suppl.), 1989, pp 50–56.
6. Grimm H, Binmoeller K, Hamper K, et al. Endosonography for pre-operative locoregional staging of esophageal and gastric cancer. Endoscopy 25:224–230, 1993.
7. Grimm H, Hamper K, Maydeo A, et al. Accuracy of endoscopic ultrasound and computed tomography in determining local/regional spread of gastric cancer: Results of a prospective controlled study. Gastrointest Endosc 37:279(abstract), 1991.

8. Murata Y, Suzuki S, Hashimoto H. Endoscopic ultrasonography of the upper gastrointestinal tract. Surg Endosc 2:180–183, 1988.
9. Ito M, Takasu S, Ikegama F, et al. Endoscopic ultrasonography in gastric cancer. Endosc 24:653(abstract), 1992.
10. Saito N, Takeshita K, Habu H, et al. The use of endoscopic ultrasound in determining the depth of cancer invasion in patients with gastric cancer. Surg Endosc 5:14–19, 1991.
11. Ziegler K, Sanft C, Zimmer T, et al. Comparison of computed tomography, endosonography, and intraoperative assessment in TN staging of gastric carcinoma. Gut 34:604–610, 1993.
12. Akahoshi H, Misawa T, Fujishima H, et al. Preoperative evaluation of gastric cancer by endoscopic ultrasound. Gut 32:479–482, 1991.
13. Tio TL, Schouwink MH, Cikot RJLM, et al. Preoperative TNM classification of gastric carcinoma by endosonography in comparison with the pathological TNM system: A prospective study of 72 cases. Hepato-gastroenterol 36:51–56, 1989.
14. Aibe T, Fujimura H, Noguchi T, et al. Endosonographic detection and staging of early gastric cancer. In Dancygier H, Classen M (eds): 5th International Symposium on Endoscopic Ultrasonography. Munich: Demeter Verlag (Z Gastroenterol suppl.), 1989, pp 71–78.
15. Froment S, Pujol B, Napoleon B, et al. Endoscopic ultrasound (EUS) and adenocarcinoma of the cardia: Results and practical usefulness. Gastrointest Endosc 39:A305(abstract), 1993.
16. Bótet JF, Lightdale CJ, Zauber AG, et al. Preoperative staging of gastric cancer: Comparison of endoscopic US and dynamic CT. Radiology 181:426–432, 1991.
17. Nattermann C, Galbenu-Grunwald R, Nier H, et al. Endoskopischer Ultracshall im TN-Staging des Magenkarzinoms. Ein Vergleich mit der Computertomographie und der konventionellen Sonographie. Z Gesamte Inn Med 48:60–64, 1993.
18. Caletti GC, Ferrari A, Brocchi E, et al. Accuracy of endoscopic ultrasonography in the diagnosis and staging of gastric cancer and lymphoma. Surgery 113:14–27, 1993.
19. Rösch T, Lorenz R, Zenker K, et al. Local staging and assessmant of resectability in carcinoma of esophagus, stomach and duodenum by endoscopic ultrasonography. Gastrointest Endosc 38: 460–467, 1992.
20. Yoshimi M, Kusuyama A, Tashiro H, et al. EUS approach to the regional lymph nodes in early gastric cancer. Abstracts of the World Congresses of Gastroenterology, Sydney 1990 Abingdon: The Medicine Group (UK) 1990; abstr. no. FP 325.(abstract)
21. Cerizzi A, Botti F, Carrara A, et al. EUS in preoperative staging of gastric cancer. Endoscopy 24 (suppl I): 380(abstract), 1992.
22. Heintz A, Junginger T. Endosonographisches Staging von Karzinomen in Speiseröhre und Magen. Bildgebung (Imaging) 58:4–8, 1991.
23. Yasuda K, Mukai H, Cho E, et al. Evaluation of the degree of gastric cancer invasion by endoscopic ultrasonography (EUS) for endoscopic treatment of early gastric cancer. Stomach Intest 221:1167–1176, 1992.
24. Kida M, Yamada Y, Sakaguchi T, et al. The diagnosis of gastric cancer by endoscopic ultrasonography. Stomach Intest 26:61–70, 1991.
25. Kimura K, Yamanaka T. Endoscopic ultrasonography in the assessment of depth of infiltration of gastric cancer. In Takemoto T, Kawai K (eds): Recent Topics of Digestive Endoscopy. Amsterdam: Exerpta Medica, 1982, pp 20–26.
26. De Angelis C, Gindro T, Recchia S, et al. Value and limitations of preoperative endoscopic ultrasonography in predicting stage and resectability of gastric cancer. Gastroenterology 106:A380(abstract), 1994.
27. Natsugoe S, Yoshinaka H, Moringa T, Shimada M, Hokita S, Baba M, Takao S, Fukumoto T, Stein HJ, Aikou ST. Assessment of tumor invasion of the distal esophagus in carcinoma of the cardia using endoscopic ultrasonography. Endoscopy 28:750–755, 1996.
28. Yoshikawa J, Matsumoto J, Saisho A, et al. Depth of gastric cancer invasion determined by endoscopic ultrasonography. Gastrointest Endosc 43:432(abstract), 1996.
29. Rösche T, Dittler HJ, Kunte M, et al. Comparison of a sector-type with a linear-type echoendoscope in the staging of GI cancer. Gastrointest Endosc 40(abstract), 1994.
30. Maruta S, Tsukamata Y, Niwa Y, et al. Endoscopic ultrasonography for assessing the horizontal spread of gastric carcinoma. Am J Gastroenterol 88:555–559, 1993.
31. Fein J, Gerdes H, Karpeh M, et al. Overstaging of ulcerated gastric cancer by endoscopic ultrasonography. Gastrointest Endosc 39:A274(abstract), 1993.
32. Niwa Y, Nakazawa S, Yoshino J, et al. Quantification of gastric ulcer healing by endoscopic ultrasonography. Gastrointest Endosc 36:116–122, 1990.
33. Ziegler K, Sanft C, Zeitz M, et al. Can endosonography differentiate benign and malignant lesions of the stomach? Gastroenterology 96:566(abstract), 1989.
34. Rösch T, Lorenz R, von Wichert A, et al. Endoscopic ultrasonography is not useful in the differential diagnosis of gastric ulcers. Gastrointest Endosc 38:241(abstract), 1992.
35. Motoo Y, Okai T, Ohta H, Satomura Y, Watanabe H, Yamakawa O, Yamaguchi Y. Endoscopic ultrasonography in the diagnosis of extraluminal compression mimicking gastric submucosal tumors. Endoscopy 26:239–242, 1994.
36. Bashir RM, Gupta PK. Endoscopic ultrasonographic diagnosis of a splenic artery aneurysm. Pract Gastroenterol 19:24, 1995.
37. Mendis RE, Gerdes H, Lightdale CJ, Bótet JF. Larger gastric folds: A diagnostic approach using endoscopic ultrasonography. Gastrointest Endosc 40:437–441, 1994.
38. Avunduk C, Navab F, Hampf F, Coughlin B. Prevalence of *Helicobacter pylori* infection in patients with large gastric folds: Evaluation and follow-up with endoscopic ultrasound before and after antimicrobial therapy. Am J Gastroenterol 90:1969–1973, 1995.
39. Songür Y, Okai T, Watanabe H, Motoo Y, Sawabu N. Endosonographic evaluation of giant gastric folds. Gastrointest Endosc 41:468–474, 1995.
40. Ferrari AP, Van Dam J, Carr-Locke DL. Endoscopic needle aspiration of a gastric duplication cyst. Endoscopy 27:270–272, 1995.
41. Faigel DO, Burke A, Ginsberg GG, Stotland BR, Kadish SL, Kochman ML. The role of endoscopic ultrasound in the evaluation and management of foregut duplications. Gastrointest Endosc 45:99–103, 1997.
42. Jacob P, Pujol B, Napoleon B, Keriven-Souquet O, Souquet JC. Accuracy of endoscopic ultrasonography (EUS) in the staging of gastric MALT lymphoma. Endoscopy 28:S38, 1996.
43. Wiersema MJ, Gatzimos K, Nisi R, Wiersema LM. Staging of non-Hodgkins gastric lymphoma with endosonography-guided fine needle aspiration biopsy and flow cytometry. Gastrointest Endosc 44:734–736, 1996.
44. Andriulli A, Recchia S, De Angelis C, et al. Endoscopic ultrasonographic evaluation of patients with biopsy negative gastric linitis plastica. Gastrointest Endosc 36:611–615, 1990.
45. Tio TL, Maas JJ, Colin EM, et al. Endosonography in diagnosing and staging gastric wall abnormalities. Gastrointest Endosc 38:A281–282(abstract), 1992.
46. Isoard B, Berger F, Napoleon B, et al. Accuracy of endosonography (ENS) for the diagnosis of gastric linitis plastica. Gastrointest Endosc 38:A242(abstract), 1992.
47. Palazzo L, Dubois C, Cellier C, et al. Is endoscopic ultrasonography a reliable tool for the diagnosis of gastric linitis? Gastrointest Endosc 39:A285(abstract), 1993.
48. Vilmann P, Hancke S, Henriksen FW, et al. Endoscopic ultrasonography with guided fine needle aspiration biopsy of malignant lesions in the upper gastrointestinal tract. Endoscopy 25: 523–527, 1993.
49. Shimizu S, Tada M, Kawai K. Endoscopic ultrasonography in early gastric cancer. Endoscopy 26:767–768, 1994.
50. Yanai H, Fujimura H, Suzumi M, et al. Delineation of the gastric muscularis propria and assessment of depth of invasion of early gastric cancer using 20-megahertz endoscopic ultrasound probe. Gastrointest Endosc 39:505–512, 1993.
51. Takemoto T, Yanai H, Tada M, et al. Application of ultrasonic probes prior to endoscopic resection of early gastric cancer. Endoscopy 24:329–333, 1992.
52. Takemoto T, Yanai H, Tada M, et al. Application of ultrasonic probes prior to endoscopic resection of early gastric cancer. Endoscopy 24:329–333, 1992.
53. Tio TL, Tytgat GNJ. Evaluation of resectability of gastrointestinal tumors. In Kawai K (ed): Endoscopic Ultrasonography in Gastroenterology. Tokyo: Igaku Shoin, 1988, pp 106–118.
54. Salmon P. Endoscopic treatment of gastrointestinal tumors: When can surgery be avoided? Endoscopy 24:229–231, 1992.

# SECTION

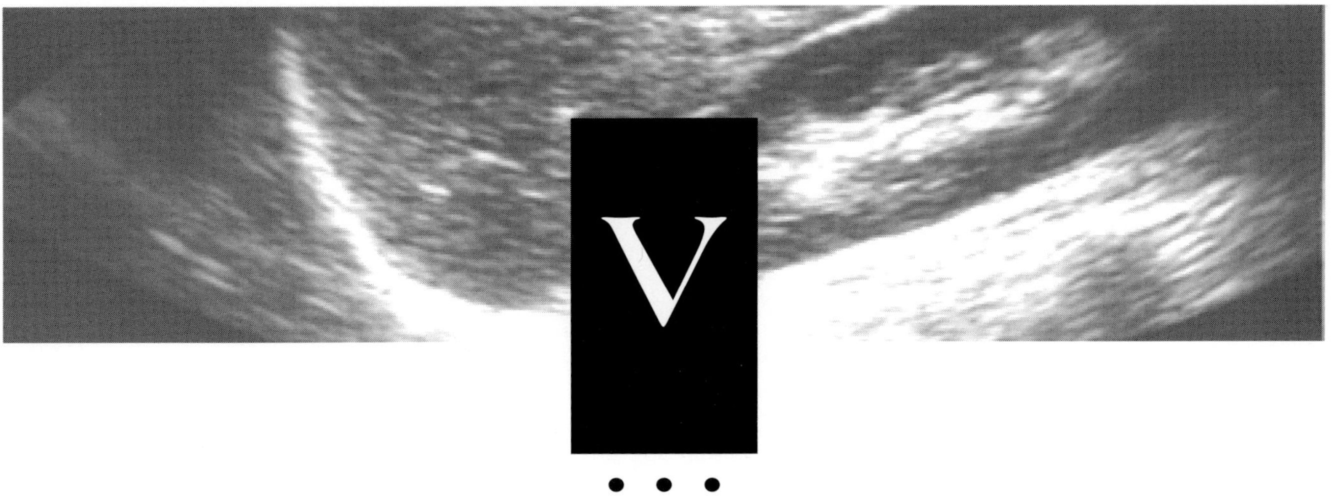


# Portal Hypertension

CHAPTER

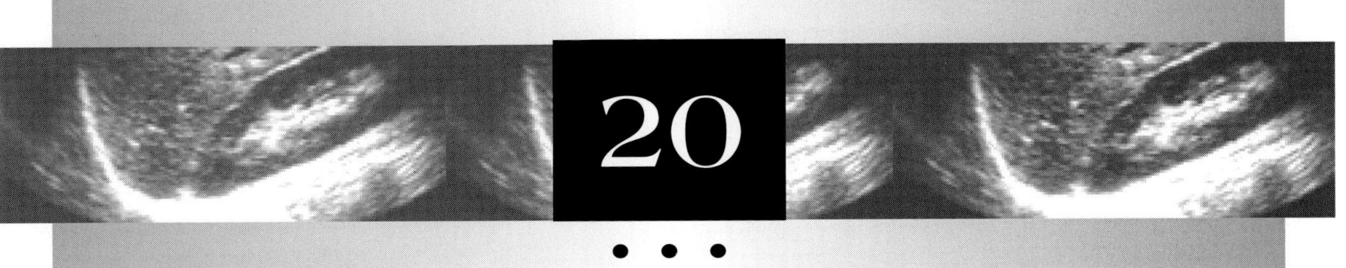


# Endosonographic Evaluation of the Patient with Portal Hypertension

## THE BOLOGNA EXPERIENCE

Giancarlo Caletti
Paolo Bocus
Thomas Togliani
Enrico Roda
Alberto Ferrari
Luigi Barbara

Endosonography of the portal venous system is performed by evaluating the esophagus and stomach. EUS examination of the esophagus and surrounding structures is performed with a water-filled balloon placed over the ultrasonic probe, while examination of the stomach and adjacent structures is performed by instillation of deaerated water (1,2). The diameter and length of the visualized vascular structures of the portal venous system can be measured and recorded. Thus, endoscopic (3) and endosonographic (4) findings may be correlated in order to determine whether EUS provides a substantial contribution to the evaluation of the patient with portal hypertension.

It is useful to visualize the portal venous system in patients with portal hypertension (PH) to evaluate the severity of the disease and to determine the best method of treatment. This may be accomplished in a number of ways. Angiography has been the principal method of evaluation, although less invasive methods have been proposed, including dynamic CT scanning (5,6) and magnetic resonance (7). Conventional transabdominal ultrasonography is also suitable as a screening method for portal hypertension (8,9); measurements of the main portal vessels are reliable and the diagnosis of portal obstruction can be made in a very high percentage of patients (8–13). Unfortunately, small tributaries are seldom visualized and no information is provided about the gastroesophageal collateral veins which anastomose with the caval system (14).

Color-flow Doppler sonography has emerged as a promising tool for flow studies (15,16). Duplex Doppler endosonography has also emerged as an important imaging technique (17,18). In one study, duplex and Doppler endosonography were used to prospectively evaluate 20 volunteers and, subsequently, 11 patients with nondiagnostic transabdominal ultrasonography in whom clinical evidence suggested thrombosis of the splenic and/or portal veins (18). While standard transabdominal ultrasound failed to make a diagnosis in 10 of 11 patients, Duplex endosonography provided the correct diagnosis: the accuracy of ultrasound was 0% and that of EUS was 91% ($p < .001$) (18).

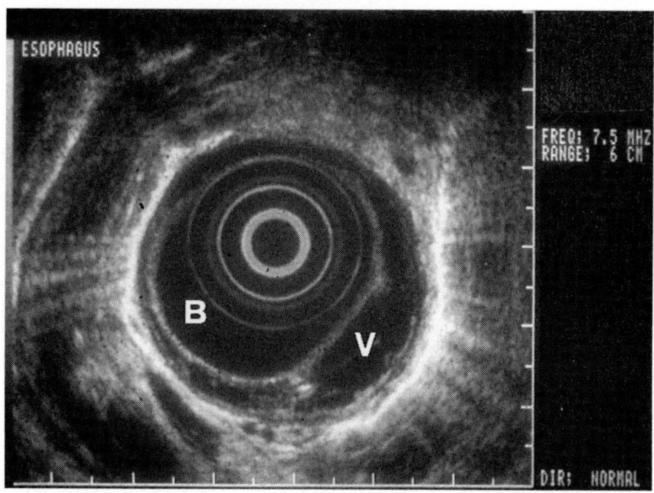


**FIGURE 20–1**

Transverse scan of the esophagus at the junction with the cardia. Large submucosal varices (V) are clearly displayed. B = balloon; V = esophageal varices.

## EUS Findings in Portal Hypertension

In preliminary reports, endosonography was shown to reveal esophageal and gastric varices while also displaying periesophageal collateral veins (1,2,19,20). Endosonography can also demonstrate small dilated vessels within the gastric walls in patients with portal hypertensive gastropathy (21). Other vascular structures of the portal venous system are also visualized by this technique in patients with and without portal hypertension.

Endosonographically, esophageal varices are displayed in transverse section as rounded, echo-free structures just beneath the mucosal and submucosal layers in only 50% of patients (Fig. 20–1). EUS demonstrated varices in 14% of patients with endoscopic grade I esophageal varices, in 78% with grade II, and in 50% with grade III (4).

Periesophageal collateral veins appear in transverse section as rounded, echo-free structures just outside the esophageal wall, and are noted in nearly 80% of patients (Figs. 20–2, 20–3). These external collateral vessels were demonstrated in 57% of patients with endoscopic grade I varices, in 89% with grade II, and in all patients with grade III esophageal varices (4). The azygous vein appears in transverse section as a rounded echo-free structure between the esophageal wall, aorta, and spine (Fig. 20–4). It is displayed in all normal patients and patients with portal hypertension. The proximal margin is established when the vein arches in a forward and slightly lateral direction at the level of the fourth thoracic vertebra to enter the superior vena cava. In control subjects the diameter at the distal and proximal margins ranged from 4 to 9 mm (mean 5.9 ± 1.2) and from 5 to 9 mm (mean 6.8 ± 1.1), respectively. In patients with portal hypertension, the diameter at the distal and proximal margins ranged from 5 to 13 mm (mean 7.9 ± 1.8) and from 5 to 14 mm (mean 9.2 ± 2.1), respectively. The mean observed length of the azygos vein ranged from 5 to 6 cm in normal subjects as well as in patients with portal hypertension.

With the ultrasound probe positioned just below the gastroesophageal junction and the stomach filled with water, EUS can display gastric varices as rounded

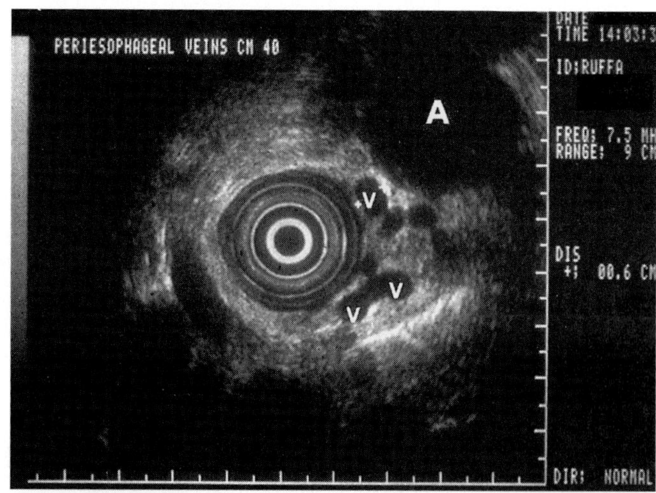


**FIGURE 20–2**

Transverse scan of the esophagus at the junction with the cardia. Dilated periesophageal veins (V) are visualized outside the wall. A = aorta.

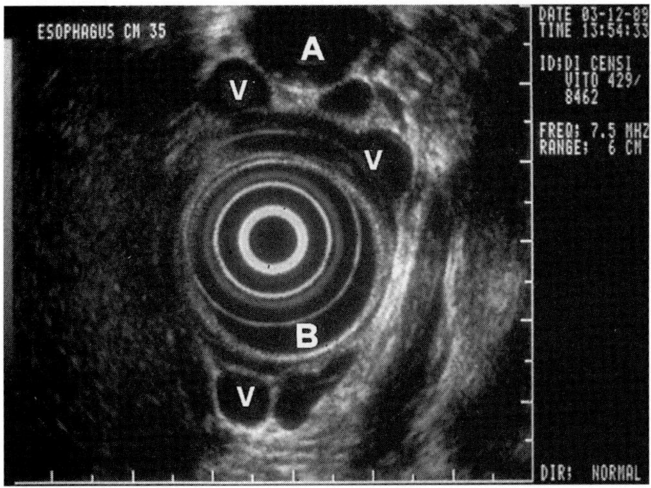


**FIGURE 20–3**

Magnification of a transverse scan of the esophagus at the junction with the cardia. Markedly dilated periesophageal veins (V) are visualized outside the wall. B = balloon; A = aorta.

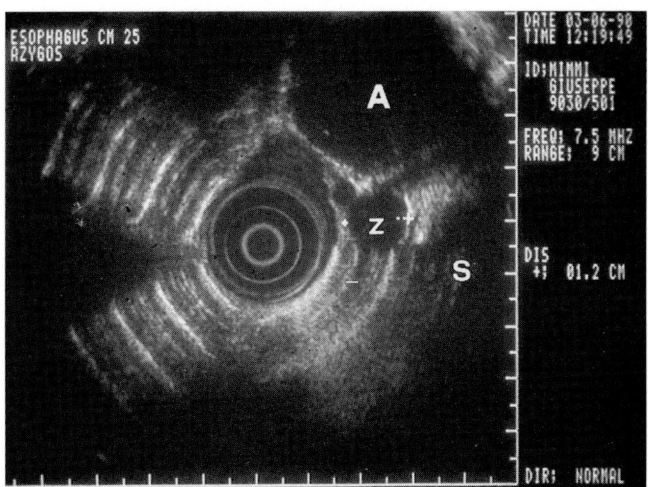


**FIGURE 20–4**

Scan of the esophagus at 25 cm from the incisor teeth in a portal hypertensive patient. The enlarged azygous vein (Z) is visualized among the esophageal wall, the aorta (A), and the spine (S).

echo-free structures beneath the mucosa and submucosa of the fundus (Fig. 20–5). EUS detected gastric varices in 29% of patients with portal hypertension with endoscopic grade I esophageal varices, in 56% of patients with grade II, and in 100% of patients with grade III. The same echo pattern may be found in patients with portal hypertension who have no endoscopic evidence of gastric varices (4).

Endosonographically visualized multiple small, rounded, echo-free structures within the submucosa of the stomach are noted in virtually all portal hypertensive patients with endoscopic findings of portal hypertensive gastropathy (4,22,23) (Figs. 20–6, 20–7). Dilated vessels can be demonstrated as numerous echo-free structures just external to the gastric wall in nearly half of portal hypertensive patients (Fig. 20–8).

A single, rounded, echo-free structure external to the greater curve of the gastric body most likely represents the gastroepiploic vein and is noted in almost half of all normal subjects (Fig. 20–9). The splenic vein is displayed as a longitudinal echo-free channel posterior to the stomach and pancreas. Its complete course from the spleen to the portal confluence (where the splenic vein joins the superior mesenteric vein to form the portal vein) can be seen in nearly all normal and portal hypertensive subjects and is an important anatomic

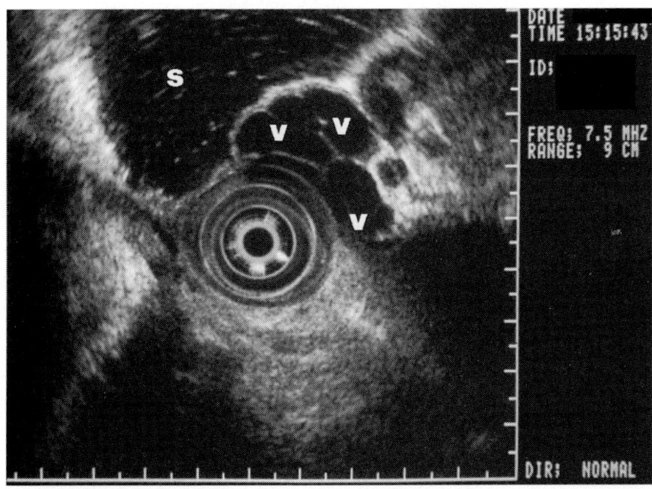


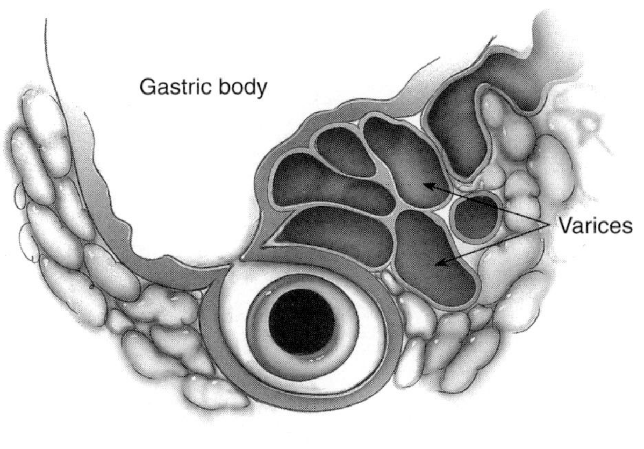


**FIGURE 20–5**

An endosonograph of the gastric fundus using the water-filled stomach technique. Gastric varices (V) are clearly visualized. S = stomach.

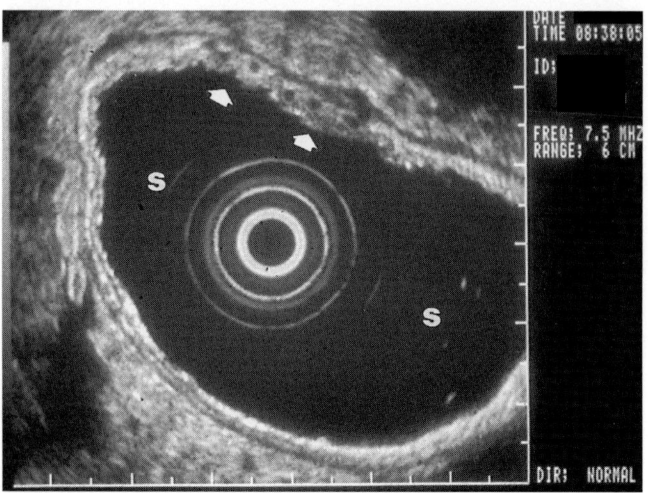


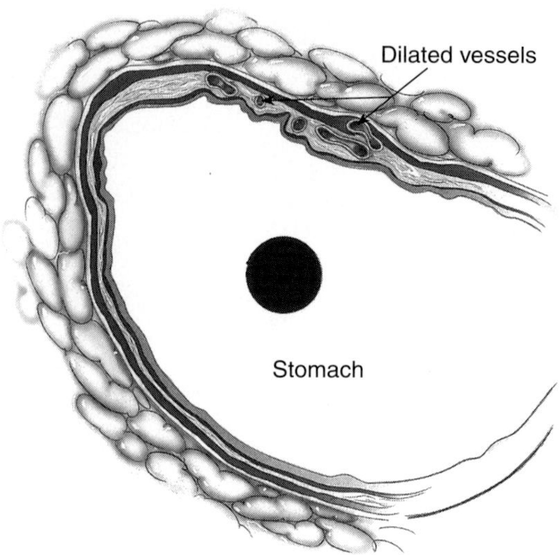


**FIGURE 20–6**

An endosonograph of a water-filled stomach (S). Dilated veins within the gastric wall (arrows) are noted. In this patient, endoscopic findings of portal hypertensive gastropathy were present.

landmark. When the ultrasonic probe is located in the proximal body of the stomach, the mesenteric vein is noted in all normal and portal hypertensive subjects as a round echo-free structure posterior to the gastric wall and pancreas (Fig. 20–10). The confluence of the splenic and superior mesenteric veins to form the portal vein can be noted external to the lesser curvature of the gastric wall in almost every examination. The portal vein can be partially visualized in just one-third of normal and portal hypertensive subjects, and its entire course is virtually never visualized.

The azygous, splenic, mesenteric, and portal veins are displayed by EUS in normal subjects and in patients with portal hypertension. Esophageal and gastric varices, periesophageal and perigastric collateral veins, and submucosal gastric venules are seen only in patients with portal hypertension as these structures are normally very small and undetectable by EUS in normal subjects.

It is thus evident that endosonography can visualize a large part of the portal venous system; however, EUS does not supplant transabdominal ultrasonography in the study of the splenic, mesenteric, and portal veins because the latter technique is less time-consuming and provides a better resolution. In fact, it is not possible to scan the entire course of the main portal vessels by EUS.

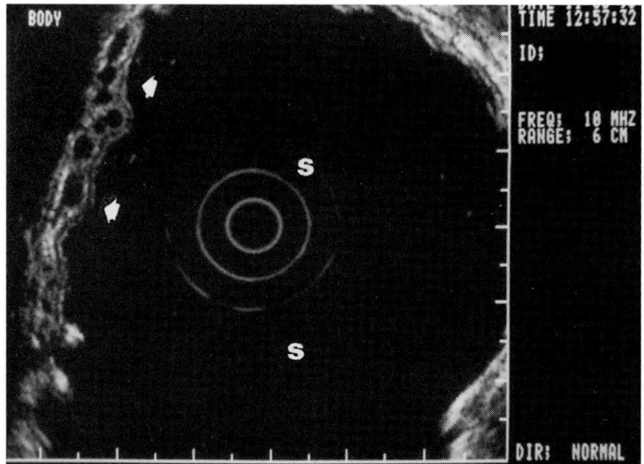


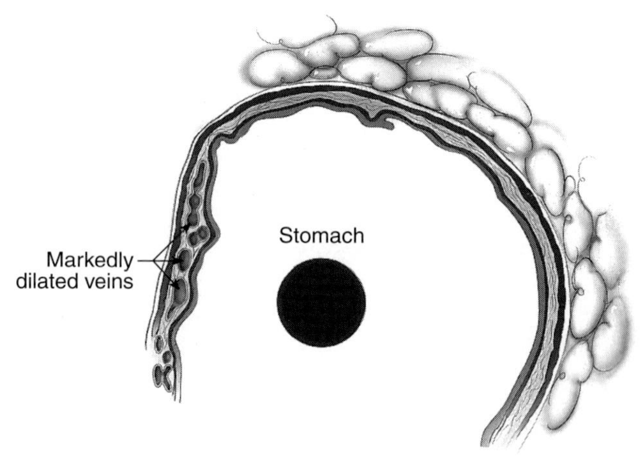


**FIGURE 20–7**

An endosonograph of a water-filled stomach (S). Markedly dilated veins within the gastric wall (arrows) are noted. Endoscopic evaluation of the patient disclosed evidence of portal hypertensive gastropathy.

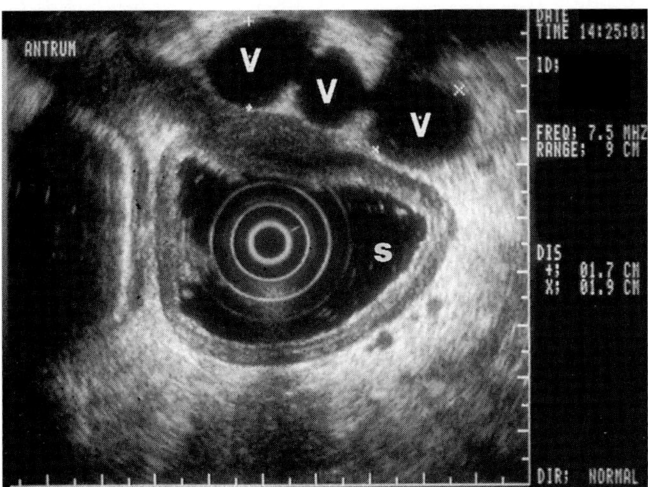


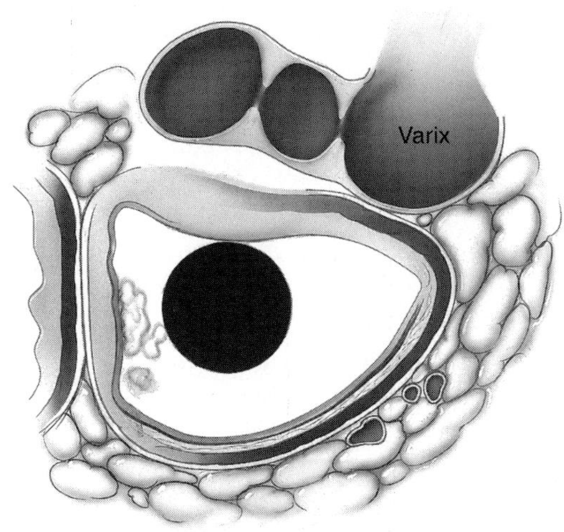


**FIGURE 20–8**

An endosonograph of a water-filled stomach, antrum (S). Markedly dilated veins are seen outside the gastric walls.

Endoscopy remains the most important technique for the assessment of esophageal varices. It is superior to EUS for detection of varices and in grading these vessels according to diameter and length. This may be partially attributable to problems with focusing the ultrasound display and to compression of the varices by the water-filled balloon at the tip of the echoendoscope. Furthermore, EUS does not demonstrate the so-called red color signs that indicate an increased risk of bleeding (3,24). In order to avoid this problem and to improve the visualization of esophageal varices, Urabe et al. (25) proposed avoiding the water-filled balloon technique, but rather filling the esophageal lumen with water and using a balloon, placed 7 cm proximal to the distal tip of the echoendoscope, to prevent reflux of injected water. With this method, the authors reported a success rate of 100% in the EUS visualization of untreated esophageal varices.

The inability of EUS to detect periesophageal veins in some patients may be related to the stage of the patient's disease. It is possible that esophageal varices are more fully developed in the early stages of the disease in the absence of dilated periesophageal veins. It is not surprising that the diameter of the azygous vein is significantly greater in cirrhotic patients because the azygous system is the main conduit from both the intra- and periesophageal collateral veins. The length of the azygous vein displayed by EUS is less than its true

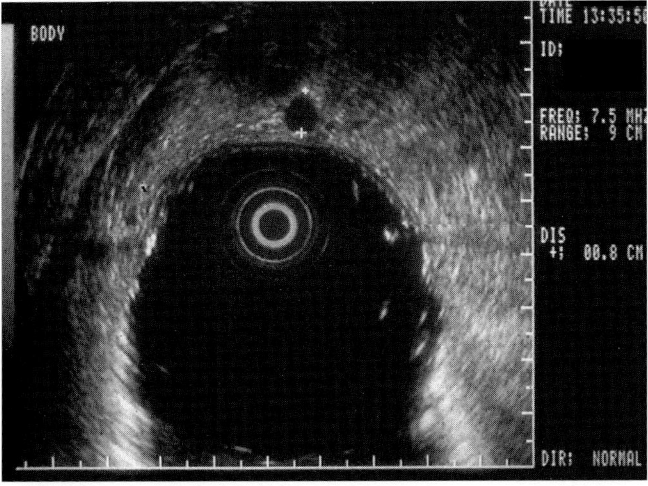


**FIGURE 20–9**

An endosonograph of a water-filled stomach. Outside the greater curve of the gastric wall the gastroepiploic vein is seen.

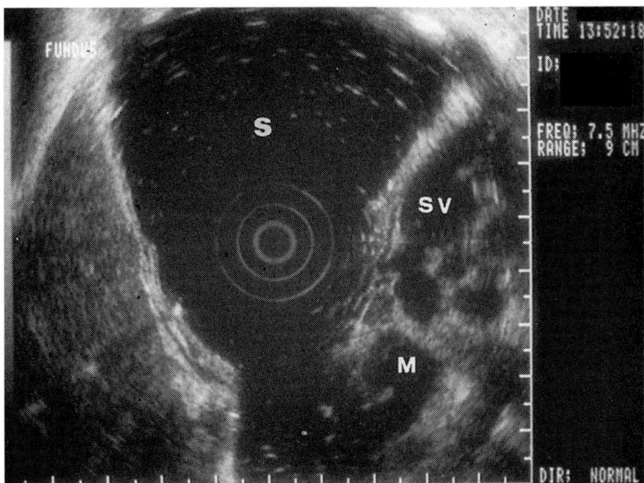


**FIGURE 20–10**

An endosonograph of a water-filled stomach, fundus (S). Dilated mesenteric (M) and splenic veins (SV) are displayed.

anatomic length. This is easily explained by anatomic factors: The azygous is in contact with the thoracic vertebrae for its full length, whereas the esophagus is near these vertebrae only in its upper part and gradually diverts anteriorly. Thus the visualized portion of the vein is only its upper aspect where the esophagus is in contact with the thoracic vertebrae (16).

It is noteworthy that EUS detects fundal varices with greater frequency than endoscopy—a phenomenon that may be related to the relative inability of endoscopy to distinguish varices from normal gastric folds. The diagnosis of fundic varices based solely on endoscopic appearance is therefore often inaccurate and is better made by endoscopic ultrasonography (26). In fact, endosonography may be the imaging method of choice for the evaluation of large gastric folds (see Chapter 17) (27–29). There was a direct correlation between esophageal variceal grade at endoscopy and the detection by EUS of gastric varices. With grade III esophageal varices, EUS always demonstrated the presence of gastric varices, even in those patients with negative endoscopic findings.

EUS can detect small dilated veins within the gastric wall in patients with portal hypertensive gastropathy. As these findings are not present in normal subjects (21), this feature may prove to be useful in the study of this poorly understood condition. EUS can reliably differentiate inflammatory gastritis from congestive gastropathy, thus avoiding the danger associated with obtaining biopsies in the latter condition. Since portal hypertensive gastropathy is a possible cause of bleeding, accurate diagnosis is essential for correct management.

## EUS For Monitoring Variceal Treatment

Ziegler et al. (30) performed EUS 4–5 days after every sclerotherapy session in an effort to evaluate the need for further injection treatment. According to these authors, endoscopy alone is not sufficient to evaluate the status of the varices after sclerotherapy, whereas EUS better demonstrates the thrombosis within the vein. Thus, the EUS method may facilitate the decision to continue or discontinue treatment, thereby diminishing the risk of rebleeding due to incomplete sclerosis of varices. However, this indication has not been firmly established and is under debate. The debate concerns two important points: one related to sclerotherapy, the other to EUS. Concerning sclerotherapy, a single procedure is usually inadequate for long-term prevention of recurrent bleeding. In the majority of reported series, a sequence of injections was utilized to achieve variceal obliteration. It is well known that in the first few weeks of endoscopic sclerotherapy, the risk of rebleeding remains high because of the lack or incomplete formation of the thrombus within the varices. For this reason, the majority of experts agree that all visible varices must be injected at each session.

The suggested interval between subsequent sclerotherapy sessions is one week. Sessions must be continued until eradication—complete disappearance of varices—is achieved. Sclerotherapy can be deferred only in the case of large esophageal ulcers and necrosis (31). Until several years ago, some authors, arguing that it was desirable to know when to conclude the series of procedures, suggested that it would be advantageous to determine when and where blood flow persists after variceal sclerosis. Such findings would permit modification of the injection pattern, allowing fewer injections without loss of effect but with, perhaps, less esophageal ulceration. For this reason, Kovacs and Jensen (32) proposed a technique able to clarify the persistence of blood flow within the varix. However, the body of experience with sclerotherapy has demonstrated that such problems are unfounded. Subsequent injections of visible vessels are not followed by serious complications, but lead to eradication in the great majority of cases.

Endosonographic evaluation of esophageal varices in an emergency is not ethical as treatment is delayed. In addition, images are not optimal as blood limits transmission of ultrasound. A few days after sclerotherapy, the esophageal wall is involved with an intense inflammatory response which lasts for several weeks. This inflammation strongly modifies the endosonographic pattern of the esophageal wall, and a correct interpretation of the images is difficult if not eccentric. Moreover, during this period, any balloon compression of the wall (and hence EUS examination) can be dangerous in the absence of visible ulcers. Despite the report by Ziegler et al. (30), it must be remembered that when esophageal varices are displayed with sector scanning echoendoscopes, no data about flow are provided. Information about the variceal flow can be obtained only with Doppler equipment and, at present, no evidence suggests that such a technique would provide useful data for sclerotherapy. Thus the routine use of EUS in monitoring the effects of variceal sclerotherapy is not recommended.

Endoscopic variceal ligation, based on the elastic banding technique initially used for treating hemorrhoids, has emerged as the alternative method for treating esophageal varices. Some investigators have proposed that endoscopic variceal ligation can be used in combination with endoscopic injection sclerotherapy. Nagamine et al. (33) used endoscopic ultrasound to evaluate the effects of endoscopic variceal ligation alone and in combination with endoscopic injection sclerotherapy. In their study, they used 15-MHz and 20-MHz ultrasound probes, passed via the accessory channel of the endoscope, to evaluate 20 patients (12 male, 8 female) with portal hypertension and esophageal varices. Although the study was limited by a short-term follow-up period, endoscopic ultrasonography was shown to be an objective and accurate adjunct to endoscopy, visualizing esophageal varices and their surrounding vessels both before and after therapy. Additionally, EUS was judged superior to endoscopy alone in determining the complete eradication of varices and hence the need for additional therapy (33).

Burtin et al. (34) confirmed our preliminary experience (19–21), showing that EUS is of limited value in the diagnosis of cirrhosis because it adds little to the information obtainable by upper gastrointestinal endoscopy. Only the visualization of perforating veins below the gastroesophageal junction was found to be clinically useful, having predictive value for the effectiveness of endoscopic sclerotherapy. This finding may also help in selecting patients for appropriate therapy (34).

## Other Indications of EUS in Portal Hypertension

In a retrospective study, EUS was used to investigate the change in collateral circulation during non-shunting operations (35). It would seem that EUS can be useful in devascularization procedures in the transabdominal approach. Real-time, intraoperative observation of the vascular structures should be helpful in assessing the adequacy of devascularization. Further prospective and comparative studies with other imaging techniques will be necessary to assess the results of these studies.

Although bleeding from gastroesophageal varices occurs commonly in patients with portal hypertension, bleeding from varices located elsewhere in the gastrointestinal tract is uncommon. Cutler et al. reported on an 81-year-old man who, having undergone surgery (including a Billroth II anastomosis) for peptic ulcer disease, presented with melena (36). The patient was found to be bleeding from endoscopically detected large serpiginous varices within the efferent limb of the Billroth II anastomosis. Endoscopic ultrasonography confirmed the presence of efferent limb varices and demonstrated small gastric varices which had not been visualized previously (35).

Endoscopic ultrasonography has also been used to detect varices in the rectum of patients with portal hypertension. Dhiman et al., who used the sector scanning echoendoscope to evaluate the rectum in 20 patients with portal hypertension, found that EUS was superior to endoscopy in detecting the presence (85% vs. 45%, $p < .01$) and number ($p < .01$) of rectal varices (37). Thus, regional vascular anatomic alterations resulting from portal hypertension not previously suspected may be detected using EUS.

Two interesting papers have been published on the use of miniature ultrasonic probes with high frequencies in the evaluation of varices. Liu et al. (38), using a 20-MHz transnasal probe, detected esophageal varices and correctly measured their size in 79% of patients, versus 94% by endoscopy. In their conclusions they suggest that this technique be used as a supplement to endoscopy, although endoluminal ultrasonography cannot enable determination of certain endoscopic criteria useful for the prediction of variceal bleeding. Kishimoto et al. (39) proposed that ultrasonic miniprobes be used to monitor the effects of endoscopic variceal ligation. They succeeded in obtaining clear ultrasonographic images without compression of the varices; their observations were similar to those reported by Liu et al. (8).

## Conclusions

It is evident that many of the reports published on this subject fail to demonstrate a useful clinical role for EUS in portal hypertension. In detail, EUS is

- not useful in the diagnosis and assessment of esophageal varices.
- possibly useful in the assessment of gastric varices.
- possibly useful in the diagnosis of portal hypertensive gastropathy.
- useful in assessing the number, size, and length of periesophageal and perforating veins. (However, no precise clinical impact is attributable to these findings.)

Concerning this last point, it must be emphasized that the presence of periesophageal and perforating veins is extremely variable from patient to patient and even in the same patient. There can be just a few or several veins present and they may be small or large. These veins can follow the external esophageal wall for few centimeters or for longer tracts. All these variables greatly influence the pressure and the flow within periesophageal and perforating veins and, consequently, within the esophageal varices. Thus, a clinically useful correlation between esophageal varices and periesophageal and perforating veins will be possible only when these structures can be accurately measured, possibly with a mathematical model.

In practice, those who perform variceal sclerotherapy or band ligation have no need for EUS before, during, or after these procedures as it does not influence the number and the timing of the sessions. In fact, sclerotherapy and ligation are widely used because they are simple to perform, easy to learn, and inexpensive. Therefore an accessory technique such as EUS—which is complex, difficult to master, and expensive—is considered nonessential.

Conceivably, it may scientifically demonstrated that the presence of periesophageal and perforating veins is correlated with higher failure rates of sclerotherapy or band ligation. We are, however, skeptical that physicians will ask for EUS before treating all their patients endoscopically. Moreover, we do not think that positive EUS findings would modify their therapeutic choice.

Finally, color Doppler endosonography has very limited clinical value as it allows the visualization of the intra-abdominal vasculature and can be considered only when transabdominal ultrasound is nondiagnostic in patients with suspected thrombosis of the splenic vein, portal vein, or porto-systemic shunt (18).

EUS in portal hypertension can therefore be considered a fascinating technique still looking for a practical application in this field (40). However, anatomic, physiologic, and pathophysiologic studies of the portal system are now possible with a safe, easy, repeatable, and well-accepted technique. Surely, in the long run, we will appreciate the contribution of EUS to the medical knowledge in this field.

In the diagnosis and treatment of patients with portal hypertension, it is vital to know, as precisely as possible, the time when a varix is prompted to bleed. Additional data are needed—pressure and blood flow within the varix, varix size and wall thickness, structure and tension of the varix wall—because the interaction among all these factors may best determine the time for variceal rupture (41).

## References


1. Caletti GC, Bolondi L, Zani L, Labo G. Technique of endoscopic ultrasonography investigation: Esophagus, stomach and duodenum. Scand J Gastroenterol 21(suppl 123):1–5, 1986.
2. Caletti GC, Bolondi L, Barbara L. Instrumentation and scanning techniques. In Kawai K (ed): Endoscopic ultrasonography in gastroenterology. Tokyo: Igaku-Shoin, 1988, pp. 1–17.
3. Beppu K, Inokuchi K, Koyanagi N, Nakayama S, Sakata H, Kitano S, Kobayashi M. Prediction of variceal hemorrhage by esophageal endoscopy. Gastrointest Endosc 27:213–218, 1981.
4. Caletti GC, Brocchi E, Zani L, Barbara L. The important role of EUS in the assessment of patient with portal hypertension. Gastrointest Endoscopy 34:154–155, 1988.
5. Waller RM III, Mc Cain AH, Oliver TW Jr, Sones PJ Jr, Bernardino ME. Computed tomography and sonography of hepatic cirrhosis and portal hypertension. Radiographics 4:677–715, 1984.
6. Clark KE, Foley WD, Lawson TL, Bertand LL, Maddison FE. CT evaluation of esophageal and upper abdominal varices. J Comput Assist Tomogr 4:510–515, 1980.
7. Torres WE, Gaylor GM, Whitmire L, Chuang VP, Bernardino ME. The correlation between MR and angiography in portal hypertension. AJR 148:1109–1113, 1987.
8. Bolondi L, Gandolfi L, Arienti V, Caletti GC, Corcioni E, Gasbarrini G, Labo G. Ultrasonography in the diagnosis of portal hypertension, diminished response of portal vessels to respiration. Radiology 1:167–172, 1982.
9. Bolondi L, Mazziotti A, Arienti V, Casanova P, Gasbarrini G, Cavallari A, Bellusci R, Gozzetti G, Possati L, Labo G. Ultrasonographic study of portal venous system in portal hypertension and after portosystemic shunt operation. Surgery 95:261–269, 1984.
10. Weinreb J, Kumari S, Phillips G, Pochaczebsky R. Portal vein measurements by real time sonography. AJR 139:497–499, 1982.
11. Zoli M, Dondi C, Marchesini G, Cordiani MR, Melli A, Pisi E. Splanchnic vein measurements in patients with liver cirrhosis. J US Med 4:641–646, 1985.
12. Pristauts H, Schrieber F, Petritsch W, Eber B, Sommergutter M, Stauber R. Comparative sonographic examination of the portal venous system before and after sclerotherapy. Wien Med Wochenschr 136:540–543, 1986.
13. Caletti GC, Brocchi E, Zani L, Bolondi L, Baraldini M, Rollo V, Barbara L. Sonographic evaluation of the portal venous system after elective endoscopic sclerotherapy of esophageal varices. Surg Endosc 1:165–167, 1987.
14. Bolondi L, Caletti GC, Brocchi E, Ferrentino M, Calcamuggi G, Casanova P, Gasbarrini G, Labo G. Ultrasonographic findings in portal hypertension: Correlation with the presence and size of esophageal varices. In Lerski AL, Morley P (eds): Ultrasound 82. Oxford: Pergamon Press, 1983, pp 499–503.
15. Zoli M, Marchesini G, Cordiani MR, Pisi P, Brunori A, Trono A, Pisi E. Echo-Doppler measurements of splanchnic blood flow in control and cirrhotic subject JCU 14:429–435, 1986.
16. Sukigara M, Komazaki T, Ohata M, Matsumoto T, Omoto R. Transesophageal real-time two dimensional Doppler echography—A new method for evaluation of azygos venous flow. Gastrointest Endosc 34:125–128, 1988.
17. Iwase H, Suga S, Morise K, Kuroiwa A, Yamaguchi T, Horiuchi Y. Color Doppler endoscopic ultrasonography for the evaluation of gastric varices and endoscopic obliteration with cyanoacrylate glue. Gastrointest Endosc 41:150–154, 1995.
18. Wiersema MJ, Chak A, Kopecky KK, Wiersema LM. Duplex Doppler endosonography in the diagnosis of splenic vein, portal vein, and portosystemic shunt thrombosis. Gastrointest Endosc 42:19–26, 1995.
19. Caletti GC, Bolondi L, Arienti V, Brocchi E, Testa S, Ferrentino M, Zani L, Passaniti A, Labò G. Assessment of gastroesophageal collateral veins in portal hypertension by means of endoscopic ultrasonography. Gut 24:A459, 1983.
20. Caletti GC, Bolondi L, Zani L, Brocchi E, Guizzardi G, Labo G. Detection of portal hypertension and esophageal varices by means of endoscopic ultrasonography. Scand J Gastroenterol 21(suppl 123):75–77, 1986.
21. Caletti GC, Brocchi E, Baraldini M, Ferrari A, Gibilaro M, Barbara L. Assessment of portal hypertension by endoscopic ultrasonography. Gastrointest Endosc 36:S21–S27, 1990.
22. McCormack TT, Sims J, Eyre-Brook I, Kennedy H, Goepel J, Johnson AG, Triger DR. Gastric lesions in portal hypertension: Inflammatory gastritis or congestive gastropathy? Gut 26:1226–1232, 1985.
23. Papazian A, Braillon A, Dupas JL, Sevenet F, Capron JP. Portal hypertensive gastric mucosa: An endoscopic study. Gut 27:1199–1203, 1986.
24. Brocchi E, Caletti GC, the NIEC (North Italian Endoscopy Club). Prediction of the first variceal hemorrhage in patients with cirrhosis of the liver and esophageal varices. N Engl J Med 329:983–984, 1988.
25. Urabe T, Yoneshima M, Oiko Y, Inagaki Y, Kanedo S, Unoura M, Kobaiashi K. Evaluation of esophago-gastric varices with endoscopic ultrasonography. Dig Endosc 2:414–423, 1990.
26. Tio TL, Kimmings N, Rauws E, Jansen P, Tytgat G. Endosonography of gastrointestinal varices: Evaluation and follow-up of 76 cases. Gastrointest Endosc 42:145–150, 1995.
27. Mendis RE, Gerdes H, Lightdale CJ. Large gastric folds: A diagnostic approach using endoscopic ultrasonography. Gastrointest Endosc 40:437–441, 1994.
28. Songur Y, Okai T, Watanabe H, Motoo Y, Sawabu N. Endosonographic evaluation of giant gastric folds. Gastrointest Endosc 41:468–474, 1995.
29. Avunduk C, Navab F, Hampf F, Coughlin B. Prevalence of *Helicobacter pylori* infection in patients with large gastric folds: Evaluation and follow-up with endoscopic ultrasound before and after antimicrobial therapy. Am J Gastroenterol 90:1969–1973, 1995.

30. Ziegler K, Gregor M, Zeitz M, Zimmer T, Habermann F, Riecken EO. Evaluation of endosonography in sclerotherapy of esophageal varices. Endoscopy 23:247–250, 1991.
31. Smith PM. Variceal sclerotherapy: Further progress. Gut 28:645–649, 1987.
32. Kovacs TOG, Jensen DM. Endoscopy of upper gastrointestinal bleeding. In Cotton PB, Tytgat GNJ, Williams CB (eds): Annual of Gastrointest Endosc 1988, ed. London: Gower Academic Journals LTD, 1988, pp 37–54.
33. Nagamine N, Ido K, Ueno N, et al. The usefulness of ultrasonic microprobe imaging for endoscopic variceal ligation. Am J Gastroenterol 91:523–529, 1996.
34. Burtin P, Calès P, Oberti F, Joundy N, Person B, Carpentier S, Boyer J. Endoscopic ultrasonograhic signs of portal hypertension in cirrhosis. Gastrointest Endosc 44:257–261, 1996.
35. Nakamura H, Endo M, Shimojuu K, Goseki N, Inoue H. Esophageal varices evaluated by endoscopic ultrasonography: Observation of collateral circulation during nonshunting operations. Surg Endosc 4:69–75, 1990.
36. Cutler CS, Rex DK, Lehman GA. Enteroscopic identification of ectopic small bowel varices. Gastrointest Endosc 41:605–608, 1995.
37. Dhiman RK, Choudhuri G, Saraswat VA, et al. Endoscopic ultrasonographic evaluation of the rectum in cirrhotic portal hypertension. Gastrointest Endosc 39:635–640, 1993.
38. Liu JB, Miller LS, Feld RI, Barbarevech CA, Needleman L, Goldberg BB. Gastric and esophageal varices: 20-MHz transnasal endoluminal US. Radiology 187:363–366, 1993.
39. Kishimoto H, Sakai M, Kajiyama T, Torii A, Kin G, Tsukada H, Okuma M, Ueda S. Miniature ultrasonic probe evaluation of esophageal varices after endoscopic variceal ligation. Gastrointest Endosc 42:256–260, 1995.
40. Caletti GC, Ferrari A, Bocus P, Togliani Th, Scalorbi C, Barbara L. Portal hypertension: Review of data and influence on management. Gastrointest Endosc Clin N Am 5:655–665, 1995.
41. Schiano TD, Adrian AL, Cassidy MJ, McCray W, Liu JB, Baranowski RJ, Bellary S, Black M, Miller LS. Use of high resolution endoluminal sonography to measure the radius and wall thickness of esophageal varices. Gastrointest Endosc 44:425–428, 1996.

CHAPTER

21

# Endosonographic Evaluation of the Patient with Portal Hypertension

## THE CLEVELAND EXPERIENCE

Marc F. Catalano

In patients with portal hypertension diagnostic imaging is essential to evaluate the severity of the sequelae of their disease. Assessment of the portal venous system allows for the appropriate implementation of available treatment options. Gastroesophageal complications arising from portal hypertension include esophageal varices, gastric varices, portal hypertensive gastropathy, and splenic vein thrombosis. Imaging currently used to evaluate these features of portal hypertension include conventional upper endoscopy (1,2), dynamic computerized tomography (3–8), magnetic resonance imaging (9–17), transabdominal ultrasonography alone (18–21) or with duplex Doppler capability (22–30), and angiography (3,10).

A few studies have investigated the role of endoscopic ultrasonography in evaluating patients with portal hypertension and the gastrointestinal manifestation of their disease (31–34). These studies have shown considerable promise in the endosonographic assessment of disease severity, although lack of control subjects has led to significant operator bias in some instances (31,32). The evaluation described below was undertaken to assess the accuracy of endoscopic ultrasonography (EUS) in evaluating the gastrointestinal features of portal hypertension. In addition to the direct evaluation of the patient using EUS, expert and inexperienced endosonographers individually reviewed videotaped examinations to determine the extent of interobserver variation and the importance of experience in endosonographic imaging of portal hypertension.

## Endosonography in Patients with Portal Hypertension: The Studies

Endosonographic evaluation of the portal venous system requires imaging the esophagus, stomach, adjacent organs and tissues, and vascular structures. This was accomplished by placing the echoendoscope within the gastric or esophageal lumen. Images were best obtained using the water-filled balloon method. The 12-MHz transducer was used to obtain detailed images of esophageal and gastric varices while the 7.5-MHz transducer was used to visualize the periesophageal collateral veins. These vascular structures were visualized in transverse section as rounded or elongated echo-free structures within and outside the esophageal wall (Fig. 21–1).

The azygous vein was shown by Caletti et al. (31) to be dilated at its distal and proximal margins in patients with cirrhosis. Endosonographically, it may be seen in transverse section as a round or elongated echo-free structure between the aorta, spine, and wall of the esophagus (Fig. 21–2).

The stomach may also be investigated for evidence of portal hypertension by advancing the echoendoscope beyond the gastroesophageal junction and orienting the image so that the liver is located on the left side of the screen (patient's right) and the spleen on the right (patient's left) (Fig. 21–3). The stomach is filled with deaerated water while the patient is in the left lateral position and in 15° of Trendelenburg to ensure filling of the fundus and cardia. Endosonography demonstrates gastric varices as rounded echo-free structures within the stomach wall, seen predominantly within the cardia and fundus (Fig. 21–4). Also, EUS can demonstrate portal hypertensive gastropathy as multiple, small (2–3 mm), rounded, echo-free structures just beneath the mucosa and submucosa (Fig. 21–5).

Endosonography can also be used to investigate the size and extent of perigastric collateral veins as well as the splenic, mesenteric, and portal veins. The splenic vein, which can be visualized in transverse section as an elongated echo-free structure posterior to the stomach and pancreas, can be traced to its origin at the splenic hilum (Fig. 21–6). The tip of the echoendoscope is initially placed parallel to the spine at the level of the gastric fundus. Slight tip deflection while advancing into the body of the stomach permits complete visualization of the splenic vein. At the level of the splenic confluence, the mesenteric vein can be seen as a round, echo-free structure posterior to the gastric wall (Fig. 21–7). The portal vein can occasionally be seen at the confluence of the splenic and superior mesenteric veins. It is best seen with the echoscope tip within the second portion of the duodenum parallel to the spine and posterior and lateral to the common bile duct.

In the early 1990s, a prospective study designed to evaluate the role of EUS in the assessment of patients with portal hypertension was undertaken at the Cleveland Clinic Foundation. In that study, 40 patients with portal hypertension and 40 patients without portal hyper-

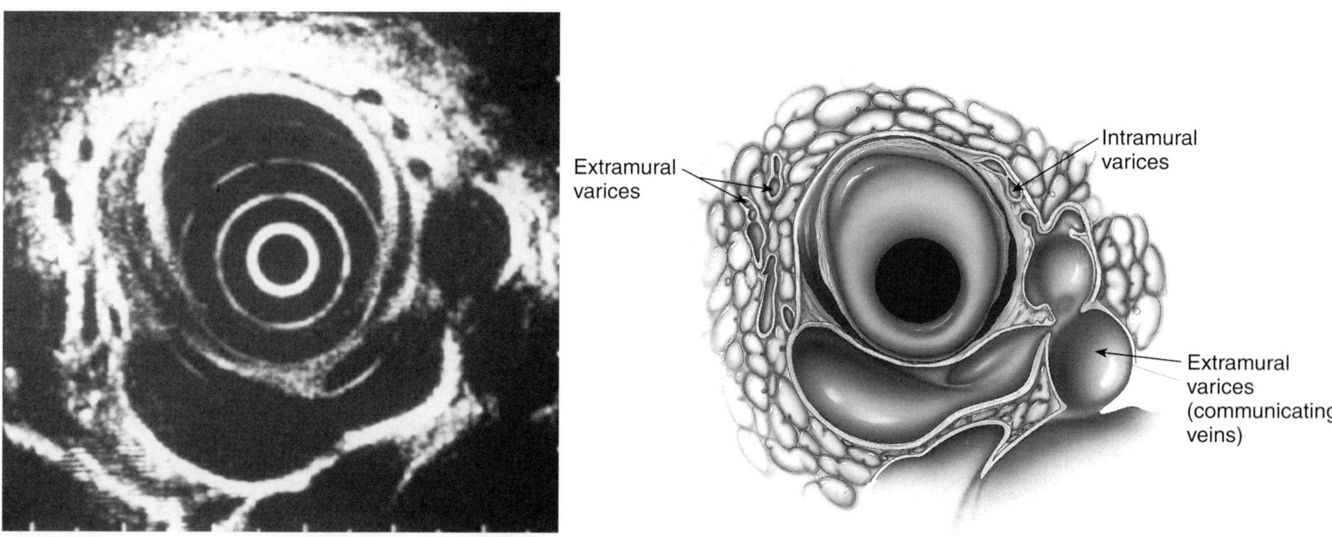


**FIGURE 21–1**

EUS image of the esophagus showing rounded echo-free structures within (esophageal varices) and outside the esophageal wall (periesophageal collateral veins).

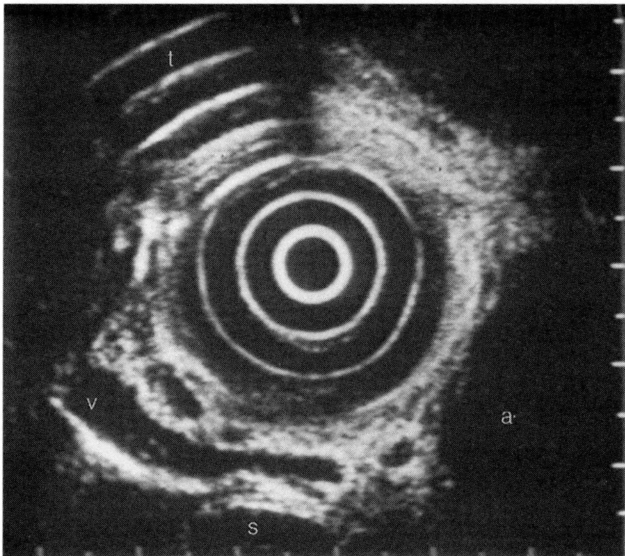


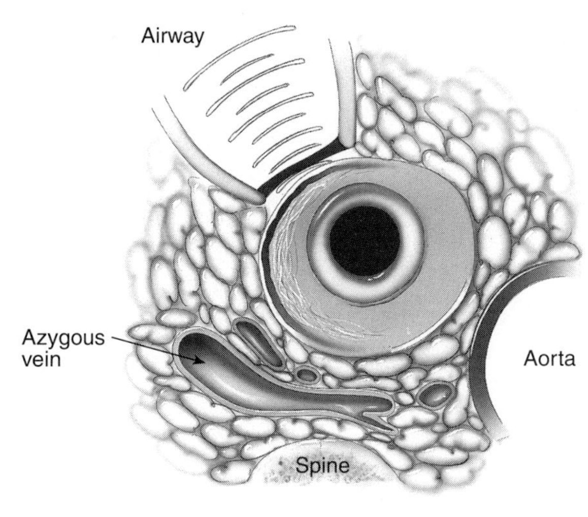


**FIGURE 21-2**

Transverse EUS image of the esophagus showing the azygous vein (v) surrounded by the aorta (a), spine (s), and esophageal wall. Also shown is the trachea (t).

tension underwent upper endoscopy and endoscopic ultrasonography. Indications for ultrasonography in the subjects without portal hypertension included Barrett's esophagus, thickened gastric folds, nonhealing gastric ulcers, and submucosal lesions. All patients underwent thorough endosonographic examination of the esophagus, mediastinum, stomach, and paragastric structures using the Olympus GF-UM3 or GF-UM20 echoendoscopes (Olympus America, Inc.; Melville, New York). All endoscopic and endosonographic examinations were videotaped in their entirety. Taped examinations were randomly arranged and reviewed by five experienced (trained in EUS) and two inexperienced endosonographers without prior knowledge of the patients' identities or diagnoses.

Experienced endosonographers were defined as having performed 50 or more endosonographic examinations; inexperienced endosonographers had a sound understanding of ultrasound principles but had performed fewer than 20 endosonographic examinations.

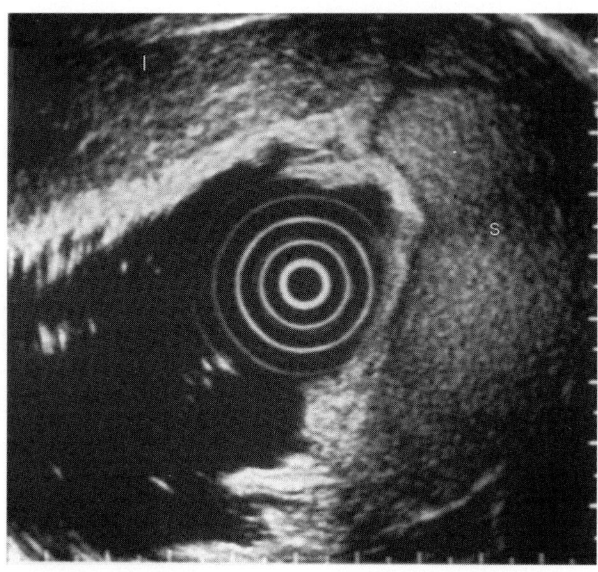


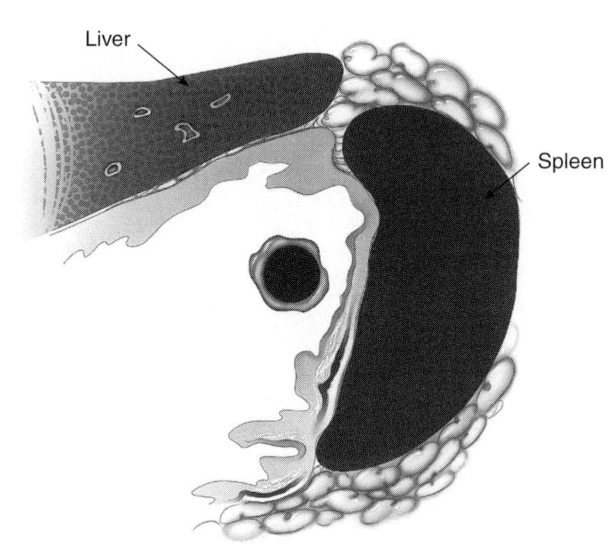


**FIGURE 21-3**

EUS image showing the probe in the proximal gastric fundus with the liver (l) in the left side of the image and spleen (s) on the right.

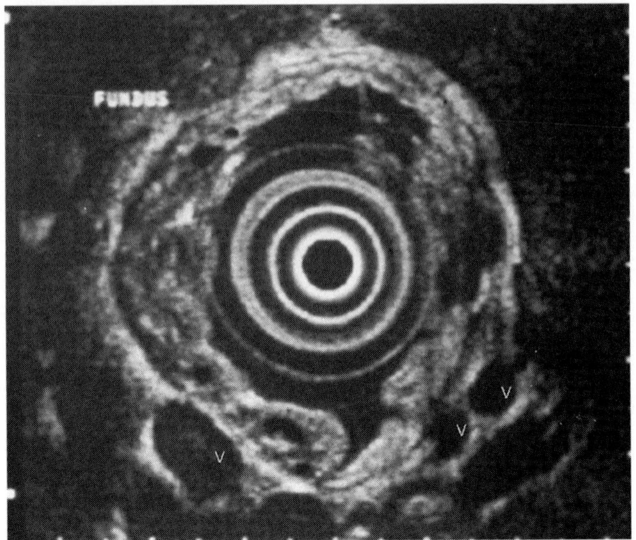


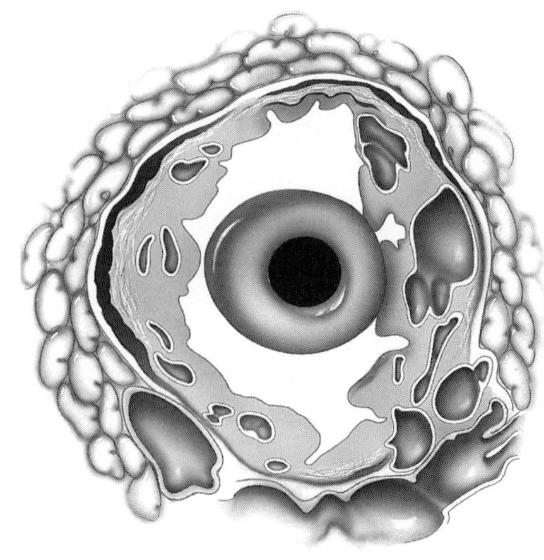

**FIGURE 21-4**

EUS showing the gastric fundus with rounded echo-free structures within the stomach wall consistent with gastric varices (v).

The two groups of endoscopists evaluated features of portal hypertension—including esophageal and gastric varices, paraesophageal and paragastric dilated vessels, portal hypertensive gastropathy, and ascites—both endoscopically and endosonographically.

Kappa statistics were used to evaluate interobserver agreement with respect to each sign of portal hypertension for both experienced and inexperienced ultrasonographers. Kappa ($\kappa$) is a measure of agreement with desirable properties. If there is complete agreement, $\kappa = 1$. If observed agreement is greater than or equal to chance agreement, $\kappa \geq 0$. For most purposes, values greater than .75 may be taken to represent excellent agreement beyond chance, values below .40 poor agreement beyond chance, and values between .40 and .75 fair to good agreement beyond chance.

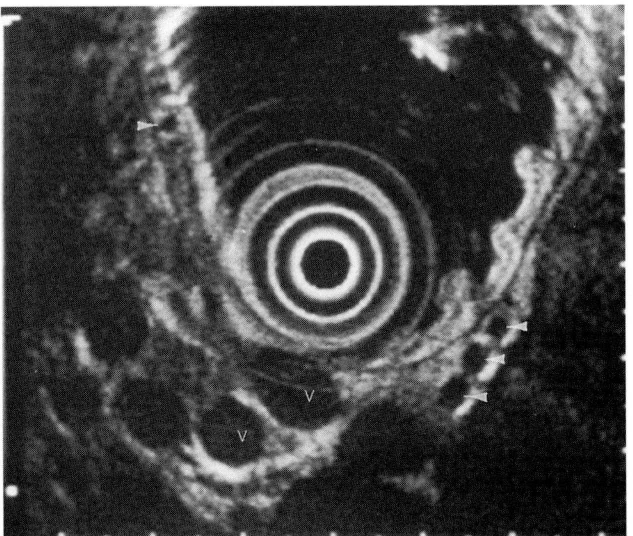


**FIGURE 21-5**

EUS image demonstrating portal hypertensive gastropathy as small, rounded echo-free structures within the wall of the stomach (arrowheads). Also shown are larger echo-free structures within the wall consistent with gastric varices (v).

Results of interobserver agreement for endoscopic interpretation are summarized in Table 21–1, while those for endosonographic evaluation are summarized in Table 21–2. All kappa indices were assessed for significant difference from zero. For all endoscopists (experienced and inexperienced), unless otherwise noted, the overall and individual kappa indices were significantly different from zero, the magnitude indicating fair to good agreement beyond random chance. In addition, the overall kappa indices were tested for each sign between type of endoscopist and compared for differences between experienced and inexperienced endoscopists. For endoscopic signs of portal hypertension, the experienced endosonographers had a significantly higher kappa score than inexperienced endosonographers for the overall endosonographic grade of esophageal varices (EV) ($p$ = .034). Similarly, for the endosonographic signs of portal hypertension, experienced endosonographers had a significantly higher kappa score than inexperienced endosonographers for the overall endosonographic grade of EV ($p$ = .0004).

## Esophagus

The first feature of portal hypertension evaluated was esophageal varices. The endoscopic grading system used for esophageal varices was as follows: Grade I = not flattened by insufflation, small, straight channels; Grade II =

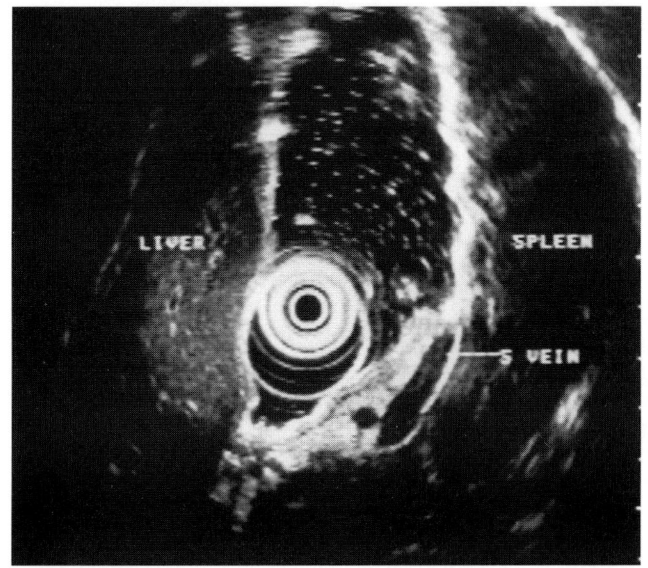


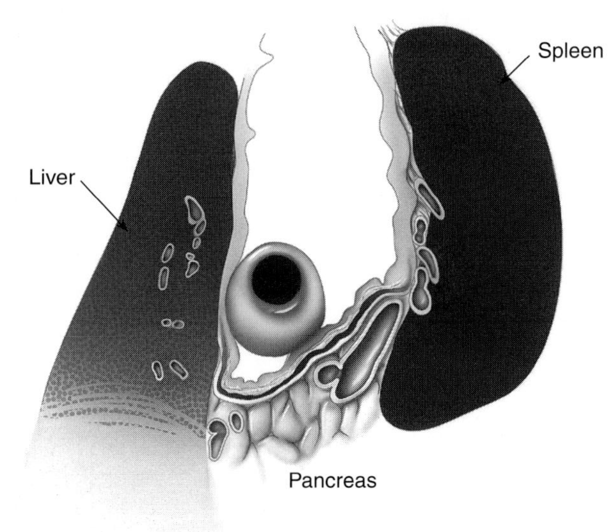


**FIGURE 21–6**

EUS image demonstrating the splenic vein as an elongated echo-free structure emanating from the splenic hilum. The left lobe of the liver can also be seen on the left portion of the image.

not flattened by insufflation, separated by normal mucosa, occupy <33.3% of lumen; Grade III = not flatened, no intervening normal mucosa, occupy >33.3% of esophageal lumen. These endoscopic features were correlated with the following endosonographic grading system: Grade I = flattened by balloon insufflation, small, nonconfluent varices (Fig. 21–8A,B); Grade II = semi-confluent (2–3 adjacent varices), not flattened by balloon insufflation, occupy <50% of wall circumference (Fig. 21–9A,B); Grade III = not flattened by balloon insufflation, confluent (>3 adjacent varices), occupy >50% of wall circumference (Fig. 21–10A,B). These grading systems are summarized in Table 21–3.

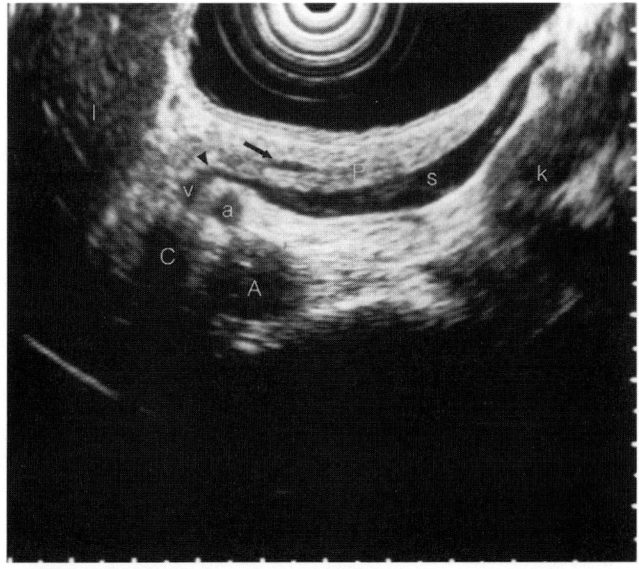


**FIGURE 21–7**

EUS image showing the splenic vein (s), splenic confluence (arrowhead), superior mesenteric vein (v) and artery (a), aorta (A), vena cava (c), left kidney (k), left lobe of the liver (l), and pancreas (p) with pancreatic duct (arrow).

Upper endoscopy revealed 4 patients with no esophageal varices, 9 with Grade I, 16 with Grade II, and 11 with Grade III varices. Esophageal varices were demonstrated endosonographically as rounded or elongated hypoechoic (echo-free) structures within the boundaries of the esophageal adventitia and mucosa. Care was taken not to overinflate the latex balloon to prevent flattening of the vascular structures during the endosonographic examination. EUS demonstrated 67% of endoscopic Grade I, 81% of Grade II, and 100% of Grade III esophageal varices.

Further investigation of the esophagus and surrounding structures revealed dilated collateral vessels by endosonography, appearing as rounded hypoechoic structures of various diameters. These were seen in 56% of endoscopic Grade I, 89% of Grade II, and 100% Grade III esophageal varices. Observer agreement ($\kappa$) was good for all grades of esophageal varices except for Grade I esophageal varices, and fair for the presence of periesophageal collaterals ($\kappa$ = .40).

To investigate the utility of the new EUS grading system of esophageal varices and to correlate it with an existing endoscopic grading system, five experienced and two inexperienced endosonographers evaluated esophageal varices of 40 patients with portal hypertension. Spearman correlation was calculated to determine if

**TABLE 21–1**

Kappa Indices for Endoscopic Signs of Portal Hypertension[1]

| Sign | *Experienced (5)* Overall | *Experienced (5)* Individual | *Inexperienced (2)* Overall | *Inexperienced (2)* Individual | *All (7)* Overall | *All (7)* Individual |
|---|---|---|---|---|---|---|
| Grade of EV | 0.52[2] | | 0.30 | | 0.47 | |
| Not present | | 0.84 | | 0.72 | | 0.81 |
| Small | | 0.53 | | 0.10 (NS) | | 0.44 |
| Medium | | 0.44 | | 0.29 (NS) | | 0.37 |
| Large | | 0.47 | | 0.29 (NS) | | 0.47 |
| Extent of EV | 0.38 | | 0.36 | | 0.38 | |
| None | | 0.77 | | 0.72 | | 0.77 |
| 1/3 | | 0.34 | | 0.21 (NS) | | 0.31 |
| 2/3 | | 0.25 | | 0.33 | | 0.26 |
| 3/3 | | 0.14 | | 0.26 (NS) | | 0.24 |
| Red color signs | 0.46 | | 0.62 | | 0.53 | |
| Size of GV | 0.38 | | 0.30 | | 0.33 | |
| Not present | | 0.50 | | 0.49 | | 0.43 |
| Small | | 0.19 | | 0.13 (NS) | | 0.18 |
| Medium | | 0.44 | | 0.33 | | 0.37 |
| Large | | 0.15 | | −0.05 (NS) | | 0.12 |
| PHG | 0.41 | | 0.67 | | 0.46 | |
| MP (Grade III) | 0.45 | | 0.77 | | 0.53 | |
| PHG, Grades IV–V | 0.52 | | 0.38 | | 0.55 | |

[1]Unless otherwise noted, all kappa indices were significantly different from 0 ($p < .05$).
[2]Experienced ultrasonographers had a significantly higher kappa score than inexperienced ultrasonographers ($p = .0342$).

the endoscopic and endosonographic grade of esophageal varices correlated among all levels of endoscopists. These correlations are summarized in Table 21–4. In all cases there was a strong positive correlation between the two grading systems, which indicated that when the endoscopic grade of esophageal varices is high, the endosonographic grade is also high.

## Gastric Varices

Endosonography was also used to compare the diagnostic accuracy of the presence of gastric varices (GV) with standard endoscopy. Videotaped recordings of endoscopic examinations were reviewed in a random sequence by five experienced and two inexperienced endoscopists. Endoscopically, gastric varices were viewed as straight, nodular, or lobulated lesions in the submucosa in the area of the cardia and fundus, although these were occasionally difficult to distinguish from prominent gastric folds (Fig. 21–11). Alternatively, gastric varices were viewed by EUS as rounded echo-free structures just beneath the mucosal and submucosal layers (Fig. 21–12A,B). Table 21–5 shows the frequency of gastric varices diagnosed by EGD and EUS in the portal hypertension and control subjects both by expert and inexperienced endosonographers. EUS was found to be superior to EGD in demonstrating gastric submucosal vessels, revealing these vascular structures in the majority of the patients with portal hypertension. There was no significant difference in the detection of

**TABLE 21–2**

Kappa Indices for Endosonographic Signs of Portal Hypertension[1]

| Sign | *Experienced (5)* Overall | *Experienced (5)* Individual | *Inexperienced (2)* Overall | *Inexperienced (2)* Individual | *All (7)* Overall | *All (7)* Individual |
|---|---|---|---|---|---|---|
| Grade of EV | 0.42[2] | | 0.07 (NS) | | 0.32 | |
| Not present | | 0.49 | | 0.05 (NS) | | 0.41 |
| Small | | 0.29 | | 0.10 (NS) | | 0.23 |
| Medium | | 0.41 | | 0.06 (NS) | | 0.26 |
| Large | | 0.51 | | 0.42 | | 0.44 |
| PEV | 0.30 | | 0.27 (NS) | | 0.28 | |
| GV | 0.51 | | 0.27 (NS) | | 0.40 | |
| PGV | 0.38 | | 0.06 (NS) | | 0.29 | |
| PHG | 0.39 | | 0.26 (NS) | | 0.32 | |
| Ascites | 0.71 | | — | | — | |

[1]Unless otherwise noted, all kappa indices were significantly different from 0 ($p < .05$).
[2]Experienced endosonographers had a significantly higher kappa score than inexperienced endosonographers ($p = .0004$).

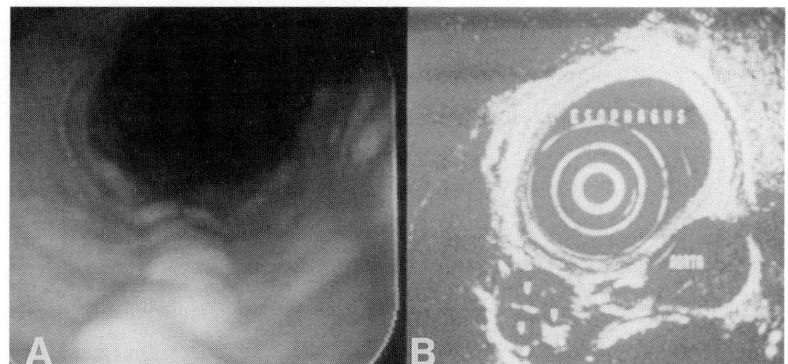

**FIGURE 21-8**

(**A**) Endoscopic image of the esophagus showing Grade I esophageal varices. (**B**) EUS image of the esophagus demonstrating Grade I esophageal varices. (*See color insert for color plate.*)

gastric varices by EUS when viewed by the inexperienced and accomplished endoscopists. The false-positive rate of gastric varices by EUS was higher in the inexperienced (12.5%) than in the experienced (9.0%) group, but was not statistically significant.

To investigate whether the advancing grade of esophageal varices (Grades I–III) was predictive of the presence of gastric varices, 40 portal hypertension patients were evaluated both by EGD and EUS (Table 21–6). EUS revealed gastric varices in 0 of 4 patients without demonstrable esophageal varices, 3 of 9 with endoscopic Grade I esophageal varices, 12 of 16 with Grade II, and 11 of 11 with endoscopic Grade III varices. EGD revealed gastric varices in 0, 1, 6, and 5, respectively, demonstrating the superiority of EUS in diagnosing gastric varices.

## Portal Hypertensive Gastropathy

Portal hypertensive gastropathy (PHG) is the term used to describe the sometimes altered endoscopic appearance of the gastric mucosa in patients with portal hypertension. PHG ranges from Grade I (punctate erythema) to Grade V (diffuse subepithelial hemorrhages). Endoscopic ultrasonography demonstrated PHG as small (2–3 mm), round, echo-free structures beneath the mucosal and submucosal layers (Fig. 21–13A,B). Of the 40 patients with portal hypertension, 30 (75%) were shown to have PHG by endoscopy. When these patients were examined by endosonography, only 12 of 40 patients (30%) were shown to have small, round echo-free structures consistent with PHG. Therefore, the diagnosis by EUS is difficult and much lower in sensitivity than is observed by endoscopy. In addition, interobserver variation with respect to the endosonographic diagnosis of PHG was poor, with a kappa score of .39.

## Other Retroperitoneal Structures

Perigastric dilated veins (PGV) were visualized in 22 of 40 patients (55%), although with poor interobserver agreement ($\kappa$ = .38). The splenic vein was well defined in all patients, and could be followed from its origin (splenic hilum) to the portal confluence in the majority of patients (see Fig. 21–6). The superior mesenteric vein could be seen in 75% of the patients studied (see Fig. 21–7) while the portal vein was visualized in approximately one-third of the patients (35%).

## Ascites

To further investigate the complications of portal hypertension, endosonography was used to evaluate the presence or absence of ascites. Five experienced endoso-

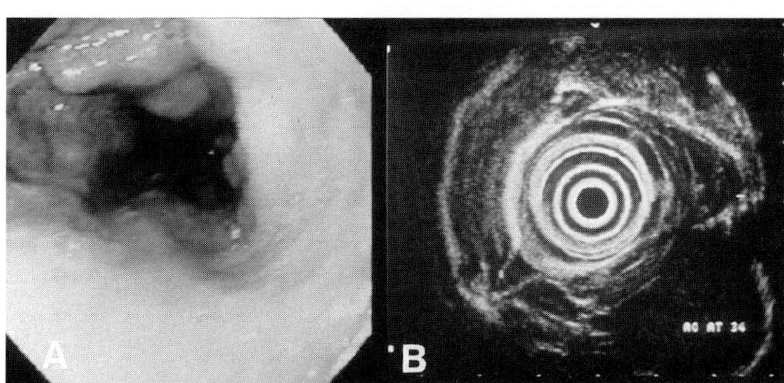

**FIGURE 21-9**

(**A**) Endoscopic image of the esophagus showing Grade II esophageal varices. (**B**) EUS image of the esophagus demonstrating Grade II esophageal varices. (*See color insert for color plate.*)

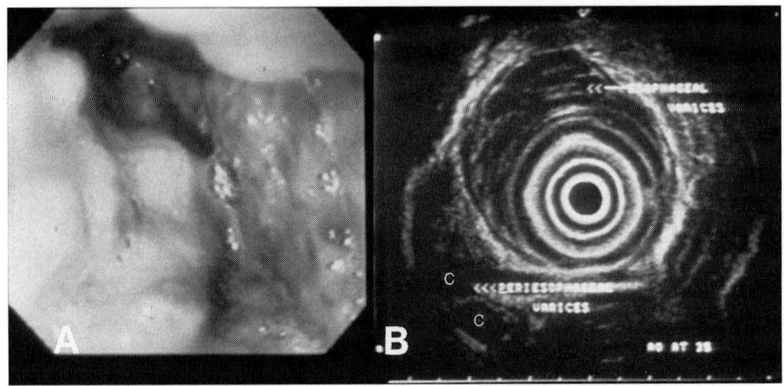


**FIGURE 21–10**

(**A**) Endoscopic image of the esophagus showing Grade III esophageal varices. (**B**) EUS image of the esophagus demonstrating Grade III esophageal varices. Also shown are periesophageal collateral veins (c). (*See color insert for color plate.*)

nographers assessed the presence or absence of ascites as a fluid-filled, echo-free cavity outside the gastric or duodenal wall (Fig. 21–14). Patients were examined in the prone position with 10–15° of Trendelenburg to ensure accumulation of ascitic fluid anteriorly and away from the pelvic floor. Kappa statistics were used to determine observer agreement. Ascites was demonstrated by EUS in 16 of 40 cirrhotics (40%) among the five endosonographers (as agreed by at least three endosonographers). The kappa score was very good ($\kappa$ = .71) for the diagnosis of ascites by EUS. Physical examination prior to EUS indicated the presence of ascites in just four patients. Computed tomography (CT) and abdominal ultrasound (US) within 72 hours of EUS was available in 21 patients (CT 8, US 13). Of the 16 patients with ascites demonstrated by EUS, CT scan was available in 6 and abdominal ultrasound in 8 patients. Using EUS as the "gold standard," the diagnostic accuracy of CT scan was positive in 5 of 8 patients (62%) and that of abdominal ultrasound was positive in 5 of 6 patients (83%).

**TABLE 21–3**

Endoscopic and Endosonographic Grading Systems for Esophageal Varices

| Grade | Endoscopic | EUS |
|---|---|---|
| I (small) | Flattened by insufflation | Flattened by balloon insufflation |
| | Small | Small |
| | Straight | Nonconfluent |
| II (medium) | Not flattened by insufflation | Not flattened by balloon insufflation |
| | Separated by normal mucosa | Semiconfluent (2–3) |
| | Occupy <33.3% of esophageal lumen | Occupy <50% of wall circumference |
| III (large) | Not flattened by insufflation | Not flattened by balloon insufflation |
| | No intervening normal mucosa | Confluent (>3) |
| | Occupy >33.3% of esophageal lumen | Occupy >50% of wall circumference |

## Summary of Findings

Patients with portal hypertension are at increased risk of hemorrhage from esophageal varices, gastric varices, and portal hypertensive gastropathy (35–40). Portal hypertension (PH) affects patients with cirrhosis in the end stage of their disease, but can also occur in the absence of cirrhosis, particularly in patients with Budd–Chiari syndrome and obstruction of the inferior vena cava as well as in patients with splenic vein thrombosis, as is seen in some patients with pancreatitis or pancreatic carcinoma. Evaluation of the gastrointestinal sequelae of portal hypertension has relied upon a variety of imaging modalities, including conventional endoscopy (1,2), angiography (3,10), dynamic CT scan (3–8), magnetic resonance imaging (9–17), transabdominal ultrasound (18–21), and duplex Doppler ultrasonography (22–30). More recently, studies utilizing endoscopic ultrasonography have shown considerable promise as an adjunctive modality in the evaluation of patients with portal hypertension (31–34).

Conventional upper endoscopy, which has been the mainstay examination for endoluminal investigation of varices (esophageal and gastric), is also useful for describing the unique feature of the gastric mucosa in patients with portal hypertension and portal hypertensive gastropathy (1,2). Endoscopy has been used to predict disease severity by describing the extent and grade of esophageal varices, assessing the presence of red color signs, assessing the size of gastric varices and their continuity with esophageal varices, and determining the presence and grade of portal hypertensive gastropathy. Although seemingly straightforward, endoscopic diagnosis has been difficult, with poor observer agreement. The study described above demonstrates that endoscopists disagree on the extent and grade of esophageal varices, the presence of gastric varices, the evaluation of red color signs, and early stages of portal hypertensive gastropathy (Grades I–III); however, there is better, but less than unanimous, agreement for the

**TABLE 21-4**

Spearman Correlation of Endoscopic Grade of Esophageal Varices (EV) with Endosonographic Grade of Esophageal Varices (EV)

| | | Endosonographic Grade of EV | | | |
|---|---|---|---|---|---|
| | | **Not present** | **Small** | **Medium** | **Large** |
| ***A. All Endosonographers (7)*** | | | | | |
| | Not present | 19 | 9 | 1 | 0 |
| ***Endoscopic*** | Small | 10 | 28 | 9 | 1 |
| ***Grade of EV*** | Medium | 3 | 18 | 93 | 18 |
| | Large | 0 | 4 | 17 | 50 |
| | | | Spearman Correlation: | .746 ($p$ = .0001) | |
| ***B. Experienced Endosonographers (5)*** | | | | | |
| | Not present | 15 | 6 | 0 | 0 |
| ***Endoscopic*** | Small | 6 | 22 | 5 | 0 |
| ***Grade of EV*** | Medium | 0 | 9 | 76 | 11 |
| | Large | 0 | 1 | 12 | 37 |
| | | | Spearman Correlation: | .824 ($p$ =0.0001) | |
| ***C. Inexperienced Endosonographers (2)*** | | | | | |
| | Not present | 4 | 3 | 1 | 0 |
| ***Endoscopic*** | Small | 4 | 6 | 4 | 1 |
| ***Grade of EV*** | Medium | 3 | 9 | 17 | 7 |
| | Large | 0 | 3 | 5 | 13 |
| | | | Spearman Correlation: | .574 ($p$ = .0001) | |

presence and size of esophageal varices and advanced portal hypertensive gastropathy (Grades IV, V) (41).

Historically, angiography has been the gold-standard imaging modality in evaluation of the portal systemic system, although it is by far the most invasive test available (3,10). Angiography analyzes the vascular anatomy with precision. The splenic, mesenteric, portal veins may be assessed for size and patency. Collateral tributaries, esophageal varices, and gastric varices can be identified and their distribution documented. However, angiography is invasive, uncomfortable, and expensive, with substantial radiation exposure. Owing to the emergence of other imaging modalities, it is no longer used as a diagnostic tool for portal hypertension, but rather for the preoperative assessment (3) in patients undergoing decompressive shunt surgery.

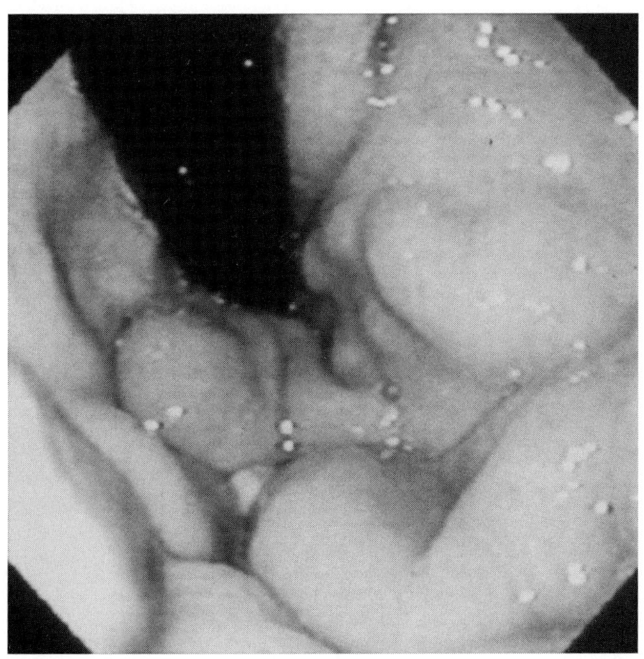

**FIGURE 21-11**

Endoscopic photograph demonstrating typical nodular varices within the gastric fundus and cardia. (*See color insert for color plate.*)

Dynamic computed tomography is a diagnostic procedure that obtains a maximum of data regarding the portal system morphology. Its sensitivity approaches 85% for advanced grade esophageal and gastric varices (8), and it demonstrates splenorenal, gastrorenal, peripancreatic, pericholecystic, retroperitoneal and omental collateral vessels, and spontaneous large portosystemic shunts with greater sensitivity than angiography. It is also able to evaluate size and patency of splenic, portal, and mesenteric veins (5). Computed tomography has widespread clinical application in the evaluation of the portal venous system, even though quantitative methods are impractical because portal flow cannot be measured separately from hepatic arterial flow. The morbidity associated with the use of large volumes of iodinated contrast, technical limitations, and significant radiation exposure make CT scan a less than optimal imaging modality in some patients with portal hypertension due to end-stage liver disease or those with related renal system compromise (7).

In contrast to CT scan, magnetic resonance imaging (MRI) may be valuable in the evaluation of patients with portal hypertension because it can image patients easily

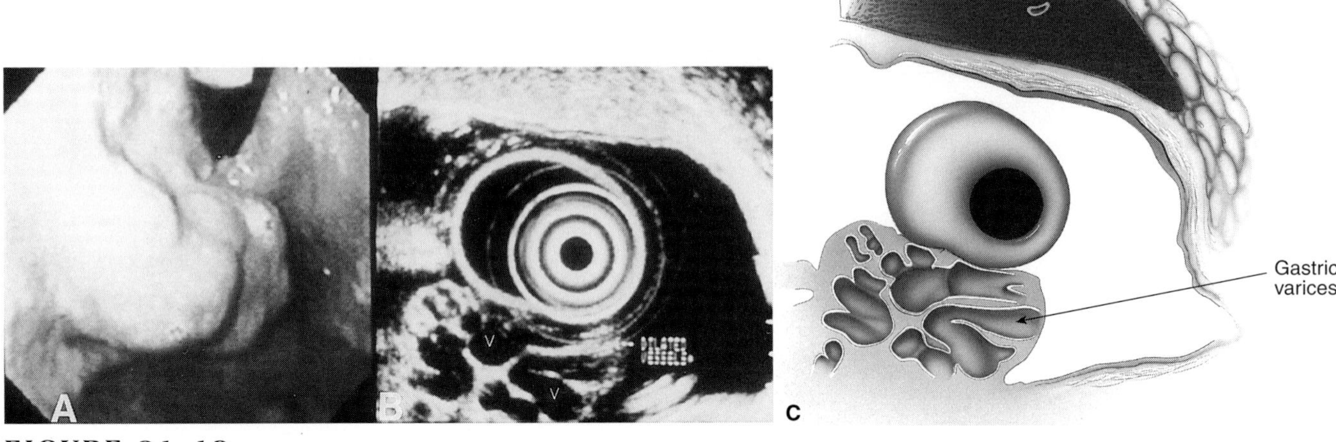


**FIGURE 21-12**

(**A**) Endoscopic image showing lobulated gastric varices in the fundus of the stomach. (**B**) EUS image of the same patient, demonstrating rounded echo-free structures beneath the mucosal and submucosal layers consistent with gastric varices (v). (*See color insert for color plate.*) (**C**) Artist's rendering of the endosonograph.

in axial, coronal, and sagittal planes. Also, because MRI images offer inherent contrast between soft tissue and flowing blood, MRI can establish flow in major abdominal vessels (14). Previous reports have shown the ability of MRI to determine the patency of the portal venous system, assess portosystemic collaterals, and evaluate the presence and patency of portosystemic shunts (15). However, in grading blood flow through a patent portal—an indirect measure of the severity of portal hypertension—MRI has not proved useful (16). Unlike CT scan, MRI involves no radiation exposure, and does not require intravenous iodine-based contrast media (problematic in patients with iodine allergy and renal failure). Disadvantages include its high expense and its lack of availability in some centers (9).

Real-time transabdominal ultrasonography has been used as a frequent diagnostic screening modality in patients with portal hypertension (18–20). It reliably diagnoses portal hypertension by accurately measuring portal systemic vessels, including splenic and mesenteric veins, the portal vein, and larger tributaries (19). Because of limited resolution, small tributaries, including gastric and esophageal varices and periesophageal and perigastric collateral veins, are rarely visualized. Ultrasonography is able to diagnose portal vein thrombosis, and it can differentiate an occluded portal vessel from a patent por-tal vessel nonvisualization attributable to hepatofugal blood flow in the presence of intrahepatic obstruction (21). The sensitivity of sonography in diagnosing portal hypertension has been reported to range from 72% to 86% with specificity approaching 100% (19). Maxwell et al. (20) attempted to correlate congestive gastropathy to wall thickness as seen by sonography. They reported a 62% increased wall thickness of the gastric antrum and 63% increase in wall thickness of the gastric body when compared to normal controls. These results have not been reproduced and cannot reliably suggest or predict portal hypertensive gastropathy.

Pulsed Doppler techniques, which add a new dimension to real-time sonographic imaging, can be used to characterize flow dynamics, particularly in evaluating the portal system (25–27). Not only can the diagnosis of portal hypertension be made, but the cause of elevated portal pressures can be located as presinusoidal, intra-

**TABLE 21-5**

Frequency of Gastric Varices Diagnosed by EGD and EUS

| | *Experienced* | | *Inexperienced* | |
|---|---|---|---|---|
| | **EUS** | **EGD** | **EUS** | **EGD** |
| Portal hypertension | 126/200 (63%) | 77/200 (38.5%) | 53/80 (66.3%) | 35/80 (44%) |
| Controls | 18/200 (9%) | 7/200 (3.5%) | 10/80 (12.5%) | 5/80 (6.3%) |

**TABLE 21-6**

The Presence of Gastric Varices as Determined by EUS and EGD

| | *GV (by EUS)* | | *GV (by EGD)* | |
|---|---|---|---|---|
| **Esophageal Varices** | **Yes** | **No** | **Yes** | **No** |
| None (4) | 0 | 4 | 0 | 4 |
| G-I (9) | 3 | 6 | 1 | 8 |
| G-II (16) | 12 | 4 | 6 | 10 |
| G-III (11) | 11 | 0 | 5 | 6 |

GV = gastric varices.

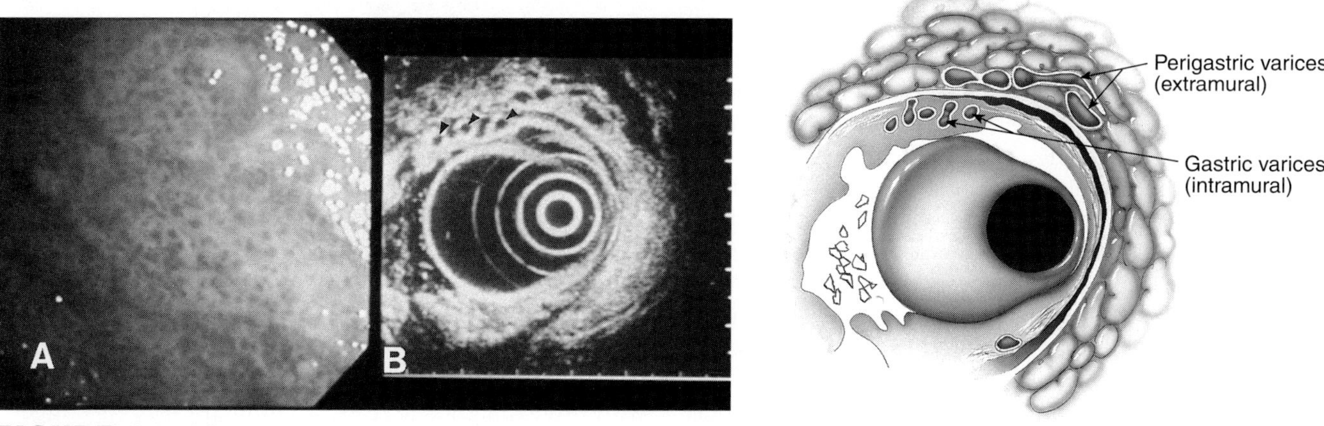


**FIGURE 21-13**

(**A**) Endoscopic image showing diffuse subepithelial hemorrhages in a patient with portal hypertension consistent with Grade V PHG. (**B**) EUS image of the same patient, demonstrating small (2–3 mm), round, echo-free structures consistent with PHG. (*See color insert for color plate.*) (**C**) Artist's rendering of the endosonograph.

hepatic, or postsinusoidal. Spontaneous shunts can be identified as well. On the basis of their location and direction of flow, portohepatic collaterals can be differentiated from portosystemic collaterals. By providing insight into portal hemodynamics, Doppler ultrasound can help to select optimal individualized treatment, and is well suited for follow-up of medical and surgical therapy. It can also reliably diagnose patency of the ligamentum teres hepatic vein, which is highly suggestive of portal hypertension (28).

Doppler ultrasonography is technically demanding, operator-dependent, and time-consuming; it is also frequently unsatisfactory owing to overlying bowel gas and obesity, complex anatomy, or postoperative alterations in the normal anatomic patterns (27). Other significant drawbacks are the limited sampling ability of pulsed-gated technology and the inability to provide a global display of Doppler information. Sonographic imaging of intra-abdominal vessels has improved markedly with the advent of color Doppler techniques (29). Its advantages reside primarily in the absence of toxicity and in the generation of physiologic as well as anatomic information. In centers with the proper instrumentation and a skilled technician, duplex examination can be useful in the diagnosis and management of abdominal vascular disease and avoids the inherent dangers of contrast angiography (27).

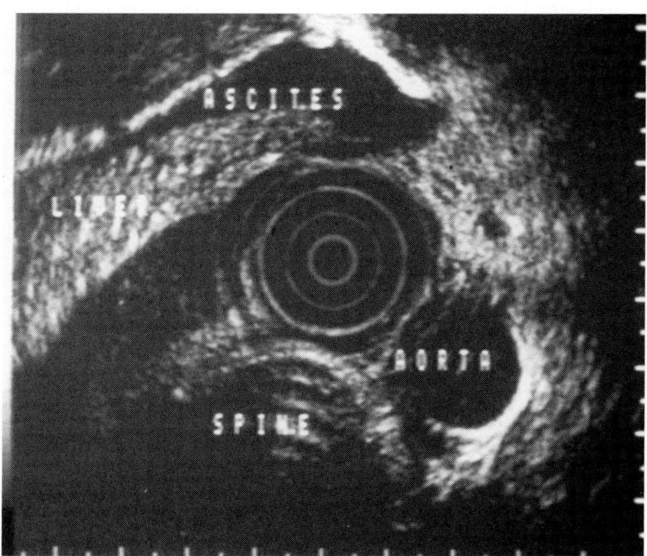


**FIGURE 21-14**

EUS image showing the echoprobe in the gastric cardia. Ascites can be clearly seen as an echo-free cavity between the liver and abdominal wall.

EUS investigation of the portal venous system has been infrequently undertaken, although it shows considerable promise (31–34). Specifically, the presence and size of esophageal and gastric varices, diameter of the azygos vein, and visualization of portal hypertensive gastropathy were evaluated with high accuracy. Other investigators have utilized endosonography to assess the effectiveness of sclerotherapy in patients with bleeding esophageal varices (33).

Thus, endosonography was determined to be an excellent adjunctive modality to existing imaging techniques. It can visualize the portal venous system extensively and it is generally well tolerated and safe, with no radiation exposure or use of potentially allergenic contrast medium. The results obtained by EUS show good interobserver agreement, which is a hallmark of reliable testing. In addition, EUS may be used to monitor the results of treatment of esophageal varices (33,42–44).

Endoscopic examination remains the technique of choice to demonstrate the size and extent of esophageal varices and stigmata of recent hemorrhage (red color signs). Although it is superior to EUS in the detection of small esophageal varices, there is a close correlation between the endoscopic grade and the new endosonographic grading system described above. Endoscopically, small (Grade I) esophageal varices were demonstrated in just 67% by endosonograhy—a finding perhaps related to compression of the vessels by the inflated water-filled contact balloon at the echoscope tip. But endosonography demonstrated 100% of the endoscopic Grade III varices. EUS cannot demonstrate the presence of red color signs; however, it was able to describe the presence and extent of periesophageal collateral feeding vessels, which were shown to be present in 89% of the endoscopic Grade II and 100% of endoscopic Grade III esophageal varices. The significance of these vessels is not entirely clear but may reflect the severity of portal hypertension and predict those individuals at higher risk of hemorrhage.

EUS was most useful in evaluating the stomach of patients with portal hypertension with respect to the detection of gastric varices. EUS revealed gastric varices in 63% of the patients with cirrhosis, compared to 38% revealed by endoscopy. The interobserver variation of gastric varices among the experienced ultrasonographers was good ($\kappa$ = .51) with a low false-positive rate (12.5%). As previously described (31), the presence of gastric varices increased with advancing grade of esophageal varices, reaching 100% in patients with endoscopic Grade III esophageal varices.

Portal hypertensive gastropathy is the unique appearance of the gastric mucosa in patients with portal hypertension. It has been suggested that patients with PHG demonstrate multiple small dilated veins (2–3 mm) within the submucosa of the stomach (31) and that this phenomenon can assist in the differentiation between inflammatory gastritis and congestive gastropathy. This finding was reported in 100% of patients with portal hypertension. The data presented above showed distinctly different and less promising results. Seventy-five percent of the patients had endoscopic evidence of PHG (30 of 40) while EUS detected the presence of small, round echo-free structures within the submucosa in only 12 of 40 patients with portal hypertension (30%).

Finally, EUS was highly sensitive in the evaluation and detection of ascites in patients with portal hypertension. EUS was more sensitive than conventional abdominal ultrasound and computed tomography. Furthermore, the interobserver agreement among the five expert ultrasonographers was very good ($\kappa$ = .71). This may be helpful in those patients with localized areas of ascites needing investigation (i.e., spontaneous bacterial peritonitis).

In summary, endoscopic ultrasonography is a promising new imaging modality in the evaluation of patients with portal hypertension. It has clear advantages in the assessment of gastric varices and periesophagogastric collateral vessels. Although endoscopic evaluation of esophageal varices is clearly superior with respect to assessment of size and extent as well as presence of red color sign, EUS visualizes the majority of endoscopic Grades II and III varices and is able to more accurately predict effectiveness of sclerotherapy. The assessment of portal hypertensive gastropathy by EUS is less sensitive than endoscopic visualization, in contrast to previous reports. Therefore, EUS does not supplant available imaging modalities (CT scan, MRI, US), but may be used in conjunction with other diagnostic tests. Preliminary reports suggest that the addition of color Doppler to EUS may enhance the diagnostic capabilities for evaluating patients with portal hypertension (45,46) and that the use of EUS probes may be helpful in assessing the results of endoscopic therapy (endoscopic variceal ligation) for patients with the gastrointestinal sequelae of portal hypertension (47,48).

## References


1. Misra SP, Divedi M, Misra V, et al. Endoscopic and histologic appearance of the gastric mucosa in patients with portal hypertension. Gastrointest Endosc 36:575–579, 1990.
2. DeWeert TM, Gostout CJ, Wiesner RH. Congestive gastropathy and other upper endoscopic findings in 81 consecutive patients undergoing orthotopic liver transplantation. Am J Gastroenterol 85:573–576, 1990.
3. Marn CS, Glazer GM, Williams DM, Francis IR. CT-angiographic correlation of collateral venous pathways in isolated splenic vein occlusion: New observation. Radiology 175(2):375–380, 1990.
4. Georgescu SA, Morsin LF, Fotiade B, et al. The value of computed tomography in the diagnosis of the prehepatic portal hypertension. Radiol Diagn 30(1):13–20, 1989.
5. Taylor CR. Computed tomography in the evaluation of the portal venous system. Clin Gastroenterol 14(2):167–172, 1992.
6. Chezmar JL, Redvanly RD, Nelson RC, Henderson JM. Persistence of portosystemic collaterals and splenomegaly on CT after orthotopic liver transplantation. Am J Radiol 159(2):317–320, 1992.
7. Waller RM III, McCain AH, Oliver TW Jr, et al. Computed tomography and sonography of hepatic cirrhosis and portal hypertension. Radiographics 4:677–715, 1984.
8. Cherk KE, Foley WD, Lawson TL, et al. CT evaluation of esophageal and upper abdominal varices. J Comput Assist Tomography 4:510–515, 1980.
9. Arai K, Matsui O, Kodoya M, et al. MR imaging in idiopathic portal hypertension. Comput Assist Tomography 15(3):405–408, 1991.
10. Vock P, Terrier F, Wegnuller H, et al. Magnetic resonance angiography of abdominal vessels: Early experience using the three-dimensional phase-contrast technique. Brit J Radiol 64(757): 10–16, 1991.
11. Finn JP, Longniaid HE. Abdominal magnetic resonance venography. Cardiovasc Interven Radiol 15(1):51–59, 1992.
12. Johnson CD, Ehman RL, Rakela J, Ilstrup DM. MR angiography in portal hypertension: Detection of varices and imaging techniques. J Comput Assist Tomography 15(4):578–584, 1991.
13. Torres WE, Gaylor GM, Vhitmire L, et al. The correlation between MR and angiography in portal hypertension. AJR 148:1109–1113, 1987.
14. Williams DM, Cho KJ, Aisen AM, Eckhauser FE. Portal hypertension evaluated by MR imaging. Radiology 157:703–706, 1985.

15. Bernardino ME, Steinberg HV, Pearson TC, et al. Shunts for portal hypertension: MR and angiography for determination of patency. Radiology 158:57–61, 1980.
16. Axel L. Blood flow effects in magnetic resonance imaging. AJR 43:1157–1166, 1984.
17. Bradley WG, Waluch V, Lai KS, et al. The appearance of rapidly flowing blood on magnetic resonance images. AJR 143:1167–1174, 1985.
18. Goyal AK, Pikharna DS, Sharma SK, Jain TC. Can sonography replace splenoportovenography in evaluation of patients with portal hypertension? Ind J Gastroenterol 8(3):157–159, 1989.
19. Goyal AK, Pokharna DS, Sharma SK. Ultrasonic measurements of portal vasculature in diagnosis of portal hypertension. A controversial topic reviewed. J Ultrasound Med 9(1):45–48, 1990.
20. Saverymuttu SH, Corbshley CM, Maxwell JD, Joseph SE. Thickened stomach—An ultrasound sign of portal hypertension. Clin Radiol 41(1):17–18, 1990.
21. Weinreb J, Kumari S, Phillips G, et al. Portal vein measurements by real-time sonography. AJR 139:497–499, 1982.
22. Sukigara M, Matsumoto T, Takeuchi M, et al. Doppler echography for hemodynamic studies of the azygos vein. Surgical Endoscopy 3(1):21–28, 1984.
23. Kawasaki T, Morigasu F, Mashida, et al. Analysis of hepatofugal flow in portal venous system using ultrasonic Doppler duplex system. Am J Gastroenterol 84(8):937–941, 1989.
24. Gibson RN, Gibson PR, Donlan JD, Clinie DA. Identification of a patient paraumbilical vein by using Doppler sonography: Importance in the diagnosis of portal hypertension. Am J Roentgenol 153(3):513–516, 1989.
25. Johansen K, Paun M. Duplex ultrasonography of the portal vein. Surg Clin NA 70(1):181–190, 1990.
26. Van Leeauven MS. Doppler ultrasound in the evaluation of portal hypertension. Clin Diagnostic Ultrasound 26:53–76, 1990.
27. Eidt JF, Harward T, Cook JM, et al. Current status of duplex Doppler ultrasound in the examination of the abdominal vasculature. Am J Surg 160(6):604–609, 1990.
28. Gibson PR, Gibson RN, Donlan JD, et al. Duplex Doppler ultrasound of the ligamentous teres and portal vein: A clinically useful adjunct in the evaluation of patients with known or suspected chronic liver disease of portal hypertension. J Gastroenterol Hepatol 6(1):61–65, 1991.
29. Grant EG, Schiller VL, Millener P, et al. Color Doppler imaging of the hepatic vasculature. Am J Roentgenol 159(5):943–950, 1992.
30. Sukigara M, Komazoki T, Ohata M, et al. Transesophageal real-time two-dimensional Doppler echography—A new method for evaluation of azygous venous flow. Gastrointest Endosc 34:125–128, 1988.
31. Caletti G, Brocchi E, Baraldini M, et al. Assessment of portal hypertension by endoscopic ultrasonography. Gastrointest Endosc 36:S21–S27, 1990.
32. Caletti G, Bolondi L, Zani L, et al. Detection of portal hypertension and esophageal varices by means of endoscopic ultrasonography. Scand J Gastroenterol 21(supp 123):74–77, 1986.
33. Ziegler K, Gregor M, Zietz M, et al. Evaluation of endosonography in sclerotherapy of esophageal varices. Endoscopy 23:247–250, 1991.
34. Nakamira H, Endo M, Shimojui K, et al. Esophageal varices evaluated by endoscopic ultrasonography: Observation of collateral circulation during non-shunting operations. Surg Endosc 4(2):69–74, 1990.
35. North Italian Endoscopic Club for the Study and Treatment of Esophageal Varices. Prediction of the first variceal hemorrhage in patients with cirrhosis of the liver and esophageal varices. A prospective multicenter study. N Engl J Med 319:983–989, 1988.
36. Bake LSA, Smith C, Lieberman G. The natural history of esophageal varices: A study of 115 cirrhotic patients in whom varices were diagnosed prior to bleeding. Am J Med 26:228–237, 1959.
37. Beppu K, Inokuchi K, Koyanagi N, Nokoyoma S, Sakata H, Kitano S, Kolayashi M. Prediction of variceal hemorrhage by esophageal endoscopy. Gastrointest Endosc 27:213–218, 1981.
38. Graham DY, Smith JL. The course of patients after variceal hemorrhage. Gastroenterology 27:213–218, 1981.
39. Binmoeller KF, Grimm H, Soehendre N. Treatment of esophageal varices. Endoscopy 24:52–57, 1992.
40. Grace ND. Prevention of initial variceal hemorrhage. Gastroenterol Clin NA 21:149–161, 1992.
41. Catalano MF, Bedford RA, Sivak MV Jr, et al. Are endoscopic features diagnostic of portal hypertension (PH)? Interobserver variation. Gastroenterology 102(4):A789, 1992.
42. Caletti GC, Brocchi E, Barbara L. Role of endoscopic ultrasonography in the treatment of esophageal varices. Endoscopy 284–285, 1991.
43. Caletti GC, Brocchi E, Ferrari A, Fiorino S, Barbara L. Value of endoscopic ultrasonography in the management of portal hypertension. Endoscopy 24(suppl 1):342–346, 1992.
44. Tio TL, Kimmings N, Rauws E, Jansen P, Tytgat G. Endosonography of gastroesophageal varices: Evaluation and follow-up of 76 cases. Gastrointest Endosc 42:145–150, 1995.
45. Iwase H, Suga S, Morise K, Kuroiwa A, Yamaguchi T, Horiuchi Y. Color Doppler endoscopic ultrasonography for the evaluation of gastric varices and endoscopic obliteration with cyanoacrylate glue. Gastrointest Endosc 41:150–154, 1995.
46. Wiersema MJ, Chak A, Kopecky KK, Wiersema LM. Duplex Doppler endosonography in the diagnosis of splenic vein, portal vein, and portosystemic shunt thrombosis. Gastrointest Endosc 42:19–26, 1995.
47. Nagamine N, Ido K, Ueno N, et al. The usefulness of ultrasonic microprobe imaging for endoscopic variceal ligation. Am J Gastroenterol 91:523–529, 1996.
48. Kishimoto H, Saka M, Kajiyama T, et al. Miniature ultrasonic probe evaluation of esophageal varices after endoscopic variceal ligation. Gastrointest Endosc 42:256–260, 1995.

SECTION

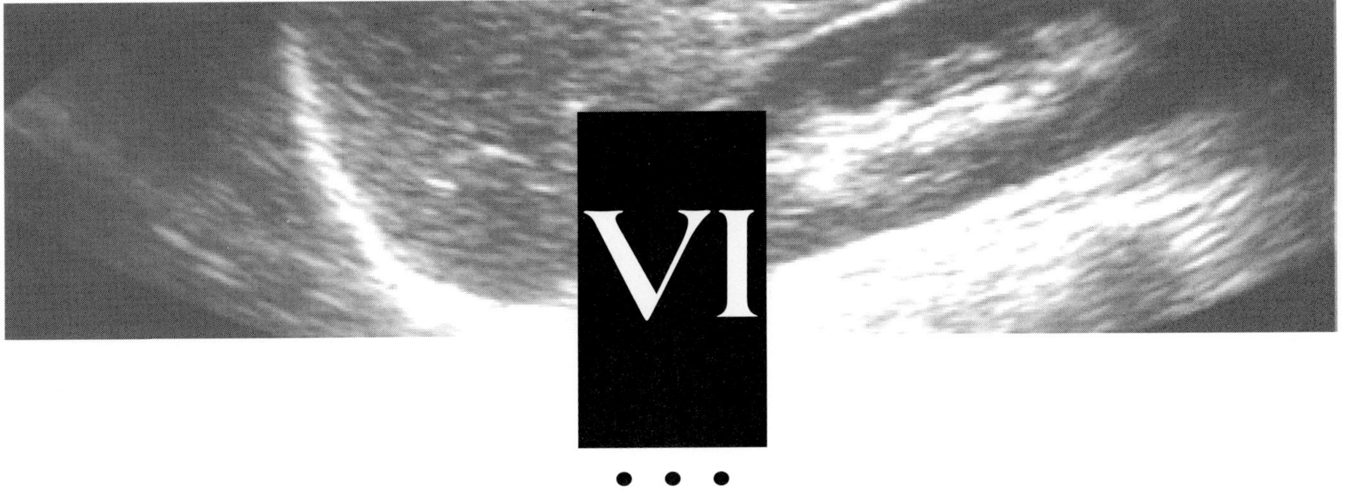


# Retroperitoneal Endosonography

CHAPTER

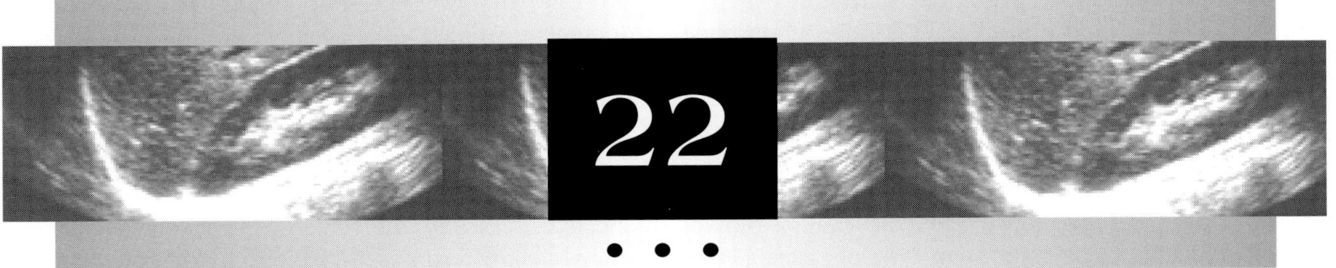


# Endosonography of the Retroperitoneum

## NORMAL ANATOMY USING THE RADIAL SCANNING ECHOENDOSCOPE

Thomas Rösch
Meinhard Classen

The advantage of endoscopic ultrasonography (EUS)—high-resolution imaging of the gastrointestinal wall and neighboring structures—is balanced by its limited penetration depth (maximum 5–6 cm). Therefore, complete endosonographic assessment of organs such as the liver, spleen, and kidneys is beyond the capability of endosonography. Fortunately, certain organs and structures of interest are near to the duodenal and gastric wall. These include the pancreas (which has been the focus of much attention during recent years), the biliary tract, and the surrounding large vessels. EUS has been shown to be useful in detecting metastatic disease in the adrenal gland of patients with lung cancer (1).

Endosonographic evaluation of the retroperitoneal organs (2–6) typically starts with the patient in a left lateral position; changing the patient's position during the examination is rarely helpful. In most cases, it is desirable to employ conscious sedation using midazolam or diazepam. Administration of an anticholinergic drug is not recommended because passage of the echoendoscope through the pylorus and imaging from the duodenum may be limited by gastric and duodenal relaxation. For pancreatobiliary endosonography, the echoendoscope must first be introduced into the descending portion of the duodenum. The technique of introduction is similar to duodenoscopy for endoscopic retrograde cholangiopancreatography (ERCP), but it requires greater skill because the rigid tip of the ultrasound endoscope restricts maneuverability. Insertion of the endoscope through the pylorus and beyond the proximal duodenal flexure can be difficult, especially when the duodenum is displaced or narrowed by inflammatory or tumorous lesions. Under most circumstances, however, an operator with adequate experience can pass the instrument beyond the pylorus in more than 95% of cases. When the level of the papilla is reached, the balloon is inflated to provide adequate ultrasound visualization by creating a fluid interface with the duodenal wall. It may be necessary to intermittently remove air from the lumen by suction.

Ultrasound scanning is primarily at 7.5 MHz. Ultrasound penetration at 12 MHz is not adequate for visualization of the entire pancreas and surrounding vessels. However, delineation of structures within the pancreas close to the duodenal wall (e.g., small endocrine tumors) may be improved by switching to 12 MHz (L. Palazzo, personal communication). Whether switching to 5 MHz (Pentax instrument) is advantageous in terms of better ultrasound penetration has not yet been established. For further examination of the pancreas, the echoendoscope is then slowly withdrawn to the duodenal bulb (for examination of the pancreatic head and biliary system). Further withdrawal causes the instrument tip to slip back into the stomach. For proper visualization of the pancreatic body and tail from the stomach, it is usually sufficient to inflate the balloon and to remove any residual air by suction. The technique of filling the stomach with water (200–400 mL) is rarely necessary. A complete ultrasound examination of the pancreas requires about 10–30 minutes depending on the indication.

## Normal Paraduodenal Anatomy

Using the radial scanning echoendoscope, at the level of the papilla, the distal common bile duct can be followed to its entrance into the ampullary region. The normal papilla usually cannot be demonstrated as a separate structure, but it may be seen in a few patients as slight localized thickening of the innermost layers of the sonographic wall pattern. The ampullary orifice of the bile duct is not visible either unless a relatively long endoscopic papillotomy has been performed. By slowly retracting the instrument and moving the ultrasound tip, the common bile duct can be followed up to the hepatic bifurcation and into both hepatic ducts. The cystic duct is sometimes demonstrable, but the gall-bladder can always be visualized adjacent to the descending duodenum or near the duodenal bulb, depending on its relative position. The gallbladder wall is seen as a three-layer structure. In one interesting report, EUS was used to document gallbladder adhesions, but this is not a standard indication for endosonography (7).

There have been few systematic studies of the ability to visualize the biliary system by EUS. In experienced hands, EUS can be an accurate means of detecting common bile duct stones (8–10). Palazzo et al. retrospectively assessed the value of EUS for detecting common bile duct stones in patients undergoing cholangio-graphy (9). Ductal stones were imaged by EUS in 168 patients, but failed in 2.3% of cases (ERCP failed in 8.3%). Comparison of EUS with surgical exploration showed a sensitivity of 94.9%, a specificity of 97.8%, and an accuracy of 95.9%. When compared with ERCP, all common bile duct stones found by EUS were also found by ERCP. Dilation of the bile duct facilitates visualization by EUS. Demonstration of the intrahepatic bile ducts, especially the right hepatic duct (and its relation to the portal venous system), may be difficult due to the limited ultrasound penetration of EUS.

The EUS examination of the pancreatic head starts at the level of the papilla. The lower part of the pancreatic head, including the uncinate process, is often difficult to visualize as a distinct structure since it is not surrounded by large vessels that facilitate orientation. Tumors of this region, however, can be identified and demonstrated near the duodenal wall. From a position inferior to the papilla, the inferior vena cava comes into view. The course of the superior mesenteric vein cannot be followed by EUS, since the vessel runs a rather parallel course to the descending duodenum. The best position for scanning the pancreatic head is usually the proximal duodenal flexure and/or the duodenal bulb. From here, the portal vein and its confluence with the splenic vein, and a short section of the superior mesenteric vein are visible (Fig. 22–1). These vessels serve as the landmarks for EUS of the pancreatic body, and the superior mesenteric artery will be visible in transverse section (as in conventional ultrasound examination) (Fig. 22–2).

Anatomic orientation of the linear array echoendoscope is different (2). However, from the duodenal bulb a similar view of the pancreatic head with a portal vein can be obtained. In the descending duodenum, the vessels and the common bile duct are mostly imaged in cross sections; the Doppler incorporated into the instrument is therefore helpful to differentiate between the bile duct and major parapancreatic vessels.

The normal pancreatic head presents as a homogeneous echo band that is usually slightly more echodense than the liver. In many patients a more or less circumscribed triangular area within the lower pancre-

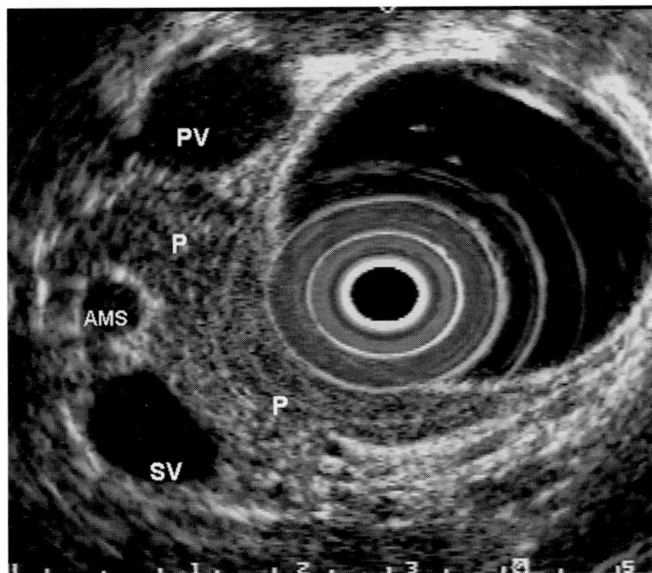


**FIGURE 22-1**

Normal pancreatic head as imaged from the duodenal bulb. The pancreatic parenchyma (P) is surrounded by landmark vessels such as the portal vein (PV), the splenic vein (SV), and the superior mesenteric artery (AMS).

atic head can be delineated which has a lower echodensity of varying degree (Fig. 22–3). Its significance remains unclear (it could be due to differences in the echopattern between the ventral and dorsal areas of the pancreatic head), but it should not be confused with a tumorous lesion (11,12). Measurements of the size of the normal pancreas are subject to interobserver variation as we demonstrated in a recent EUS study of the normal pancreas (12). This probably results from using different (and nonstandardized) positions for the ultrasound transducer in relation to the region of the pancreatic head. It is therefore not especially useful for clinical purposes to have a normal range of size in pancreatic endosonography. Tumorous lesions leading to pancreatic enlargement are usually well identified by their characteristic echopattern. Therefore, size is not an important criterion with EUS (as opposed to computed tomography) for differentiating pancreatic tumors from the normal pancreas.

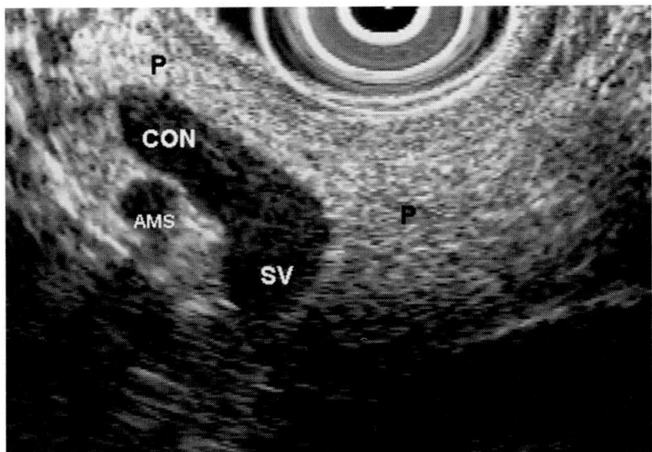


**FIGURE 22-2**

Endosonographic image of the pancreatic head/body transition area (P) from the postpyloric bulb with the portal confluence (CON), the splenic vein (SV), and the superior mesenteric artery (AMS) observed in cross section.

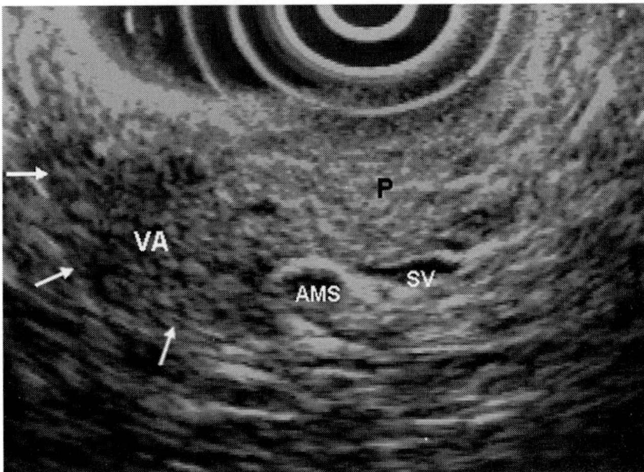


**FIGURE 22-3**

Ventral anlage of the pancreas imaged as a relatively hypoechoic triangular area (VA, arrows) in the lateral pancreatic head. The remaining portion of the pancreatic parenchyma (P) is relatively hyperechoic. (AMS = superior mesenteric artery; SV = splenic vein)

The common bile duct can be seen at its entrance into the ampullary region with the instrument positioned at and slightly above the level of the papilla. It can then be traced on withdrawal of the instrument into the duodenal bulb (Fig. 22–4). The hepatic bifurcation can be scanned from the duodenal bulb; but although no systematic studies exist on common bile duct visualization, the hepatic bifurcation is not always accessible by EUS. The gallbladder can be seen endosonographically from the descending duodenum, the proximal bulb, or the gastric antrum.

## Normal Paragastric Anatomy

When the instrument is pulled back from the duodenal bulb into the stomach with the balloon inflated, it usually slips all the way back to the gastric fundus and must be reintroduced into the gastric body. Using the radial scanning echoendoscope, a longitudinal section through the pancreatic body and tail is usually achieved when

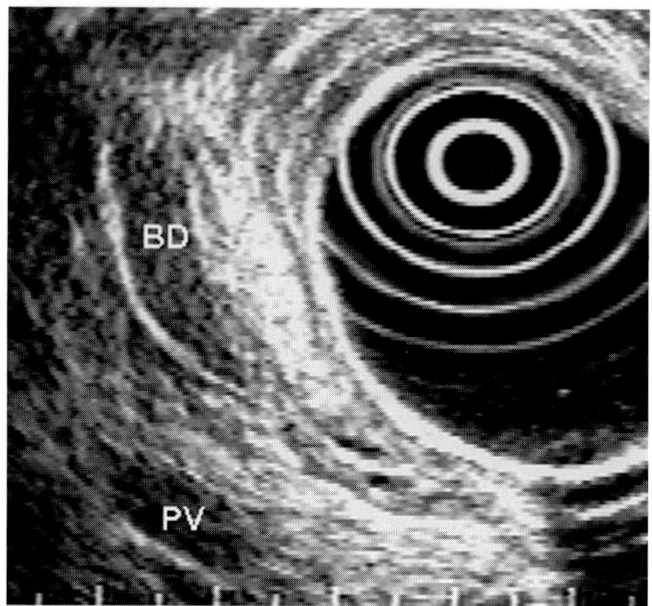


**FIGURE 22–4**

Common bile duct (BD) as imaged from the proximal duodenum. (PV = portal vein)

the ultrasound tip is (to a variable degree) angulated upward or downward. Using the linear array echoendoscope, the pancreas with the splenic vein is usually visualized in a rather straight position of the instrument's tip, and the instrument eventually has to be torqued around its axis for full visualization of the organ. The splenic vein serves as a landmark for general orientation. It is located with the echoendoscope positioned somewhere in the middle of the gastric body and slowly moving the instrument back and forth. Once the splenic vein is located, only minor adjustments in the instrument's position are necessary, and the respiratory movements of the patient frequently bring the pancreas into view. It is located between the gastric wall and the splenic vein, but in full extent it is seen somewhat ventrally to the splenic vessels. The pancreatic body and tail are scanned by slowly withdrawing the instrument toward the gastric fundus where the tail region can be visualized between the upper pole of the left kidney and the spleen (2,3) (Figs. 22–5, 22–6).

The echostructure of the pancreas in the body and tail region is homogeneous and the borders are distinct because they are marked by the gastric wall and the splenic vein. The pancreatic duct can be seen in the pancreatic body and tail and in the pancreatic head in up to 80% of cases (2,12). Since the duct does not take a straight course, it can be visualized only partially in any single ultrasound view. Therefore, the pancreatic duct must be defined section by section by means of slight changes in the position of the ultrasound transducer. The splenic vein can be followed into the splenic hilum. The splenic artery is seen between the vein and the stomach wall, and it runs an arch-like course to the celiac trunk. Again, the vessel in its full course can be defined only by slight changes in the position of the transducer. The hepatic artery can be delineated originating from the celiac arch, but its further course into the liver is difficult to follow.

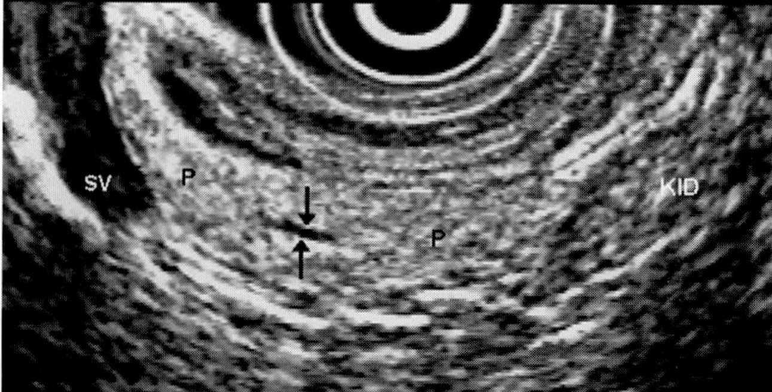


**FIGURE 22–5**

Pancreatic body (P) as imaged from the gastric body with a small section of the pancreatic duct (arrows) and the splenic vein (SV). The upper pole of the left kidney (KID) is also shown.

## Endoscopic Ultrasound in Pancreatic Disease

Endoscopic ultrasound has been clinically useful in the evaluation of patients with pancreatic disease (13). The resolution of EUS has been shown to be sensitive

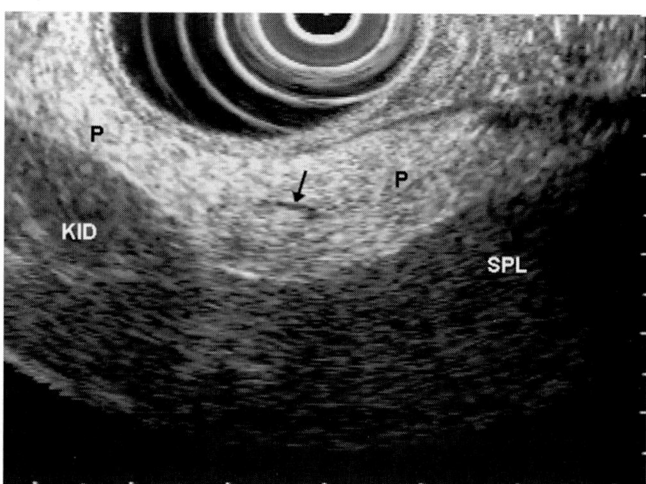


**FIGURE 22–6**

Pancreatic body and tail (P) with a small portion of the pancreatic duct (arrow). Also shown are portions of the adjacent left kidney (KID) and the spleen (SPL). Neither organ is fully visible due to the limited penetration depth.

enough to detect such subtle findings as the embryologic ventral pancreatic parenchyma and annular pancreas (14,15). EUS has been applied for diagnosing and staging of pancreatic and biliary carcinoma (16–19). However, its value in the differential diagnosis between malignant and inflammatory masses appears to be limited if fine-needle aspiration is not employed (18). Because endoscopic ultrasonography provides detailed images of the pancreatic parenchyma, lesions as small as 2–3 mm can be delineated. This may be especially useful in the preoperative localization of pancreatic endocrine tumors (20–29). Snady et al. showed that in patients with (predominantly malignant) biliary disease, EUS supplements the information available from ERCP and CT in 75% of cases, leading to a change in management in 32% (30).

The value of EUS in benign pancreatic diseases is uncertain. Discrete variations in the parenchymal pattern might reflect early inflammatory changes or changes associated with pancreatic trauma (31). However, if other imaging methods such as endoscopic retrograde pancreatography (ERP) and CT scan are normal, the significance of these EUS changes must remain obscure, although it might be possible to clarify this issue by meticulous follow-up studies. Compared to ERP, the discrete changes of early chronic pancreatitis involving only the side branches of the main duct will not be detected by EUS (when performed prospectively and blindly) if these are the only features of chronic pancreatitis (12), but a variable percentage of these cases will have discrete parenchymal abnormalities on EUS. In one recent study, EUS was shown to be 100% sensitive in detecting chronic pancreatitis compared to ERP, also including first-degree disease. EUS also showed parenchymal irregularities in 3 of 6 cases with normal ERP but decreased secretory function (32). Endoscopic ultrasonography is especially useful in evaluating patients with cystic disorders of the pancreas and in guiding some forms of endoscopic therapy (33,34). EUS has been used to clarify anomalous connections between the pancreatic and the biliary duct in one recent study (35). However, EUS was obtained after ERCP in this study, so the examiners were probably biased in their evaluations. Generally, the accuracy of EUS in detecting discrete changes of the pancreatic duct and the parenchyma can be assessed only if endosonography is evaluated in prospective, blinded trials. Without such studies, the role of EUS in pancreatic disease and in relation to ERP will remain undefined.

## References


1. Chang KJ, Erickson RA, Nguyen P. Endoscopic ultrasound (EUS) and EUS-guided fine-needle aspiration of the left adrenal gland. Gasrointest Endosc 44:568–572, 1996.
2. Rösch T, Classen M. Gastroenterologic Endosonography. Stuttgart: Thieme, 1992.
3. Snady H. Endoscopic ultrasonography images of the normal retroperitoneum. Gastrointest Endosc Clin North Am 2:637–656, 1992.
4. Lux G, Heyder N. Endoscopic ultrasonography of the pancreas. Technical aspects. Scand J Gastroenterol 21(suppl 123):112–118, 1986.
5. Yasuda K, Nakajima M, Kawai K. Technical aspects of endoscopic ultrasonography of the biliary system. Scand J Gastroenterol (suppl 123):143–150, 1986.
6. Rösch T, Dancygier H, Lorenz R, Classen M. Endosonographic imaging of the biliary tract and the pancreas. In Dancygier H, Classen M (eds): 5th International Symposium on Endoscopic Ultrasonography. Munich: Demeter Verlag (Z Gastroenterol suppl) 1989, pp 26–28.
7. Dill JE, Henretta TR, Berkhouse L. Endoscopic ultrasound in the diagnosis of gallbladder adhesions. Am J Gastroenterol 90:855–856, 1995.
8. Canto M. Endoscopic ultrasonography and gallstone disease. Gastrointest Endosc 43:S37–S42, 1996.
9. Palazzo L, Girollet PP, Salmeron M, et al. Value of endoscopic ultrasonography in the diagnosis of common bile duct stones: Comparison with surgical exploration and ERCP. Gastrointest Endosc 42:225–231, 1995.
10. Sugiyama M, Atomi Y. Endoscopic ultrasonography for diagnosing choledocholithiasis: A prospective study with ultrasonography and computed tomography. Gastrointest Endosc 45:143–146, 1997.
11. Lees WR. Endoscopic ultrasonography of the pancreas. In Sivak MV (ed): Endoscopic Ultrasonography Symposium. Syllabus Cleveland Clinic 1989, pp 197–208.
12. Rösch T, Lorenz R, Birkenfeld G, Nehaus H, Classen M. The normal pancreas in endoscopic ultrasound. Gastrointest Endosc 37:255(abstract), 1991.
13. Tenner SM, Banks PA, Wiersema MJ, Van Dam J. Evaluation of pancreatic disease by endoscopic ultrasonography. Am J Gastroenterol 92:18–26, 1997.
14. Savides T, Gress F, Zaidi S, Ikenberry SO, Hawes RH. Detection of embryologic ventral pancreatic parenchyma with endoscopic ultrasound. Gastrointest Endosc 43:14–19, 1996.
15. Gress F, Yiengpruksawan A, Sherman S, Ikenberry S, Kaster S, Ng RY, Cerulli MA, Lehman GA. Diagnosis of annular pancreas by endoscopic ultrasound. Gastrointest Endosc 44:485–489, 1996.
16. Yasuda K, Mukai H, Fujimoto S, Nakajima M, Kawai K. The diagnosis of pancreatic cancer by endoscopic ultrasonography. Gastrointest Endosc 34:1–8, 1988.
17. Tio TL, Tytgat GNJ, Cikot RJLM, Houthoff HJ, Sars PRA. Ampullopancreatic carcinoma: Preoperative TNM classification with endosonography. Radiology 175:455–461, 1990.
18. Rösch T, Lorenz R, Braig C, Feuerbach S, Siewert JR, Schusdziarra V, Classen M. Endoscopic ultrasound in pancreatic tumor diagnosis. Gastrointest Endosc 37:347–352, 1991.
19. Tio TL, Cheng J, Wijers OB, Sars PRA, Tytgat GNJ. Endosonographic TNM staging of extrahepatic bile duct cancer: Comparison with pathological staging. Gastroenterology 100:1351–1361, 1991.
20. Rösch T, Lightdale CJ, Bótet JF, Boyce GA, Sivak MV, Yasuda K, Heyder N, Palazzo L, Dancygier H, Schusdziarra V, Classen M. Endosonographic localization of pancreatic endocrine tumors. New Engl J Med 36:1721–1726, 1992.
21. Lightdale CJ, Bótet JF, Woodruff JM, Brennan MF. Localization of endocrine tumors of the pancreas with endoscopic ultrasound. Cancer 68:1815–1820, 1991.
22. Glover JR, Shover PJ, Lees WR. Endoscopic ultrasound for localization of islet cell tumors. Gut 33:108–110, 1992.
23. Yamada M, Komoto E, Naito Y, Tsukamoto Y, Mitake M. Endoscopic ultrasonography in diagnosis of pancreatic islet cell tumors. J Ultrasound Med 23:85–87, 1991.
24. Palazzo L, Roseau G, Siegel JH. Endoscopic ultrasonography in the preoperative localization of pancreatic endocrine tumors. Endoscopy 24:350–353, 1992.
25. Cadiot G, Lebtahi R, Sarda L, et al. Preoperative detection of duodenal gastrinomas and peripancreatic lymph nodes by somatostatin receptor scintigraphy. Gastroenterology 111:845– 854, 1996.

26. Wiersema MJ. Insulinoma: Finding the needle in a haystack. Endoscopy 28:310–11, 1996.
27. Ueno N, Tomiyama T, Tano S, Wada S, Aizawa T, Kimura K. Utility of endoscopic ultrasonography with color Doppler function for the diagnosis of islet cell tumor. Am J Gastroenterol 91: 772–776, 1996.
28. Fahmy N, Wassef W, Brewer W, Clore J, Newsome H, Zfass A. Endosonography may be the only test needed to preoperatively localize pancreatic insulomas. Am J Gastroenterol 91:2013A, 1996.
29. Schumacher B, Lübke HJ, Frieling T, Strohmeyer G, Starke AAR. Prospective study on the detection of insulomas by endoscopic ultrasonography. Endoscopy 28:273–276, 1996.
30. Snady H, Cooperman A, Siegel JH. Endoscopic ultrasonography compared with computed tomography with ERCP in patients with obstructive jaundice or small peripancreatic mass. Gastrointest Endosc 38:27–34, 1992.
31. Sugiyama M, Atomi Y, Kuroda A, Muto T, Wada N. Endoscopic ultrasonography for diagnosing blunt pancreatic trauma. Gastrointest Endosc 44:723–725, 1996.
32. Wiersema MJ, Hawes RH, Lehman GA, Sherman S, Kopecky KK. Prospective evaluation of endosonography compared to ERP in patients with chronic abdominal pain of potential pancreatic origin. Endoscopy 25:555–564,1993.
33. Chan AT, Heller SJ, Van Dam J, Carr-Locke DL, Banks PA. Endoscopic cystgastrostomy: Role of endoscopic ultrasonography. Am J Gastroenterol 91:1622–1625, 1996.
34. Wiersema MJ. Endosonography-guided cystoduodenostomy with a therapeutic ultrasound endoscope. Gastrointest Endosc 44:614–617, 1996.
35. Mitake M, Nakazawa S, Naitoh Y, Kimoto E, Tsukamoto Y, Yamao K, Inui K. Value of endoscopic ultrasonography in the detection of anomalous connections of the pancreatobiliary duct. Endoscopy 23:177–220, 1991.

CHAPTER

# Endosonography in Pancreatic Disease

## DIFFERENTIAL DIAGNOSIS

Gregory Zuccaro, Jr.
Mark J. Sterling

Endoscopic ultrasound imaging of the pancreas has several important advantages: It is generally well tolerated, it is performed with standard conscious sedation, and it avoids exposure to radiation. Endosonography provides close-proximity imaging of the entire pancreas and adjacent structures. Cystic lesions are readily distinguished from solid lesions. Anatomic features of chronic pancreatitis can be identified. Local spread, lymph node involvement, and vascular invasion from pancreatic tumors can be detected.

The retroperitoneum is the most technically demanding area to visualize with EUS. Even in the best of hands, it may be difficult to ensure that the entire gland is imaged adequately. Extrinsic compression of the duodenum by a pancreatic or peripancreatic mass lesion may limit movement of the echoendoscope. In patients with prior gastric surgery, such as a Billroth II anastomosis, imaging of the pancreatic head may be problematic.

The utility of endoscopic ultrasonography must be compared with conventional imaging for the evaluation of suspected pancreatic disease, including transabdominal ultrasonography, CT scanning, and endoscopic retrograde pancreatography (ERP). These techniques generally provide adequate information to guide clinical decision making. However, each modality has its limitations.

Transabdominal ultrasound is highly operator-dependent. Campbell and Wilson identified pancreatic masses in 50 of 51 patients using ultrasonography (1).

Lindsell reported an 84% sensitivity for ultrasound in patients with pancreatic abnormalities found on subsequent ERCP (2). However, Nix et al. reported diagnostic accuracy of only 54% for ultrasound in patients with adenocarcinoma of the head of the pancreas (3). Our experience is that ultrasound examination of the pancreas is often limited due to technical difficulty, including overlying bowel gas, and is not as reliable as CT scan or ERCP when pancreatic disease is suspected clinically.

Computerized tomography (CT) with thin cuts through the pancreas is a commonly utilized imaging technique. Among its advantages are the delineation of the extent and contiguous spread of pancreatic tumors, the identification of prominent lymph nodes or metastatic lesions, the differentiation of solid versus cystic lesions, and the identification of anatomic changes of chronic pancreatitis. The limitations of CT include an inability to identify small lesions (especially those <3 cm), and difficulty in differentiating pancreatic from surrounding tissue (Fig. 23–1). This may result in an inconclusive CT scan, where the presence or absence of pancreatic pathology is not definitively established. Disparate reports on the accuracy of CT scan in the evaluation of pancreatic disease are available in the literature. Freeny et al. found CT scan provided a correct diagnosis in 91% of patients with pancreatic adenocarcinoma (4). However, in the study by Nix et al., the accuracy of CT scanning in the diagnosis of pancreatic adenocarcinoma was 59%, not much improved over ultrasonography.

Spiral CT scan is an advancement in CT technology that has been used to image the pancreas. To date, no large-scale studies have directly compared spiral CT scan to endoscopic ultrasound (EUS) for diagnosing pancreatic disease; however, preliminary reports suggest that EUS will be superior to spiral CT scan for detecting and staging biliary and pancreatic cancers (5). Dupuy et al. compared spiral CT with conventional dynamic CT in two groups of 30 patients with sus-

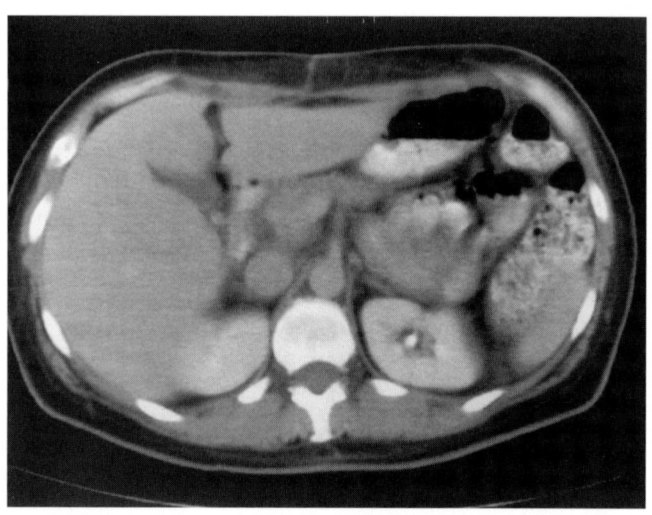
A

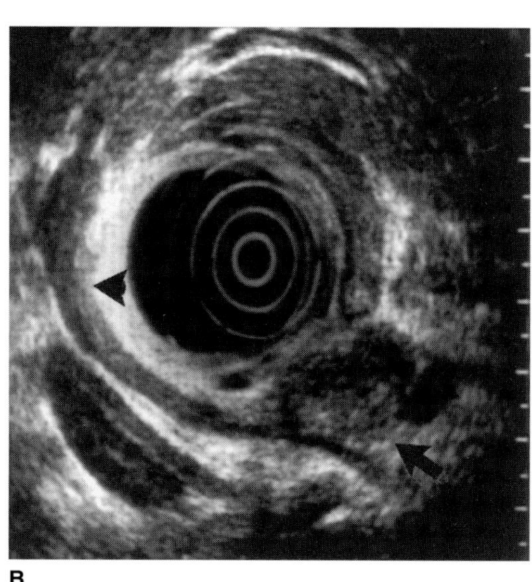
B

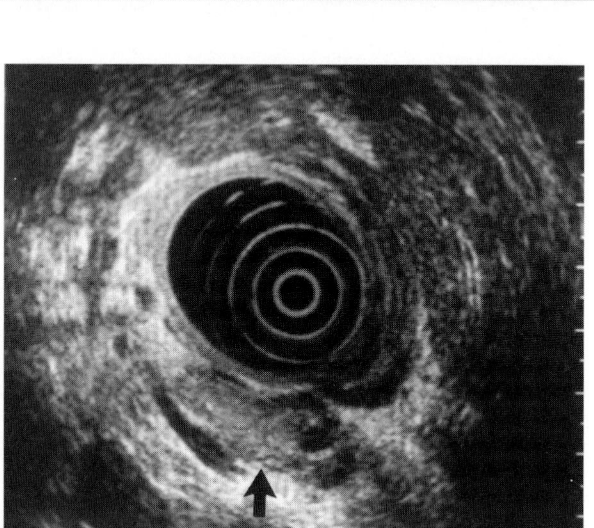
C

**FIGURE 23–1**

(**A**) CT scan of the pancreas indefinite for mass lesion. (**B–C**) EUS examination demonstrates a mass lesion within the pancreas (black arrow). The portal vein is also identified (arrowhead). An islet cell tumor of the pancreatic body, near the pancreatic head, was identified at laparotomy.

pected pancreatic disease (6). As compared with conventional CT, images obtained with spiral CT showed superior vascular opacification, had reduced respiratory artifact, and required less examination time and smaller amounts of contrast agent. Bluemke et al. detected 89% of small pancreatic carcinomas using spiral CT and found that the overall accuracy for assessing resectability was 70% (7). Lu et al. utilized a two-phase helical CT protocol in 27 patients with pathologically proven pancreatic adenocarcinoma and found that the pancreatic phase (40–70 sec after contrast infusion) provided better pancreatic, arterial, and portal venous enhancement than did hepatic phase imaging, with improved tumor–pancreas contrast (8). Van Hoe et al. were able to detect 9 of 11 islet cell pancreatic tumors using two-phase helical CT (9). Scanning in both the arterial and parenchymal phases serves to enhance detection of these hypervascular tumors. Finally, Zeman et al. utilized three-dimensional rendering of spiral CT data to evaluate vascular encasement in patients with pancreatic neoplasms (10–11). They suggested that interpretation of three-dimensional views in conjunction with axial images accurately shows vascular encasement and may be superior to conventional arteriography by virtue of better detection of portal vein involvement.

The pancreas may also be studied by magnetic resonance imaging (MRI). Vellet et al., in a prospective evaluation, report that small intrapancreatic carcinomas were identified more reliably with MRI than CT. More accurate local staging of the tumors was also provided (12). Cost and patient tolerance issues have limited the routine use of this modality.

Endoscopic retrograde pancreatography (ERP) provides a radiograph of the main pancreatic duct and its branches as well as the intrapancreatic portion of the bile duct. Although an excellent diagnostic method in experienced hands, it is not always possible to obtain a retrograde pancreatogram. Some pancreatic lesions, such as an islet cell tumor, may not affect the pancreatic duct, and therefore are not detectable by ERP. Obstruction of the main pancreatic duct is a relatively common but nonspecific finding that may occur in both benign and malignant conditions. ERP does not usually provide information on local or distant spread of pancreatic tumors. It is, however, highly accurate in the diagnosis of pancreatic disease. Accuracy rates of diagnosis of adenocarcinoma of the pancreas are greater than 90%. Endoscopic ultrasound can serve as a diagnostic adjunct to ERP in the investigation of pancreatic ductal obstruction of indeterminate etiology, or in cases where the pancreatogram is unobtainable.

Published reports regarding the utility of endoscopic ultrasound for the evaluation of patients with pancreatic disease indicate a diagnostic accuracy for pancreatic cancer of 90%, and for chronic pancreatitis 89% (13–14). Lux and Heyder report successful EUS detection of pancreatic cancer in 73% of cases (15). Dancygier and Classen found EUS 100% accurate in the diagnosis of chronic pancreatitis (16). Lees has found EUS to be helpful in distinguishing chronic pancreatitis from normal in cases where ultrasound, CT scan, and ERP were inconclusive (17). Amouyal et al. reported EUS to be more accurate than transabdominal ultrasound or CT scan in establishing the etiology of extrahepatic biliary obstruction (18).

## Evaluation of Acute Pancreatitis

Sugiyama et al. assessed the diagnostic utility of EUS in patients with acute pancreatitis (19). Twenty-three patients with acute pancreatitis were evaluated with EUS, conventional ultrasound, CT scan and ERCP. EUS was found to be equivalent to CT scan, but superior to conventional ultrasound in differentiating edematous from necrotizing pancreatitis and in identifying peripancreatic involvement. EUS was also more sensitive than CT scan or conventional ultrasound and was equivalent to ERCP for detecting common bile duct stones in biliary pancreatitis. The authors suggest that EUS allows excellent visualization of the pancreas, peripancreatic tissue, and bile duct. Moreover the equipment is mobile, the procedure is relatively noninvasive, and there is no radiation exposure or need for contrast material. But duodenal edema or gastric outlet obstruction might preclude endosonographic evaluation of the pancreatic head in patients with acute pancreatitis.

## Evaluation of Chronic Pancreatitis

Endoscopic ultrasonography is highly accurate in detecting pancreatic parenchymal changes in patients with chronic pancreatitis (13,14,16,20). The pancreatic parenchyma normally has a homogeneous, smooth appearance when imaged endosonographically. The parenchyma in advanced chronic pancreatitis is typically irregular or heterogeneous. Hyperechoic foci may be scattered throughout the gland. Lees has reported that these changes may represent hyperechoic fibrous walls separating areas of hypoechoic lobular inflammatory change (17). The changes seen on plain film representing calcific pancreatitis may also be responsible for the hyperechoic areas noted on EUS. Pseudocysts are seen as cystic structures that may be anechoic or of mixed echogenicity; contiguity with the main pancreatic duct (MPD) or its branches may or may not be apparent (21). Bhutani et al. have shown that most patients who do not abuse alcohol do not have endosonographic changes consistent with chronic pancreatitis; but alcohol abusers, both symptomatic and asymptomatic for chronic pancreatitis, have EUS changes with nearly equal frequency (22). Thus, EUS may be a sensitive method for detecting early pancreatic damage in individuals who abuse alcohol.

In patients with early chronic pancreatitis, a significant change of the main pancreatic duct may not be appreciated. In more advanced disease, the main pancreatic duct may be dilated or ectatic, with dilated side branches. Concretions or stones may be identified (Fig. 23–2). Ductal stricturing with or without proximal dilation may also be appreciated.

Deviere et al. suggested that EUS is a useful adjunct to other imaging techniques for the diagnosis of chronic pancreatitis (23). Possible findings on EUS include ductal enlargement, with irregular and hyperechoic walls, and heterogeneous and hypoechoic parenchyma in which small calcifications can be identified. EUS can be helpful for precise localization of main pancreatic duct stones and for differentiating between intraductal stones and strictures in patients with pancreatographic ductal cutoff. It can be difficult to detect tumor in patients with chronic pancreatitis. Multiple heterogeneous or hypoechoic areas may be seen in both. Also, small tumors can be missed because of artifacts secondary to multiple calcifications. EUS can detect pseudocysts as small as 1 cm in diameter, but may miss a fluid collection remote from the digestive tract wall.

Buscail et. al looked at 81 patients with suspected chronic pancreatitis, all of whom underwent EUS, abdominal ultrasound, and CT scan (24). Fifty-five patients also underwent ERCP. In diagnosing chronic pancreatitis, EUS, abdominal ultrasound, ERCP, and CT scan had respective sensitivities of 88%, 58%, 74%, and 75%, while the specificities were 100%, 75%, 100%, and 95%. The most significant changes seen on EUS in chronic pancreatitis were dilatation of the pancreatic duct, heterogeneous echogenicity of the pancreatic parenchyma, cysts <20 mm in diameter and microcalcifications. Sherman et al. suggested that ERCP could itself account for ductal and parenchymal changes that have the endosonographic appearance of chronic pancreatitis (25). That is, ERCP with short-term pancreatic duct stenting induced both ductal and characteristic parenchymal changes in more than 50% of patients.

Pancreatic pseudocysts can occur in 20–40% of patients with chronic pancreatitis. Endoscopic drainage of pseudocysts is well described. EUS may be used to locate—and hence avoid—intramural or perigastric vessels, thereby reducing the risk of bleeding secondary to incision with electrocautery (26,27,28). Etzkorn et al. described the use of EUS to guide the endoscopic drainage of pancreatic pseudocysts (29). In two patients, EUS assisted in successful cystgastrostomy drainage; in the third patient, EUS fitted with Doppler ultrasound detected a large venous structure between the gastric wall and pseudocyst, thereby preventing possible hemorrhage. Chan et al. used EUS guidance to perform

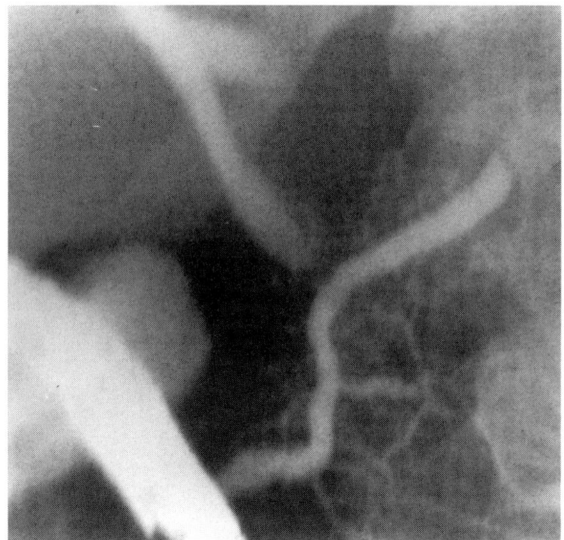

A

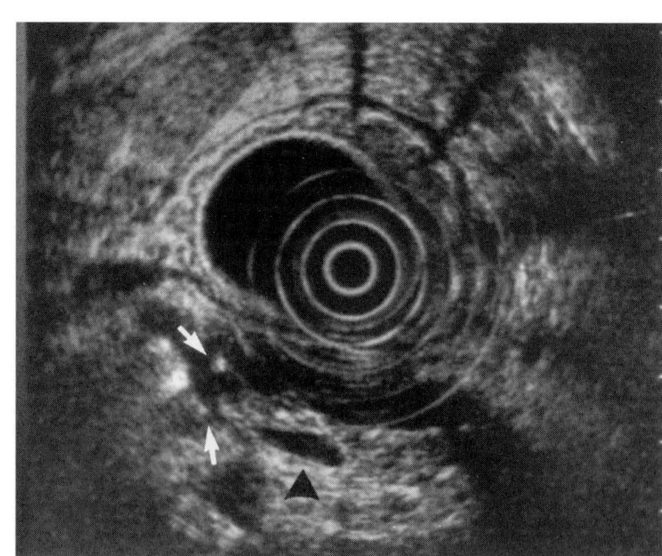

B

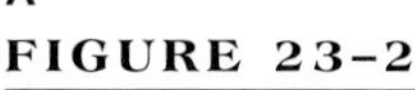

**FIGURE 23–2**

(**A**) Retrograde pancreatogram shows obstruction of the main pancreatic duct. (**B**) EUS examination identifies stone material (white arrows) within the main pancreatic duct. The splenic vein (black arrowhead) is identified just below the main pancreatic duct. The main pancreatic duct is dilated and ectatic. These changes of chronic pancreatitis were confirmed atlaparotomy.

endoscopic cystgastrostomy after the procedure had failed without cyst localization (27). The authors suggested that EUS guidance be used when the cyst fails to produce a gastric "bulge" that aids in localizing the cyst for puncture, or when the procedure fails because the cyst cavity cannot be entered transgastrically. Savides et al. used a 20-MHz ultrasound catheter probe to determine the optimal site for cystgastrostomy drainage of a pancreatic pseudocyst (30). The probe allows detection of intramural vessels and determines if the pseudocyst is within 1 cm of the lumen. It also obviates the need for exchange of endoscopes over a catheter—an exchange needed for stent placement when the linear array echoendoscope is used for cystenterostomy.

CT has generally been considered the "gold standard" for diagnosing pancreatic pseudocysts. EUS has an 83–92% accuracy rate for the diagnosis of pancreatic pseudocysts, and is especially useful for pseudocysts of less than 2 cm. Cystic tumors account for 10–13% of cystic pancreatic lesions. EUS has utility in distinguishing pseudocysts from cystic tumors. Cystic neoplasm typically exhibits wall irregularities, solid areas within the cyst, and septation or lobulation; but pseudocysts usually appear as round or oval, with a smooth contour, thin wall, and no intracystic structure (31). EUS-guided fine-needle aspiration (FNA) has also been found to be useful in distinguishing pseudocysts from cystic neoplasms.

Endoscopic ultrasonography also has the potential to provide therapy (see Chapter 25: Interventional Endosonography). EUS-guided celiac plexus neurolysis has been shown to be safe and effective for providing pain control in patients with chronic pancreatitis (32) as in patients with pancreatic cancer (33).

## Distinguishing Benign from Malignant Pancreatic Disease

The differentiation of benign from malignant pancreatic lesions with endoscopic ultrasound is problematic. Fukuda et al. examined several criteria—parenchymal pattern, glandular enlargement, and presence of a cyst—and found that none reliably distinguished benign from malignant disease (34). Hyashi et al. reported that benign pancreatic nodules typically possessed a smooth contour, while the contour of a pancreatic adenocarcinoma was irregular. Internal echopatterns and characteristics of the lesion border were less specific (35). Yasuda studied internal echopatterns and border characteristics in an attempt to distinguish benign from malignant lesions; this was somewhat successful for masses greater than 30 mm. Smooth-bordered lesions with a homogeneous echopattern were likely benign. However, prediction was less accurate for smaller lesions (36). Jones et al. used EUS to detect a large mass arising from the head of the pancreas (37). ERCP was unsuccessful due to extrinsic compression and distortion of the second portion of the duodenum. The mass was subsequently diagnosed as non-Hodgkin lymphoma by CT-guided true-cut needle biopsy (37). As lesions greater than 30 mm are often visible on other imaging modalities (such as CT scan), a definitive advantage for EUS for this purpose has yet to be established. And, although EUS is highly sensitive in detecting abnormal masses in cases of chronic pancreatitis, the positive predictive value of the diagnosis of pancreatic cancer is weak (38).

Endoscopic ultrasound has been reported to be the single best modality for diagnosing small carcinomas of the pancreas, but it is currently incapable of distinguishing malignant from inflammatory pancreatic lesions. With the new generation of curved linear array echoendoscopes, further diagnostic capability is provided by EUS-guided fine-needle aspiration. With this technique, the endoscopist is able to directly guide the needle into the target lesion using real-time ultrasonography. Additionally, color flow mapping and Doppler can be applied so as to decrease the likelihood of puncturing a vessel or a vascular lesion. Chang et al. used EUS-guided FNA to definitely diagnose a 1.6-cm carcinoma in the head of the pancreas (39). Using transabdominal ultrasound or conventional CT-guided FNA, the success rate for detecting pancreatic carcinomas less than 2 cm is in the 20–25% range. Chang et al. utilized EUS-guided FNA in 38 patients with various submucosal and extraluminal lesions, of which 12 were pancreatic masses (40). Adequate specimens were obtained in 91% of targeted lesions, with an accuracy of 87%. Sensitivity was 91% and specificity was 100% for patients with malignant lesions. EUS influenced the decision not to proceed with surgery in 26% of patients with a primary malignancy. No complications were reported.

Wiersema et al. prospectively looked at EUS-guided FNA in 26 patients with abdominal masses or nodes (41). This technique had an accuracy of 90% for detecting malignancy. EUS-guided FNA was diagnostic in 9 lesions in which other modalities were unsuccessful. Giovannini et al. evaluated EUS-guided FNA using the curved-array transducer in 141 patients with various types of abdominal or mediastinal masses or lymph nodes. EUS-guided FNA was possible in 85 cases, and the sensitivity and specificity for the diagnosis of malignancy were 77% and 100%, respectively (42).

Gress et al. utilized EUS to provide TNM staging in 99 patients with pancreatic cancer, 59 of whom went on to surgical resection (43). In these 59 patients, the accuracy of EUS for determining T stage, N stage, and vascular invasion was 87%, 80%, and 95%, respectively. EUS is felt to be useful as a staging technique for patients with documented pancreatic adenocarcinoma. But, with the exception of advanced disease, there are no pathognomonic features that allow differentiation of malignant from benign disease (e.g., portal vein or SMV obstruction or double duct sign). These and other ancillary signs in advanced pancreatic adenocarcinoma (enlarged lymph nodes, visible metastases, and vascular encasement) can often be diagnosed with conventional diagnostic tests, rendering EUS unnecessary in these patients (44).

Another area of utility for EUS is in the diagnosis of pancreatic endocrine tumors, such as insulinomas and gastrinomas. Endosonographically, these tumors are usually round and hypoechoic, with a surrounding hyperechoic rim. Rösch et al. studied 37 patients with pancreatic endocrine tumors undetected by conventional ultrasound and CT (45). Using EUS, they were able to localize 32 of the 39 tumors, with a sensitivity of 82%. EUS was negative in 18 out of 19 control patients without pancreatic endocrine tumors, such that specificity was 95%. Twenty-two of the patients also underwent selective angiography, but the sensitivity was only 27%. The authors suggested the use of EUS early in the preoperative localization of pancreatic endocrine tumors, once the diagnosis has been established by laboratory testing.

Bansal et al. evaluated linear array endosonography for the localization of pancreatic endocrine tumors in 12 patients (46). Linear array EUS had a 75% accuracy in the preoperative localization of the pancreatic endocrine tumors. EUS produced two false-negative results; both of the lesions were insulinomas that were confirmed by surgical exploration.

Resectability in pancreatic cancer is dictated by the presence or absence of distal metastasis or local invasion of surrounding vessel or nodes. Unfortunately, resection is feasible in just 5–10% of patients. The efficacy of EUS in assessing vascular invasion by tumor has been demonstrated by several authors. Snady et al. used EUS to evaluate 38 patients with pancreatic cancer (47). They suggested that three EUS signs were reliable criteria for identifying vascular invasion of the portal confluence: (1) peripancreatic venous collaterals in the area of a mass that obliterates the normal location of a portal confluence vessel, (2) tumor within the vessel lumen, and (3) abnormal vessel contour with loss of the vessel–parenchymal sonographic interface. At least one of the criteria was present in each of the 21 patients with vascular invasion, while none was present in the 21 patients without vascular invasion. In 12 of 13 patients EUS accurately demonstrated vascular invasion of tumors smaller than 3 cm. They concluded that by using these criteria, detection of vascular invasion by pancreatic neoplasms smaller than 3 cm is more accurate by EUS than by either CT or venous phase angiography.

Brugge et al. compared the utility of EUS with angiography in diagnosing portal, splenic, and superior mesenteric vein invasion in patients with pancreatic cancer (48). They used four EUS criteria to aid in diagnosis: irregular venous wall, lack of hyperechoic interface between the vein and tumor, proximity of the mass to the vein, and the size of the mass. They also used three angiographic criteria to assess sensitivity, specificity, and overall accuracy in detecting malignant venous invasion. It was concluded that EUS is highly sensitive and superior to angiography for detecting portal and splenic vein invasion, but is insensitive for detecting superior mesenteric vein involvement. In addition, Hoffman et al. found EUS to be superior to CT scan for localizing pancreatic tumors and determining resectability based on vascular invasion (49).

## Endoscopic Ultrasound as an Adjunct to Conventional Imaging

Few studies have addressed the proper utilization of endoscopic ultrasound in the evaluation of patients with suspected pancreatic disease. Rösch et al. studied 132 patients with suspected pancreatic tumors with transabdominal ultrasound, CT scan, ERCP, and EUS. EUS was superior to transabdominal ultrasound and CT scan in the accurate identification of pancreatic tumors, and was approximately equal to ERCP. However, as noted in other series, differentiation of malignant from benign masses was problematic (50). The authors advocate early use of endoscopic ultrasound in this clinical situation. Snady et al. evaluated 60 patients with pancreaticobiliary masses using CT, ERCP, and EUS. Compared to a combination of CT and ERCP, EUS more accurately determined the nature of the disease, and cancer resectability. EUS frequently provided additional detail pertinent to patient care, and in 32% of cases affected patient management (51). EUS may aid in the diagnosis of annular pancreas (52), and in rare instances, EUS may be used to perform retrograde pancreatography (53).

EUS can be a useful adjunct to CT scan or ERCP in the diagnosis of pancreatic disease. It potentially provides additional diagnostic information to CT scan in cases indefinite for mass lesions, and can identify small lesions not seen on CT scan. It appears likely that CT scan will continue to be important both as a screening tool pancreatic disease and to rule out distant metastases in patients with pancreatic cancer (54). EUS detects many early changes of chronic pancreatitis. Its primary diagnostic role as an adjunct to ERCP is further characterization of ductal obstructions, or it may be used when the pancreatogram is unobtainable (Figs. 23–3 and 23–4). In addition to diagnostic information, local extension of pancreatic malignancies (adenocarcinoma or islet cell tumors) can be assessed with EUS using either the radial or linear array echoendoscopes (55).

Newer applications of EUS include the use of high-frequency endosonographic probes, which are passed

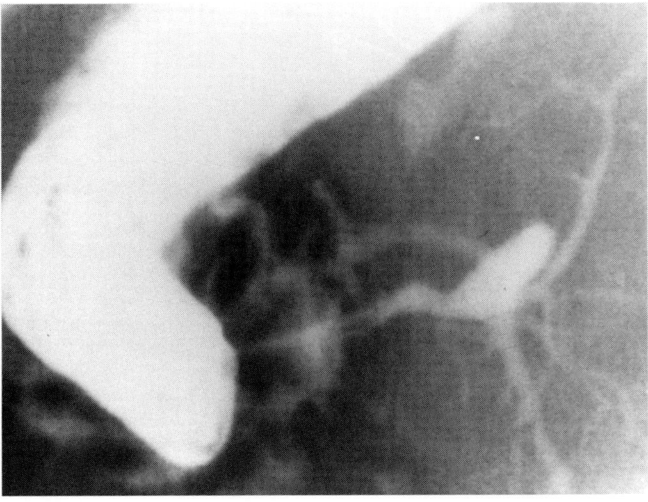

A

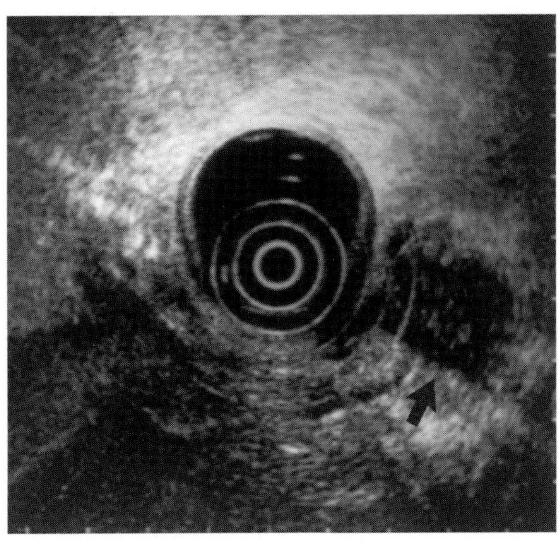

B

**FIGURE 23-3**

(**A**) A retrograde pancreatogram with obstruction of the main pancreatic duct. (**B**) EUS demonstrates a mass lesion within the pancreas (black arrow). This was confirmed as an adenocarcinoma at laparotomy.

through the accessory channel of a standard endoscope; thus they have potential utility intraductally or in areas of stricture. Menzel et al. utilized high-resolution EUS intraductal probes (20 MHz, 4.8 and 6.0 in diameter) to evaluate the pancreatic duct in 7 ex vivo specimens (6 autopsy and 1 surgical specimen). By comparing their ultrasound images to the respective histopathologic cross sections, they were able to differentiate blood vessels, ductal system elements, fibrotic tissue, and fatty tissue; and at an average distance of 5.5 mm, they could discriminate structures as small as 0.1 mm. They postulated that this technique would be useful in the evaluation of indeterminate ductal strictures and in diagnosis of small hormone-active tumors or ampullary tumors (56).

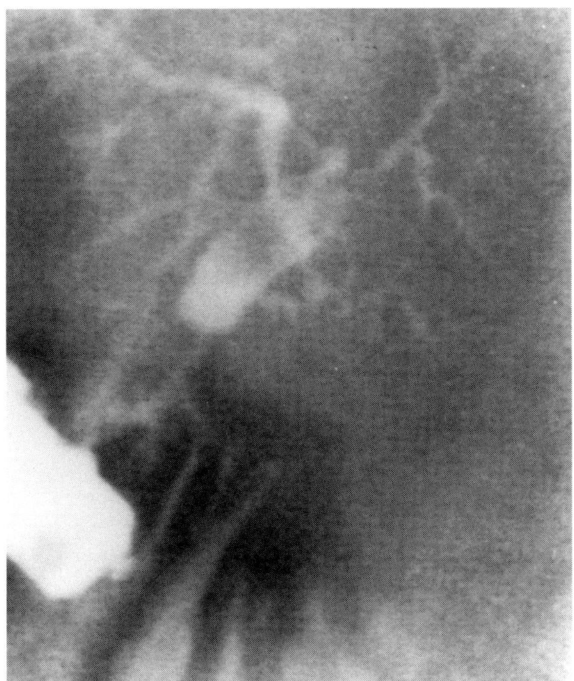

A

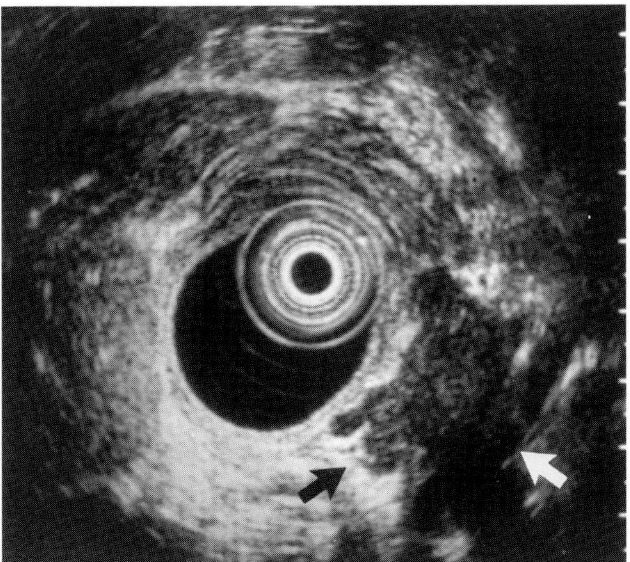

B

**FIGURE 23-4**

(**A**) A retrograde pancreatogram with obstruction of the main pancreatic duct. (**B**) EUS demonstrates an irregularly shaped pancreatic mass lesion (black arrow). The splenic vein, near the portal vein confluence, is also shown (white arrow). A large islet cell tumor was found at laparotomy.

Furukawa et al. used a 30-MHz intraductal ultrasound (IDUS) probe to evaluate 26 patients with localized stenosis of the MPD as seen on ERP (57). They classified the IDUS images in two types: type I showed an echo-rich area surrounded by an echo-poor margin and was characteristic of pancreatic cancer; type II showed a ring-like echolucent band surrounded by a fine reticular pattern and was characteristic of chronic pancreatitis. They compared IDUS to EUS, CT, and ERP, and found the following sensitivities/specificities: EUS 92.9%/58.3%; CT 64.3%/66.7%; ERP 85.7%/66.7%; IDUS 100%/91.7%. Since all 26 patients then underwent surgical resection, specific histologic results could be correlated with the findings on IDUS characteristic for pancreatic cancer and chronic pancreatitis.

Gress et al. used a 6.2 Fr, 12.5-MHz IDUS probe to evaluate 36 patients who underwent ERCP for pancreatobiliary disorders, which mostly included bile duct and pancreatic duct strictures (58). The depth of penetration of the probe is up to 2 cm. Although they could detect no obvious difference between benign and malignant biliary strictures, they could easily discern characteristics of chronic pancreatitis, such as nonhomogeneous parenchymal changes. However, of their 7 pancreatic ductal evaluations, none involved patients with pancreatic carcinoma. Though IDUS may potentially be useful in conjunction with ERP in differentiating chronic pancreatitis from carcinoma in indeterminate MPD strictures, current limitations include the probe's poor maneuverability, its fragility, and its limited tissue penetration depth.

In conclusion, potential applications for endoscopic ultrasound in patients with pancreatic disease continue to unfold, but future research will need to address specifically where EUS will fit in among the other available modalities for the diagnosis and treatment of such patients (59). Endoscopic ultrasound likely will serve as an adjunct to the more established modalities, where it can yield information not provided by these other diagnostic tests. Currently, EUS has established utility for local disease staging in pancreatic cancer, detecting early chronic pancreatitis and localizing islet cell tumors. Some of the limitations of EUS include the following: the steep learning curve for this technically challenging procedure; the mildly invasive nature of the procedure, which requires conscious sedation; and the difficulty in distinguishing an inflammatory mass from a neoplastic process. The advent of technologies such as FNA of masses or lymph nodes, EUS-guided pseudocyst drain-age, and high-frequency/intraductal probes signals the future of endosonography, suggesting an increasing interventional role in addition to a diagnostic one.

## References


1. Campbell JP, Wilson SR. Pancreatic neoplasms: How useful is evaluation with US? Radiology 167:341–344, 1988.
2. Lindsell DRM. Ultrasound imaging of the pancreas and biliary tract. Lancet 335:390–393, 1990.
3. Nix Gajj, Schmitz PIM, Wilson JPH, Van Blankenstein M, Groeneveld CPM, Hofwijk R. Carcinoma of the head of the pancreas. Gastroenterology 87:37–43, 1984.
4. Freeny PC, Marks WM, Ryan JA, Traverso WL. Pancreatic ductal adenocarcinoma: Diagnosis and staging with dynamic CT. Radiology 166:125–133, 1988.
5. Jellouli F, Keriven-Souquet O, Henry L, Napoléon B, Pujol B, Valette PJ, Ponchon T, Souquet JC. Endoscopic ultrasound and helical CT-scan for bilio-pancreatic cancer: A prospective study of 40 patients. Endoscopy 28:S5(abstract), 1996.
6. Dupuy DE, Costello P, Ecker CP. Spiral CT of the pancreas. Radiology 183:815–818, 1992.
7. Bluemke DA, Cameron JL, Hruban RH, Pitt HA, Siegelman SS, Soyer P, Fishman EK. Potentially resectable pancreatic adenocarcinoma: Spiral CT assessment with surgical and pathologic correlation. Radiology 197:381–385, 1995.
8. Lu DSK, Vedantham S, Krasny RM, Kadell B, Berger WL, Reber HA. Two-phase helical CT for pancreatic tumors: Pancreatic versus hepatic phase enhancement of tumor, pancreas, and vascular structures. Radiology 199:697–701, 1996.
9. Van Hoe L, Gryspeerdt S, Marchal G, Baert AL, Mertens L. Helical CT for the preoperative localization of islet cell tumors of the pancreas: Value of arterial and parenchymal phase images. AJR 165:1437–1439, 1995.
10. Zeman RK, Davros WJ, Berman P, Weltman DI, Silverman PM, Cooper C, Evans SRT, Buras RR, Stahl TJ, Nauta RJ, Al-Kawas F. Three-dimensional models of the abdominal vasculature based on helical CT: Usefulness in patients with pancreatic neoplasms. AJR 162:1425–1429, 1994.
11. Zeman RK, Silverman PM, Ascher SM, Patt RH, Cooper C, Al-Kawas F. Helical (spiral) CT of the pancreas and biliary tract. Radiol Clin N Am 33(5):887–902, 1995.
12. Vellet AD, Romano W, Bach DB, Passi RB, Taves DH, Munk PL. Adenocarcinoma of the pancreatic ducts: Comparative evaluation with CT and MR imaging at 1.5 $T_1$. Radiology 183:87–95, 1992.
13. Sivak MV Jr, Kaufman A. Endoscopic ultrasonography in the differential diagnosis of pancreatic disease. A preliminary report. Scand J Gastroenterol 21(suppl 123):130–134, 1986.
14. Kaufman AR, Sivak MV Jr. Endoscopic ultrasonography in the differential diagnosis of pancreatic disease. Gastrointest Endosc 35:214–219, 1989.
15. Lux G, Heyder N. Endoscopic ultrasonography of the pancreas, technical aspects. Scand J Gastroenterol 21(suppl 123):112–118, 1986.
16. Dancygier H, Classen M. Endosonographic diagnosis of benign pancreatic and biliary lesions. Scand J Gastroenterol 21(suppl 123):119–123, 1986.
17. Lees WR. Endoscopic ultrasonography of chronic pancreatitis and pancreatic pseudocysts. Scand J Gastroenterol 21(suppl):123–129, 1986.
18. Amouyal P, Amouyal, Mompoint D, Gayet B, Palazzo L, Ponsot P, Vilgrain V, Flejou JP, Paolaggl JA. Endosonography: Promising method for diagnosis of extrahepatic cholestasis. Lancet 2:1195–1198, 1989.
19. Sugiyama M, Wada N, Atomi Y, Kuroda A, Muto T. Diagnosis of acute pancreatitis: Value of endoscopic sonography. AJR 165:867–872, 1995.
20. Zuccaro G Jr, Sivak MV Jr. Endosonographic ultrasonography in the diagnosis of chronic pancreatitis. Endoscopy 24(suppl):347–349, 1992.
21. Classen M Strohm WD, Kurtz W. Pancreatic pseudo cysts and tumors in endosonography. Scand J Gastroenterol 19(suppl 94): 77–84, 1984.
22. Bhutani MS, Markert RJ. Endoscopic ultrasound detects changes of chronic pancreatitis in asymptomatic alcohol abusers. Am J Gastroenterol 91:1929(abstract), 1996.

23. Deviere J, Finet L, Dunham F, Cremer M. Endosonographic changes in chronic pancreatitis. Endoscopy 26:808–809, 1994.
24. Buscail L, Escourrou J, Moreau J, Delvaux M, Louvel D, Lapeyre F, Tregant P, Frexinos J. Endoscopic ultrasonography in chronic pancreatitis: A comparative prospective study with conventional ultrasonography, computed tomography, and ERCP. Pancreas 10(3):251–257, 1995.
25. Sherman S, Hawes RH, Savides TJ, Gress FG, Ikenberry SO, Smith MT, Saidi S, Lehman GA. Stent-induced pancreatic ductal and parenchymal changes: Correlation of endoscopic ultrasound with ERCP. Gastrointest Endosc 44:276–282, 1996.
26. Smits ME, Rauws AJ, Tytgat GNJ, Huibregtse K. The efficacy of endoscopic treatment of pancreatic pseudocysts. Gastrointest Endosc 42(3):202–207, 1995.
27. Chan AT, Heller SJ, Van Dam J, Carr-Locke DL, Banks PA. Endoscopic cystgastrostomy: Role of endoscopic ultrasonography. Am J Gastroenterol 91:1622–1625, 1996.
28. Wiersema MJ. Endosonography-guided cystduodenostomy with a therapeutic ultrasound endoscope. Gastrointest Endosc 44:614–618, 1996.
29. Etzkorn KP, DeGuzman LJ, Holderman WH, Abu-Hammour A, Schlesinger PK, Harig JM, Watkins JL. Endoscopic drainage of pancreatic pseudocysts: Patient selection and evaluation of the outcome by endoscopic ultrasonography. Endoscopy 27:329–333, 1995.
30. Savides TJ, Gress F, Sherman S, Rahaman S, Lehman GA, Hawes RH. Ultrasound catheter probe-assisted endoscopic cystgastrostomy. Gastrointest Endosc 41(2):145–148, 1995.
31. Binmoeller KF, Soehendra N. Endoscopic ultrasonography in the diagnosis and treatment of pancreatic pseudocysts. Gastrointest Endosc Clin N Am 5(4):805–816, 1995.
32. Faigel DO, Veloso KM, Long WB, Kochman ML. Endosonography-guided celiac plexus injection for abdominal pain due to chronic pancreatitis. Am J Gastroenterol 91:1675, 1996.
33. Wiersema MJ, Wiersema LM. Endosonography-guided celiac plexus neurolysis. Gastrointest Endosc 44:656–662, 1996.
34. Fuduka M, Nakano Y, Saito K, Hirata K, Terada S, Urushizaki I. Endoscopic ultrasonography in the diagnosis of pancreatic carcinoma. Scand J Gastroenterol 19(suppl 94):65–76, 1984.
35. Hayashi Y, Nakazawa S, Kimoto E, Naito Y, Morita K. Clinicopathologic analysis of endoscopic ultrasonograms in pancreatic mass lesions. Endoscopy 21:121–125, 1989.
36. Yasuda K, Mukai H, Fujimoto S, Nakajima M, Kawai K. The diagnosis of pancreatic cancer by endoscopic ultrasonography. Gastrointest Endosc 34:1–8, 1988.
37. Jones WF, Sheikh MY, McClave SA. AIDS-related non-Hodgkin's lymphoma of the pancreas. Am J Gastroenterol 92:335–338, 1997.
38. Barthet M, Portal I, Boujaoude J, Bernard J-P, Sahel J. Endoscopic ultrasonographic diagnosis of pancreatic cancer complicating chronic pancreatitis. Endoscopy 28:487–491, 1996.
39. Chang KJ, Albers CG, Erickson RA, Butler JA, Wueker RB, Lin F. Endoscopic ultrasound-guided fine needle aspiration of pancreatic carcinoma. Am J. Gastroenterol 89(2):263–266, 1994.
40. Chang KJ, Katz KD, Durbin TE, Erickson RA, Butler JA, Lin F, Wueker RB. Endoscopic ultrasound-guided fine-needle aspiration. Gastrointest Endosc 40(6):694–699, 1994.
41. Wiersema MJ, Kochman ML, Cramer HM, Tao LC, Wiersema LM. Endosonography-guided real-time fine-needle aspiration biopsy. Gastrointest Endosc 40(6):700–707, 1994.
42. Giovannini M, Seitz JF, Monges G, Perrier H, Rabbia I. Fine-needle aspiration cytology guided by endoscopic ultrasonography: Results in 141 patients. Endoscopy 27:171–177, 1995.
43. Gress F, Savides T, Zaidi S, Sherman S, et al. Endoscopic ultrasound (EUS) staging correlates with survival in patients with pancreatic cancer. Gastrointest Endosc 41:423, 1995.
44. Forsmark CE. Differential diagnosis of pancreatic tumors. Gastrointest Endosc Clin N Am 5(4):713–721, 1995.
45. Rösch T, et al. Localization of pancreatic endocrine tumors by endoscopic ultrasonography. New Engl J Med 326(26):1721–1726, 1992.
46. Bansal R, Kochman, Bude R, Nostrant TT, Elta GH, Thompson NW, Scheiman JM. Localization of neuroendocrine tumors utilizing linear-array endoscopic endosonography. Gastrointest Endosc 42(1):76–79, 1995.
47. Snady H, Bruckner H, Siegel J, Cooperman A, Neff R, Kiefer L. Endoscopic ultrasonographic criteria of vascular invasion by potentially resectable pancreatic tumors. Gastrointest Endosc 40(3):326–333, 1994.
48. Brugge WR, Lee MJ, Kelsey PB, Schapiro RH, Warshaw AL. The use of EUS to diagnose malignant portal venous system invasion by pancreatic cancer. Gastrointest Endosc 43(6):561–750, 1996.
49. Hoffman BJ, Aabakken L, Cole DJ, Baron LF, Daniel DM, Hawes RH, Baron PL. Endoscopic ultrasound (EUS) can effectively diagnose and predict resectability of pancreatic cancers. Am J Gastroenterol 91:1987(abstract), 1996.
50. Rösch T, Lorenz R, Braig C, Feuerbach S, Siewert JR, Schusdziarra V, Classen M. Endoscopic ultrasound in pancreatic tumor diagnosis. Gastrointest Endosc 37(3):347–352, 1991.
51. Snady H, Cooperman A, Siegel J. Endoscopic ultrasonography compared with computed tomography with ERCP in patients with obstructive jaundice or small peripancreatic mass. Gastrointest Endosc 38(1):27–34, 1992.
52. Gress F, Yiengpruksawan A, Sherman S, Ikenberry S, Kaster S, Ng RY, Cerulli MA, Lehman G. Diagnosis of annular pancreas by endoscopic ultrasound. Gastrointest Endosc 44:485–489, 1996.
53. Gress F, Ikenberry S, Sherman S, Lehman G. Endoscopic ultrasound-directed pancreatography. Gastrointest Endosc 44:736–739, 1996.
54. Faigel DO, Kochman ML. The role of endoscopic ultrasound in the preoperative staging of pancreatic malignancies. Gastrointest Endosc 43:626–628, 1996.
55. Gress F, Savides T, Cummings O, Sherman S, Lehman G, Zaidi S, Hawes R. Radial scanning and linear array endosonography for staging pancreatic cancer: A prospective randomized comparison. Gastrointest Endosc 45:138–145, 1997.
56. Menzel J, Foerster EC, Ubrig B, Keller R, Kerber S, Domschke W. Ex vivo examination of the pancreas by intraductal ultrasonography (IDUS). Endoscopy 25:571–576, 1993.
57. Furukawa T, Tsukamoto Y, Naitoh Y, Hirooka Y, Hayakawa T. Differential diagnosis between benign and malignant localized stenosis of the main pancreatic duct by intraductal ultrasound of the pancreas. Am J. Gastroenterol 89(11):2038–2041, 1994.
58. Gress F, Sherman S, Savides T, Zaidi S, Jaffe P, Lehman G, Wonn MJ, Hawes R. Experience with a catheter-based ultrasound probe in the bile duct and pancreas. Endoscopy 27:178–184, 1995.
59. Tenner SM, Banks PA, Wiersema MJ, Van Dam J. Evaluation of pancreatic disease by endoscopic ultrasonography. Am J Gastroenterol 92:18–26, 1997.

CHAPTER

# Endosonographic Staging of Pancreatic Cancer

Thomas Rösch
Meinhard Classen

Endoscopic ultrasonography (EUS) using high ultrasonic frequencies permits high-resolution imaging of intra- and paramural structures and such organs as the pancreas when the ultrasonic transducer at the tip of the instrument is placed into the duodenum and stomach (47). Due to the limited penetration depth, only the pancreas and the biliary tract and the surrounding large vessels are in the focus of endosonographic imaging (1,2). It has been shown by several groups that EUS is a highly sensitive method for the diagnosis of pancreatic tumors, whether exocrine (3–5), endocrine (6–10, 53–57), or lymphomatous (51). Since EUS is also able to visualize the parapancreatic vessels (1,11,12), it can be used in the local staging of pancreatic and periampullary carcinoma.

## Staging Systems for Pancreatic and Ampullary Carcinoma

The modified TNM system, together with the stage grouping system for pancreatic carcinoma, is shown in Table 24–1. Note that stage T2 specifies resectability, whereas in the original form of the TNM classification (13), stage T3 included both resectable and nonresectable tumors. For example, the splenic vessels are usually removed together with pancreatic body and tail tumors irrespective of tumor infiltration; however, resection of a pancreatic head carcinoma involving the portal vein, while technically possible, is not clinically feasible. The involvement of the portal vein, the confluence, the

**TABLE 24–1**

**TNM Staging Systems for Pancreatic Carcinoma**

| | | | |
|---|---|---|---|
| ***Modified TNM System*** | | | |
| T1 | No extension beyond pancreas | | |
| T1a | <2 cm | | |
| T1b | >2 cm | | |
| T2 | Limited extension into duodenum, bile duct, stomach | | |
| T3 | Advanced local extension, especially into major vessels; incompatible with resection | | |
| N0 | No nodal involvement | | |
| N1 | Regional lymph nodes involved | | |
| M0 | No distant metastases | | |
| M1 | Distant metastases | | |
| R0 | Complete resection | | |
| R1 | Microscopic residues after resection (i.e., resection margins not tumor-free) | | |
| R2 | Macroscopic tumor residues after resection (i.e., macroscopically palliative resection) | | |
| ***Group Staging Criteria*** | | | |
| Stage I | T1–2 | N0 | M0 |
| Stage II | T3 | N0 | M0 |
| Stage III | any T | N1 | M0 |
| Stage IV | any T | any N | M1 |

superior mesenteric vessels, and the celiac trunk usually precludes resectability, so the integrity of these vessels should be assessed separately. Thus more recent descriptions of the TNM system for the pancreas use a more practical description for stages T2 and T3 ("limited extension" and "advanced extension incompatible with resection") (14). The R classification was introduced (Table 24–1) for the determination of resectability. It has been shown that only patients with complete tumor removal (R0) benefit from surgery. The TNM system for staging tumors of the papilla of Vater is shown in Table 24–2.

## Visualization of Tumor Extent by Endoscopic Ultrasonography

On EUS, pancreatic carcinoma presents as a mainly echo-poor/inhomogeneous-mass lesion with irregular margins (3,4,15) (Fig. 24–1 through 24–3). Periampullary carcinomas and those of the uncinate process are examined from the descending duodenum at the level of the papilla of Vater, whereas pancreatic head carcinomas and their relation to such vascular structures as the portal vein and the confluence are best visualized from the duodenal bulb. Scanning of pancreatic body and tail tumors and the celiac trunk/splenic vessels is done from the gastric body and fundus. Examination of the tumor—and especially the tumor–vessel relation—assuming different ultrasonic positions must be careful in order to avoid artifacts arising from insufficient or oblique ultrasound scanning. Peritumorous lymph nodes are visualized as roundish, more or less echo-poor structures of different sizes, but it is not clear whether certain

**TABLE 24–2**

**TNM Staging of Ampullary Carcinoma and Carcinoma of the Papilla of Vater**

| | |
|---|---|
| T1 | Tumor limited to the ampulla of Vater |
| T2 | Tumor invasion into the duodenal wall |
| T3 | Tumor invasion into pancreas, but by >2 cm |
| T4 | Tumor invasion into pancreas or adjacent organs/vessels >2 cm |
| N0 | No nodal involvement |
| N1 | Regional lymph nodes involved |
| M0 | No distant metastases |
| M1 | Distant metastases |

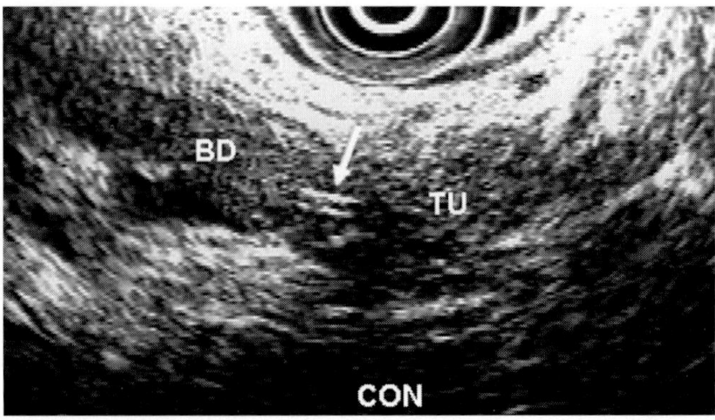


**FIGURE 24–1**

Pancreatic head cancer (TU) with infiltration into the distal common bile duct (BD) in which an endoprosthesis is seen (arrow); CON = confluence. (radial echoendoscope)

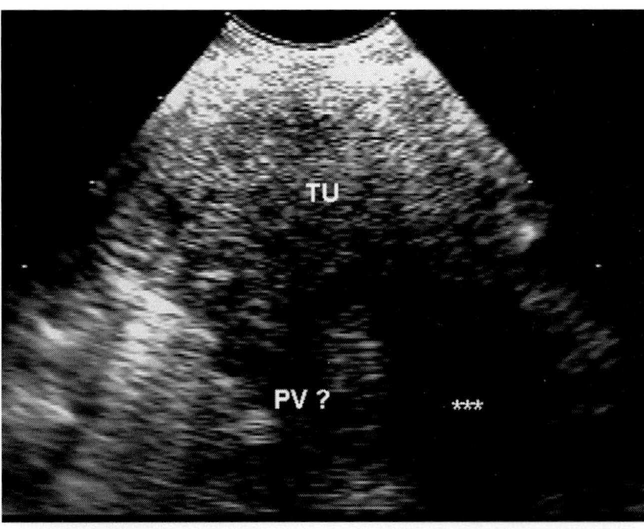


**FIGURE 24–2**

Large pancreatic head tumor (TU); due to the limited penetration depth of EUS, the outer margins of the mass cannot be properly delineated (***). Therefore, it cannot be decided whether the echo-free structure (PV ?) represents the portal vein. (linear echoendoscope)

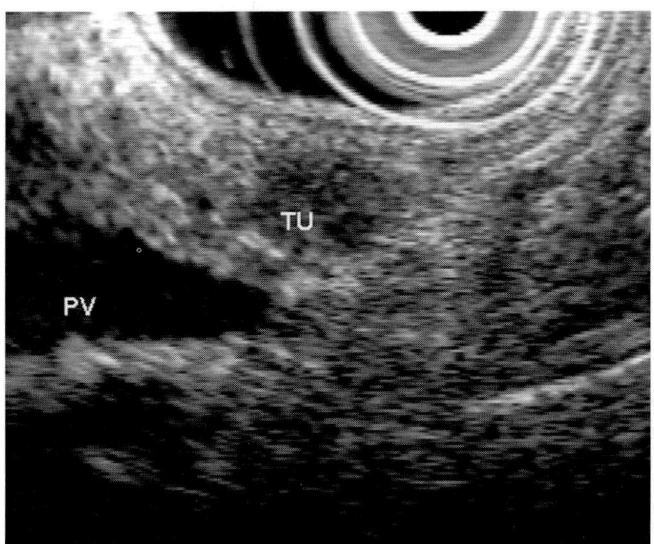


**FIGURE 24-3**

Small pancreatic cancer (TU) in the pancreatic head; PV = portal vein. (radial echoendoscope)

features are indicative of malignancy or not (1,16). The complete assessment of the N-staging accuracy is furthermore highly dependent on the performance of a radical surgical lymphadenectomy. Given these precautions, vascular infiltration via pancreatic tumor should be assumed (39) if one or more of the following criteria are found (Fig. 24–3, 24–4):

- Direct visualization of tumor ingrowth or complete vascular obstruction.
- Loss of the echo-rich vascular wall echo and an irregular interface between the tumor and the vessel when they are in direct contact.
- Presence of paratumorous collateral vessels, which are a reliable indirect sign of vascular infiltration or obstruction if concomitant portal hypertension is excluded.

The nonvisibility of major vessels is, in our and others' experience (5), not a reliable sign of vascular involvement. This is because the vessel can leave a single ultrasonic section, thus giving a false impression of vessel obstruction (Fig. 24–5). Therefore, different ultrasonic sections must be assumed as described above. Loss of the echo-rich interface between tumor and vessel (without direct visualization of tumor within the lumen) is, in our experience, the most sensitive but least specific criterion; however, this opinion still lacks systematic evaluation.

In tumors of the papilla of Vater, endosonographic staging is reported according to the TNM classification. Tumor growth through the duodenal wall in the pancreatic head can be visualized. Principally, adenomas and T1 carcinomas are not discernible when the balloon is overly inflated, leading to a compression of underlying wall layers by the tumor. In such cases, overstaging (T2 instead of T1) can occur. Infiltration into the pancreas is diagnosed when the wall layers are interrupted and tumorous growth is seen within the pancreatic head.

Because its penetration depth is limited, EUS can provide information only about the local tumor stage, not about distant metastates. In one report, EUS with fine-needle aspiration was shown to be useful for diagnosing metastatic adenocarcinoma in an adrenal gland in a patient with lung cancer (48). However, such reports are rare, and the utility and reliability for diag-

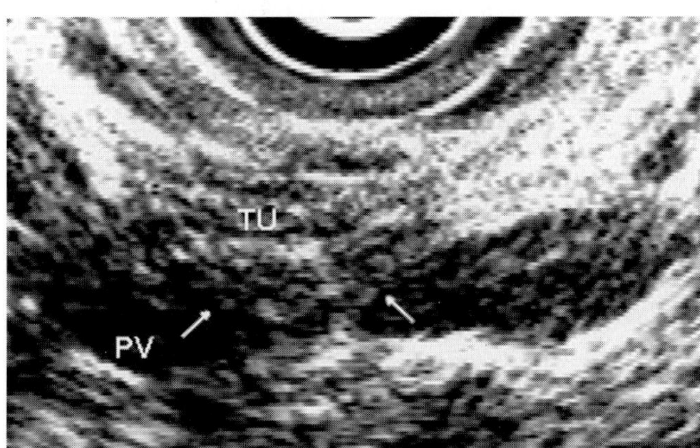


**FIGURE 24-4**

Pancreatic head carcinoma (TU) leading to an infiltration and almost complete obstruction (arrows) of the portal vein (PV) at the level of the confluence. (radial echoendoscope)

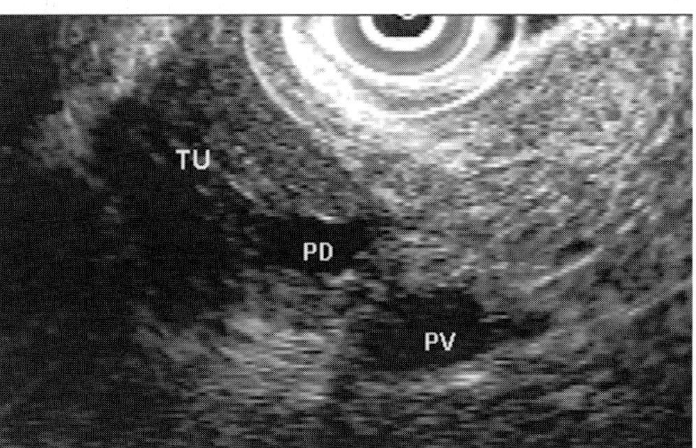


**FIGURE 24-5**

Pancreatic head carcinoma (TU) with a dilated pancreatic duct (PD). Only a part (cross section) of the portal vein (PV) is shown. This phenomenon should not be misinterpreted as venous obstruction. (radial echoendoscope)

nosing adrenal gland lesions remains to be proved. Although the full extent of the liver cannot be delineated by EUS and the first results from EUS diagnosis of liver metastases were poor (17), careful endosonographic screening of the accessible parts of the liver may reveal small metastases undetectable by US and CT scan; but this has not yet been evaluated. In patients with advanced pancreatic cancer, small amounts of ascites are often seen adjacent to the duodenum or stomach (lesser sac), indicating peritoneal metastases. The value of EUS in this regard has not yet been examined systematically.

## Accuracy of EUS in Staging Ampullopancreatic Carcinomas

Several studies have shown that EUS is highly accurate in the local staging of pancreatic and ampullary carcinomas. High accuracy rates were found when the T and the N stages were evaluated as well as when vascular involvement was assessed (3,5,18–28) (Table 24–3). This also applied to the use of linear EUS instruments (40). In contrast to the good EUS staging results achieved for the assessment of the portal venous system, results for assessment the celiac axis are less satisfactory (21,29). Yasuda et al. showed that EUS was also accurate in determining gastric wall, duodenal wall, and posterior (mainly intravascular) extension of pancreatic carcinoma (27). With respect to resectability, EUS was shown to be reliable in predicting resectability when the somewhat arbitrary curative/palliative and nonresectability criteria were used (4). EUS was also shown to be 80% accurate in the prediction of R0 versus R1/R2 resectability (30) (Table 24–3). In the case of ampullary carcinoma, EUS was also shown to be highly accurate in the local staging in a variety of studies (21,23,31–35) (Table 24–4).

More recent work, however, has shown less convincing results (42–44). Blinded videotape analysis could not confirm our initial positive results (44). In addition, others found a low accuracy of EUS in predicting resectability (42). In ampullary tumors, the value of EUS to guide treatment was also doubtful (45). This is in contrast to recent excellent results of other groups, showing a superiority of EUS over CT technology, such as spiral CT (46).

## Clinical Usefulness of EUS

A continued limitation of endoscopic ultrasonography is the detection of pancreatic cancer in patients with chronic pancreatitis (49). In patients with pancreatic and ampullary carcinoma, endoscopic ultrasonography provides only local staging information. For patients with such tumors, surgery represents the only chance for potential cure. Radiotherapy and chemotherapy are largely ineffective. However, only patients in whom complete tumor removal (R0 resection) can be expected benefit from surgery. From these facts it is evident that only patients fit for major surgery, showing no evidence of distant metastases as judged on ultrasonography and CT, should undergo preoperative evaluation by EUS. The contribution of EUS for this select group of patients is currently under discussion, as recent results have reassessed downward the initial conclusions.

Whether or not preoperative angiography in patients lacking evidence of vascular involvement on EUS remains indicated is therefore not clear. In most instances, obtaining angiography depends on whether the surgeon wishes to have information about the vascular anatomy. Among the staging procedures, laparoscopy should also be included since it has been shown that it reveals small hepatic and peritoneal metastases not detectable by any of the other imaging procedures (36). At present, EUS is

**TABLE 24–3**

**Results in the Local Staging and Assessment of Resectability of Pancreatic Cancer**

| Parameter Assessed | $n$[1] | EUS(%) | US(%) | CT(%) | Angiography(%) |
|---|---|---|---|---|---|
| T stage | 250 | 80 | 35 | 44 | — |
| N stage | 327 | 72 | 42 | 48 | — |
| Vascular involvement[2] | 333 | 83 | 52 | 62 | 81 |
| Portal venous involvement[2] | 256 | 85 | 49 | 69 | 81 |
| Arterial involvement[2] | 40 | 78 | 55 | 83 | 95 |
| Resectability[3] (R0 vs. R1/R2) | 35 | 80 | 24 | 36 | 52 |

[1] The number of patients ($n$) is the maximum number reached when all EUS cases are included; the numbers for US, CT, and angiography are lower since not all methods were performed in all studies included. [Data from refs. (3,5,18–30,40)]

[2] Vascular involvement means all (venous and arterial) involvement not specified in all studies included; portal venous and arterial involvement are subgroups from studies where this is specified in detail; data from arterial involvement are from just one study (21).

[3] For definitions see Table 24–1; these data are for pancreatic head cancers (30).

TABLE 24-4

Accuracy of EUS in the Local Staging of Carcinoma of the Papilla of Vater

| Stage | $n^1$ | Accuracy of EUS Compared to Histopathology |
|---|---|---|
| T stage | 98 | 86% |
| N stage | 87 | 70% |

[1]Data from refs. (21,23,31–35).

considered of clinical benefit because it decreases the need for laparotomy for staging purposes. When determining resectability of tumors of the papilla of Vater, the extent of tumor penetration determines the prognosis of patients. This determination can, in large part, be made preoperatively by EUS.

There are additional problems in the endosonographic staging of pancreatic and ampullary cancer. In ampullary tumors, the question whether these are benign or malignant cannot be satisfactorily answered by EUS (37). Large pancreatic masses may be beyond the ultrasound penetration depth of EUS, so the tumor–vessel relationship cannot be visualized. Tumors of the uncinate process with a distal growth direction and infiltration exclusively into the superior mesenteric vein may also escape endosonographic detection. The combined information by radial and linear EUS scanning and the possibilities of color Doppler ultrasound are currently being explored and evaluated. In the first comparative study of radial scanning and linear array endosonography for staging pancreatic cancer, both echoendoscopes appear equivalent for staging pancreatic cancer and assessing vascular invasion (50). However, the capability for ultrasound-directed fine-needle aspiration with the linear array echoendoscope suggests that this may be the preferred instrument for evaluating patients with pancreatic cancer.

## Conclusions

Pancreatic cancer has a very poor prognosis even after surgery (38), and surgery is the only therapy offering a potential cure albeit for a small percentage of patients. A meticulous selection of patients for either surgery or palliation is therefore mandatory, since only patients with an expected complete tumor removal will benefit from surgery in terms of survival. In the remaining patients laparotomy, possibly with palliative resection procedures, only diminishes the quality of their remaining life span. The degree to which EUS is helpful in identifying tumors that are nonresectable, thus improving the selection of patients for surgery, is currently under discussion. EUS has been found to be superior to other imaging modalities, and could therefore be used early in the staging of patients with limited disease. The specific limitations of EUS—such as poor visualization of the superior mesenteric vein—should, however, be kept in mind. Another indication for EUS in patients with pancreatic cancer is EUS-guided celiac plexus neurolysis as a method to palliate the pain associated with pancreatic cancer (52). The role of other new imaging methods, such as angio-CT, spiral CT scan, or MRI (MR angiography), may limit the need for EUS; for final evaluation, however, prospective controlled studies are needed.

## References


1. Rösch T, Classen M. Gastroenterologic Endosonography. Stuttgart: Thieme, 1992.
2. Rösch T, Classen M. Endoscopic ultrasonography in pancreatobiliary disease: Just another imaging modality? In Herlinger H, Megibow AJ (eds): Advances in Gastrointestinal Radiology, Vol II. Chicago: Mosby-Year Book, 1991.
3. Yasuda K, Mukai H, Fujimoto S, et al. The diagnosis of pancreatic cancer by endoscopic ultrasonography. Gastrointest Endosc 34:1–8, 1988.
4. Rösch T, Lorenz R, Braig C, et al. Endoscopic ultrasound in pancreatic tumor diagnosis. Gastrointest Endosc 37:347–352, 1991.
5. Palazzo L, Roseau G, Gayet B, et al. Endoscopic ultrasonography in the diagnosis and staging of pancreatic adenocarcinoma. Results of a prospective study with comparison to ultrasonography and CT scan. Endoscopy 25:143–150, 1993.
6. Rösch T, Lightdale CJ, Bótet JF, et al. Endosonographic localization of pancreatic endocrine tumors. New Engl J Med 326: 1721–1726, 1992.
7. Lightdale CJ, Bótet JF, Woodruff JM, et al. Localization of endocrine tumors of the pancreas with endoscopic ultrasound. Cancer 68:1815–1820, 1991.
8. Palazzo L, Roseau G, Salmeron M. Endoscopic ultrasonography in the preoperative localization of pancreatic endocrine tumors. Endoscopy 24:350–353, 1992.
9. Yamada M, Komoto E, Naito Y, et al. Endoscopic ultrasonography in the diagnosis of pancreatic islet cell tumors. J Ultrasound Med 23:85–87, 1991.
10. Glover JR, Shover PJ, Lees WR. Endoscopic ultrasound for localization of islet cell tumors. Gut 33:108–110, 1992.
11. Caletti GC, Brocchi E, Baraldini M, et al. Assessment of portal hypertension by endoscopic ultrasonography. Gastrointest Endosc 36:S21–S27, 1990.
12. Kaufman AR, Sivak MV. Endoscopic ultrasonography in the differential diagnosis of pancreatic disease. Gastrointest Endosc 35: 214–219, 1989.
13. Sobin LH, Hermanek P, Hutter RP. TNM classification of malignant tumors. Cancer 61:2310–2314, 1988.
14. Ahlgren JD, Hill MC, Roberts IM. Pancreatic cancer: Patterns, diagnosis and approaches to treatment. In Ahlgren JD, Macdonald JS (eds): Gastrointestinal Oncology. Philadelphia: J.B. Lippincott, 1992, pp 197–207.
15. Hayashi Y, Nakazawa S, Kimoto E, et al. Clinicopathological analysis of endoscopic ultrasonograms in pancreatic mass lesions. Endoscopy 21:121–125, 1989.
16. Tio TL, Tytgat GNJ. Endoscopic ultrasonography in analyzing peri-intestinal lymph node abnormality. Preliminary results of studies in vitro and in vivo. Scand J Gastroenterol 21(suppl 123): 158–163, 1986.
17. Gandolfi L, Rossi A, Solmi L, et al. Endoscopic ultrasonography in liver disease. Ann Radiol 28:28–30, 1985.
18. Sugiyama S, Asada M, Fujita R, et al. Endoscopic ultrasonography for the diagnosis of pancreas carcinoma. Endoscopy 20:94 (abstract), 1988.

19. Amouyal P, Amouyal G, Mompoint D, et al. Endosonography: Promising method for diagnosis of extrahepatic cholestasis. Lancet II:1195–1198, 1989.
20. Snady H, Cooperman A, Siegel JH. Assessment of vascular involvement by pancreatic disease—A comparison of endoscopic ultrasonography to computerized tomography and angiography. Gastrointest Endosc 36:197(abstract), 1990.
21. Rösch T, Braig C, Gain T, et al. Staging of pancreatic and ampullary carcinoma by endoscopic ultrasonography. Gastroenterology 102:188–199, 1992.
22. Grimm H, Maydeo A, Soehendra N. Endoluminal ultrasound for the diagnosis and staging of pancreatic cancer. Baillière's Clin Gastroenterol 4:869–887, 1990.
23. Tio TL, Tytgat GNJ, Cikot RJLM, et al. Ampullopancreatic carcinoma: Preoperative TNM classification with endosonography. Radiology 174:455–461, 1990.
24. Rösch T, Dittler HJ, Lorenz R, et al. Endosonographisches Staging des Pankreaskarzinoms. Dtsch med Wschr 117:563–569, 1992.
25. Kalantzis N, Kallimanis G, Laoudi F, et al. Endoscopic ultrasonography and computed tomography in preoperative (TNM) classifications of pancreatic carcinoma. Endoscopy 24:653(abstract), 1992.
26. Wiersema MJ, Chak A, Hawes RH, et al. Evaluation of endosonography in distinguishing malignant from inflammatory pancreatic masses. Gastrointest Endosc 39:A336(abstract), 1993.
27. Yasuda K, Mukai H, Nakajima M, et al. Staging of pancreatic carcinoma by endoscopic ultrasonography. Endoscopy 25:151–155, 1993.
28. Kobayashi G, Fujita N, Noda Y, et al. The evaluation of portal venous invasion of pancreatic cancer by endoscopic ultrasonography. Jpn J Gastroenterol 90:49–56, 1993.
29. Kallimanis G, Axiotis E, Papantoniou P, et al. Endoscopic ultrasonography in preoperative TNM classification of pancreatic cancer. Endoscopy 24:656(abstract), 1992.
30. Rösch T, Dittler HJ, Lorenz R, et al. Endosonographic assessment of resectability of pancreatic head carcinoma. Gastrointest Endosc 38:259(abstract), 1992.
31. Fujino MA, Morozumi A, Ikeda M, et al. Diagnosis of carcinoma of the major duodenal papilla by endoscopic ultrasonography. Gastroenterology 100:316(abstract), 1991.
32. Barkun AN, Jones S, Bowie J, et al. The assessment of ampullary tumors by endoscopic ultrasonography. Gastrointest Endosc 36: 207(abstract), 1990.
33. Mukai H, Cho E, Yasuda K, et al. Evaluation of endoscopic ultrasonography in the diagnosis of cancer extension of the papilla of Vater and common bile duct. Gastrointest Endosc 36:201(abstract), 1990.
34. Mukai H, Nakajima M, Yasuda K, et al. Evaluation of endoscopic ultrasonography in the pre-operative staging of carcinoma of the ampulla of Vater and common bile duct. Gastrointest Endosc 38:676–683, 1992.
35. Mitake M, Nakazawa S, Tsukamoto Y, et al. Endoscopic ultrasonography in the diagnosis of depth invasion and lymph node metastasis of carcinoma of the papilla of Vater. J Ultrasound Med 9:645–683, 1990.
36. Warshaw AL, Tepper JE, Shipley WU. Laparoscopy in the staging and planning of therapy for pancreatic cancer. Am J Surg 151: 76–80, 1986.
37. Rösch T, Dittler HJ, Lorenz R, et al. The role of endoscopic ultrasonography in the diagnosis and staging of tumors of the papilla of Vater. Gastrointest Endosc 38:259–260(abstract), 1992.
38. Baylor SM, Berg JW. Cross-classification and survival characteristics of 500 cases of cancer of the pancreas. J Surg Oncol 4:335–358, 1972.
39. Brugge WR. Pancreatic cancer staging: Endoscopic ultrasonography criteria for vascular invasion. Gastrointest Endosc Clin North Am 5:741–754, 1995.
40. Giovannini M, Seitz JF. Endoscopic ultrasonography with a linear-type echoendoscope in the evaluation of 94 patients with pancreatobiliary disease. Endoscopy 26:579–85, 1994.
41. Müller MF, Meyenberger C, Bertolringer P, et al. Pancreatic tumors: Evaluation with endoscopic US, CT and MR. Radiology 190:745–757, 1994.
42. Pager P, Buscail L, Berthélémy P, et al. Evaluation of endoscopic ultrasonography for prediction of pancreatic carcinoma resectability. Gastrointest Endosc 43:427(abstract), 1996.
43. Aubertin JM, Bouillot JL, Bloch F, et al. Endosonography and computed tomography in evaluation of vascular involvement in malignant pancreatic tumors. Gastroenterology 110:486A, 1996.
44. Rösch T, Dittler HJ, Lorenz R, et al. Endoscopic ultrasound is less accurate in pancreatic cancer staging than previously thought: A blind analysis of videotapes. Gastrointest Endosc 43:429A, 1996.
45. Cahen DL, Fockens P, Tio TL, et al. Endosonography of villous adenomas of the ampulla of Vater. Gastrointest Endosc 41:391A, 1995.
46. Gress F, Ikenberry S, Sherman S, et al. A prospective comparison of endoscopic ultrasound versus spiral computed tomography for pancreatic, biliary and ampullary cancer staging and determination of vascular invasion and resectability. Gastrointest Endosc 43:422A, 1996.
47. Tenner SM, Banks PA, Wiersema MJ, Van Dam J. Evaluation of pancreatic disease by endoscopic ultrasonography. Am J Gastroenterol 92:18–26, 1997.
48. Chang KJ, Erickson RA, Nguyen P. Endoscopic ultrasound (EUS) and EUS-guided fine-needle aspiration of the left adrenal gland. Gasrointest Endosc 44:568–572, 1996.
49. Barthet M, Portal I, Boujaoude JP, Sahel J. Endoscopic ultrasonographic diagnosis of pancreatic cancer complicating chronic pancreatitis. Endoscopy 28:487–491, 1996.
50. Gress F, Savides T, Cummings O, Sherman S, Lehman G, Zaidi S, Hawes R. Radial scanning and linear array endosonography for staging pancreatic cancer: A prospective randomized comparison. Gastrointest Endosc 45:138–142, 1997.
51. Jones WF, Sheikh Y, McClave SA. AIDS-related non-Hodgkin's lymphoma of the pancreas. Am J Gastroenterol 92:335–338, 1997.
52. Wiersema MJ, Wiersema LM. Endosonography-guided celiac plexus neurolysis. Gastrointest Endosc 44:656–662, 1996.
53. Cadiot G, Lebtahi R, Sarda L, et al. Preoperative detection of duodenal gastrinomas and peripancreatic lymph nodes by somatostatin receptor scintigraphy. Gastroenterology 111:845–854, 1996.
54. Wiersema MJ. Insulinoma: Finding the needle in a haystack. Endoscopy 28:310–311, 1996.
55. Ueno N, Tomiyama T, Tano S, Wada S, Aizawa T, Kimura K. Utility of endoscopic ultrasonography with color Doppler function for the diagnosis of islet cell tumor. Am J Gastroenterol 91:772–776, 1996.
56. Fahmy N, Wassef W, Brewer W, Clore J, Newsome H, Zfass A. Endosonography may be the only test needed to preoperatively localize pancreatic insulomas. Am Gastroenterol 91:2013A, 1996.
57. Schumacher B, Lübke HJ, Frieling T, Strohmeyer G, Starke AAR. Prospective study on the detection of insulomas by endoscopic ultrasonography. Endoscopy 28:273–276, 1996.

CHAPTER

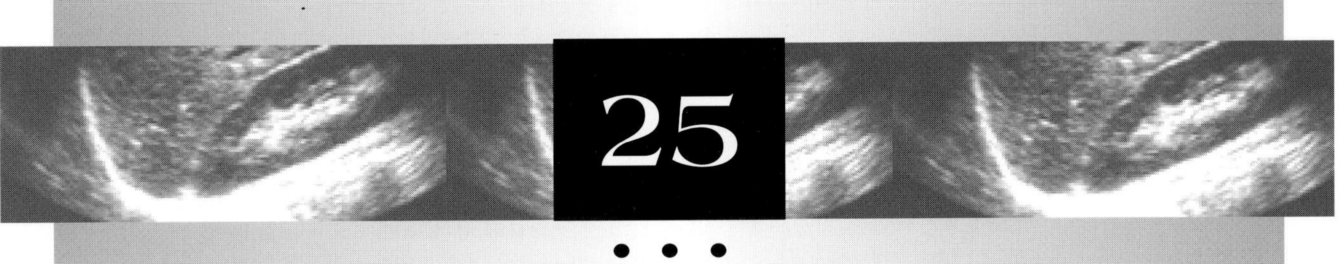


# Endosonography in Pancreatic Disease

## INTERVENTIONAL ENDOSONOGRAPHY

Kenneth F. Binmoeller
Hans Seifert
Nib Soehendra

Percutaneous fine-needle biopsy of the pancreas and drainage of pancreatic fluid collections under ultrasonography (US) and computer tomography (CT) guidance are well established techniques. A logical extension of the percutaneous approach is the use of endoscopic ultrasonography (EUS) to guide fine-needle procedures through the bowel wall. EUS has the advantages of better resolution of the pancreas and a direct route of access to the organ through the duodenal or gastric wall.

Although EUS has been in clinical use for more than a decade, interventional applications such as fine-needle aspiration biopsy have only recently been described. This has been due to the inability to visualize an accessory passed into the imaging plane using the conventional radial scanning echoendoscope (Fig. 25–1). Guided instrumentation became feasible with the development of the curved linear array echoendoscope, which produces a sector image in the long axis of the echoendoscope. The operator can visualize an accessory lengthwise as it enters the imaging field (Fig. 25–2).

## Curved Linear Array Echoendoscopes

Linear array echoendoscopes are available from the Pentax and Olympus corporations (Fig. 25–3). Technical specifications of the instruments are detailed in

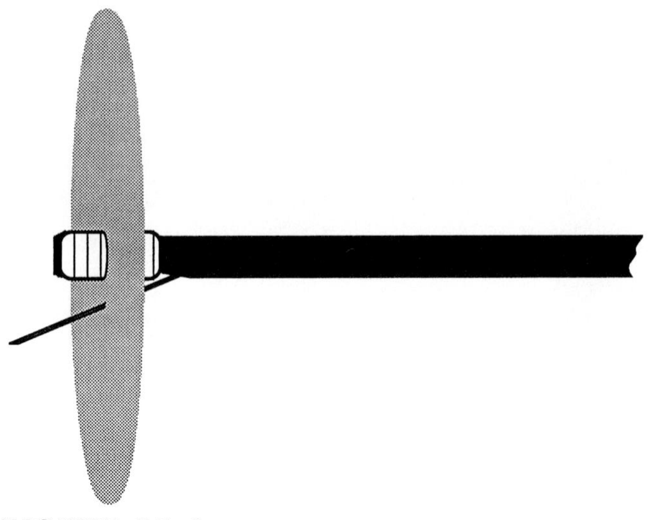

**FIGURE 25-1**

Schematic representation of the radial mode of endosonographic scanning. A single transducer mechanically rotates to produce a 360° image perpendicular to the long axis of the echoendoscope. A needle inserted into the imaging plane appears as a dot.

Table 25–1. The echoendoscopes are completely immersible, oblique-viewing fiberscopes that incorporate an electronic curved linear array transducer. A latex balloon is mounted over the transducer housing and filled with water for acoustic coupling. A working channel allows the passage of accessories into the scanning plane. The Pentax FG-32UA has a fixed angle (25°) at which the accessory exits, whereas the Olympus GF-UC30P has an elevator which allows adjustment of the exit angle (up to 40°). The accessory can also be endoscopically visualized as it exits the working channel. A recently introduced prototype linear scanning echoendoscope with a 2.4-mm instrument channel and elevator is now available (Pentax FG-36UA, Pentax Precision Instruments, Inc.; Orangeburg, New York).

The Pentax and Olympus echoendoscopes are connected to their respective console units with a B-mode sector display. The Pentax FG-32UA is used with an Hitachi/Picker ultrasound console, and the Olympus prototype is used with the Acoustic Imaging Ultrasound System. These consoles provide several unique features. The focal length of the ultrasound beam is adjustable to provide optimal resolution of a specific region of interest. Color and pulsed Doppler capability are available. After freezing an image, a cine-loop memory function allows the examiner to scroll through preceding images frame by frame. The consoles can also be used with other ultrasound probes such as transducers for standard transabdominal scanning.

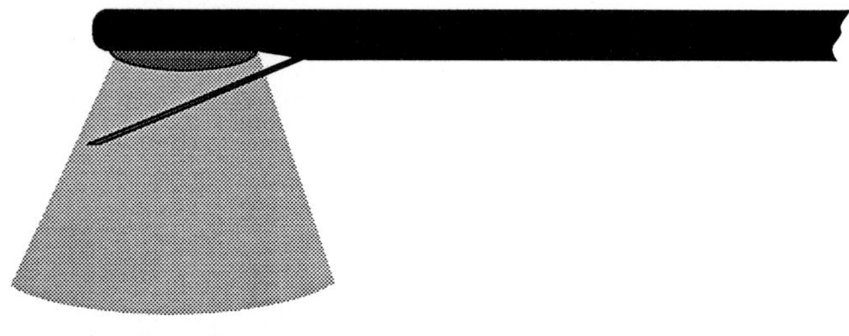

**FIGURE 25-2**

Schematic representation of the curved linear mode of endosonographic scanning. A series of transducers is electronically triggered in sequence to produce a sector image parallel to the axis of the echoendoscope. A needle inserted into the imaging plane is visualized lengthwise.

## Doppler

The reliable differentiation of vascular from nonvascular structures is imperative when performing EUS-guided interventional procedures. Doppler technology assists in this differentiation. Various Doppler imaging modes are available on the Pentax and Olympus processor units. Color Doppler flow imaging highlights vascular structures during real-time EUS examination (Fig. 25–4). By convention, flow toward the transducer is represented in shades of red, whereas flow away from the transducer is represented in shades of blue. Pulsed Doppler, which is a spectral waveform (time– velocity) representation of blood flow, provides a quantitative discrimination of arterial and venous flow. Duplex imaging allows continuous display of the B-mode image and Doppler waveform side by side (Fig. 25–5). Doppler scanning should be routinely performed prior to FNA to identify vessels interposed between the needle and target lesion (Fig. 25–6).

## Imaging Technique

The patient is positioned in the left lateral position and sedated. Insertion of the echoendoscope is relatively blind due to the oblique-viewing optics. Special care must be taken when negotiating the oropharynx, cardia, and pylorus, especially since the distal segment of the echoendoscope containing the transducer is rigid. The pancreatic head is best visualized from the second portion of the duodenum and the duodenal bulb, whereas the pancreatic body and tail are best visualized from the gastric body and fundus. Acoustic contact with the bowel wall is established by removing air from the lumen and filling the balloon with water. Instillation of water into the bowel is a further option to improve acoustic contact, but is usually unnecessary.

Anatomic orientation using the curved linear array system is different from that of radial scanning instruments. The normal pancreas is recognized by its typical granular parenchymal echotexture (Fig. 25–7). Landmark vessels that border the pancreas, such as the su-

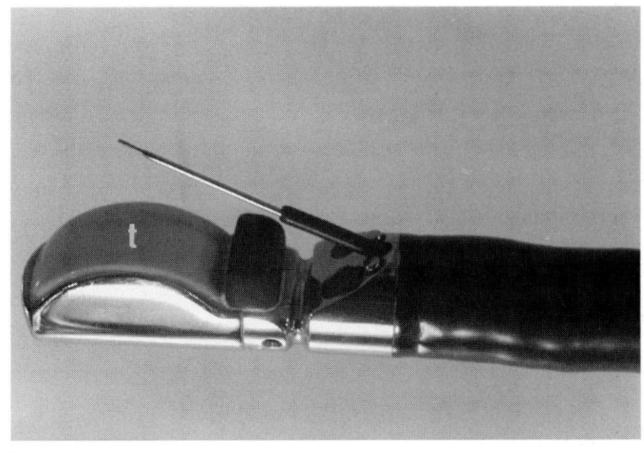


A

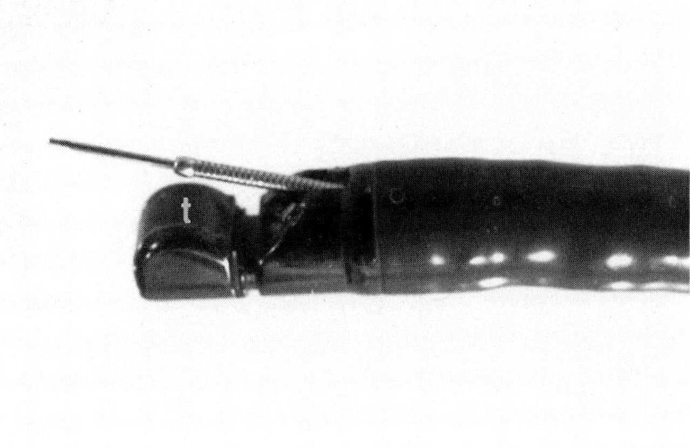


B

**FIGURE 25-3**

Distal end of the curved linear array echoendoscope with needle exiting through the biopsy channel for EUS-guided fine-needle aspiration. (**A**) Pentax FG-32UA; (**B**) Olympus GF-UC30P. t=transducer.

perior mesenteric vein and artery, inferior vena cava, portal vein, and the splenic vein and artery, will assist in orientation. The common bile and pancreatic ducts are seen as either circular or tubular structures depending on the position of the transducer. Color Doppler is very helpful when differentiating ducts from vessels.

## Endoscopic Ultrasound Guided Fine-Needle Aspiration

EUS was developed to overcome the limitations of transabdominal ultrasonographic examination of the pancreas. Subcutaneous fat, air in the bowel, and ascites can impair transabdominal imaging. The superior image quality afforded by EUS has led to its increased use in the diagnostic evaluation of pancreatic disease. However, EUS is limited in its ability to differentiate between inflammatory and malignant diseases. Rösch et al. (1) reported an overall accuracy of 76% for malignant and 46% for focal inflammatory disease. Fine-needle aspiration, by providing a tissue specimen for cytologic and/or histologic examination, aids in establishing a diagnosis.

**TABLE 25-1**

Comparative Product Specifications for Curved Array Echoendoscopes

| | Pentax FG-32UA | Olympus GF-UC30P |
|---|---|---|
| Angle of view | 105° | 85° |
| Distal outer diameter | 12 mm | 12.8 mm |
| Tip deflection | | |
| up/down | 160/160 | 130/90 |
| right/left | 100/100 | 90/90 |
| Working length | 1250 mm | 1255 mm |
| Total length | 1600 mm | 1570 mm |
| Working channel diameter | 2.0 mm | 2.8 mm |
| Elevator | No | Yes (approx. 40° range) |
| Scanning angle | 100° | 180° |
| Frequency | 5 and 7.5 MHz | 7.5 MHz |
| Display mode | M, B, Doppler | M, B, Doppler |

## Needles and Technique

The needle catheters for EUS-guided FNA have gone through several developmental stages. Initially, a stan-

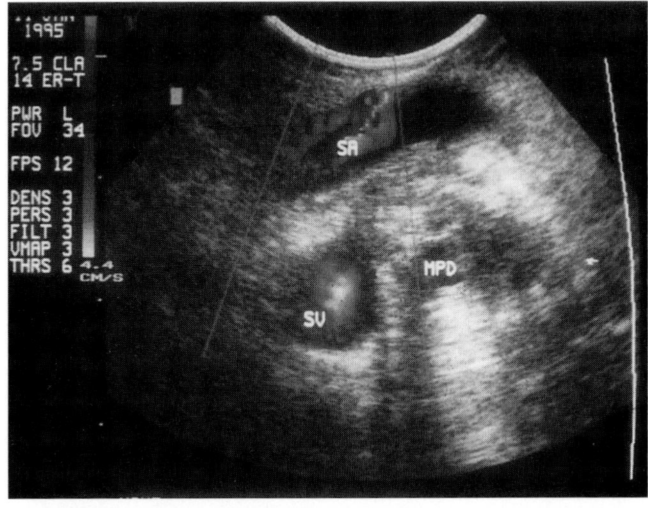


**FIGURE 25-4**

Endosonographic image demonstrating the use of color Doppler to identify vascular structures. SA = splenic artery, SV = splenic vein, MPD = main pancreatic duct (dilated). (*See color insert for color plate.*)

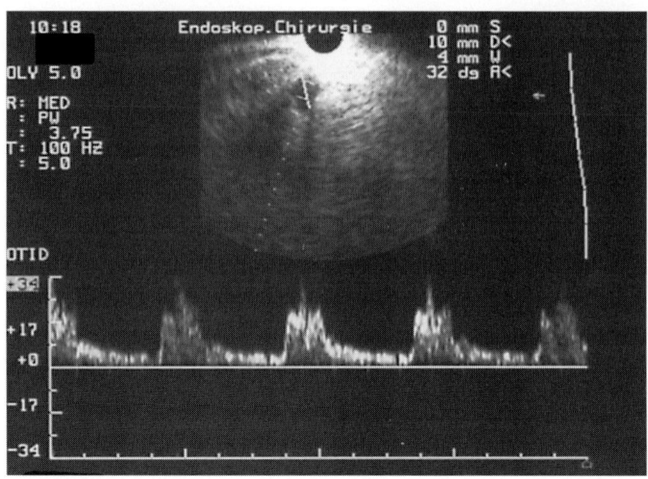


A

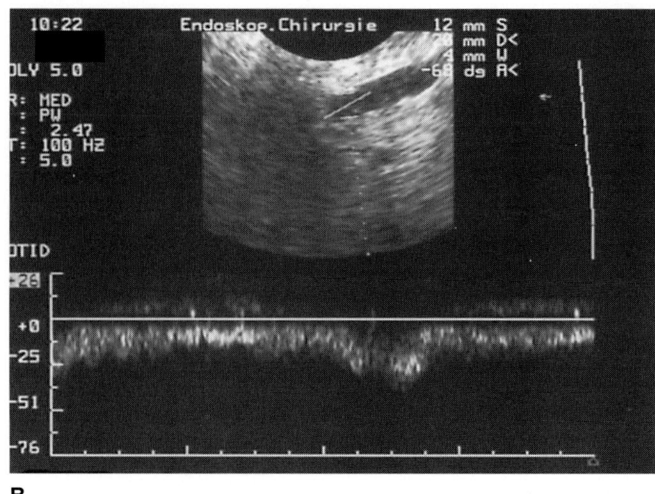


B

**FIGURE 25–5**

Pulsed (duplex) Doppler images. (**A**) High-velocity, pulsatile signal recorded from the splenic artery. (**B**) Low-velocity, broad-spectrum signal recorded from the splenic vein.

dard needle catheter resembling a conventional sclerotherapy needle mounted on an inner plastic catheter was used. This construction lacked adequate transfer of force to the needle tip and was subsequently replaced by a continuous stainless steel needle. However, being substantially stiffer, this needle is capable of perforating the protective Teflon sheath and the working channel of the echoendoscope. Vilmann and co-workers at the Gentofte University Hospital designed a needle catheter (GIP Medizin Technik, Germany) for the Pentax FG-32UA echoendoscope with features that safeguard against damage to the echoendoscope (Fig. 25–8). First, the Teflon sheath is replaced by a protective metal spiral coil sheath. Second, the metal sheath is secured at the inlet of the biopsy port by Luer lock to ensure that the full length of the working channel is protected and the sheath does not slip back into the working channel. Third, a safety catch on the handle locks the position of the retracted needle, ensuring that the needle is protected during advancement through the working channel. We have developed a needle of similar design to the GIP needle for use with the Olympus echoendoscope (Fig. 25–9). The technique of FNA using these needles is detailed below.

**FIGURE 25–6**

Doppler imaging showing a small vessel interposed between the needle (arrow) and target lesion (pancreatic head tumor), illustrating the importance of Doppler scanning prior to FNA. (*See color insert for color plate.*)

1. The lesion is endosonographically visualized and the transducer is positioned to allow optimal needle access. Color Doppler is used to scan the area for vessels. The needle catheter is passed through the instrumentation channel with the needle fully retracted within the protective metal coil sheath (safety catch on, handle is used to lock the position).
2. The handle of the needle catheter is Luer-locked to the inlet of the biopsy channel (see Fig. 25-9). The needle is advanced approximately 1 cm beyond the sheath until the needle is sonographically visualized against the bowel wall. The needle will appear as a hyperechoic linear density and is readily identified by the artifactual acoustic reflections produced by metal.
3. The stylet is withdrawn several millimeters to allow the needle tip to become sharp, after which the needle is advanced into the target tissue under endosonographic guidance (see Fig. 25–10). Stabbing movements may be required to penetrate indurated tissue.
4. Once the lesion has been penetrated, the stylet is advanced to the original position to "unplug" the needle, then fully removed. Suction is applied using a 10- or 20-mL syringe, and the needle is moved to and fro within the target tissue several times.

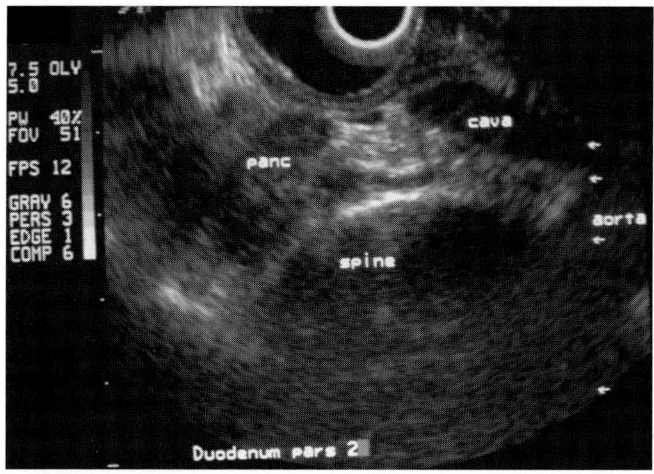


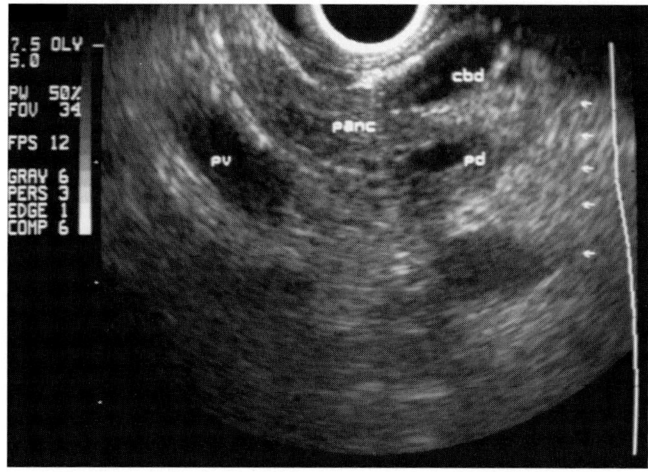


A B

**FIGURE 25–7**

Endosonographic images of the pancreatic head in relation to surrounding anatomy. (**A**) panc = pancreas; cava = inferior vena cava. (**B**) panc = pancreas; CBD = common bile duct; PD = pancreatic duct, PV = portal vein.

5. Before removing the needle, suction is released by disconnecting the syringe. The core specimen is placed in formalin for cell block; the remaining contents are expelled from the needle with a syringe and smeared onto slides for cytologic study (Figs. 25–11, 25–12).

## Results

EUS-guided FNA of a pancreatic lesion was first reported by Vilmann et al. in 1992 (2). The authors biopsied a 3-cm tumor in the head of the pancreas which revealed mucin-secreting columnar epithelial cells suggestive of a mucinous cystadenoma. In a follow-up series the authors reported pancreatic FNA in seven patients, of whom a conclusive cytologic diagnosis was possible in five.

Chang et al. (3) reported EUS-guided FNA of pancreatic tumors in 12 patients, of whom 10 had adequate specimens. Three of the patients had lesions in the body or tail of the pancreas. Wiersema et al. (4) reported EUS-guided FNA in 14 patients, of whom 11 had malignant lesions. The sensitivity of EUS-guided FNA in diagnosing malignancy was 82%. In the largest series published to date, Giovannini et al. (5) performed EUS-guided FNA in 43 patients with pancreatic tumors, of whom 27 had adenocar-

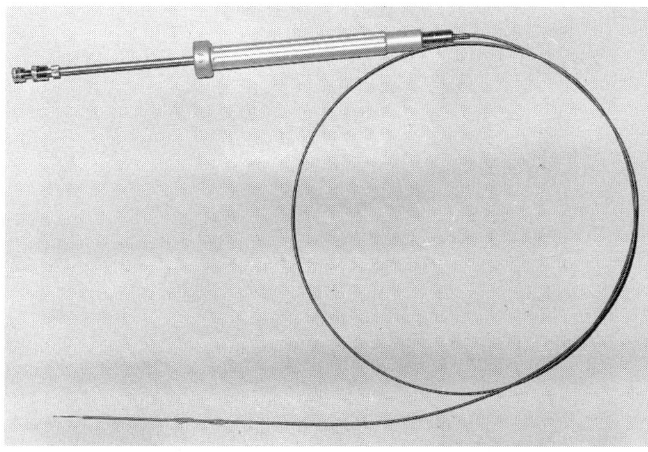

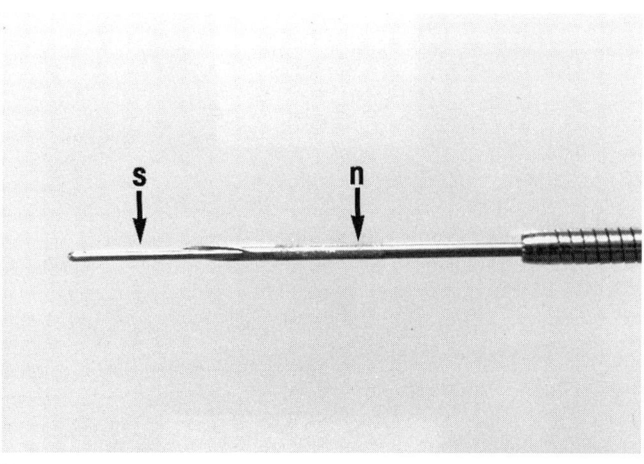


A B

**FIGURE 25–8**

Needle catheter for FNA (Type Hancke/Villmann, GIP Medizin Technik). (**A**) Overview of instrument showing handle with locking piston and metal spiral sheath housing the needle. (**B**) Tip of catheter showing stylet (s) and needle (n) extending from the metal spiral sheath. The end of the needle is sandblasted to enhance echogenicity.

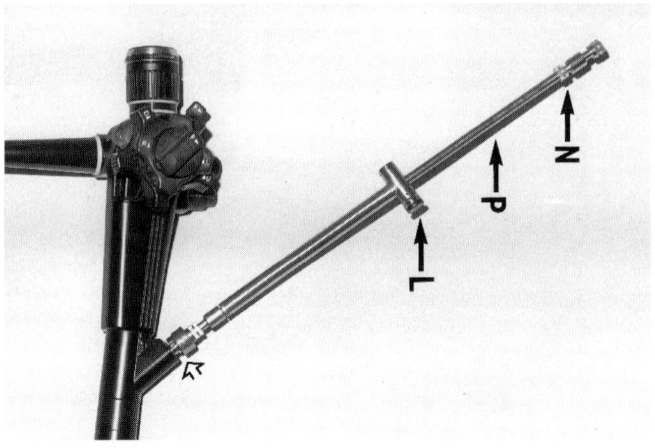


**FIGURE 25-9**

Needle catheter for FNA (prototype) attached to the working channel of the echoendoscope by Luer lock mechanism (open arrow). P = piston; L = lock for piston; N = needle attached to piston.

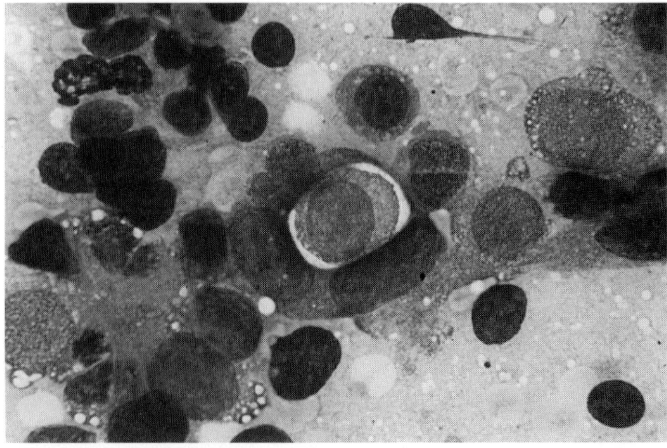

**FIGURE 25-11**

Cytologic smear of a pancreatic fine-needle aspirate showing enlarged, polymorphic nuclei diagnostic of a pancreatic malignancy (adenocarcinoma). (Hematoxylin–esosin, ×400) (*See color insert for color plate.*)

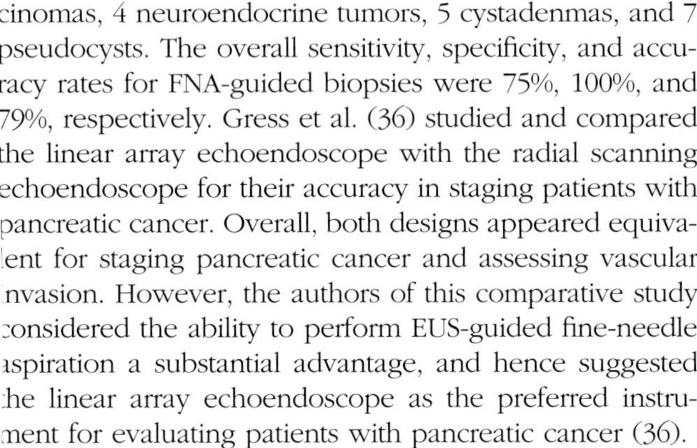

cinomas, 4 neuroendocrine tumors, 5 cystadenmas, and 7 pseudocysts. The overall sensitivity, specificity, and accuracy rates for FNA-guided biopsies were 75%, 100%, and 79%, respectively. Gress et al. (36) studied and compared the linear array echoendoscope with the radial scanning echoendoscope for their accuracy in staging patients with pancreatic cancer. Overall, both designs appeared equivalent for staging pancreatic cancer and assessing vascular invasion. However, the authors of this comparative study considered the ability to perform EUS-guided fine-needle aspiration a substantial advantage, and hence suggested the linear array echoendoscope as the preferred instrument for evaluating patients with pancreatic cancer (36).

We have performed EUS-guided FNA of solid pancreatic tumors using an 18G needle in 45 patients (39). FNA provided an adequate yield for cytologic diagnosis in 34 patients, and a core specimen for histologic diagnosis in 31 patients. Histocytology was positive for malignancy in 13 of 17 patients ultimately diagnosed to have malignant tumors (sensitivity of 76%). FNA demonstrated adenocarcinomas in eleven patients, an anaplastic carcinoma in one patient, and a neuroendocrine tumor in one patient. Of the four patients with false-negative aspirates, adenocarcinomas were diagnosed at surgery in three patients and one patient died two months after FNA.

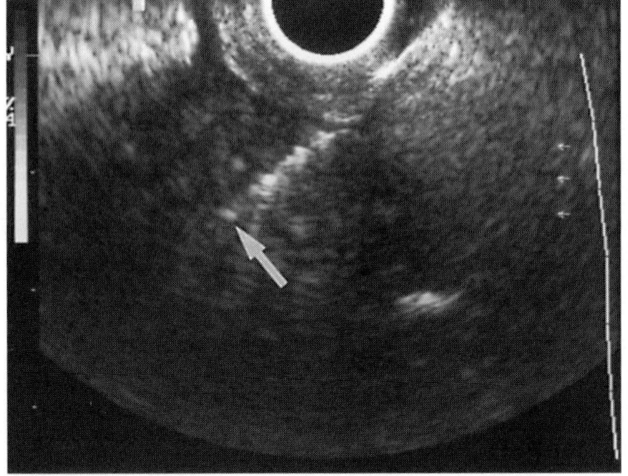

A

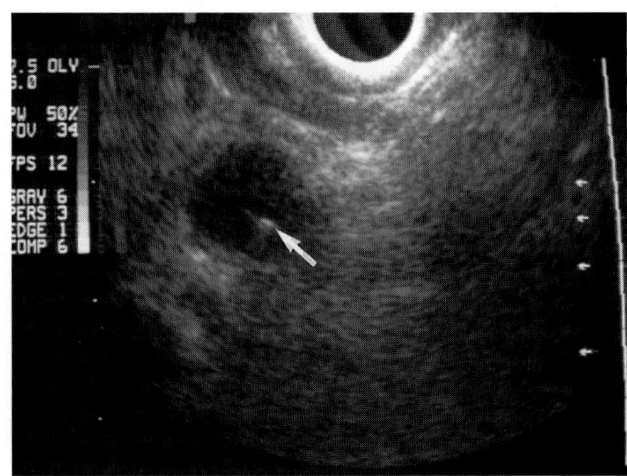

B

**FIGURE 25-10**

Endosonographic images of FNA. (**A**) Tumor in the pancreatic tail. (**B**) Peripancreatic lymph node. The needle is seen lengthwise entering the sonographic field from the right (arrow shows needle tip).

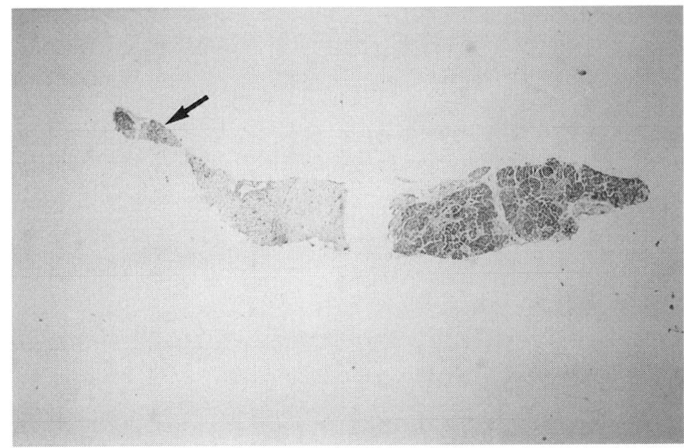

A

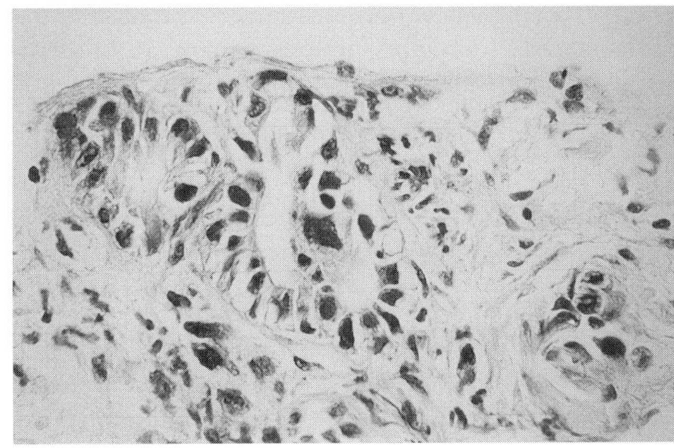

B

**FIGURE 25–12**

Histologic sections of a pancreatic fine-needle biopsy. (**A**) 3-cm core specimen, fragmented in the middle. Histology shows adenocarcinoma (left fragment, arrow) accompanied by changes of chronic pancreatitis (right fragment). (Hematoxylin–eosin ×50) (**B**) Magnified view of area below arrow shows highly atypical epithelial cells forming primitive glandular structures diagnostic of adenocarcinoma. (Hematoxylin–eosin, ×400) (*See color insert for color plates.*)

## Risks and Complications

Major complications resulting from EUS-guided FNA have not been reported; however, experience is still limited. An obvious risk is hemorrhage; this can be minimized if precautions are taken to identify and avoid vascular structures. The application of Doppler is indispensable in this respect (see Fig. 25–6).

Experience with percutaneous fine-needle biopsy has demonstrated extremely low complication rates, usually of minor importance (6–8). Some of the severe complications reported include pancreatitis, peritonitis, ascites, and fistula formation (9–12). Tumor seeding of the percutaneous needle tract and peritoneum is rare, but has aroused significant concern (13–15). Warshaw (15) has cautioned against preoperative percutaneous biopsies in patients with potentially resectable pancreatic tumors. The risk of tumor dissemination with EUS-guided FNA of the pancreas is unknown, but it is likely to be negligible since the peritoneal cavity is not violated and the target organ is directly adjacent to the bowel wall. Lesions in the head of the pancreas are sampled through the duodenum, which is removed if the patient undergoes surgery. In a report on more than 200 consecutive patients in whom EUS-guided fine-needle aspiration biopsy was performed using linear array and radial scanning endosonography, immediate complications were noted in 2% (4 of 208 patients) (30). All complications occurred in patients undergoing EUS-guided fine-needle aspiration of pancreatic lesions and consisted of bleeding and pancreatitis in two patients each.

## Clinical Ultility of Interventional Endosonography

The clinical utility of EUS-guided FNA is a complex issue (33). A tissue diagnosis of malignancy should allow more accurate therapeutic planning. Information regarding the histologic type of malignancy may have direct bearing on treatment strategy; for example, a lymphoma would warrant chemotherapy, whereas an adenocarcinoma would be treated surgically (or palliatively). FNA of a metastatic lymph node (see Fig. 25–10) may establish unresectability and thereby avoid the risks of surgical exploration.

The clinical utility of FNA is more controversial when negative for malignancy. It could be argued that, since a benign tissue diagnosis does not exclude malignancy, any mass lesion suspicious of malignancy warrants surgery. This is particularly true for pancreatic adenocarcinoma, which is typically accompanied by a marked desmoplastic reaction. Percutaneous biopsy has been reported to miss a diagnosis of adenocarcinoma in 50% or more of cases (16,17). In our series of 30 patients who underwent EUS-guided FNA of the pancreas, 3 patients with adenocarcinomas had a false-negative diagnosis of chronic pancreatitis.

EUS-guided FNA may be indicated for reasons not related to management. The patient suspected of having malignant disease may desire the certainty of a tissue diagnosis. The documentation of pancreatic malignancy is generally required prior to palliative chemotherapy or radiation therapy. Some surgeons prefer documentation of malignancy prior to surgery because intraoperative frozen sections prolong surgery and the differentiation of inflammation from malignancy can be problematic.

Indications for interventional endosonography under investigation include EUS-guided celiac plexus neurolysis as a method for improving pain control in patients with intra-abdominal malignancy (32), EUS-guided FNA of the adrenal gland as a method for evaluating adrenal metastases (35), and EUS-guided cholangiopancreatography in patients for whom ERCP is unsuccessful (29,37). Just as the technical aspects of endosonography are in a state of development, so too are the indications for the procedure. Similarly, the interventional aspects of the procedure are in a period of expansion and evolution.

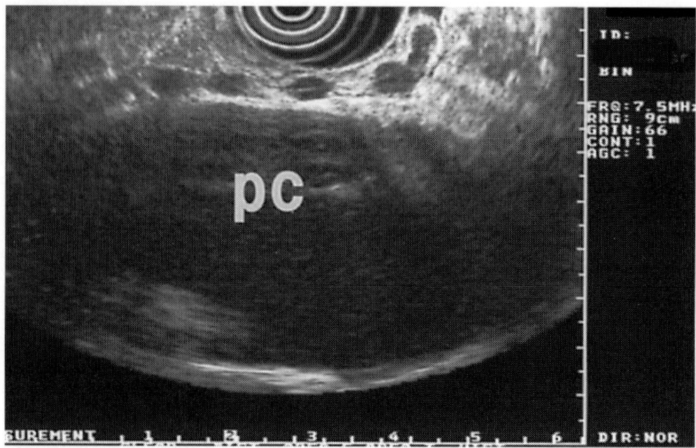


**FIGURE 25–13**

Endosonographic radial scanning image showing multiple vessels sandwiched between the bowel wall and a pseudocyst (PC) in a patient with portal hypertension.

## Pseudocyst puncture and drainage

The management of pancreatic pseudocysts has traditionally been surgical. Although highly effective, surgery may be associated with an average complication rate of 35% and a mortality of 9% (18). This has encouraged the development of nonsurgical approaches. Percutaneous puncture and aspiration under ultrasonographic or CT guidance has been used. Aspiration alone has been found to be ineffective owing to high recurrence rates of up to 71% (18–20). Continuous percutaneous drainage with indwelling catheters reduces the relapse rates, but may be associated with a complication rate ranging from 5% to 60%. Complications include fistula formation, infection, and bleeding (18,21).

Endoscopic transmural drainage of pseudocysts is an alternative nonsurgical approach (22–25). This entails the creation of a fistulous tract between the pseudocyst and the gastric lumen (cystogastrostomy) or duodenal lumen (cystoduodenostomy). Having established endoscopic access to the pseudocyst, a nasocystic catheter or stent can be placed for continuous drainage.

The obvious limitation of endoscopic transmural drainage of pseudocysts is its relatively "blind" approach. In the series by Sahel et al. (24), perforation occurred in two patients in whom no endoscopically visible intraluminal bulging was evident. Consequently, these and other authors have recommended that transmural drainage be restricted to patients with prominent intraluminal bulging on upper endoscopy. Diagnostic EUS prior to endoscopic puncture or EUS-guided cystgastrostomy/cystduodenostomy has been used in some studies to measure intervening wall thickness and to look for vessels that may be interposed between the pseudocyst and bowel lumen (Fig. 25–13) (28,31,38). The ideal approach would be pseudocyst puncture under EUS guidance (31). This should improve the safety of pseudocyst puncture, and increase the number of patients eligible for endoscopic transmural drainage.

### Needle and Technique

Among current commercially available accessories, the "needle knife" catheter is probably best suited for EUS-guided pseudocyst puncture. It consists of a retractable needle catheter housed in an outer Teflon catheter. Current can be applied to the needle to facilitate penetration of the cyst wall, and contrast can be injected through the needle catheter. After puncturing the pseudocyst, the outer sheath is advanced into the pseudocyst and the inner needle catheter is exchanged for a guidewire. The Wilson-Cook needle knife has a detachable handle for removal of the inner needle catheter.

The needle knife catheter was not designed for pseudocyst puncture and has limitations. First, its relatively short needle length (5 mm) and fine caliber may not suffice to penetrate a thick intervening wall. Second, there is a relatively large step-off between the diameters of the needle and outer sheath that may hinder advancement of the sheath into the pseudocyst. We developed a needle catheter for pseudocyst puncture with a longer, thicker needle (15 mm, 20 gauge) and an outer sheath that tapers toward the tip (7 Fr to 4 Fr), thus minimizing any gap between the needle and sheath (26) (see Fig. 25–15). The technique of pseudocyst puncture using this needle is detailed below.

1. After the echoendoscope is introduced, the pseudocyst is localized endosonographically in the stomach or duodenum. Doppler ultrasound is used to identify neighboring vessels (Fig. 25–14).
2. Having determined the optimal site for puncture, the puncture device (Fig. 25–15) is passed through the

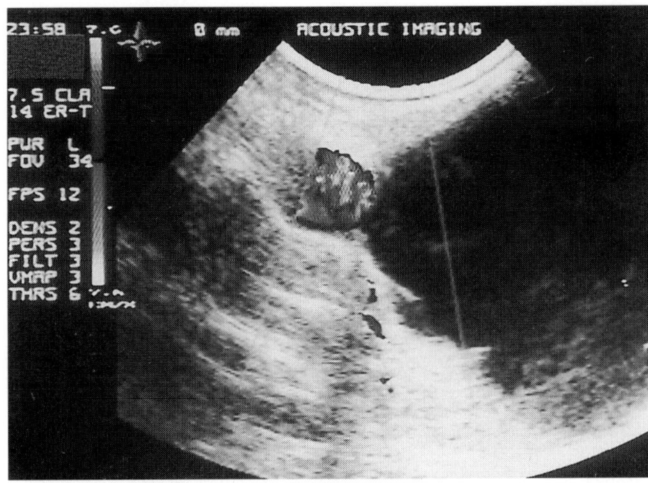


**FIGURE 25–14**

Endosonographic image with Doppler showing a large vessel adjacent to a pseudocyst. (*See color insert for color plate.*)

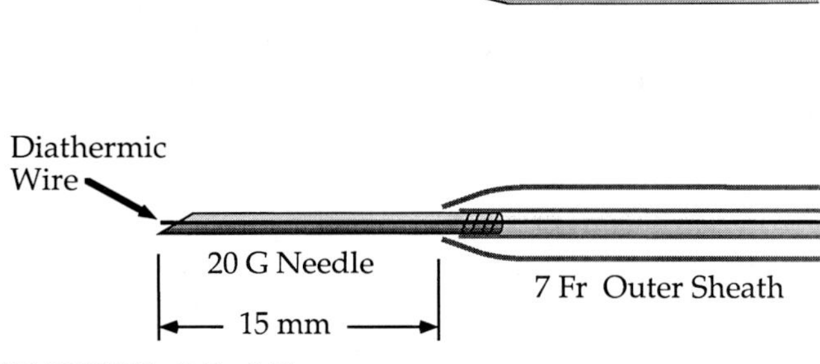


**FIGURE 25–15**

Instrument (prototype) for transmural pseudocyst puncture consisting of a retractable injection catheter contained in an outer 7 Fr Teflon sheath. Current is applied to the injection needle via a diathermic wire which runs through the inner catheter. Note tapering of the outer sheath toward the tip, eliminating step-off between sheath and needle.

instrumentation channel with the injection needle retracted within the outer sheath.

3. The needle is advanced from the sheath and identified on the imaging screen. Pure cutting current is applied to the needle as the pseudocyst is punctured (Fig. 25–16). Cyst entry is usually signaled by a sudden "give" in resistance.
4. Pseudocyst entry is confirmed fluoroscopically by contrast filling of the pseudocyst through the injection catheter (Fig. 25–17A). Injecting fluid into the

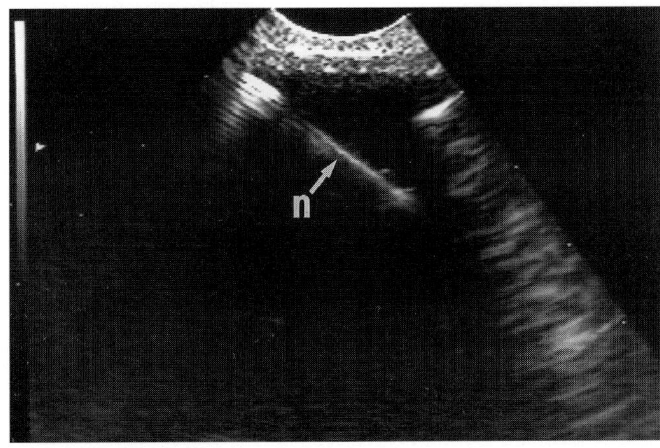


A

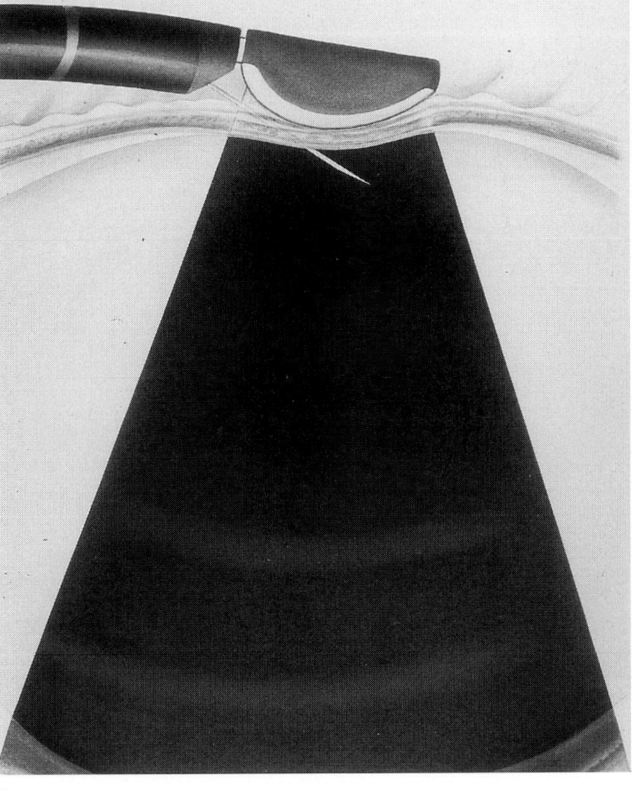

B

**FIGURE 25–16**

Endosonography guided pseudocyst puncture and drainage. (**A**) Endosonographic image of pseudocyst puncture. n = needle. (**B**) Corresponding schematic diagram. (*See color insert for color plate.*)

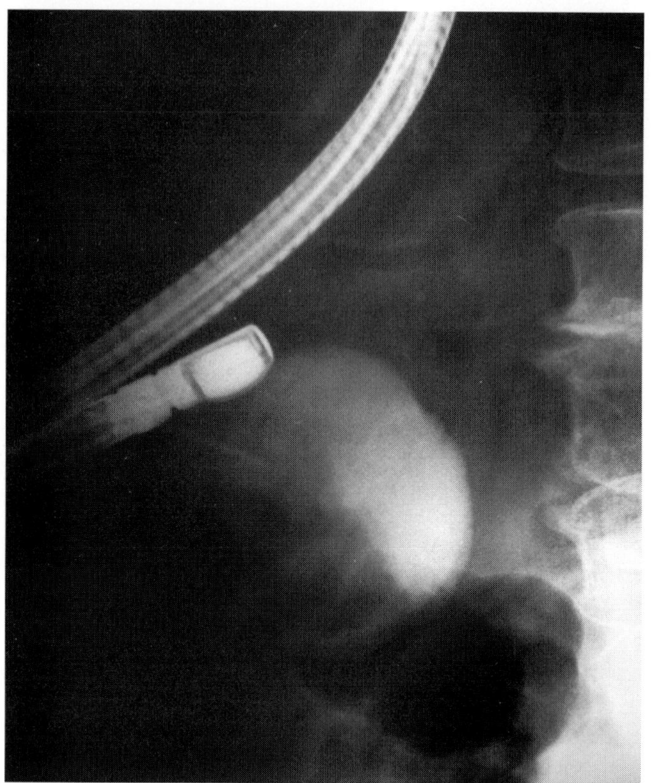

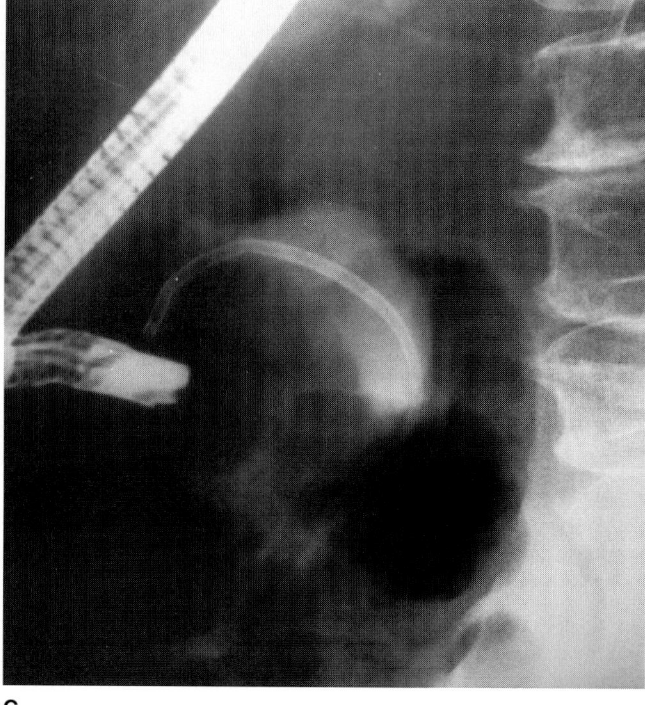

C

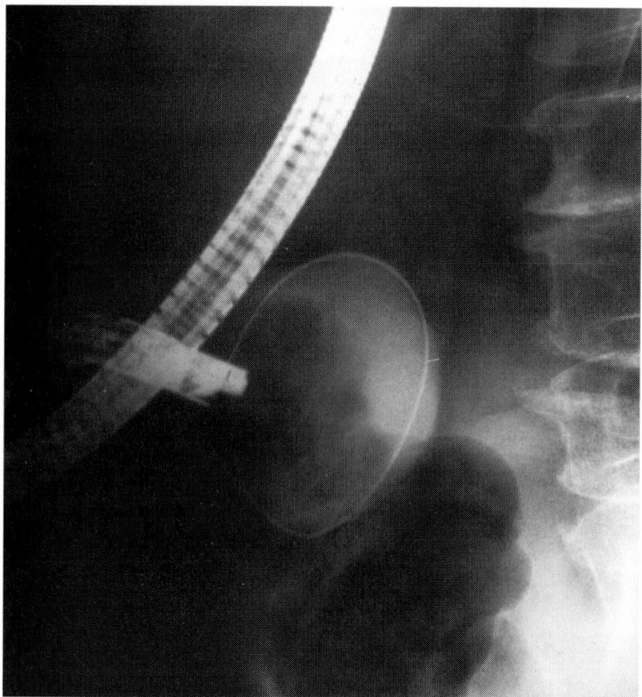

B

**FIGURE 25–17**

Radiologic views of EUS-guided pseudocyst puncture and drainage. (**A**) Contrast filling of pseudocyst. (**B**) Guidewire placement. (**C**) 10 Fr stent draining the pseudocyst.

pseudocyst will also produce a sonographically visible streamline effect.

5. The outer sheath is advanced over the needle catheter into the cyst cavity. Leaving the outer sheath in place, the needle catheter is withdrawn. Pseudocyst contents are aspirated for biochemical analysis and cytology.
6. A conventional 0.035-inch Teflon-coated guidewire is passed into the pseudocyst via the outer sheath. The guidewire should coil several times in the cyst (Fig. 25–17B).
7. A stent or nasocystic catheter is coaxially inserted over the guidewire for continous drainage (Fig. 25–17C). This may require an exchange of the echoendoscope for a duodenoscope. The Olympus convex array echoendoscope (GF-UC30P) has a 2.8-mm working channel and an elevator assembly for insertion of a 7 Fr stent or nasocystic catheter.

## Results

The first case of pseudocyst drainage under EUS-guidance was reported by Grimm et al. in 1992 (27). We have since extended our experience to 27 additional patients with symptomatic pseudocysts (Table 25–2). Pseudocysts were associated with an episode of acute necrotizing pancreatitis in 10 patients and chronic pancreatitis in the remainder. The mean cyst diameter measured by transabdominal sonography or computed tomography was 11 cm. Visible mural bulging on endoscopy was absent in 12 patients. The primary puncture route was transgastric in 23 patients and transduodenal in 4. Pseudocyst puncture was successful in 25 patients and failed in 2 patients due to procedure-related bleeding. In both cases interposed vessels were not endosonographically seen, but Doppler ultrasound was not used to exclude the presence of vessels. We now routinely apply Doppler ultrasound prior to pseudocyst puncture. No other procedure-related complications were observed.

**TABLE 25-2**

**Results of EUS-Guided Pseudocyst Puncture in 27 Patients**

| | |
|---|---|
| Study period | 2/1993–12/1995 |
| Sex | 15 males, 12 females |
| Mean age | 49 (range 22–71) |
| Mean cyst diameter | 11 cm (range 7–20) |
| Technical success | 24 patients |
| Median hospital stay post drainage | 14 days |
| Complications | Procedural bleeding: 2<br>Delayed bleeding: 2<br>Infection due to stent clogging: 13 |
| Cyst resolution | 21 patients |

Of the 25 patients who had successful pseudocyst punctures, stent or nasocystic catheter placement for continuous drainage succeeded in 24. Delayed bleeding occurred in 2 patients and was treated by surgery. Pseudocysts became infected due to stent clogging in 13 patients; infection resolved with stent exchange and nasocystic catheter irrigation in all but 2 patients. Pseudocysts resolved completely in 11 patients and partially (>50% size reduction) in 10. Cyst resolution was accompanied by symptomatic improvement in all patients. During a median follow-up of 140 days cyst recurrence was observed in just one patient.

Because of the high rate of pseudocyst infection, a nasocystic catheter should be placed for 3–5 days, then exchanged for a 10 Fr stent for longer-term drainage. If the pseudocyst contents appear inspissated or already infected, both a stent and nasocystic catheter should be inserted for continuous saline irrigation.

## Conclusion

EUS is a well established modality for imaging of the gastrointestinal tract wall and adjacent structures, especially the pancreas (34). The mainstay of its application has been for diagnostic imaging using radial scanning instruments. Convex linear array instruments have ushered in the potential for interventional applications of EUS analogous to interventional percutaneous procedures under sonographic and CT guidance. Two applications currently undergoing investigation are EUS-guided fine-needle biopsy and drainage of pancreatic pseudocysts. Experience is still limited, but early results are encouraging. Compared to percutaneous intervention, EUS-guided intervention promises to be more accurate and safer owing to the immediate proximity of the target organ.

### References

1. Rösch T, Lorenz R, Braig C, et al. Endoscopic ultrasound in pancreatic tumor diagnosis. Gastrointest Endosc 37:347–352, 1991.
2. Vilmann P, Jacobsen GK, Henriksen FW, Hancke S. Endoscopic ultrasonography with guided fine needle aspiration biopsy in pancreatic disease. Gastrointest Endosc 38:172–173, 1992.
3. Chang KJ, Albers CG, Erickson RA, et al. Endoscopic ultrasound-guided fine needle aspiration of pancreatic carcinoma. Am J Gastroenterol 89:263–266, 1994.
4. Wiersema MJ, Wiersema LM, Khusro Q, et al. Combined endosonography and fine-needle aspiration cytology in the evaluation of gastrointestinal lesions. Gastrointest Endosc 40:199–206, 1994.
5. Giovannini M, Seitz JF, Monges G, et al. Fine-needle aspiration cytology guided by endoscopic ultrasonography: Results in 141 patients. Endoscopy 27:171–177, 1995.
6. Livraghi T, Damascelli B, Lombardi C, et al. Risk in fine-needle abdominal biopsy. J Clin Ultrasound 11:77–81, 1983.
7. Fornari F, Civardi G, Cavanna L, et al. Complications of ultrasonically guided fine-needle abdominal biopsy: Results of a

multicenter Italian study and review of the literature. Scand J Gastroenterol 24:949–955, 1989.
8. Smith EH. Complications of percutaneous abdominal fine-needle biopsy: Review. Radiology 78:253–258, 1991.
9. Dzieniszewski GP, Neher M, Linhart P, et al. Necrotising pancreatitis after ultrasonography guided fine-needle aspiration biopsy. Dtsch Med Wochenschr 107:1438–1440, 1982.
10. Mueller PR, Miketic LM, Simeone JF, et al. Severe acute pancreatitis after percutaneous biopsy of the pancreas. Am J Roentgenol 151:493–494, 1988.
11. Rosenbaum DA, Frost DB. Fine-needle aspiration biopsy of the pancreas complicated by pancreatic ascites. Cancer 65:2537–2538, 1990.
12. Simms MH, Tindall N, Allan RN. Pancreatic fistula following operative fine-needle aspiration. Br J Surg 69:548, 1982.
13. Rashleigh BH, Russell R, Lees WR. Cutaneous seeding of pancreatic carcinoma by fine-needle aspiration biopsy. Br J Radiol 59:182–183, 1986.
14. Lundstedt C, Stridbeck H, Andersson R, et al. Tumor seeding occurring after fine-needle biopsy of abdominal malignancies. Acta Radiol 32:518–520, 1991.
15. Warshaw AL. Implications of peritoneal cytology for staging of early pancreatic cancer. Am J Surg 161:26–30, 1991.
16. Mitchell ML, Bittner CA, Wills JS, et al. Fine needle aspiration cytology of the pancreas. A retrospective study of 73 cases. Acta Cytol 32:447–451, 1988.
17. Parsons LJ, Palmer CH. How accurate is fine-needle biopsy in malignant neoplasia of the pancreas? Arch Surg 124:681–683, 1989.
18. Gumaste VV, Dave PB. Editorial: Pancreatic pseudocyst drainage—The needle or the scalpel? J Clin Gastroenterol 13:500–505, 1991.
19. Torres WE, Evert MB, Baumgartner BR, et al. Percutaneous aspiration and drainage of pancreatic pseudocysts. Am J Roentgenol 147:1007–1009, 1986.
20. Grosso M, Gandini G, Cassinis MC, et al. Percutaneous treatment (including pseudocystogastrostomy) of 74 pancreatic pseudocysts. Radiology 173:493–497, 1989.
21. Gerzof SG, Johnson WC, Robbins AH, et al. Percutaneous drainage of infected pancreatic pseudocysts. Arch Surg 119:888–893, 1984.
22. Kozarek RA, Brayko CM, Harlan J, et al. Endoscopic drainage of pancreatic pseudocysts. Gastrointest Endosc 31:322–328, 1985.
23. Cremer M, Deviere J, Engelholm L. Endoscopic management of cysts and pseudocysts in chronic pancreatitis: Long-term follow-up after 7 years of experience. Gastrointest Endosc 35:1–9, 1989.
24. Sahel J. Endoscopic treatment of pancreatic cysts and pseudocysts. In Beger HG, Buechler M, Malfertheine P (eds): Standards in Pancreatic Surgery. Berlin: Springer Verlag, 1993, pp 526–532.
25. Binmoeller KF, Seifert H, Walter A, et al. Transpapillary and transmural drainage of pancreatic pseudocysts. Gastrointest Endosc 42:219–224, 1995.
26. Binmoeller KF, Seifert H, Soehendra N. Endoscopic pseudocyst drainage: A new instrument for simplified cystoenterostomy. Gastrointest Endosc 40:112, 1994.
27. Grimm H, Binmoeller KF, Soehendra N. Endosonography-guided drainage of a pancreatic pseudocyst. Gastrointest Endosc 38:170–171, 1992.
28. Chan AT, Heller SJ, Van Dam J, Carr-Locke DL, Banks PA. Endoscopic cystgastrostomy: Role of endoscopic ultrasonography. Am J Gastroenterol 91:1622–1625, 1996.
29. Gress F, Ikenberry S, Sherman S, Lehman G. Endoscopic ultrasound-directed pancreatography. Gastrointest Endosc 44:736–739, 1996.
30. Gress FG, Hawes RH, Savides TJ, Ikenberry SO, Lehman GA. Endoscopic ultrasound-guided fine-needle aspiration biopsy using linear array and radial scanning endosonography. Gastrointest Endosc 45:243–250, 1997.
31. Wiersema MJ. Endosonography-guided cystoduodenostomy with a therapeutic ultrasound endoscope. Gastrointest Endosc 44:614–617, 1996.
32. Wiersema MJ, Wiersema LM. Endosonography-guided celiac plexus neurolysis. Gastrointest Endosc 44:656–662, 1996.
33. Cahn M, Chang K, Nguyen P, Butler J. Impact of endoscopic ultrasound with fine-needle aspiration on the surgical management of pancreatic cancer. Am J Surg 172:470–472, 1996.
34. Tenner SM, Banks PA, Wiersema MJ, Van Dam J. Evaluation of pancreatic disease by endoscopic ultrasonography. Am J Gastroenterol 92:18–26, 1997.
35. Chang KJ, Erickson RA, Nguyen P. Endoscopic ultrasound (EUS) and EUS-guided fine-needle aspiration of the left adrenal gland. Gasrointest Endosc 44:568–572, 1996.
36. Gress F, Savides T, Cummings O, Sherman S, Lehman G, Zaidi S, Hawes R. Radial scanning and linear array endosonography for staging pancreatic cancer: A prospective randomized comparison. Gastrointest Endosc 45:138–142, 1997.
37. Wiersema MJ, Sandusky D, Carr R, Wiersema LM, Erdel WC, Frederick PK. Endosonography-guided cholangiopancreatography. Gastrointest Endosc 43:102–106, 1996.
38. Gerolami R, Giovannini M, Laugier R. Endoscopic drainage of pancreatic pseudocysts guided by endosonography. Endoscopy 29:106–108, 1997.
39. Binmoeller KF, Thul R, Rathod V, et al, Endoscopic ultrasound-guided, 18-gauge, fine needle aspiration biopsy of the pancreas using a 2.8 mm channel convex array echoendoscope. Gastrointest Endos 47:123–129, 1998.

CHAPTER

# Neuroendocrine Tumors

Charles J. Lightdale
Frank Van de Mierop

The diagnosis of functional neuroendocrine tumor is made on the basis of symptoms, signs, and laboratory tests. Of the various neuroendocrine tumors affecting the pancreas, insulinomas and gastrinomas are much more common than somatostatinomas, VIPomas, or glucagonomas. Insulinomas are located in the pancreas 99% of the time, whereas gastrinomas, either single or multiple, are located in peripancreatic sites in 30–45% of cases, particularly in the duodenum, lymph nodes, and liver (in the setting of metastases from an unknown primary gastrinoma) (1,2). The diagnosis of gastrinoma warrants a thorough endoscopic examination of the stomach and duodenum, using both forward and side viewing instruments (1,2). About 90% of insulinomas can be localized at surgery by palpation and intraoperative ultrasonography (IOUS), whereas up to 30% of gastrinomas remain occult, even after selective angiography with venous sampling and transduodenal illumination. If the precise location of a pancreatic neuroendocrine tumor can be determined preoperatively, it serves to confirm the diagnosis and facilitate surgery.

## Noninvasive Localization

Noninvasive imaging studies should be performed first. Transabdominal ultrasonography, CT (with intravenous contrast and dynamic technique), and MRI have all been utilized. However, small insulinomas and gastrinomas often cannot be identified (3). Noninvasive imaging at best locates only 40–60% of functional neuroendocrine tumors (percentages prior to octreotide scanning studies) (4). Whether technical advances such as spiral CT imaging, CT angiography, or MRI will improve the detection rate remains to be shown. Gastrinomas have recently been localized using radionuclide somatostatin receptor imaging (5). Octreotide (somatostatin-analog) scanning uses iodine-123 or indium-111–labeled octreotide. Sensitivity for gastrinoma with octreotide scanning varies in different studies between 80% and 90% (6). However, insulinomas have fewer somatostatin receptors compared to gastrinomas, accounting for a lower sensitivity for insulinoma detection.

## Invasive Tests

Upper gastrointestinal endoscopy in Zollinger-Ellison syndrome should include a careful search for duodenal and gastric tumors, which may even be amenable to endoscopic removal (7). Selective angiography may demonstrate small tumors not evident on dynamic CT, and, while technically demanding, transhepatic portal venous sampling may help localize tumors to one region of the pancreas. However, a frustrating minority of tumors remain occult.

## Endoscopic Ultrasonography

It has been well demonstrated that EUS can localize small cancers of the pancreas not detected by other imaging tests; it allows careful imaging of the pancreas through the wall of the duodenum and stomach as well as imaging of the duodenal wall (looking for submucosal gastrinomas) (8,9). Thus, it was logical to apply this method for localization of pancreatic neuroendocrine tumors. It was found that small endocrine tumors of the pancreas, even those in the 0.5-cm range seen in multiple endocrine neoplasia (MEN) syndrome type I, could be imaged by EUS (10) (Figs. 26–1 through 26–5). Larger tumors, of course, were easier to image (11).

In a multicenter study (12), it was decided to specifically address the issue of the ability of EUS to detect pancreatic endocrine tumors in patients where transabdominal ultrasonography and CT were negative. There were 39 tumors in 37 patients studied, all of whom underwent EUS, with 22 having selective angiography. All the tumors were confirmed by surgical excision and by immunohistologic examination. They consisted of 31 insulinomas, 7 gastrinomas, and 1 glucagonoma. The patients all had negative CT scans and transabdominal ultrasounds. The tumors were small, ranging in size from 0.5 to 2.5 cm in diameter, with a mean diameter of 1.4 cm. All but one of the patients were cured of their disease, as determined by at least six months of clinical and laboratory follow-up.

EUS localized 32 of the 39 tumors (sensitivity 82%), and no tumor was incorrectly localized. The size of the tumor imaged on EUS was within 2 mm of the size found at pathology. EUS was significantly more sensitive than angiography in the 22 patients who had both procedures (82% vs. 27%, $p < .05$). In 19 patients evaluated for pancreatic endocrine tumors who were subsequently determined not to have this condition (controls), EUS was negative in 18 (specificity 95%).

In most cases, endocrine tumors appeared as homogeneous, relatively hypoechoic masses with smooth margins (see Figs. 26–1, 26–2, and 26–3); but there were exceptions, with some tumors being relatively echo-rich or exhibiting an echopattern similar to that of the sur-

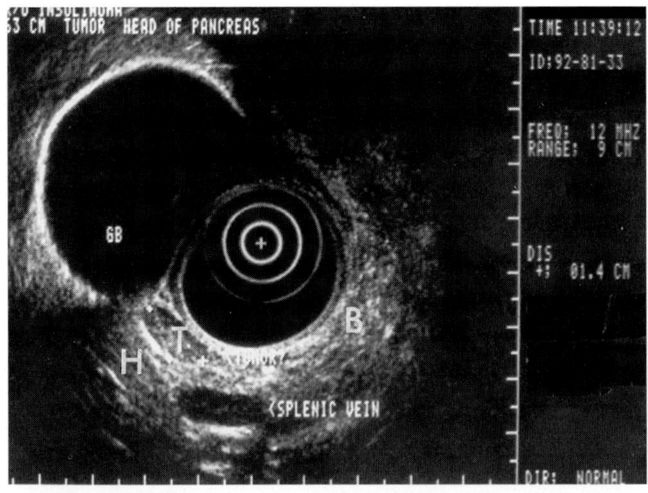


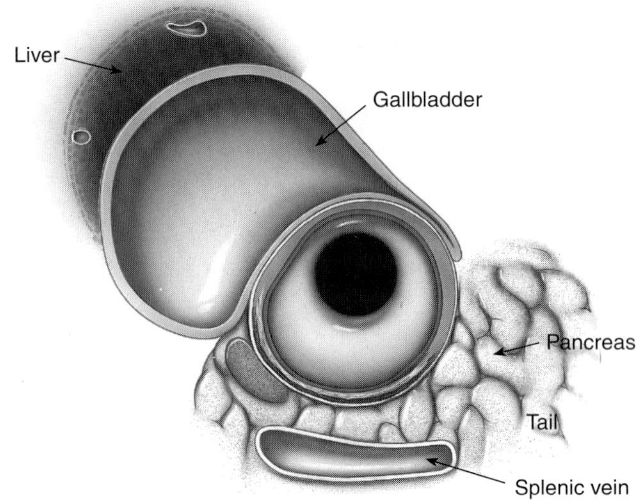


**FIGURE 26–1**

EUS of endocrine tumor in the head of the pancreas. The transducer is in the duodenal bulb. GB is the gallbladder, T is the tumor in the head of the pancreas seen just above the splenic vein.

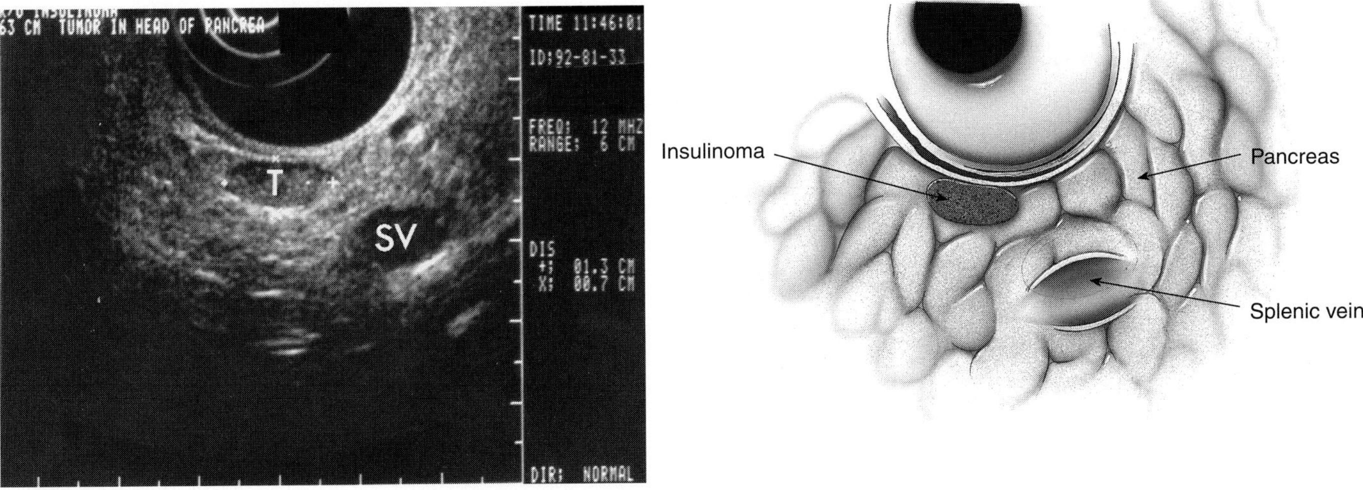


**FIGURE 26–2**

View of the head of the pancreas, showing the same tumor (T) as in Figure 26–1, demonstrating it to be 1.3 × 0.7 cm in size with decreased echogenicity compared to the surrounding pancreas above the splenic vein (SV).

rounding pancreas. Cystic areas and calcification were also seen, as were irregular or echo-poor margins. No differences were found between functional and nonfunctional neuroendocrine tumors (13). Some authors have described an echo-free halo around the tumor or central echo-rich foci (14).

In the one false-positive patient in the multicenter study, a hyperplastic lymph node on the surface of the pancreas was misinterpreted (12). It can be difficult to distinguish such lymph nodes from polyploid endocrine tumors emerging from the pancreatic surface. Duodenal wall tumors are similar in appearance to other tumors localized in the mucosa and submucosa (relatively hypoechoic, homogeneous, and well defined). As in other tumors, especially gastrinomas, infiltration into adjacent organs or vessels should be looked for as well as lymph node metastasis.

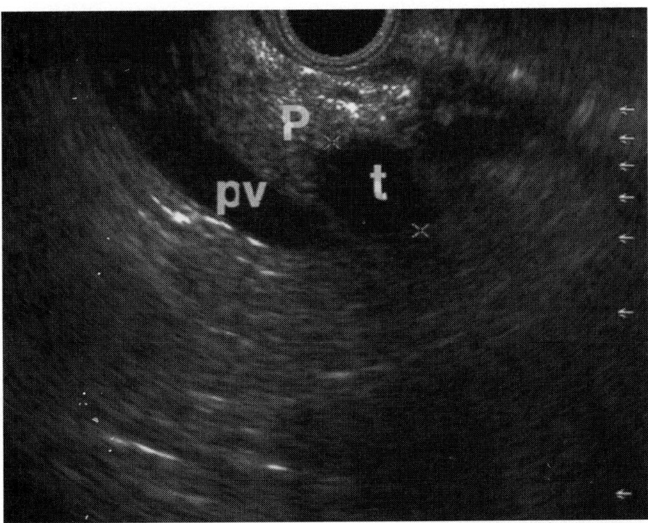


**FIGURE 26–3**

EUS of endocrine tumor (t) in the head of the pancreas (p) imaged from the duodenal bulb using the Olympus GF-UC30P electronic echoendoscope. The lesion near the portal vein (pv) is measured between the cursors at 13 mm. Linear technology allows EUS-guided fine needle aspiration of such lesions for cytology confirmation.

Other recent studies have shown similar results for EUS in imaging pancreatic neuroendocrine tumors. Yamada et al. (15) were able to localize 10 of 10 tumors less than 2.0 cm in size with EUS. Glover et al. (16) used EUS to successfully localize 12 of 15 insulinomas, one glucagonoma, and a diffuse pancreatic abnormality in a patient with MEN I syndrome. Again, in these reports EUS was more sensitive than transabdominal ultrasound (15,16) and abdominal CT scan (16). In 23 patients operated on for pancreatic endocrine tumors reported by Palazzo et al. (17), EUS localized 85% of the tumors compared to only 8.5% with transabdominal ultrasound and 17% with CT scan. Zimmer et al. (4) found an overall sensitivity of 88% for EUS in 18 patients studied. When the location of the neuroendocrine tumors was related to the sensitivity, it appeared that the sensitivity was different: 94% for pancreatic compared to 75% for extrapancreatic tumors. Sensitivities were also related to size and type of tumor (see Table 26–1).

It seems clear from a number of reports that EUS can localize small neuroendocrine tumors that cannot be imaged by other methods. The advantages of EUS imaging preoperatively will need to be compared with preoperative and intraoperative stimulated venous sampling

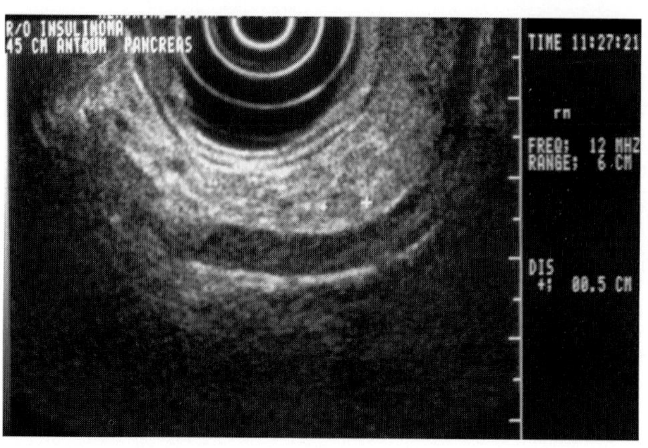


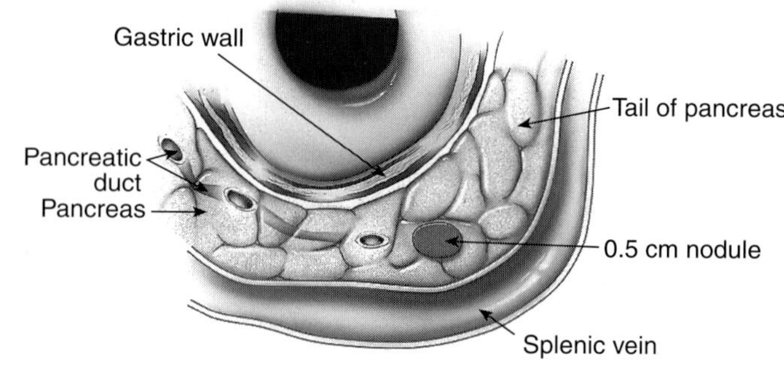


**FIGURE 26–4**

EUS through the posterior wall of the stomach in a patient with MEN I syndrome shows a 0.5-cm nodule in the tail of the pancreas above the splenic vein. Multiple small pancreatic nodules were evident in this patient.

methods and intraoperative ultrasound (1,2). The data so far indicate that with EUS small insulinomas are more easily imaged than gastrinomas, probably because of the possible extrapancreatic location of gastrinomas (see Fig. 26–5) (6). Because of the high specificity of EUS, a negative pancreatic EUS with biochemical evidence of gastrinoma points strongly toward an extrapancreatic location (13,18). Octreotide scanning should be performed in this setting. Its sensitivity for extrapancreatically located gastrinomas is 62% compared to 47% for pancreatic gastrinomas (4). Hypoechoic tumors are more easily detected than more echogenic tumors, and the distinction between a pedunculated tumor and a peripancreatic lymph node can be difficult, especially for insulinomas (12,15–17). In a recent report of 12 patients, endoscopic ultrasound scanning of the pancreas with a linear array echoendoscope (see Fig. 26–3) yielded similar results, with a sensitivity of 86% in localizing pancreatic islet cell tumors (18). Bansal et al. found no difference between linear and radial scanning EUS in this regard.

EUS is complex and can be tedious. Yet, in experienced hands, EUS has been found to be a highly sensitive and specific procedure for the localization of pancreatic endocrine tumors. It should be used following noninvasive imaging tests when these are not definitive.

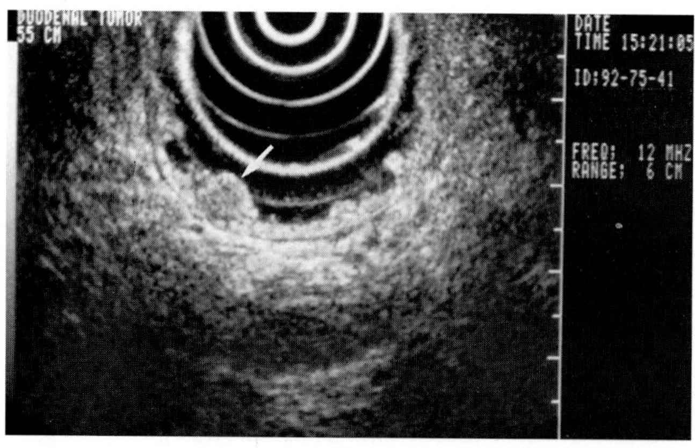


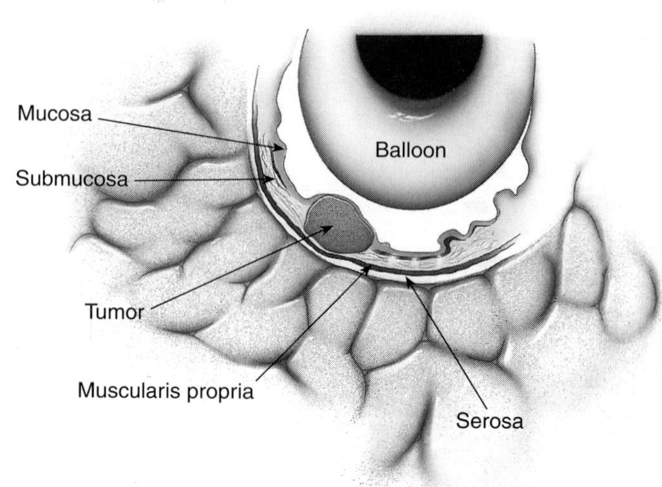


**FIGURE 26–5**

EUS showing a 0.6-cm neuroendocrine tumor localized to the deep mucosa and submucosa of the descending duodenum.

TABLE 26-1

Sensitivities of EUS Compared to SRS and MRI (n = 25)

| Sensitivity | EUS | MRI | SRS |
|---|---|---|---|
| Gastrinoma | 80 | 60 | 100 |
| Insulinoma | 87 | 0 | 12 |
| < 2 cm | 88 | 0 | 35 |
| Pancreatic lesion | 94 | 29 | 47 |
| Extrapanc. lesion | 75 | 12 | 62 |
| TOTAL | 88 | 24 | 52 |

[1]Data from ref. 17.

## References


1. Krudy AG, Doppman JL, Jensen RT, et al. Localization of islet cell tumors by dynamic CT: Comparison with plain CT, arteriography, sonography, and venous sampling. Am J Roentgenol 143:585–589, 1984.
2. Galiber AK, Reading CC, Charboneau JW, et al. Localization of pancreatic insulinoma: Comparison of pre- and intraoperative US with CT and angiography. Radiology 166:405–408, 1988.
3. Frucht H, Doppman JL, Norton JA, et al. Gastrinomas: Comparison of MR imaging with CT, angiography, and US. Radiology 171: 713–717, 1989.
4. Zimmer T, Ziegle K, Bader M, Fett U, Hamm B, Riechen EO, Wiedenmann B. Localization of neuroendocrine tumors of the upper gastrointestinal tract. Gut 35:471–475, 1994.
5. Lamberts SWJ, Bakker WH, Reubi JC, Krenning EP. Somatostatin receptor imaging in the localization of endocrine tumors. N Engl J Med 323:1246–1249, 1990.
6. Krenning EP, Kwekkeboom DJ, Oei HY, de Jong RJB, Dop FJ, de Herder JC, Reubi JC, Lanberts SWJ. Somatostatin-receptor scintigraphy in carcinoids, gastrinomas and Cushing's syndrome. Digestion 55(suppl 3):54–59, 1994.
7. Straus E, Raufman JP, Samuel S, Waye JD, Metz DC, Pisegna JR, Jensen RT. Endoscopic cure of the Zollinger-Ellison syndrome. Gastrointest Endosc 38:709–711, 1992.
8. Yasuda K, Mukai H, Fujimoto S, Nakajima M, Kawai K. The diagnosis of pancreatic cancer by endoscopic ultrasonography. Gastrointest Endosc 34:1–8, 1988.
9. Rösch T, Lorenz R, Braig C, Feuerbach S, Siewert JR, Schusdziarra V, Classen M. Endoscopic ultrasound in pancreatic tumor diagnosis. Gastrointest Endosc 37:347–352, 1991.
10. Lees WR. The pancreas: Differential diagnosis and pancreatitis. In Lightdale CJ (ed): Endoscopic Ultrasonography. Gastrointestinal Endoscopy Clinics of North America, Philadelphia: W.B. Saunders, 1992, pp 657–672.
11. Lightdale CJ, Bótet JF, Woodruff JM, Brennan MF. Localization of endocrine tumors of the pancreas with endoscopic ultrasonography. Cancer 68:1815–1820, 1991.
12. Rösch T, Lightdale CJ, Bótet JF, et al. Localization of pancreatic endocrine tumors by endoscopic ultrasonography. N Engl J Med 326:1721–1726, 1992.
13. Fishbeyn VA, Norton JA, Benya RV, et al. Assessment and prediction of long-term cure in patients with the Zollinger-Ellison syndrome: The best approach. Ann Intern Med 119:199–206, 1993.
14. Hayashi Y, Naburawa S, Kinoto E. Clinicopathological analysis of endoscopic ultrasonograms in pancreatic mass lesions. Endoscopy 21:121–125, 1989.
15. Yamada M, Komoto E, Naito Y, Tsukamoto Y, Mitake M. Endoscopic ultrasonography in the diagnosis of pancreatic islet cell tumors. J Ultrasound Med 10:271–276, 1991.
16. Glover JR, Shorvon PJ, Lees WR. Endoscopic ultrasound for localization of islet cell tumors. Gut 33:108–110, 1992.
17. Palazzo L, Roseau G, Salmeron M. Endoscopic ultrasonography in the preoperative localization of pancreatic endocrine tumors. Endoscopy 24(suppl 1):350–353, 1992.
18. Bansal R, Kochman ML, Bude R, Nostrant TT, Elta GH, Thompson NW, Scheiman JM. Localization of neuroendocrine tumors utilizing linear array endoscopic ultrasound. Gastrointest Endosc 42(1): 76–79, 1995.

SECTION

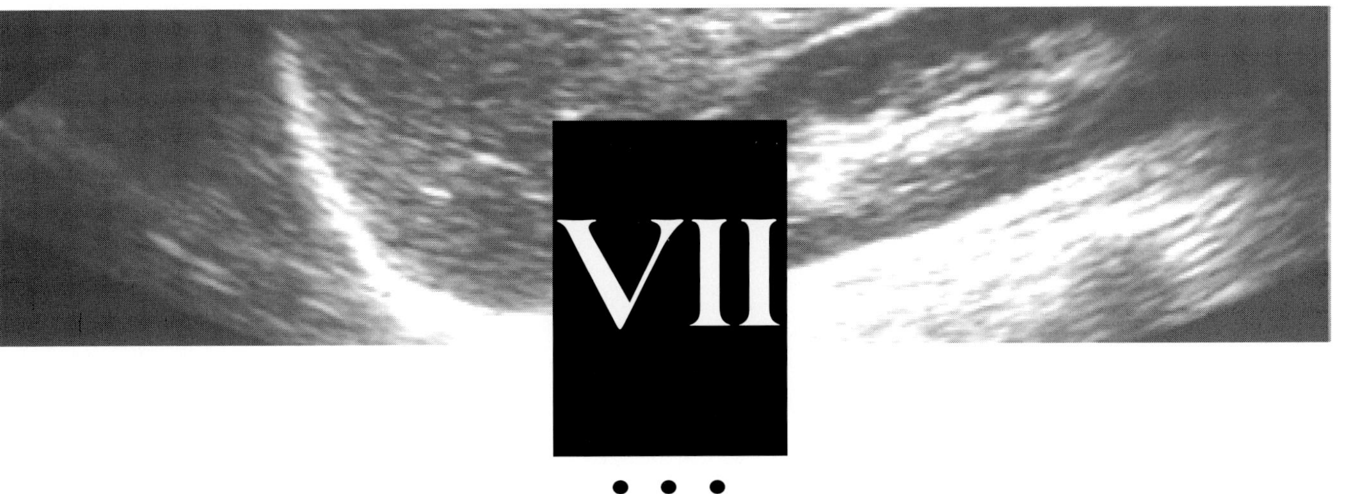


# Endosonography of the Colon and Rectum

CHAPTER

# Endosonography of the Colon and Rectum

## NORMAL ANATOMY USING THE RADIAL SCANNING ECHOENDOSCOPE

Thomas Rösch
Meinhard Classen

Endoluminal ultrasound of the rectum via rigid ultrasound probes has been an established technique for several years. Its main clinical application has been for staging rectal cancer. However, it has also been used in various benign diseases (1–3). Recently, an ultrasound colonoscope (echocolonoscope) has been developed which allows for a combined endoscopic and endosonographic evaluation throughout the large intestine (4). Experience with this new instrument and technique is growing.

## Technique

The echocolonoscope is a flexible, forward-viewing instrument (Fig. 27–1). The rigid distal tip of the insertion tube contains the ultrasound transducer which produces a radial sector scan at an ultrasound frequency of 7.5 MHz. Using the most recently modified echocolonoscope, the CF-UM3 and CF-UM20, there are two methods of establishing the necessary fluid interface between

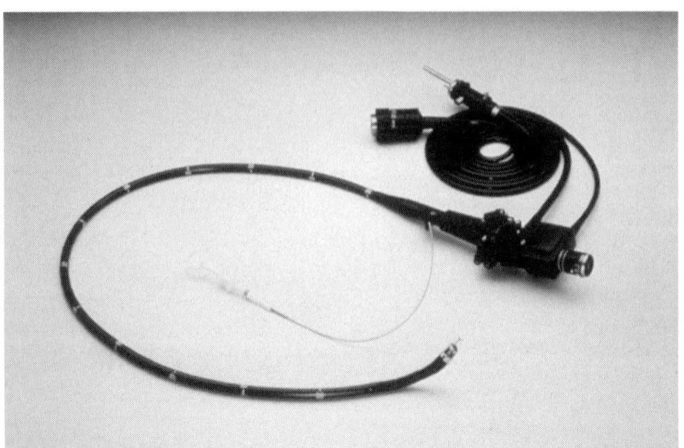

**FIGURE 27-1**

Echocolonoscope (Olympus CF-UM3).

the transducer and colonic wall: water filling of the respective bowel segment and the balloon method, similar to that in upper gastrointestinal endosonography. The two methods are complementary because the balloon may not be large enough to fill the entire lumen and filling the bowel with water may be insufficient to provide the proper acoustic interface.

The preparation for colonic endosonography is conventional (e.g., lavage with a balanced electrolyte solution). Midazolam or diazepam are commonly used for premedication. In a preliminary study, we found that additional analgesic and/or sedative drugs were not required (4). We reached the cecum in 19 of the first 20 patients we examined. The time required to reach the cecum was slightly longer than that for conventional colonoscopy (4,5). Shimizu and colleagues also reported rapid achievement of instrument passage into the descending or transverse colon (6). A complete examination of the colon can be performed and biopsies can be obtained, but there are not enough data on the safety of electrosurgical snare polypectomy with this instrument. It must be stated, however, that the rigid tip of the instrument restricts maneuverability to some degree. This might limit the use of the echocolonoscope for more difficult therapeutic procedures.

In clinical practice, many of the patients examined by colonoscopic ultrasonography have already undergone colonoscopy in which a lesion was detected. In general, colonic EUS should be restricted to the lesion and region of the colon of interest because it is very time-consuming to achieve the necessary fluid interface in the entire colon. This makes complete EUS examination of the entire large bowel impractical.

## The Rectum

Cancer staging is the main indication for endorectal ultrasonography, although larger adenomas, perimural inflammatory lesions, and anal sphincter morphology have been investigated by EUS (1,4,7,8). In colonic EUS, which may be applied for all of these indications, intraluminal lesions are targeted under visual control. However, the cost of flexible endoluminal ultrasound of the colon greatly exceeds that of ultrasonography with a rigid endorectal probe. This raises the question of which type of instrument, an echoendoscope or nonoptical rigid probe, should be used in the rectum.

Tio and Tytgat (9) compared a rigid echoprobe (5 MHz) with a side-viewing echoendoscope (7.5 MHz) intended for upper gastrointestinal EUS in 20 patients with rectal and perirectal diseases. The flexible instrument was superior with respect to visualization of small tumors and lymph nodes adjacent to the rectal wall and for differentiating adenoma from carcinoma. However, the detection of more distant lymph nodes and perirectal lesions (e.g., abscesses), was better with the rigid instrument. These differences are probably at least in part due to the different ultrasound frequencies of the two systems. Similar results were obtained in a recent study comparing the rigid probes with the flexible ultrasound colonoscope in patients with colorectal carcinoma (10).

## Normal Colonic and Pericolonic Anatomy

The normal colonic wall consists of five different echolayers (Fig. 27–2), although in some in vitro studies seven or even nine layers have been described, depending on the ultrasound frequency and examination technique used (1,4). Colonic specimens from humans have been shown to exhibit five echolayers (11) and the relationship of these to the actual anatomic features of the bowel wall is thought to be very similar to that for the upper gastrointestinal tract. For clinical purposes, the second hyperechoic layer corresponds to the submucosa and the outer hypoechoic band to the muscularis propria.

The pericolonic structures and organs that are visualized by colonic EUS while withdrawing the instrument from the cecum are portions of both kidneys, liver, pancreas, and spleen as well as pelvic organs such as urinary bladder, prostate, and uterus (Figs. 27–3 through 27–5).

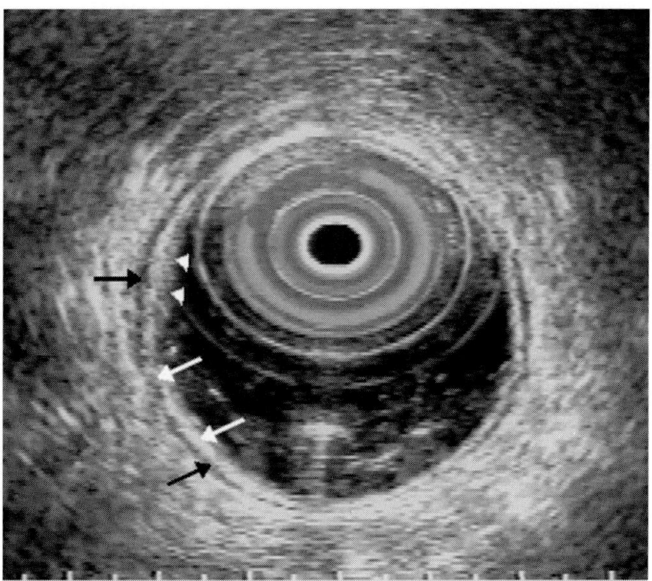

**FIGURE 27-2**

Normal colonic wall with five-layer structure (white arrows: submucosa; black arrows: muscularis propria). Due to balloon compression, the mucosa is only partly visible (arrowheads).

## Potential Indications for Colonic EUS

### Colorectal Cancer Staging

There are only limited data on colonic cancer staging by echocolonoscopy (Figs. 27–6 through 27–9). Tio et al. (12) assessed the accuracy of colorectal cancer staging using rigid probes and flexible echoendoscopes. The accuracy for depth of tumor invasion (T stage) in the rectum and colon was 80% and 96%, respectively. The presence or absence of lymph node metastases was correctly predicted in 60% of patients (for colonic and rectal cancer together). Visualization of colonic tumors was successful in just 74% of 72 colorectal cancers, including 35 suprarectal tumors, in the series of Shimizu et al. (6). For the tumors that could be visualized, EUS correctly estimated the depth of tumor penetration in 85%. If all patients are considered, including those in whom the tumor could not be visualized, the overall accuracy was 63%. The reasons for the relatively low rate of visualization were not given. Metastatic lymph nodes were recognized in only 38% of cases. This might be expected since radical lymphadenectomy often discloses lymph node metastases along vascular structures at sites distant from the primary cancer and therefore beyond the scope

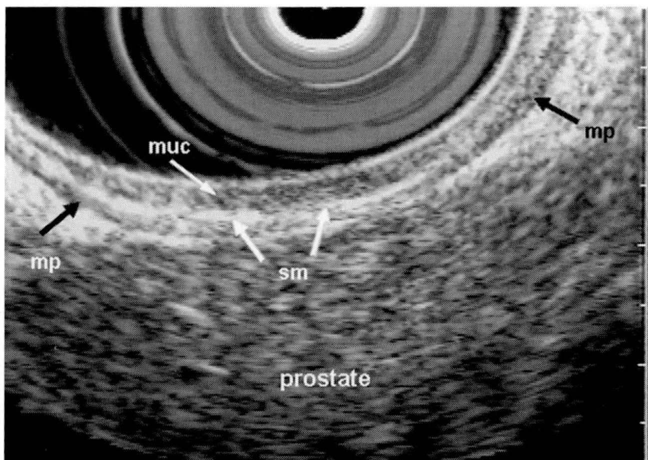


**FIGURE 27-3**

Normal colonic wall on EUS consisting of mucosa (muc), submucosa (sm), and muscularis propria (mp). The surrounding hyperechoic serosa cannot be distinguished from the hyperechoic perirectal tissue. The prostate gland is also seen.

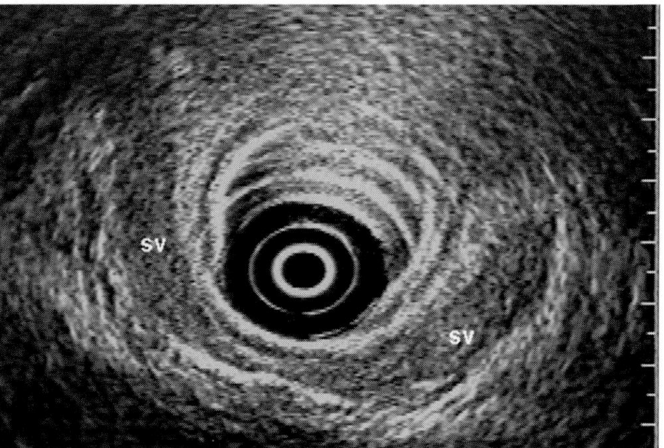


**FIGURE 27-4**

Pararectal anatomy: The seminal vesicles (sv).

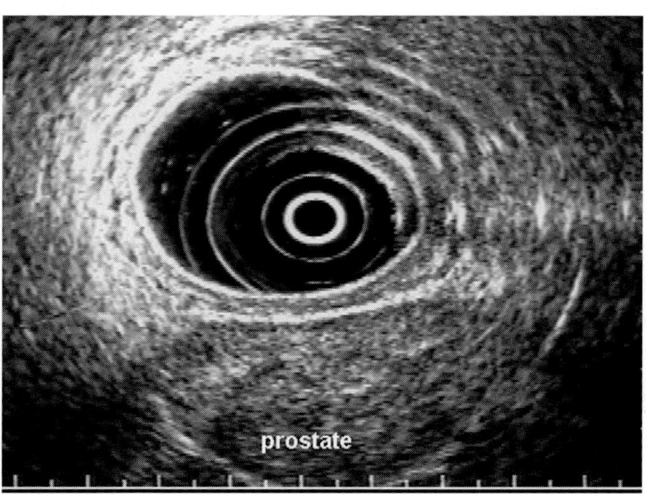


**FIGURE 27-5**

Pararectal anatomy: The prostate gland.

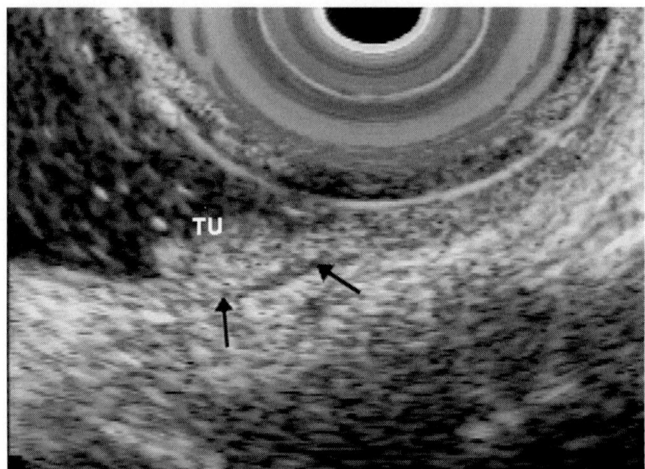


**FIGURE 27-6**

Early colonic cancer (stage T1), visible as echo-rich tumor with contact to the submucosa; the underlying muscularis propria is preserved (arrows).

of EUS. The same group recently reported on 164 colonic tumors with an accuracy in T staging of 83% and a sensitivity and specificity of 67% and 70%, respectively, in the diagnosis of lymph node metastases (13). Comparable results seem to be achievable with small US miniprobes as shown in 29 colonic cancers (accuracy of conventional EUS 85%, with mini-probes 83%). In a small number of patients in another study, staging accuracy was only 71% (14).

EUS may be useful in predicting local tumor extent in colonic carcinoma. Differentiation between early and advanced cancer was achieved in 96% of the cases properly visualized in the study of Shimizu et al. (95). EUS was 94% accurate in the assessment of the integrity of the muscular layer, thus differentiating adenomas/T1 carcinomas from T2-4 tumors (15). However, the value of this information and its implications for treatment remain uncertain. With improvements in technique and experience, early cancers, as demonstrated by EUS, might be amenable to endoscopic or laparoscopic therapy (16). However, clinical trials are needed before this approach can be recommended.

Wiersema et al. reported on two rare cases of colonic linitis plastica (17). In the first case, a 32-year-old man presented with intermittent hematochezia and rectal

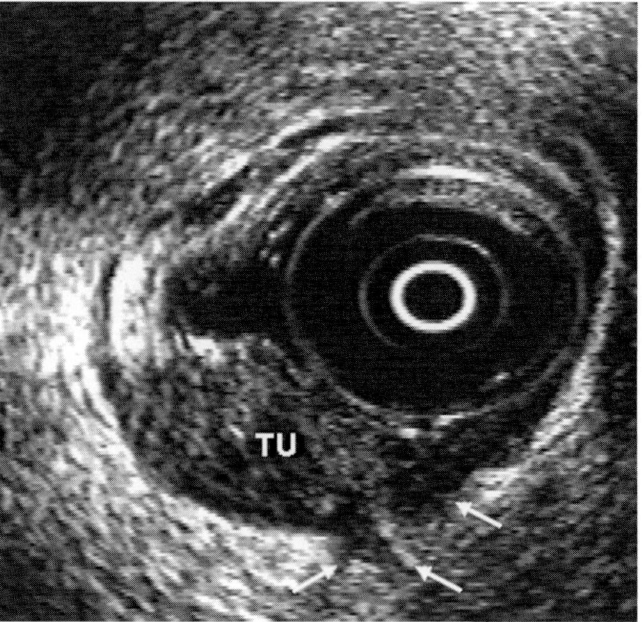


**FIGURE 27-8**

Cancer of the descending colon (TU) with irregular outer margins due to tumorous pseudopodia (stage T3).

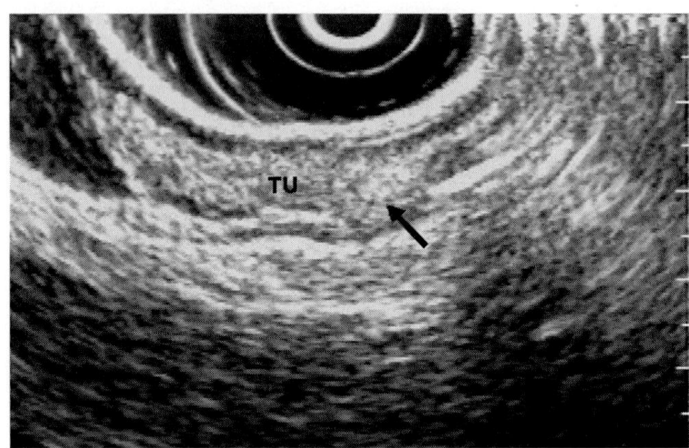


**FIGURE 27-7**

Cancer in the transverse colon (TU), infiltrating through the submucosa (arrow); the outer margin is smooth (stage T2).

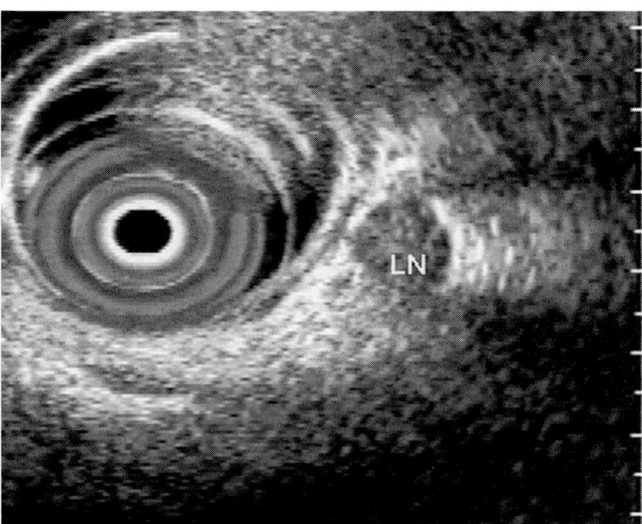


**FIGURE 27-9**

Metastatic lymph node (LN) proximal to a sigmoid cancer.

pain. Endoscopic evaluation was remarkable for luminal narrowing with submucosal rediges and edema. Endoscopic ultrasound demonstrated a circumferential infiltration of the bowel wall by a hypoechoic mass. Pseudoposia were present, indicating transmural infiltration. In the second case, a 20-year-old woman presented with two months of diarrhea, hematochezia, and rectal pain. Again, endoscopic ultrasonography demonstrated the hypoechoic tumor infiltrating the submucosa. Both patients underwent abdominal perineal resection after receiving adjuvant therapy (radiation and chemotherapy). These cases demonstrate the ability of EUS to detect intramural tumor infiltration within the colonic wall in a manner similar to that obtained when performed in the stomach for gastric lymphoma or gastric linitis plastica (17).

Whether the inability to pass the ultrasound colonoscope through a tumor-induced stenosis limits the value of EUS for cancer staging is unknown. By extrapolation from experience with EUS in esophageal carcinoma, evaluation of the distal margin of the tumor alone may provide accurate tumor staging at least in some cases (1). In a group of patients with stenotic rectal tumors which were nontraversable to the rigid US probe, staging accuracy was still 82%, five of these tumors being stage T2 (17).

EUS in suprarectal colonic cancer is unlikely to provide reliable information on lymph node involvement (N stage) because of the extended nature of the routes of tumor spread into lymph nodes. However, T stage (which can be determined accurately by EUS) correlates reasonably well with the presence of lymph node metastases. Studies of the ability of EUS to detect metastatic lymph nodes must rely on operative procedures with radical lymphadenectomy in order to avoid understaging.

## Evaluation of Colonic Adenomas

EUS can detect transmural tumor growth in large colonic adenomas when biopsy specimens are negative for cancer. Experience in this area is still limited; however, EUS of large adenomas might facilitate therapeutic decisions, especially in elderly patients at increased risk for surgery in whom the choice is between endoscopic treatment and surgery. In three reports including a total of 96 patients with villous adenomas and carcinomas of the large bowel, the sensitivity of EUS in diagnosing carcinoma ranged from 73% to 91%, specificity being 86% to 100% (18–20). However, EUS cannot detect focal malignancy that is restricted to the mucosa and muscularis mucosae. In such cases, histologic assessment after endoscopic polypectomy is the only way to determine whether the polypectomy can be considered curative. Of 25 rectal adenomas thought to be benign by clinical and endoscopic criteria, superficial endoscopic biopsy showed carcinoma in three, two of which were correctly staged by EUS. Of the remaining lesions, ten were benign adenomas and twelve were early carcinomas which could not be differentiated on EUS (21,22). The influence of EUS results in sessile, but biopsy-negative colonic adenomas may increase if the selection of patients for either endoscopic/minimally invasive (adenomas, T1 carcinomas) or conventional surgical (T2–T4 carcinomas) treatment becomes an established therapeutic concept. EUS could be helpful in making this treatment decision since it accurately predicts the involvement of the muscularis propria, thus differentiating between localized and advanced tumors (15) (Fig. 27–10). Using such an approach, Manoury et al. treated patients with biopsy-negative colonic adenomas in whom EUS showed an intact muscularis propria with endoscopic laser irradiation; during follow-up, two carcinomas (in stages Dukes A and C) were found (23).

## Evaluation of Colonic Anastomoses

A variety of studies showed rectal EUS using rigid probes to be quite sensitive in the detection of anastomotic recurrence after tumor resection; data on specificity are lacking in most of these studies [for review see (1)]. More recent preliminary work suggests that EUS may be inferior to CT scan (24) or nuclear magnetic resonance (25) in the detection of anastomotic

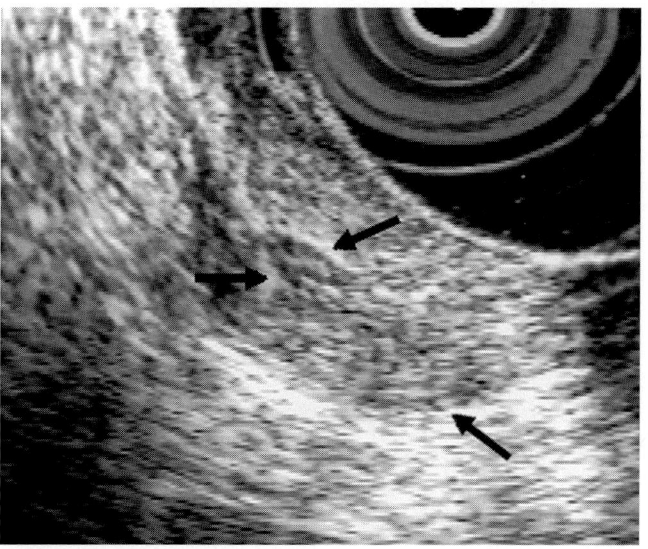

**FIGURE 27-10**

Biopsy-negative sessile adenoma in the sigmoid colon with infiltration and breakage through the submucosa (arrows); the outer margins are smooth. Resection confirmed a T2 carcinoma.

recurrence (Figs. 27–11 and 27–12). Preliminary data (26) show that colon EUS was very sensitive in the detection of postoperative recurrence in colonic carcinoma (100%) (see Fig. 27–7) and is superior to endoscopy alone (50%) and CT scan (33%). However, false-positive results, presumably due to the presence of inflammation and/or fibrosis, are problematic and limit the clinical value of EUS for this indication. If EUS is suspicious for tumor recurrence, close follow-up and attempts at histologic confirmation (transmural puncture, CT-guided puncture) but not re-operation on the basis of EUS results alone, are warranted. Generally, the value of colorectal EUS and the diagnosis of anastomotic recurrence and its clinical benefit for the patient in comparison to hitherto used procedures such as endoscopy with biopsy and CT are not yet established. The advantage of colon EUS is that it allows for combined endoscopic and endosonographic evaluation of the entire large bowel during the same procedure.

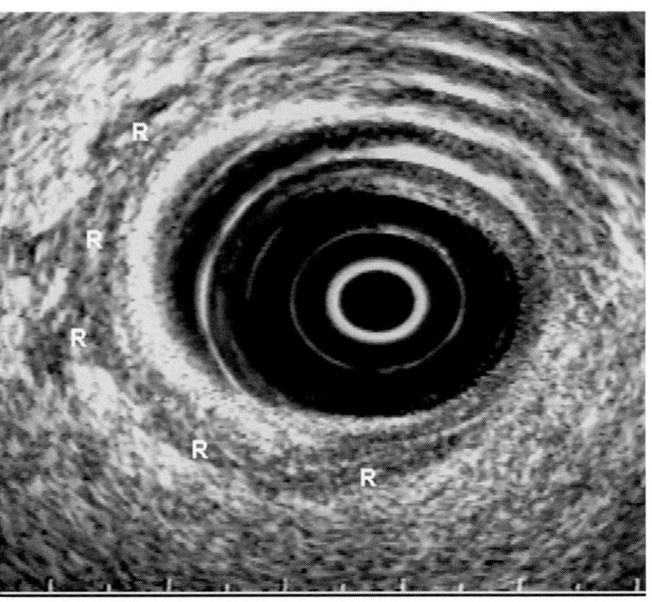


**FIGURE 27–12**

Anastomotic recurrence (R) in the sigmoid colon, visible as a hypoechoic and irregular wall thickening.

## Evaluation of Patients with Inflammatory Bowel Disease

The EUS appearance of inflammatory bowel disease is that of wall thickening and consecutive loss of the normal layer structure as the inflammatory process advances. Whether EUS can differentiate ulcerative colitis from Crohn's disease is uncertain. Whether this is necessary in a medically treatable disease is also unclear. Although ulcerative colitis is usually regarded as involving mainly the mucosa in contrast to the transmural inflammation of Crohn's disease, Shimizu et al. (27) recently reported that changes in the echopattern extended into the submucosal layer in patients with active ulcerative colitis. This observation suggests that it may be difficult to differentiate the active inflammatory process of ulcerative colitis from Crohn's disease by EUS. The study of Shimizu (27) also found a correlation between the extent of echo changes by EUS and endoscopic and clinical grading of severity of the colitis. The significance of these findings for clinical practice is unknown. Hilderbrandt et al. showed that EUS was reliable in differentiating between mucosal and transmural inflammation in patients with total colitis who had to undergo colectomy due to medical failure. This differentiation is of practical import in this special situation since transmural inflammation ileoanal pouch reconstruction is not feasible (28). Another interesting use for EUS in inflammatory bowel disease is the demonstration of perirectal and pericolonic pathology such as fistulas and abscesses, as reported in several studies (3,29–32) in which mostly rigid probes were used. It is clear, however, that more data and prospective studies of EUS in inflammatory bowel disease are needed and the procedure should be considered investigative at the present time.

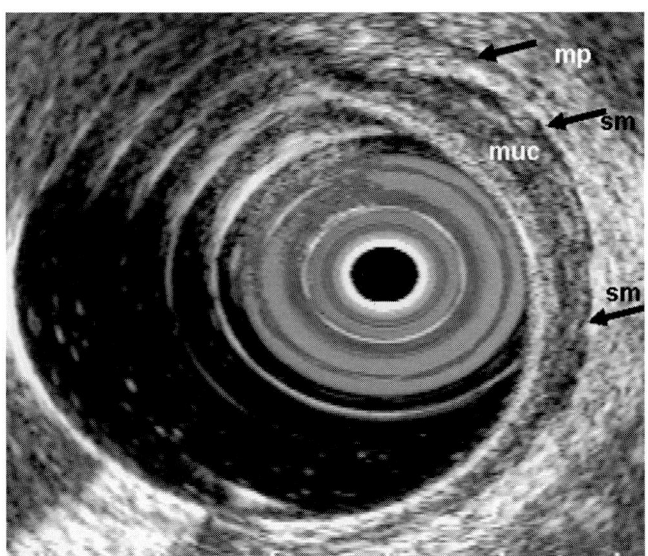


**FIGURE 27–11**

Normal colonic anastomosis with the layers being discernible (muc = mucosa, sm = submucosa, mp = muscularis propria); the thickened mucosa should not be misinterpreted as recurrence.

## Conclusions

The future of colonic EUS is difficult to predict based on the preliminary nature and limited data of currently available reports. In general, EUS will not be clinically useful if surgery is considered to be the only form of therapy for benign and malignant colonic tumors irrespective of tumor extent. However, EUS might prove valuable if an endoscopic or minimally invasive surgical approach is adopted for the treatment of large sessile adenomas and early-stage malignancy. In that regard, high-frequency ultrasound probes may be useful for detecting invasion depth of flat or depressed colorectal cancers (33). Data concerning follow-up by EUS after tumor resection are equivocal. The contribution of EUS to diagnosis and staging of inflammatory bowel disease is also uncertain.

## References


1. Rösch T, Classen M. Gastroenterologic Endosonography. Stuttgart: Thieme, 1992.
2. Rösch T, Lorenz R, Classen M. Endoscopic ultrasonography in the evaluation of colon and rectal disease. Gastrointest Endosc 36: S33–S39, 1990.
3. Schratter-Sehn AU, Lochs H, Handl-Zeller L, Tscholakoff D, Schratter M. Endosonographic features of the lower pelvic region in Crohn's disease. Am J Gastroenterol 88:1054–1057, 1993.
4. Rösch T, Lorenz R, Suchy R, et al. Colonic endoscopic ultrasonography: First results of a new technique. Gastrointest Endosc 36: 382–386, 1990.
5. Rifkin MD, Wechsler RJ. A comparison of computed tomography and endorectal ultrasound in staging rectal cancer. Int J Colorect Dis 1:219–223, 1986.
6. Shimizu S, Tada M, Kawai K. Use of endoscopic ultrasonography for the diagnosis of colorectal tumors. Endoscopy 22:31–34, 1990.
7. Rösch T. Endoscopic ultrasonography. Endoscopy 26:148–168, 1994.
8. Hildebrandt U, Schüder G, Feifel G. Preoperative staging of rectal and colonic cancer. Endoscopy 26:810–812, 1994.
9. Tio TL, Tytgat GNJ. Comparison of blind transrectal ultrasonography with endoscopic transrectal ultrasonography in assessing rectal and perirectal diseases. Scand J Gastroenterol 21(suppl 123): 104–111, 1986.
10. Laoudi F, Farmakis N, Kallimanis G, et al. Comparative study of BUS and EUS in the diagnosis and staging of rectal cancer. Endoscopy 24:658(abstract), 1992.
11. Kimmey MB, Martin RW, Haggitt RC, et al. Histologic correlates of gastrointestinal ultrasound images. Gastroenterology 96:433–441, 1989.
12. Tio TL, Coene PPLO, van Delden OM, et al. Colorectal carcinoma: Preoperative TNM classification with endosonography. Radiology 179:165–170, 1991.
13. Cho E, Nakajima M, Yasuda K, et al. Endoscopic ultrasonography in the diagnosis of colorectal cancer invasion. Gastrointest Endosc 29:521–527, 1993.
14. Gabriel P, Laoudi F, Kallimanis G, et al. Endoscopic ultrasonography in staging cancer of the descending colon. Endoscopy 24: 658(abstract), 1992.
15. Napoleon B, Valette PJ, Pujol B, et al. Echocoloscopy for the pretherapeutic evaluation of adenomas of the rectum and sigmoid. Gastrointest Endosc 38:A268–A269(abstract), 1992.
16. Buess G, Wohlrab S, Lirici MM. EUS-guided therapy in rectal tumors and other fields of minimal invasive surgery. Endoscopy 24:334–337, 1992.
17. Nielsen MB, Pedersen JF, Christiansen J. Rectal endosonography in the evaluation of stenotic rectal tumors. Dis Colon Rectum 36: 275–279, 1993.
18. Glaser F. Stellungnahme zum Kommentar von A. Heintz und T. Junginger. Chirurg 61:740–741, 1990.
19. Mosnier H, Guivarc'h M, Meduri B, et al. Endorectal sonography in the management of rectal villous tumors. Int J Colorect Dis 5:90–93, 1990.
20. Tio TL, Weijers OB, Hulsman F, et al. Endosonography of colorectal diseases. Endoscopy 24:309–314, 1992.
21. Roseau G, Palazzo L, Rahme T, et al. Role of rectal endoscopic ultrasonography in the pre-therapeutical study of villous tumors (in French). Gastroenterol Clin Biol 16:787–790, 1992.
22. Roseau G, Palazzo L, Rahme T, et al. Endoscopic ultrasonography in the staging of rectal villous adenomas. Endoscopy 24(suppl I): 380(abstract), 1992.
23. Maunoury V, Cortot A, Brunetaud JM, et al. Is endoscopic ultrasonography useful to laser management of benign villous adenomas? Gastroenterology 102:A376(abstract), 1992.
24. Romano G, Santangelo M, Esercizio L, et al Intrarectal ultrasound in the diagnosis of locally recurrent rectal cancer. Endoscopy 24 (suppl I):382(abstract), 1992.
25. Waizer A, Powsner E, Russo I, et al. Prospective comparative study of magnetic resonance imaging versus transrectal ultrasound for preoperative staging and follow up of rectal cancer. Preliminary report. Dis Colon Rectum 34:1068–1072, 1992.
26. Rösch T, Lorenz R, Classen M. Colonic endosonography is superior to computed tomography and endoscopy in detecting positive recurrence in colorectal cancer. Gastrointest Endosc 36:207 (abstract), 1990.
27. Shimizu S, Tada M, Kawai K. Value of endoscopic ultrasonography in the assessment of inflammatory bowel diseases. Endoscopy 24: 354–358, 1992.
28. Hildebrandt U, Kraus J, Ecker KW, et al. Endosonographic differentiation of mucosal and transmucosal non-specific inflammatory bowel disease. Endoscopy 24:359–363, 1992.
29. Van Outryve MJ, Pelckmans PA, Michielsen PP, et al. Value of transrectal ultrasonography in Crohn's disease. Gastroenterology 100:1171–1177, 1991.
30. Choen S, Burnett S, Bartram CI, et al. Comparison between anal endosonography and digital examination in the evaluation of anal fistulae. Br J Surg 78:445–447, 1991.
31. Grant TH, Eisenstein MM, Brandt T, et al. Supralevator abscess: Evaluation with transrectal sonography. Gastrointest Radiol 14: 354–356, 1989.
32. Tio TL, Mulder CJJ, Wijers OB, et al. Endosonography of peri-anal and peri-colorectal fistula and/or abscess in Crohn's disease. Gastrointest Endosc 36:331–336, 1990.
33. Saitoh Y, Obara T, Dinami K, Nomura M, Taruishi M, Ayabe T, Ashida T, Shibata Y, Kohgo Y. Efficacy of high-frequency ultrasound probes for the preoperative staging of invasion depth in flat and depressed colorectal tumors. Gastrointest Endosc 44:34– 39, 1996.
34. Wiersema MJ, Wiersema LM, Kochman ML. Primary linitis plastica of the colon. Gastrointest Endosc 39:716–718, 1993.

CHAPTER

# Endoscopic Ultrasound Staging of Rectal Cancer

Thomas J. Savides
Robert H. Hawes

The incidence of rectal cancer in the United States is 5–15 cases per 100,000 population. Virtually all malignant tumors of the rectum are adenocarcinomas, which presumably arise from prior adenomas. Patients typically present with hematochezia or a change in bowel habits, and diagnosis is made by endoscopy with biopsy.

Surgical resection is the primary treatment for rectal adenocarcinoma. The surgical treatment differs from that for colon cancer because most of the rectum is located beneath the peritoneal reflection and is surrounded by perirectal fat, rather than serosa. Therefore, any tumor invading through the rectal wall and below the peritoneal reflection is treated with a combined abdominoperineal resection and colostomy. Lesions located high in the rectum (6–10 cm above the dentate line) may lie above the peritoneal reflection and be amenable to a sphincter-sparing low anterior resection.

Transanal local resection of superficial rectal tumors confined to the mucosa/submucosa is gaining popularity because it causes substantially less morbidity and mortality, and avoids a colostomy. Lesions ideal for this approach are small (less than one-third of the circumference) and easily mobile (suggesting no deep invasion). One drawback to the transanal approach is the inability to remove and obtain pathologic evaluation of perirectal lymph nodes.

Outcomes of patients who are treated surgically for rectal cancer reveal that approximately 75% of patients with node-negative rectal cancer will be cured, while surgical resection results in cure in only 33% of patients with metastases to local lymph nodes (1,2). Local recurrence of tumor occurs in approximately 15% of patients after surgical resection of rectal cancer using either abdominoperineal resection or anterior resection (3). The risk of local recurrence increases with advanced tumor stage at the time of resection. Various preoperative and/or postoperative chemoradiation strategies look promising to help downstage tumors prior to resection and decrease local recurrence rates (4,5).

The optimal use of therapies such as transanal surgery or adjuvant chemoradiation depends on the precise assessment of local spread. Various means have been used to clinically stage tumors before surgery, including digital examination, computerized tomography (CT), magnetic resonance imaging (MRI), and most recently endoscopic ultrasonography (EUS). EUS appears to be the most accurate means of clinical staging of rectal tumors.

Wild and Reid in 1956 were the first to visualize the rectal wall with an ultrasound probe, but the images were not of sufficient quality to be clinically useful (6). By the early 1980s, ultrasound imaging technology had advanced to the point where rigid probes for scanning the prostate were being developed. In 1983, Dragsted and Gammelgaard, as well as Hildebrandt et al., first published applications of this technology to image rectal tumors for staging purposes (7,8). Since then, numerous reports have described EUS for staging rectal tumors. Initially, most reports came from Europe where surgeons and gastroenterologists with interests in colorectal cancer performed their own ultrasound. In contrast, in the United States most rectal ultrasound was performed by urologists or radiologists, and only for prostate imaging. With the advent of endoscopic ultrasound, awareness of the utility of ultrasound for evaluating patients with fecal incontinence (9,10,11), evaluating patients before and after ilio-anal anastomosis (12), and for staging patients with rectal tumors increased, resulting in more widespread use of this technology to stage rectal malignancy. Anal endosonography has also been shown to be useful in evaluating patients with solitary rectal ulcer syndrome (13) and anal defects after anorectal surgery (14,15).

## Ultrasound Instrumentation

Ultrasound evaluation of rectal lesions can be performed either with rigid, nonfiberoptic probes or with flexible fiberoptic endoscopes into which ultrasound transducers have been incorporated.

Commercially available rigid rectal imaging probes take two forms: either a rotating mechanical scanner, that produces a 360° image perpendicular to the long axis of the probe; or linear array transducer, which produces a 90° sector scan parallel to the long axis of the probe. Brüel and Kjaer (Denmark) manufactures a 24-cm, nonoptical, rigid probe fitted with a 7-MHz radially scanning transducer. A balloon fits around the transducer and can be filled with water. Several companies, including Acuson (Mountain View, California) and Hitachi (Terrytown, New York), manufacture nonoptical rigid rectal probes that use electronic array technology and scan at 3–7 MHz. The linear array probes have been designed primarily for imaging the prostate gland, and have the capacity to perform Doppler imaging and ultrasound-guided fine-needle aspiration. Rigid probes have been used in Europe by gastroenterologists and surgeons to image the rectum; but in the United States, they are used primarily by urologists and radiologists to image the prostate.

Flexible endosonography of the rectum is typically performed using echoendoscopes designed for the upper gastrointestinal tract. Olympus (Olympus America, Inc., Melville, New York) manufactures an echoendoscope, the GF-UM20 (or GF-UM130), with oblique optical viewing and a mechanically rotating sector scanner that provides a 360° imaging plane perpendicular to the long axis of the scope. Ultrasound imaging is performed at 7.5 and 12 MHz. Pentax (Pentax Precision Instruments, Orangeburg, New York) manufactures a flexible fiberoptic endoscope system using electronic array technology (FX32-UM, FX-36UX) that provides a 100° sector scan parallel with the long axis of the scope. Imaging is performed at 5 and 7.5 MHz. The Pentax instrument has the advantage of color Doppler and EUS-guided FNA capabilities.

Olympus also manufactures a dedicated colonic echoendoscope (Olympus CF-UM20) which has forward-viewing optics and is 133 cm long. The design requires that the light and optical bundles pass adjacent to the ultrasound transducer, which results in a 290° (rather than 360°) radial scanning plane. The echocolonoscope has a large (18-mm) rigid tip; however, its overall tip deflection is good, and it can be advanced to the cecum in more than 80% of cases in which stenosis is not significant.

The advantage of flexible echoendoscopes over the rigid probe is threefold, including the ability 1) to confirm location of the tumor by direct optical visualization, 2) to manuever around a partially obstructing tumor under direct visualization, and 3) to determine the exact distance of the tumor from the dentate line. Its disadvantages include price and time required for cleaning (Table 28–1).

The newest ultrasound device for rectal imaging is the high-frequency ultrasound probe (16). The system consists of an ultrasound transducer with a frequency of 12.5 MHz or 20 MHz (Olympus America, Inc., Melville, New York). The probe provides a 360° real-time image, perpendicular to the shaft of the probe. The probe can be passed via the accessory channel of a conventional videoendoscope, thus permitting the probe to be posi-

TABLE 28-1

Comparison of Rigid and Flexible Endoscopic Ultrasound Probes for Staging Rectal Cancer

| | Rigid Probe | Flexible EUS Scope |
|---|---|---|
| Initial cost | low | high |
| Directly visualize tumor | no | yes |
| Easy to clean | yes | no |
| Ability to FNA | some | some |

tioned within the rectum under direct, endoscopic vision. Using a catheter probe, one study evaluated 51 patients with colorectal carcinoma and 16 patients with rectal carcinoid. The accuracy of preoperative assessment of depth of tumor penetration for tumors limited to the mucosa and tumors invading the submucosa was 83% and 90%, respectively. The probe was found to be useful in assessing invasion of colorectal tumors, especially small and flat lesions limited to the mucosa or submucosa (16).

## Patient Preparation and Technique

Patient preparation for rectal endosonography typically requires two tapwater or phosphasoda enemas one hour prior to the procedure. If patients cannot tolerate this type of bowel preparation, oral laxatives may be used the night before. Patients should be asked to avoid urination immediately prior to EUS, to enhance the detection of the urinary bladder.

During the procedure, the patient is placed in the left lateral decubitus position. Standard forward-viewing endoscopy is often performed first in order to identify the location of the lesion and determine if the echoendoscope can pass proximal to the lesion. Assessing the exact location of the tumor aids in positioning the patient so that the tumor is in the dependent portion of the rectum. In this position, when water is instilled, it will cover the tumor to assist in imaging. If there is still residual stool in the rectum, another enema is given before endosonography. Patients usually require no medication, although rarely mild conscious sedation may be necessary or glucagon administration to decrease contractility.

The technique with all types of rectal endosonography probes involves placing the probe adjacent to the tumor, separated by a water-filled acoustic window. This window can be achieved by filling the rectum with water and/or using a water-filled balloon around the transducer. Using the echoendoscope, the tumor position is visually confirmed prior to ultrasonic imaging. With nonoptical probes, the lesion is identified by ultrasonography alone. Imaging is generally performed at the highest frequency possible to increase resolution. The transducer should be kept in the middle of the lumen as much as possible, as this will keep all wall layers in focus. If the lesion is small (i.e., less than 3 cm sessile mass), the water-filled–rectum technique should be used. If the balloon is filled with water, care should be taken not to overinflate the balloon and compress the tumor so much that staging may be distorted. The best imaging occurs when the transducer is perpendicular to the lumen of the bowel. The ultrasound probe is moved in small increments back and forth across the tumor, such that the layer of deepest tumor penetration can be imaged.

Attention is given to image not only the tumor, but also the organs adjacent to the rectum to determine extent of disease. In males, the prostate and seminal vesicles always should be seen along the anterior wall, and the bladder may also be visualized. In women, the vagina, cervix, and uterus may be visualized, as well as the bladder. In both men and women, the internal and external anal sphincters can be identified. The ultrasound image can be electronically rotated such that either the prostate or the vagina is in the 12 o'clock position.

A complete rectal ultrasound examination usually can be performed in 15–20 minutes. If flexible sigmoidoscopy is performed prior to the procedure, the total time should be approximately 30 minutes.

Probe cleaning is performed as with other endoscopic equipment. The latex balloons are discarded after each examination.

## Sonographic Anatomy of the Normal Rectum

The rectum is approximately 15 cm long. The middle and lower thirds are located below the peritoneal reflection. The normal thickness of the rectal wall is 2–4 mm.

As with other parts of the gastrointestinal tract, the rectal wall appears as five alternating hyper- and hypoechoic layers. Beynon et al. have performed experimental studies in which fresh operative specimens of the rectum were suspended in saline and imaged with ultrasound probes. Sharp dissection of the wall layers indicated that the echoimages represented the wall layers (17–19). Wang et al. confirmed these findings with resected colon and rectal walls, using a micropositioner to ensure that the location for the ultrasound imaging and tissue cutting for histologic analysis was exactly the same (20). The histologic correlation of the echolayers is as follows: **First hyperechoic layer**—interface between water and mucosal surface; **Second hypoechoic layer**—mucosa; **Third hyperechoic layer**—submucosa; **Fourth hypoechoic layer**—muscularis propria; **Fifth hyperechoic layer**—interface between muscularis propria and perirectal fat.

## TNM Rectal Cancer Staging

Prognosis of rectal cancer depends on its local, nodal, and distant tumor status. Rectal cancer is staged using the tumor–node–metastasis (TNM) staging system, as per the American Joint Committee on Cancer and the TNM Committee of the International Union against Cancer (AJCC/UICC) (21) (Table 28–2). The TNM system replaces the previously used staging systems, the Dukes staging system and its various modifications (22,23). (Tables 28–3 and 28–4). When preoperative ultrasound staging occurs, the prefix "u" is often added before the stage (e.g., stage uT2, N1).

## EUS Appearance of Rectal Malignancy

Tumors generally appear as hypoechoic masses with loss of the normal echolayer pattern on EUS (Figs. 28–1 through 28–3). Longitudinal and circumferential tumor extent can be determined. Irregularity at a border suggests involvement of both layers, although this can be misleading if inflammation is present. Involvement of adjacent organs appears as a continuation of the hypoechoic mass from the rectal wall into the adjacent structure.

Lymph nodes appear as round or oval structures which are hypoechoic compared to the surrounding perirectal fat. These lymph nodes can be assessed in terms of short- and long-axis dimensions, relative echogenicity, and shape. Often, lymph nodes that harbor cancer are rounded, anechoic, and have a short-axis dimension of at least 5mm.

**TABLE 28–2**

**AJCC/UICC TNM Staging System for Colorectal Cancer**

| | |
|---|---|
| ***Primary Tumor (T)*** | |
| T0 | No evidence of primary tumor |
| Tis | Carcinoma in situ: intramucosal |
| T1 | Tumor invades the submucosa |
| T2 | Tumor invades the muscularis propria |
| T3 | Tumor invades the subserosa or perirectal tissue |
| T4 | Tumor directly invades other organs (e.g., vagina, uterus, prostate, seminal vesicles, bladder) |
| ***Regional Lymph Nodes (N)*** | |
| N0 | No regional lymph nodes involved |
| N1 | Metastasis to 1–3 perirectal lymph nodes |
| N2 | Metastasis to ≥4 perirectal lymph nodes |
| ***Distant Metastasis (M)*** | |
| M0 | No distant metastasis |
| M1 | Distant metastasis |

*Source:* Data from ref. 21.

**TABLE 28–3**

**Dukes Classification**

| | |
|---|---|
| Stage A: | Cancer limited into the rectal wall (T1–2, N0, M0) |
| Stage B: | Cancer penetrating through the rectal wall (T3–4, N0, M0) |
| Stage C: | Cancer with lymph node involvement (T1–4, N1–2) |

*Source:* Data from ref. 22.

## Accuracy of EUS in Staging Rectal Cancer

Table 28–5 shows multiple studies supporting the high accuracy of transrectal ultrasonography in staging rectal cancer, with overall accuracy rates of 85% for T stage and 77% for N stage. Most of this literature is based on rigid ultrasound probe systems using radial scanners at 5–7.5 MHz. In the few studies reported using flexible endoscopic ultrasound, the results seem comparable and, given the ability to image at the higher frequency of 12 MHz, would be expected to have better resolution for superficial tumors (16,23–29,41,66,67).

## Limitations of EUS in Staging Rectal Cancer

When EUS staging is incorrect for depth of penetration, it is usually because of overstaging rather than understaging (19,25,26,30–33) (Table 28–6). EUS tends to overstage cancers because high-resolution ultrasound can detect, but not separate, hypoechoic inflammation adjacent to the malignancy from the tumor itself. This is especially true for Stage T2 tumors, which can be overstaged as T3 tumors. Yamashita et al. demonstrated that the incidence of overstaging increased in proportion to the degree of inflammation associated with the tumor (31). When understaging occurs, it is usually because of microscopic invasion of cancer cells into the next layer (31). This is especially true when an entire layer is dis-

**TABLE 28–4**

**Dukes Classification with Astler-Coller Modification**

| | |
|---|---|
| Stage A: | Cancer limited to mucosa, submucosa (T1, N0, M0) |
| Stage B1: | Cancer into the muscularis propria (T2, N0, M0) |
| Stage B2: | Cancer into the perirectal fat (T3, N0, M0) |
| Stage C1: | Cancer limited to rectal wall,with lymph node involvement (T1–2, N1–2, M0) |
| Stage C2: | Cancer through rectal wall, with lymph node involvement (T3–4, N1–2, M0) |
| Stage D: | Distant metastasis (T1–4, N1–2, M1) |

*Source:* Data from ref. 23.

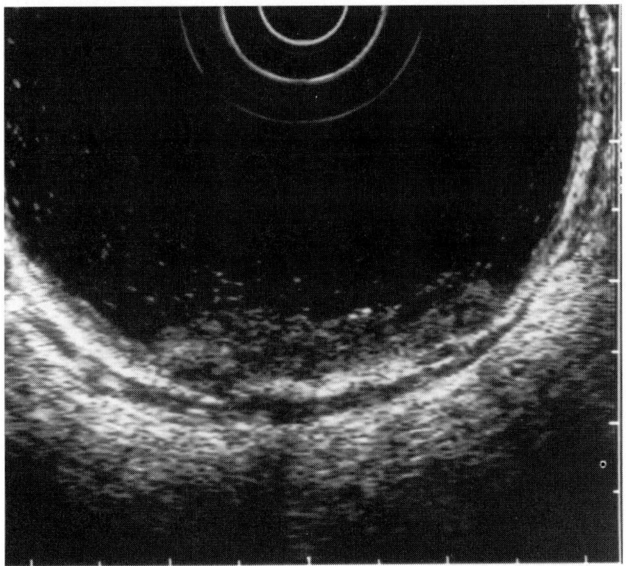

**FIGURE 28–1**

EUS stage T1, N0 rectal tumor contained within the mucosa/submucosa.

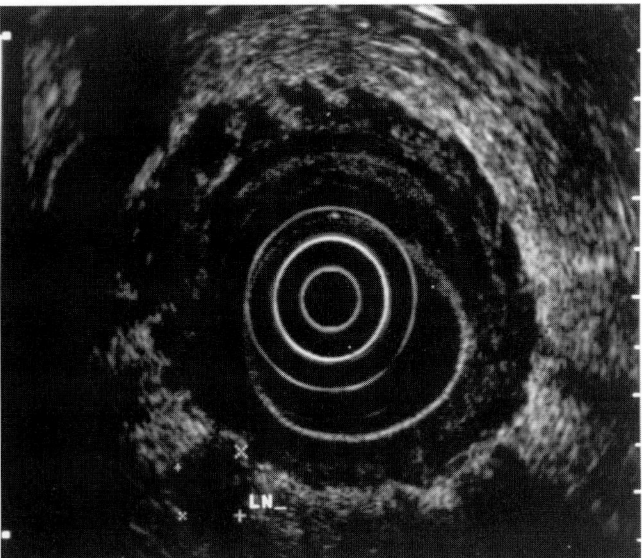


**FIGURE 28–3**

EUS stage T3, N1 rectal tumor penetrating into the perirectal fat with an adjacent anechoic, round lymph node with well demarcated borders.

tended with tumor, abutting against the next layer, but does not have any definite invasion.

Overstaging can also occur when imaging tumors located on a haustral fold or a sharp angulation, which can result in tangential imaging. For example, the prominent valves of Houston can mimic lesions because the mucosal/submucosal thickening evident on endosonography is artifactual—the product of tangential imaging.

Determination of lymph node involvement is less accurate than T staging because of difficulty in discriminating between inflammatory and metastatic lymph nodes, as well as in identifying small or distant lymph nodes. Accurate criteria for defining malignant lymph nodes do not exist. Suspicious lymph nodes for metastatic involvement have been described as rounded, echo-poor lymph nodes, with short-axis diameters greater than 5 mm (34, 35). However, most metastatic colon cancer lymph nodes are less than 5 mm in size (36).

Hulsmans et al. performed an in vitro study of perirectal lymph nodes after rectal cancer surgery, comparing the ultrasound findings with histology (37). Using univariate analysis, they showed that two sonographic findings—inhomogeneity (representing necrosis within the node) and short-axis diameter >9 mm—were most associated with malignant nodes. Hilar reflection—a single sharp central echo that represents fat deposition—was associated with benign nodes. Multivariate analysis showed only inhomogeneity (associated with malignancy) and hilar reflection (associated with benign nodes) to be significant. However, when applying these two criteria to their data, the accuracy in predicting malignant lymph nodes was just 47% (17 of 36). They also found that no nodes with a short-axis diameter greater than 9 mm were benign, but some lymph nodes with short-axis diameters of 3–5 mm were malignant.

In addition to problems with defining the sonographic appearance of perirectal lymph nodes, Nielsen et al. have suggested that transrectal ultrasound using a rigid 7-MHz probe will identify only 50% of malignant perirectal lymph nodes, and may not detect any lymph nodes when metastatic lymph nodes are present (38). With in vitro testing, they found that only 16% of small

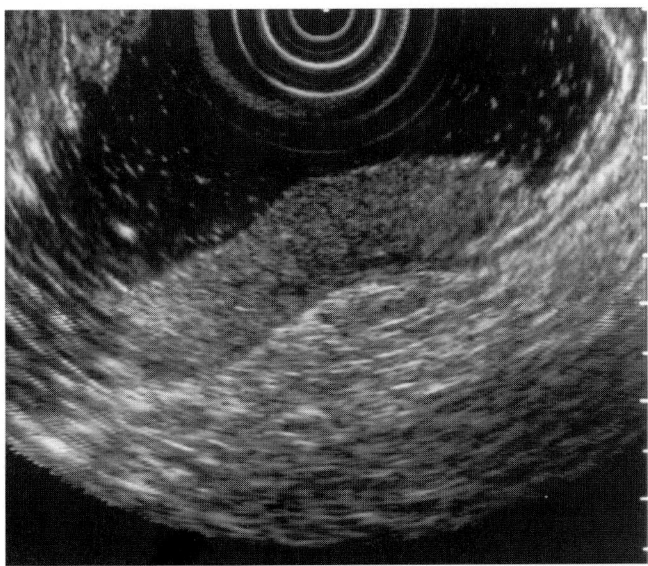

**FIGURE 28–2**

EUS stage T2, N0 rectal tumor penetrating into, but not through, the muscularis propria.

**TABLE 28-5**

Accuracy of Rectal Ultrasound in Staging Rectal Cancer Compared to Surgical Pathology

| Reference | Year | *n* | T stage | N stage | Type of US probe |
|---|---|---|---|---|---|
| Saitoh (24) | 1986 | 88 | 90%[1] | 75% | flexible, radial (7 MHz) |
| | | | | | rigid, radial (5–7.5 MHz) |
| Di Candio (67) | 1987 | 55 | 91%[1] | 75% | rigid, linear (5 MHz) |
| Feifel (30) | 1987 | 79 | 89%[2] | — | rigid, radial (3–7 MHz) |
| Beynon (19) | 1988 | 100 | 93%[2] | 83% | rigid, sector/linear (5.5–7 MHz) |
| Yamashita (31) | 1988 | 122 | 78%[2] | — | rigid, radial (7.5 MHz) |
| Rifkin (45) | 1989 | 102 | 72%[1] | 81% | rigid, radial (7 MHz) |
| | | | | | linear (5–7.5 MHz) |
| Jochem (68) | 1990 | 50 | 80%[1] | 72% | rigid, radial (7 MHz) |
| Hildebrandt (69) | 1990 | 113 | — | 78% | rigid, radial (7 MHz) |
| Boyce (25) | 1992 | 45 | 89%[2] | 79% | flexible, radial (7.5, 12 MHz) |
| Cho (32) | 1993 | 76 | 82%[2] | 70% | flexible, radial (7.5 MHz) |
| Herzog (26) | 1993 | 118 | 89%[2] | 80% | rigid, radial (7 MHz) |
| Glaser (33) | 1993 | 154 | 86%[2] | 81% | rigid, radial (7 MHz) |
| Total | | 1102 | 85% | 77% | |

[1]T staging to determine confinement of tumor to rectal wall or extension beyond wall.
[2]T staging according to the TNM system.

lymph nodes less than 5 mm were detected, while 56% of lymph nodes between 6 and 10 mm, and 82% of lymph nodes larger than 10 mm were detected.

Fourteen percent of rectal cancers cannot be staged accurately because tumor stenosis prevents passage of the ultrasound probe (Table 28–7). As most studies exclude patients with obstructing tumors, there are no published reports about the accuracy of EUS in these patients. In these cases the probe can be wedged into the tumor and may still provide important information about depth of penetration and lymph nodes. Just as with esophageal cancer, however, if a tumor is near-obstructing, it is most likely an advanced tumor which would not be amenable to local resection. If lymph nodes are visualized, this may be helpful; but if no lymph nodes are seen, one cannot rule out an N1 tumor.

Imaging in the anal canal can be difficult because of tight stenoses that may not allow the probe to pass proximal to the tumor. In addition, the tumor may lie inside the focal zone of the ultrasound probe, thereby limiting the image.

Accuracy of staging also depends on operator experience. Orrom et al. showed significant improvement in accuracy between novice and experienced endosonographers (84% vs. 95%) (39).

## Interobserver Agreement for EUS Rectal Cancer Staging

Palazzo and Burtin examined interobserver agreement in staging of rectal cancer in 37 patients (40). They found that agreement was fair for T1 tumors, poor for T2 tumors, but good for T3 and T4 tumors. They also found intraobserver agreement was good with respect to the subjective appearance of a malignant perirectal lymph node. Roubein et al. found that interobserver accuracy was good for both T and N stage; however, nearly all of their tumors were uT3 (41). Hulsmans, using an in vitro model, found that interobserver agreement on perirectal lymph nodes was poor for determining subjective ultrasound characteristics such as

**TABLE 28-6**

Accuracy of Rectal Cancer T-Staging by EUS Compared to Pathologic Stage[1]

| Pathology | *n* | *EUS Stage* uT1 | uT2 | uT3 | uT4 | Accuracy |
|---|---|---|---|---|---|---|
| pT1 | 91 | 73 | 17 | 1 | — | 80% |
| pT2 | 158 | 5 | **108**[2] | 44 | 1 | 68% |
| pT3 | 408 | — | 13 | **384**[2] | 11 | 94% |
| pT4 | 37 | — | — | 4 | 33[2] | 89% |
| Total | 694 | | | | | 83% |

[1]Compiled from references (19,25,26,31–33).
[2]Pathologic and EUS stages agree.

**TABLE 28-7**

Failure Rate of Rectal Ultrasound Probes to Adequately Stage Tumor Because of Inability to Traverse Stenotic Tumor

| Reference | Patients Included | *Patients Excluded* Number | Percentage |
|---|---|---|---|
| Glaser (33) | 86 | 6 | 7% |
| Feifel (30) | 79 | 21 | 27% |
| Herzog (26) | 125 | 7 | 6% |
| Saitoh (24) | 88 | 11 | 13% |
| Yamashita (31) | 122 | 23 | 19% |
| Total | 500 | 68 | 14% |

inhomogeneity and hilar reflection, but good for short-axis diameters (37).

## Accuracy of Rectal EUS Compared to Digital Exam, CT Scan, and MRI

Preoperative staging of rectal cancer can be performed with digital examination, abdominal/pelvic computerized tomography (CT), MRI, and transrectal ultrasound.

Digital examination can evaluate tumor mobility to help determine invasion through the rectal wall. Occasionally, perirectal lymph nodes can be palpated. Nicholls et al. reported that for experienced consultants, the accuracy for detection of moderate extrarectal spread was 80%, and for perirectal lymph nodes was 65% (42). Studies that have directly compared EUS to digital exam alone suggest EUS staging is more accurate for depth penetration (43,44). Beynon et al. showed that if one included tumors that cannot be palpated, the accuracy for digital exam was 52% compared to 91% for EUS (43). Hildebrandt and Feifel showed that the accuracy of digital exam was 60% if rectal tumors not within manual reach were included, compared to 92% for EUS (44). If the tumors not within reach were excluded in both studies, the accuracy rate of digital exam is higher, but still not as high as with EUS. Although not compared, EUS would also be expected to have much higher accuracy for lymph node assessment.

CT scan has been considered the standard for the noninvasive staging of rectal cancer. Depth of penetration is estimated by wall thickness, and lymph node involvement by size greater than 1 cm (19). Overall, EUS appears to be superior to CT in terms of both T and N staging (19,26,43,45–48) Table 28–8 shows that among several comparative studies, EUS has a greater accuracy than CT scan; 87% versus 76% for T stage, and 78% versus 62% for N stage. CT cannot discriminate between wall layers of the rectum, and therefore is not helpful in determination of T1 versus T2 tumors for local resection. CT scan is still important, however, in evaluating for distant metastasis, such as to the liver.

Magnetic resonance imaging (MRI) has been compared to EUS in a few small studies and appears to be similar in accuracy (49–51). Waizer et al. found that, in 13 patients with rectal cancer who had preoperative staging with EUS and MRI, the accuracy of MRI was 77% compared to 85% for EUS (49). Thaler et al. showed that there was no statistically significant difference in staging accuracy between MRI and EUS, as the accuracy of T staging for MRI was 82% compared to 88% for EUS, and for N staging 60% for MRI compared to 80% for EUS (50). Schäfer et al. showed that endorectal ultrasound was correct in determining the depth of rectal tumor invasion in 17 of 19 patients while rectal MRI was correct in 16 of 19 (51). However, as Schäfer et al. point out, although the accuracy rates for both imaging techniques are similar, MR imaging is more expensive than transanal ultrasound. Future technologic improvements using endorectal coil MRI may result in increased use of MRI for staging transmural or recurrent tumors, but at a much higher cost than EUS (52). However, MRI, like CT scan, is at this time still unable to distinguish between T1 and T2 lesions.

**TABLE 28-8**

**Accuracy of Rectal Endosonography Compared to CT Scan in Staging Rectal Cancer**

| | | | *T-Stage Accuracy* | | *N-Stage Accuracy* | |
|---|---|---|---|---|---|---|
| **Reference** | **Year** | **Number** | **EUS** | **CT** | **EUS** | **CT** |
| Romano (47) | 1985 | 23 | 87[1] | 83 | — | — |
| Kramann (46) | 1986 | 29 | 93[1] | 79 | — | — |
| Beynon (43) | 1986 | 44 | 91[1] | 82 | — | — |
| Rifkin (45) | 1989 | 81 | 67[2] | 53 | 80 | 72 |
| Beynon (19) | 1989 | 46 | — | — | 87 | 57 |
| Pappalardo (48) | 1990 | 14 | 93[1] | 86 | 86 | 57 |
| Herzog (26) | 1993 | 87 | 91[1] | 75 | 80 | — |
| Total | | 324 | 87 | 76 | 78 | 62 |

[1]T staging according to the TNM system.
[2]T staging to determine confinement of tumor to rectal wall or extension beyond wall.

## Rectal EUS after Radiation Therapy

Radiation to the rectum results in inflammation and thickening of the rectal wall with circumferential loss of normal echolayers and increased echogenicity, which may lead to overstaging of the T stage by EUS. Napoleon, Vallas, and colleagues performed a nonrandomized, observational study of 109 patients with stage uT2 tumors that went to surgery. They found that 69 patients who underwent EUS after preoperative radiation therapy had T-stage accuracy of only 52% and N-stage accuracy of 62%, as compared with 40 patients who had EUS without preoperative radiation therapy, whose T- and N-stage accuracies were 75% and 77%, respectively (53,54). They found that significant EUS overstaging occurred after irradiation, with rates of overstaging 44% after radiation treatment versus 18% for no radiation; and for lymph nodes, overstaging of 36% in patients who received radiation versus 13% for those who did not. They speculated that the post-radiotherapy inflammation and/or fibrosis altered accurate T staging, especially the distinction between T2 and T3. These results suggest that radiation caused downstaging of rectal tumor penetration and lymph node status, but that the EUS exam may not give an accurate estimate of tumor stage after irradiation because of overstaging.

In contrast, a prospective study by Glaser et al. showed that EUS stage did not change after radiation in 17 patients undergoing EUS both before and after radiation therapy for preoperative EUS stage T3 or T4 rectal tumors (55). They found that the EUS appearance showed shrinkage of the tumor, with change of echopattern to more hyperechoic levels in the tumor, and loss of normal rectal wall layers. Lymph nodes either disappeared or became more echogenic. There was no EUS downstaging of their tumors after radiation, with a T-stage accuracy of 88%, and an N-stage accuracy of 82%.

## EUS Tumor Stage and Impact on Treatment of Rectal Cancers

Centers that perform a large number of rectal cancer surgeries are now incorporating EUS tumor staging into their decision algorithms for treatment. Hildebrandt et al. recommend the following for tumors of the lower two thirds of the rectum: uT1, N0 tumors should undergo transanal resection, and uT1–2 should undergo either anterior resection or intersphincteric resection (56). uT3 tumors of the lower third of the rectum should undergo abdominoperineal repairs. Using these guidelines, they note that in a four-year period the proportion of abdominoperineal excisions declined from 46% to 15%.

EUS stage T3 tumors have been treated with preoperative chemoradiation with good responses, allowing two-thirds of patients to have anal-sphincter–sparing procedures (4). In these cases, more than 64% of the patients had pathologic tumor stage T1 or T2, compared to preradiation therapy uT3. This suggests that, in a sizable number of patients, chemoradiation resulted in tumor downstaging.

## Rectal EUS Follow-up after Surgical Resection for Detection of Recurrence

Local recurrence of rectal cancer occurs in at least 10–15% of cases after 'curative' surgery with abdominoperineal resection or anterior resection, usually within the first two years after surgery (57,58). Therefore it is hoped that early detection of recurrent local tumor might result in earlier treatment to improve survival.

Beynon et al. described 85 patients with resected rectal tumors who underwent postoperative rectal exam, rigid sigmoidoscopy, and endorectal sonography every 3–6 months (59). Of the 85 patients, 22 (26%) were diagnosed with recurrent rectal cancer, 3 being diagnosed by endosonography alone while 19 were diagnosed by rectal exam or sigmoidoscopy as well as by EUS. No long-term prospective data were provided, and it is unclear whether endosonography allowed any curative resection to these patients or changed outcome in any other way.

Feifel and Hildebrandt described 123 patients who were followed with EUS every 3 months after surgery for 3 years (60). Women who had undergone abdominoperineal resection were examined with transvaginal ultrasound. Suspicious abnormalities either underwent ultrasound-guided FNA or repeat ultrasound 6 weeks later. Twenty-two patients (18%) developed local recurrence. Ultrasound showed recurrence in all 22 patients, and was the only study which detected tumor recurrence in 6 of the patients.

Romano et al. detected 8 local recurrences in 42 patients within 2 years of follow-up (47). There were also 2 cases that appeared to be local recurrences, however, fine-needle aspiration showed only fibrosis, suggesting that these were false-positive results.

It is possible that rectal EUS may allow earlier detection of recurrent rectal cancer in some patients, thereby prolonging survival with additional surgery or radiation. However, clinical trials will need to further assess this possibility, as well as the frequency of false-positive EUS studies.

## Other EUS Uses and Recommendations

### EUS and Rectal Adenomas

EUS can be useful in distinguishing an adenomatous polyp from a T2 or greater lesion. However, it cannot distinguish between a benign adenoma and a T1 lesion. The ability to determine the extent of penetration may be important if considering local resection of a large adenoma, either endoscopically or with transanal resection.

### EUS and Colon Cancer

Colon cancers above the rectum and peritoneal reflection allow primary anastamoses to be performed in most cases, obviating the need for colostomy as in abdominoperineal resections. These patients will need surgery anyway; therefore, no technically less invasive therapy is available to them. As the outcome would not be modified by accurate preoperative staging, EUS is of little use in such cases.

### Recommendations for Use of EUS in Rectal Cancer Staging

If the tumor is located in the lower two-thirds of the rectum, EUS should be performed. If the tumor is a

T1 N0 tumor, perform a transanal resection. If the tumor is staged as T2 N0, consider a low anterior resection. For T2 N1, T3 N1, or T4 tumors, consider preoperative chemoradiation. See Table 28–9.

## Future Technologic Advances

A limitation of endosonographic staging is the accuracy for determining lymph node metastases. This problem is partly due to difficulty in detecting small lymph nodes (i.e., <5 mm) and partly due to the fact that EUS criteria for determining if an identified lymph node is benign or malignant are themselves inaccurate. Accuracy may, however, be improved by performing transrectal FNA of lymph nodes. Preliminary results suggest that this is safe, but it is unclear if any tumor spread is associated with this technique or if the risk of infection is high enough to warrant antibiotics. Trans-rectal EUS-guided FNA was first reported by Andersson and Aus in 1990 (61). They used the rigid 7-MHz multiplane ultrasound probe normally used for prostate imaging, and obtained biopsies with a special Biopty gun attached to the probe. Transrectal EUS-guided has also been performed using the Pentax flexible fiberoptic EUS scope (62).

Approximately 14% of rectal tumors cannot be traversed with standard rectal ultrasound probes due to tumor obstruction. It is possible that catheter-based probes could provide more successful imaging by passing through the obstruction. Currently, catheter probes are available that can pass through an endoscope and image in 12.5 and 20 MHz. Preliminary results by Cho et al. show T-stage accuracy of 85% and N-stage accuracy of 59% using these probes. These findings suggest that catheter probes may be equal to standard EUS probes for T stage, but not as good for lymph nodes because of limited ultrasound penetration (63). As their image quality and depth of penetration improve with technologic advances, these probes may become the preferred imaging modality for endoscopists because of their lower cost, ease of cleaning, and ability to traverse tight strictures. Higher-frequency ultrasound probes (25–50 MHz) may also allow better resolution of tumors, but such frequencies inherently limit depth of penetration.

Ultrasonic treatment of rectal tumors may be possible in the future using high-intensity focused ultrasound (HIFU). Ultrasonic energy is focused at a discrete point, which results in focal thermal destruction of tissue without causing injury to the tissue lying in the path of the ultrasound beam. HIFU transducers are unique in that they can image as well as focus the ultrasound energy to ablate tissue. Recent studies have shown this to be safe and effective in transrectal treatment of benign prostate hypertrophy (64). Animal studies involving pseudotumors of the rectum have shown the feasibility of using this technology to treat rectal tumors (65).

**TABLE 28-9**

**Possible Treatment Options Based on Rectal EUS for Rectal Cancer**

| EUS stage | Therapy |
|---|---|
| T1, N0 | Transanal resection |
| T2, N0 | Consider anterior resection |
| T2–3, N1 | Consider preoperative chemoradiation therapy |

## Conclusions

Rectal endosonography for staging rectal tumors is the most accurate method for preoperative staging, with T-stage accuracy of 90% and N-stage accuracy of 80%. Interobserver variation has been assessed only in small studies and results of larger prospective analyses are anticipated (41). The main limitations to accuracy are that tumors tend to be overstaged (especially T2 tumors) and good criteria for determining malignant lymph nodes are lacking. The potential risks of overstaging are generally lower than those of understaging, because understaging could result in patients' receiving inadequate therapy for their tumors. Increasing numbers of cancer centers are now incorporating EUS to help determine the optimal treatment for rectal tumors, whether it be transanal excision, sphincter-preserving surgery, or preoperative chemoradiation followed by abdominoperineal resection with colostomy. EUS also appears useful in early detection of recurrent local disease. Future trials of therapy for rectal cancer will need to include EUS staging to fully evaluate outcomes after accurate preoperative staging or in the postoperative follow-up period.

## References

1. Ransohoff DF. Colorectal cancer. In Everhart JE (ed): Digestive Diseases in the United States: Epidemiology and Impact. US Department of Health and Human Services, Public Health Service, National Institutes of Health, National Institute of Diabetes and Digestive and Kidney Diseases. Washington, DC: US Government Printing Office, 1994; NIH publication no. 94-1447:207–224.
2. Cohen AM, Minsky BD, Friedman MA. Rectal Cancer. In DeVita VT, Hellman S, Rosenberg SA (eds): Cancer: Principles and Practice of Oncology, 4th Ed. Philadelphia: J.B. Lippincott, 1993, pp 978–1005.
3. Phillips RKS, Hittinger R, Blesovsky L, et al. Local recurrence following 'curative' surgery for large bowel cancer: II. The rectum and sigmoid. Br J Surg 71:17–20, 1984.
4. Rich TA, Skibber JM, Ajani JA, et al. Preoperative infusional chemoradiation therapy for stage T3 rectal cancer. Int J Radiation Oncol Biol Phys 32:1025–1029, 1995.
5. O'Connell MJ, Martenson JA, Wieand HS, et al. Improving adjuvant therapy for rectal cancer by combining protracted infusion fluorouracil with radiation therapy after curative surgery. N Engl J Med 331:502–507, 1994.
6. Wild JJ, Reid JM. Diagnostic use of ultrasound. Br J Phys Med 19:248–57, 1956.

7. Dragsted J, Gammelgaard J. Endoluminal ultrasonic scanning in the evaluation of rectal cancer. Gastrointest Radiol 8:367–369, 1983.
8. Hildebrandt U, Feifel G, Zimmermann FA, et al. Significant improvement in clinical staging of rectal carcinoma with a new intrarectal ultrasound scanner. J Exp Clin Cancer Res 2(suppl):53, 1983.
9. Bartram CI, Sultan AH. Anal endosonography in faecal incontinence. Gut 37:4–6, 1995.
10. Bartram CI. Anal sphincter disorders. Gastrointest Endosc 43:S32–S34, 1996.
11. Bartram CI. Anal endosonography in faecal incontinence. Endoscopy 28:259–260, 1996.
12. Silvis R, van Eekelen JW, Delemarre JBVM, Gooszen HG. Endosonography of the anal sphincter after ileal pouch-anal anastomosis. Dis Colon Rectum 38:383–388, 1995.
13. Petritsch W, Hinterleitner TA, Aichbichler B, Denk H, Hammer HF, Krejs GJ. Endosonography in colitis cystica profunda and solitary rectal ulcer syndrome. Gastrointest Endosc 44:746–751, 1996.
14. Felt-Bersma RJF, van Baren R, Koorevaar M, Strijers RL, Cuesta MA. Unsuspected sphincter defects shown by anal endosonography after anorectal surgery. Dis Colon Rectum 38:249–253, 1995.
15. Meyenberger C, Bertschinger P, Zala GF, Buchmann P. Anal sphincter defects in fecal incontinence: Correlation between endosonography and surgery. Endoscopy 28:217–224, 1996.
16. Yoshida M, Tsukamoto Y, Niwa Y, Goto H, Hase S, Hayakawa T, Okamura S. Endoscopic assessment of invasion of colorectal tumors with a new high-frequency ultrasound probe. Gastrointest Endosc 41:587–592, 1994.
17. Beynon J, Mortensen NJM, Foy DMA, et al. Endorectal sonography: Laboratory and clinical experience in Bristol. Int J Colorectal Dis 1:212–215, 1986.
18. Beynon J, Foy DMA, Channer JL, et al. The ultrasonographic anatomy of the normal colon and rectum. Dis Colon Rectum 29:810–813, 1986.
19. Beynon J. An evaluation of the role of rectal endosonography in rectal cancer. Ann R Coll Surg Eng 71:131–139, 1989.
20. Wang KY, Kimmey MB, Nyberg DA, et al. Colorectal neoplasms: Accuracy of US in demonstrating the depth of invasion. Radiology 165:827–829, 1987.
21. Colon and Rectum. American Joint Committee on Cancer. Manual for Staging of Cancer, 4th Ed. Philadelphia: J.B. Lippincott, 1992, pp 75–79.
22. Dukes CE. The classification of cancer of the rectum. J Pathol 35:323–332, 1932.
23. Aster VB, Coller FA. The prognostic significance of direct extension of carcinoma of the colon and rectum. Ann Surg 139:846–851, 1954.
24. Saitoh N, Okui K, Sarashina H, et al. Evaluation of echographic diagnosis of rectal cancer using intrarectal ultrasonic examination. Dis Colon Rectum 29:234–242, 1986.
25. Boyce GA, Sivak MV, Lavery IC, et al. Endoscopic ultrasound in the pre-operative staging of rectal cancer. Gastrointest Endosc 38:468–471, 1992.
26. Herzog U, von Flue M, Tondelli P, Schuppisser JP. How accurate is endorectal ultrasound in the preoperative staging of rectal cancer? Dis Colon Rectum 36:127–134, 1993.
27. Hizawa K, Suekane H, Aoyagi K, Matsumoto T, Nakamura S, Fujishima M. Use of endosonographic evaluation of colorectal tumor depth in determining the appropriateness of endoscopic mucosal resection. Am J Gastroenterol 91:768–771, 1996.
28. Hünerbein M, Dohmoto M, Haensch W, Schlag PM. Evaluation and biopsy of recurrent rectal cancer using three-dimensional endosonography. Dis Colon Rectum 39:1373–1378, 1996.
29. Neilson MB, Qvitzau S, Pedersen JF, Christiansen J. Endosonography for preoperative staging of rectal tumors. Acta Radiologica 37:799–803, 1996.
30. Feifel G, Hildebrandt U, Dhom G. Assessment of depth of invasion of rectal cancer by endosonography. Endoscopy 19:64–67, 1987.
31. Yamashita Y, Machi J, Shirouzu K, et al. Evaluation of endorectal ultrasound for the assessment of wall invasion of rectal cancer: Report of a case. Dis Colon Rectum 31:617–623, 1988.
32. Cho E, Nakajima M, Yasuda K, et al. Endoscopic ultrasonography in the diagnosis of colorectal cancer invasion. Gastrointest Endosc 39:521–527, 1993.
33. Glaser F, Kuntz C, Schlag P, Herfarth C. Endorectal ultrasound for control of preoperative radiotherapy of rectal cancer. Ann Surg 217:64–71, 1993.
34. Tio TL, Tytgat GNJ. Endoscopic ultrasonography in analyzing peri-intestinal lymph node abnormality. Preliminary results of studies in vitro and in vivo. Scand J Gastroenterol 21(suppl 123): 158–163, 1986.
35. Hildebrandt U, Klein T, Feifel G, et al. Endosonography of pararectal lymph nodes. In vitro and in vivo evaluation. Dis Colon Rectum 33:863–868, 1990.
36. Herrera-Ornelas S, Justiniano J, Catillo N, et al. Metastases in small lymph nodes from colon cancer. Arch Surg 122:1253–1256, 1987.
37. Hulsmans FJH, Bosma A, Mulder PJJ, et al. Perirectal lymph nodes in rectal cancer: In vitro correlation of sonographic parameters and histopathologic findings. Radiology 184:553–560, 1992.
38. Nielsen MB, Qvitzau S, Pedersen JF. Detection of pericolonic lymph nodes in patients with colorectal cancer: An in vitro and in vivo study of the efficacy of endosonography. AJR 161:57–60, 1993.
39. Orrom WJ, Wong WD, Rothenberger DA, et al. Endorectal ultrasound in the preoperative staging of rectal tumors: A learning experience. Dis Colon Rectum 33:654–9, 1990.
40. Palazzo L, Burtin P. Interobserver variation in tumor staging. Gastrointest Endosc Clin North Am 5:559–567, 1995.
41. Roubein LD, Lynch P, Glober G, Sinicrope FA. Interobserver variability in endoscopic ultrasonography: A prospective evaluation. Gastrointest Endosc 44:573–577, 1996.
42. Nicholls RJ, York Mason A, Morson BC, et al. The clinical staging of rectal cancer. Br J Surg 69:404–409, 1982.
43. Beynon J, Mortensen NJMC, Foy DMA, et al. Pre-operative assessment of local invasion in rectal cancer: Digital examination, endoluminal sonography or computed tomography? Br J Surg 73:1015–1017, 1986.
44. Hildebrandt U, Feifel G. Preoperative staging of rectal cancer by intrarectal ultrasound. Dis Colon Rectum 28:42–46, 1985.
45. Rifkin MD, Ehrlich AM, Marks G. Staging of rectal carcinoma: Prospective comparison of endorectal US and CT. Radiology 170:319–322, 1989.
46. Kramann B, Hildebrandt U. Computed tomography versus endosonography in the staging-of rectal carcinoma: A comparative study. Int J Colorect Dis 1:216–218, 1986.
47. Romano G, deRosa P, Vallone G, et al. Intrarectal ultrasound and computed tomography in the pre- and postoperative assessment of patients with rectal cancer. Br J Surg 72:S117–S119, 1985.
48. Pappalardo G, Reggio D, Frattaroli FM, et al. The value of endoluminal ultrasonography and computed tomography in the staging of rectal cancer: A preliminary study. J Surg Oncol 43:219–222, 1990.
49. Waizer A, Powsner E, Russo I, et al. Prospective comparative study of magnetic resonance imaging versus transrectal ultrasound for preoperative staging and follow-up of rectal cancer. Dis Colon Rectum 34:1068–1072, 1991.
50. Thaler W, Watzka S, Martin F, et al. Preoperative staging of rectal cancer by endoluminal ultrasound vs. magnetic resonance imaging: Preliminary results of a prospective, comparative study. Dis Colon Rectum 37:1189–1193, 1994.
51. Schäefer H, Gossmann A, Heindel W, Lackner K, Hölscher AH. Comparison of endorectal MR imaging and transrectal ultrasound with pathology in rectal tumors. Endoscopy 28:S9, 1996.
52. Meyenberger C, Huch Boni RA, Bertschinger P, et al. Endoscopic ultrasound and endorectal magnetic resonance imaging: A prospective, comparative study for preoperative staging and follow-up of rectal cancer. Endoscopy 27:469–479, 1995.
53. Napoleon B, Pujol B, Berger F, et al. Accuracy of endosonography in staging of rectal cancer treated by radiotherapy. Br J Surg 78:785–788, 1991.
54. Vallas M, Napoleon B, Pujol B, et al. Endosonographic evaluation of the downstaging effect of preoperative radiotherapy on the N stage in rectal carcinoma [Abstract]. Gastroenterology 40:P97, 1994.
55. Glaser F, Kuntz D, Schlag P, Herfarth C. Endorectal ultrasound for control of preoperative radiotherapy of rectal cancer. Ann Surg 217:64–71, 1993.
56. Hildebrandt U, Schuder G, Feifel G. Preoperative staging of rectal and colonic cancer. Endoscopy 26:810–812, 1994.

57. Phillips RKS, Hittinger R, Blesovsky L, Fry JS, Fielding LP. Local recurrence following 'curative' surgery for large bowel cancer: II. The rectum and rectosigmoid. Br J Surg 71:17–20, 1984.
58. Williams NS, Johnston D. Survival and recurrence after sphincter saving resection and abdominoperineal resection for carcinoma of the middle third of the rectum. Br J Surg 71:278–282, 1984.
59. Beynon J, Mortensen NJMC, Foy DMA, et al. The detection and evaluation of locally recurrent rectal cancer with rectal endosonography. Dis Colon Rectum 32:509–517, 1989.
60. Feifel G, Hildebrandt U. Diagnostic imaging in rectal cancer: Endosonography and immunoscintigraphy. World J Surg 16:841–847, 1992.
61. Andersson R, Aus G. Transrectal ultrasound-guided biopsy for verification of lymph-node metastasis in rectal cancer. Acta Chir Scand 156:659–660, 1990.
62. Chang K, Katz KD, Durbin TE, et al. Endoscopic ultrasound-guided fine-needle aspiration. Gastrointest Endosc 40:694–699, 1994.
63. Cho E, Hirano S, Ashihara T, et al. Clinical usefulness of ultrasonic probes in the diagnosis of colorectal cancer invasion [Abstract]. Gastrointest Endosc 41:300, 1995.
64. Bihrle R, Foster RS, Sanghvi NT, et al. High intensity focused ultrasound for the treatment of BPH: Early U.S. clinical experience. J Urol 151:1271–1275, 1994.
65. Zaidi S, Gress F, Kopecky K, et al. High intensity focused ultrasound (HIFU) ablation of experimental rectal pseudotumors in the canine model. World Congress of Gastroenterology 1995:2900P.
66. Di Candio G, Mosca F, Campatelli A, et al. Endosonographic staging of rectal carcinoma. Gastrointest Radiol 12:289–295, 1987.
67. Jochem RJ, Reading CC, Dozois RR, et al. Endorectal ultrasonographic staging of rectal carcinoma. Mayo Clin Proc 65:1571–1577, 1990.

# INDEX

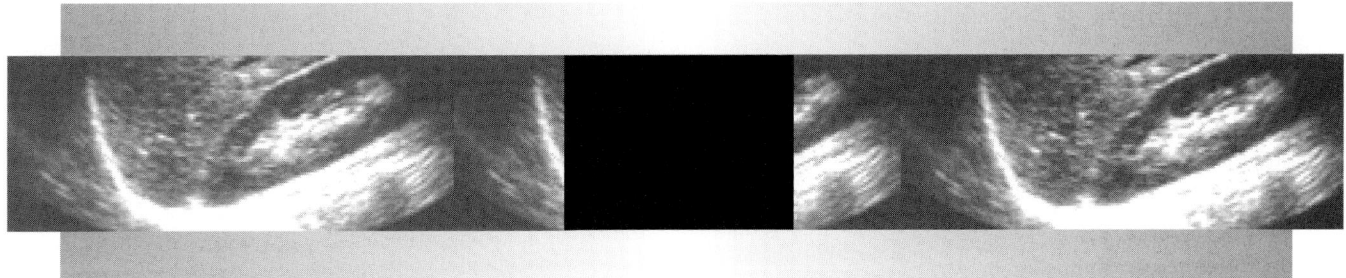

Entries followed by "f" refer to figures; entries followed by "t" refer to tables.


**A**

Abdominal aorta, linear array echoendoscopy of, 48f, 52f
  anatomy of, 110, 111f
Abdominal pain, intractable, endosonography-guided celiac plexus neurolysis for, 39–41, 41f–42f
Achalasia, radial endoluminal ultrasonography of, 86–88, 88f, 88t
Acoustic coupling agent(s), 5
Acoustic impedance, 5, 5f
Acoustic shadowing, 7f
Adenocarcinoma, pancreatic, 241f
  fine-needle aspiration biopsy of, 256f
    with Pentax/Hitachi FG-32UA linear array echo-endoscope, 35f
Adenoma, of colon, endoscopic ultrasonography of, 275, 275f
  rectal, endoscopic ultrasonography of, 286
Adrenal gland, linear array echoendoscopy of, 56, 57f
AJCC/UICC tumor staging system, 115–120. *See also* TNM staging system
Amplitude, 6
Ampulla of Vater, cancer of, endoscopic ultrasonography of, accuracy of, 248, 249t
  carcinoma of, TNM staging of, 119, 119t
  linear array echoendoscopy of, 51f–57f, 51–56
  radial endoluminal ultrasonography of, 99f
Angiography, in portal hypertension, 221
Aorta, abdominal, linear array endosonography of, 48f, 52f
  anatomy of, 110, 111f
"Aorto-pulmonary window," in linear array endosonography of mediastinum, 49, 50f
Artifacts, 13–17, 14f–17f
  enhancement, 15f, 15–16
  mirror-image, 17, 17f
  off-axis, 16, 16f
  refraction, 16, 17f
  reverberation, 13–14, 14f
  ring-down, 14, 15f
  section-thickness, 16
  shadowing, 7f, 14–15, 15f
Ascites, in portal hypertension, 219–220, 223f
Aspiration biopsy, fine-needle. *See* Fine-needle aspiration biopsy
Attenuation, 6
Axial resolution, 12–13, 13f
  of endoluminal transducers, 68, 68f
Azygous vein, imaging of, 110, 111f
  linear array echoendoscopy of, 48f
  in portal hypertension, 204, 205f, 207–208, 214, 215f

**B**

Balloon, water-filled, examination of esophagus with, 109
  for recurrence of cancer, 148–149
Barium studies, of subepithelial lesions, 153, 154f
  *vs.* endoscopic ultrasonography, 156
Barrett's esophagus, linear array endoluminal ultrasonography of, 70f
  postoperative surveillance of, 136
Bile ducts, endoscopic ultrasonography of, 230–231, 232f
  extrahepatic, linear array endosonography of, 57–58, 58f–59f
  linear array endoluminal ultrasonography of, 76–77, 78f
Biopsy, fine-needle aspiration. *See* Fine-needle aspiration biopsy
  guillotine needle, of subepithelial lesions, 170f–172f, 170–171
Bleeding, from esophageal varices, risk factors for, 89

**C**

Carcinoids, rectal, 163
Catheter probe, for EU-M20 radial scanning echoendoscope, 23
  for linear array endoluminal ultrasonography
    application of, 70–72, 71f–72f
    development of, 68–70, 69f–70f
Catheters, needle knife, for drainage of pancreatic pseudocysts, 258, 259f
Celiac artery, color flow endosonography of, 63f
  linear array endosonography of, 50f
Celiac axis, endosonography of, 114f

Celiac plexus neurolysis, endosonography-guided, with Pentax/Hitachi FG-32UA linear array echoendoscope, 39–41, 41f–42f
Chemotherapy, staging of esophageal carcinoma after, 133–135, 134f–135f
Cholangiocarcinoma, radial endoluminal ultrasonography of, 98f, 98–99
Cholangiography, retrograde, linear array endoluminal, 78f
Cholangiopancreatography, endosonography-guided, with Pentax/Hitachi FG-32UA linear array echoendoscope, 37, 38f
Circulation, collateral, in portal hypertension, 209
Collateral veins, periesophageal, in portal hypertension, 204, 205f
Colon, adenoma of, endoscopic ultrasonography of, 275, 275f
  endoscopic ultrasonography of
    indications for, 273–276, 274f–276f
    normal anatomy of, 272, 273f
    technique of, 271–272, 272f
  sigmoid, leiomyoma in, linear array endoluminal ultrasonography of, 74f
  wall of, endoscopic ultrasonography of, 107, 107f
Colonic anastomosis, tumor recurrence at, 275–276, 276f
Colorectal cancer, recurrence of, at anastomosis, 275–276, 276f
  staging of, 273–275, 274f, 286–287
    TNM, 119–120, 120f, 120t
Color flow Doppler sonography, in portal hypertension, 204
Color flow endosonography, linear array, 59–60, 60f–62f
Computed tomography (CT), of pancreas, 236, 236f
  in portal hypertension, 221
  for staging of rectal cancer, 285
  *vs.* endoscopic ultrasonography
    for staging of esophageal carcinoma, 141–142, 142t
    of subepithelial lesions, 156
Contrast sensitivity, 11–12, 12f
Contrast studies, of subepithelial lesions, 153, 154f
  *vs.* endoscopic ultrasonography, 156
Control panel, for EU-M20 radial scanning echoendoscope, 20–21, 21f
Convex array endosonography, of pancreas, interventional, 251–252, 253t
Core biopsy, of subepithelial lesions, 164
Crohn's disease, endoscopic ultrasonography of, 276
Cysts, 159–160, 160f–161f

**D**

Decibels, 6
Depth controls, 10–11
Diaphragm, radial endoluminal ultrasonography of, 85f
Diffuse reflectors, 6
Digital scan converter, 9, 9f
Doppler endosonography, linear array, 59–60, 60f–62f
Doppler sonography, color flow, in portal hypertension, 204
Doppler ultrasonography, of pancreas, interventional, 252, 253f–254f
  with Pentax/Hitachi FG-32UA linear array echoendoscope, 31, 31f
  in portal hypertension, 222–223
Dukes classification, of colorectal cancer, 119–120, 282t
Duodenofiberscope, Olympus IF-UM20, 21, 21f, 22t
Duodenum, color flow endosonography of, 60f
  lipoma in, linear array endoluminal ultrasonography of, 74, 74f
  neuroendocrine tumors, 266f
  wall of, endosonography of, 106–107
Duplex endosonography, with Pentax/Hitachi FG-32UA linear array echoendoscope, 38–39, 39f–40f

**E**

Echocolonoscopes, Olympus CF-UM3, 272f
Echoendoscopes, linear array, Pentax/Hitachi FG-32UA, 29–42. *See also* Linear array echoendoscopes, Pentax/Hitachi FG-32UA
  Olympus GF-UM20, for imaging of rectal cancer, 280
  radial scanning, EU-M20, 19–27. *See also* EU-M20 radial scanning echoendoscope
Echoes, formation of, 8, 8f
Electronic array transducers, 9f, 9–10
Endocrine tumors, 240
Endoluminal ultrasonography, of upper gastrointestinal tract, linear array, 67–78. *See also* Linear array endoluminal ultrasonography
  radial, 81–94. *See also* Radial endoluminal ultrasonography
Endoscopic retrograde cholangiopancreatography (ERCP), with Pentax/Hitachi FG-32UA linear array echoendoscope, 37, 38f
  *vs.* endoscopic ultrasonography, 240
Endoscopic retrograde pancreatography (ERP), 237
Endoscopic ultrasonography (EUS), in Barrett's esophagus, for postoperative surveillance, 136
  of bile ducts, 230–231, 232f
  of cancer of ampulla of Vater, acuracy of, 248, 249t
  of colon wall, 107, 107f
  colorectal, 271–277. *See also* Colon; Colorectal cancer; Rectum
  Doppler, linear array, 59–60, 60f–62f
  for drainage of pancreatic pseudocysts, 258f–260f, 258–261, 261t
  of duodenal wall, 106–107
  duplex, with Pentax/Hitachi FG-32UA linear array echoendoscope, 38–39, 39f–40f
  of enlarged gastric folds, 182
  of esophageal carcinoma, for treatment planning, 139–141
  of esophageal wall, 106, 106f
  examiner bias in, 123–124, 124f
  fine-needle aspiration biopsy with
    of subepithelial lesions, 169–173
    technique of, 60–63, 63f–64f
  of gut wall, 103–108. *See also* Gut wall, endosonography of
  of inflammatory bowel disease, 276
  lack of histologic diagnosis in, 124–125, 125f
  of neuroendocrine tumors, 264f–266f, 265–266, 267t
  of pancreas, 230–232, 231f–232f. *See also* Pancreas, endoscopic ultrasonography of
  of pancreatic cancer, 246f–247f, 246–248
    accuracy of, 248, 248t–249t
  pitfalls in, 123–127
  in portal hypertension. *See* Portal hypertension

Endoscopic ultrasonography (EUS) (*cont.*)
of rectal wall, 107
of retroperitoneum, 229–233
sector scanning, instruments for, 19
for staging of esophageal carcinoma. *See* Esophageal carcinoma
for staging of gastric cancer. *See* Gastric cancer
of stomach wall, 106–107
Endosonography-guided cholangiopancreatography, with Pentax/Hitachi FG-32UA linear array echoendoscope, 37, 38f
Energy, sound waves as, 6–7, 7f
Enhancement artifacts, 15f, 15–16
ERCP. *See* Endoscopic retrograde cholangiopancreatography (ERCP)
ERP (endoscopic retrograde pancreatography), 237
Esophageal carcinoma, with high-grade strictures, 133
linear array endoluminal ultrasonography of, 76f–77f
with nontraversable tumor stenosis, endoscopic ultrasonography in, 142, 142t
overstaging of, 143
postoperative recurrence of, 147–149, 148f–149f, 148t–149t
postoperative surveillance of, 135f–136f, 135–136
radial endoluminal ultrasonography of, 92, 93f, 96–97, 97f
staging of, 116t–117t, 116–117
endoscopic ultrasonography in
accuracy of, 141t
*vs.* computed tomography, 141–142, 142t
and postoperative surveillance, 135f–136f, 135–136, 139, 140f
pretreatment, 131–133, 132
retreatment, 133–135, 134f–135f
using TNM system, 139, 140f–141f
*vs.* computed tomography, 141–142, 142t
treatment planning in, 139–141
Esophageal strictures, high-grade, with carcinoma, 133
Esophageal varices, endoscopic ultrasonography of, 158–159
grading of, 217, 219f–220f, 220t
in portal hypertension, 204, 204f, 207, 216–218, 218t, 219f
radial endoluminal ultrasonography of, 88–91, 89f–90f
treatment of, monitoring of, 208–209
Esophageal wall, endosonography of, 106, 106f
layers of, 111
Esophagitis, ulcerative, radial endoluminal ultrasonography of, 92, 92f
Esophagogastric junction, cancer of, 188f
Esophagoprobe, for EU-M20 radial scanning echoendoscope, 23
Esophagus, adenocarcinoma of, fine-needle aspiration biopsy of, with Pentax/Hitachi FG-32UA linear array echoendoscope, 35f
anatomy of, radial endoluminal ultrasonography of, 84–86, 85f–86f, 86t
collateral veins in, in portal hypertension, 204, 205f
distal, para-aortic tissue in, 127f
endosonography of, 109–112, 110f–111f
stations in, 110
fibrous wall thickening of, after radiation therapy, 149
leiomyoma of, guillotine needle biopsy of, 170f
leiomyosarcoma of, guillotine needle biopsy of, 170f
linear array echoendoscopy of, 48f–50f, 48–50
pseudotumor of, 125f
radial endoluminal ultrasonography of
in humans, 84, 85f
in sheep, 83f, 83–84
strictures of, linear array endoluminal ultrasonography of, 71f, 74f
EU-M20 radial scanning endosonographic system, 19–27
attachments for, 24
balloons for, 24
camera unit for, 27
care of, 27
catheter probes for, 23
components of, 20f–21f, 20–21
duodenofiberscope for, 21, 21f, 22t
electronic controls on, 22f, 22–23
esophagoprobe for, 23
examination procedure using, 25–27
freeze feature of, 26
gastrofibroscope for, 21, 21f, 22t
image recording with, 26–27
measurements with, 26
pre-examination preparation for, 23–24
setup of, 23–24
trolley-based, 20f
uses of, 23
valve features on, 22
water pump for, 24–25
EUS. *See* Endoscopic ultrasonography (EUS)
EUS-CPN. *See* Endosonography-guided celiac plexus neurolysis
EUS FNA. *See* Fine-needle aspiration biopsy
Extrahepatic bile duct, linear array echoendoscopy of, 57–58, 58f–59f

**F**

Fine-needle aspiration biopsy, endosonographic, of pancreas, 239, 253–258, 255f–257f
clinical usefulness of, 257–258
complications of, 257
histologic examination of, 257f
needles for, 253–254, 255f–256f
results of, 255–256
technique of, 253–254, 255f
with Pentax/Hitachi FG-32UA linear array echoendoscope, 34–37, 35f–37f, 36t–37t
performance of, 36t–37t, 36–37
of subepithelial lesions, 168–173
technique of, 60–63, 63f–64f
Focal depth, 11, 13f
Foregut, cysts of, 159
Frequency, of sound waves, 3
absorption of, 7
Fujinon Sonoprobe, 77

**G**

Gain control, 10f–11f, 10–11
on EUB-515 ultrasound console, 46
on EU-M20 radial scanning ultrasound console, 24

Gallbladder, endosonography of, 113f
linear array echoendoscopy of, 58–59, 59f
Gallstones, endosonography of, 113f
Gastric artery, left, linear array echoendoscopy of, 54f
Gastric cancer, diagnosis of, 186
in fundus, 187f
invasive, 188f–189f
with lymph node metastasis, 187–188, 189f, 190
recognition of, 197–198
prognosis in, 185
radial endoluminal ultrasonography of, 98f
staging of
clinical, 186–187
endoscopic ultrasonography in, 187f–189f, 187–188
early, 190
limitations of, 189–190
with local invasion, 195–196, 197t
preoperative, 189
problems with, 198
results of, 190–191, 191f
and treatment planning, 198
*vs.* histopathology, 197t
TNM, 118, 118t, 186
Gastric folds, enlarged, 176–177, 182
Gastric ulcers, differential diagnosis of, 196–197
Gastric varices, in portal hypertension, 205, 205f, 214, 215f, 218–219, 221f–222f, 222t
radial endoluminal ultrasonography of, 88–91, 90f
Gastric veins, dilated, in portal hypertension, 205, 206f–207f
Gastric wall, layers of, 112, 112t
Gastrinoma, endoscopic ultrasonography of, 266f
Gastroepiploic vein, in portal hypertension, 205, 207f
Gastroesophageal anastomosis, recurrence of cancer at, 148, 148f–149f
Gastrofiberscope, Olympus GF-UM20, 21, 21f, 22t
Gastrointestinal tract, normal anatomy of, misinterpretation of, 126–127, 127f
Gastrointestinal wall, layers of, 177, 177f–178f
thickness of, measurement of, 125–126, 126f
Gastropathy, in portal hypertension, 219, 223f, 224
Gel, and acoustic impedance, 5
GIP/Mediglobe needle, 60, 63f–64f
Guillotine needle biopsy, of subepithelial lesions, 170f–172f, 170–171
Gut wall, endosonography of, 103–108
interfaces in, 103–104
layers in, 103–105, 104f–105f
reflection coefficient in, 104
scattering in, 104
sensitivity of, 107–108
thickness in, 105
transducers for, 106

**H**

Hemiazygous vein, imaging of, 110, 111f
Hemorrhage, subepithelial, in portal hypertension, 223f
Hepatic veins, imaging of, with Pentax/Hitachi FG-32UA linear array echoendoscope, 33, 33f
High-frequency ultrasound probes, for imaging of rectal cancer, 280
High-resolution endoluminal ultrasonography (HRUS), of upper gastrointestinal tract, linear array, 67–78. *See also* Linear array endoluminal ultrasonography
radial, 81–92. *See also* Radial endoluminal ultrasonography
Histologic diagnosis, lack of, as pitfall of endoscopic ultrasonography, 124–125, 125f
Histopathology, in staging of gastric cancer, *vs.* endoscopic ultrasonography, 197t
Hypertension, portal. *See* Portal hypertension

**I**

Image, production of, 7–11, 8f–12f
quality of, 11–13, 12f–13f
Image contrast, 11–12, 12f
Inferior vena cava, color flow endosonography of, 62f
Inflammatory bowel disease, endoscopic ultrasonography of, 276
Insulinomas, endoscopic ultrasonography of, 266
Interfaces, in endosonography, of gut wall, 103–104
Interventional endosonography, of pancreas, technique of, 252–253, 255f
Intraductal ultrasonoraphy (IDUS), of pancreas, 242
Islet cell tumors, 236f, 241f

**K**

Kidneys, linear array echoendoscopy of, 56, 57f

**L**

Laparoscopy, radial endoluminal ultrasonography during, 93–94
Lateral resolution, 12, 13f
of endoluminal transducers, 68, 68f
Leiomyoma, 154f, 156t, 156–157, 157f
of esophagus, guillotine needle biopsy of, 170f
fine-needle aspiration biopsy of, with Pentax/Hitachi FG-UA linear array echoendoscope, 34f
gastric, 168f
linear array endoluminal ultrasonography of, 74f–75f, 74–75
Leiomyosarcoma, 160, 162
esophageal, guillotine needle biopsy of, 170f
LES. *See* Lower esophageal sphincter (LES)
Linear array echoendoscopes, Pentax/Hitachi FG-32UA, 29–42
celiac plexus neurolysis with, 39–41, 41f–42f
cholangiopancreatography with, 37, 38f
components of, 30f–31f, 30–31, 45–46, 46f
Doppler imaging with, 31, 31f
Duplex endosonography with, 38–39, 39f–40f
fine-needle aspiration biopsy with, 34–37, 35f–37f, 36t–37t
imaging of normal anatomy with, 31, 32f, 33
tumor staging with, 33f–34f, 33–34
*vs.* radial echoendoscopes, 47t, 47–48
Linear array echoendoscopy, aorto-pulmonary window in, 49, 50f
color flow, 59–60, 60f–62f

Linear array echoendoscopy (*cont.*)
Doppler endosonography with, 59–60, 60f–62f
of esophagus, 48f–50f, 48–50
of gallbladder, 58–59, 59f
intubation for, 47
of mediastinum, 48f–50f, 48–50
of pancreas, interventional, 251–252, 253t
patient preparation for, 46–47
transabdominal, 50–59, 51f–57f
of adrenal gland, 56, 57f
of extrahepatic bile duct, 57–58, 58f–59f
of kidney, 56, 57f
of liver, 51, 51f
of pancreas and ampulla, 51f–57f, 51–56
of spleen, 56, 57f
Linear array endoluminal ultrasonography, of bile ducts, 76–77, 78f
retrograde cholangiography with, 78f
for staging of malignancy, 75–76, 76f
of upper gastrointestinal tract, 67–78
development of probe for, 68–70, 69f–70f
indications for, 73–77, 74f–78f
interpretation of, 72–73, 73f–74f
M-mode, 72, 72f
probes for
application of, 70–72, 71f–72f
development of, 68–70, 69f–70f
transducers for, 67–68, 68f
water for, 71–73, 73f
Linitis plastica, 176, 181f
diagnosis of, 197
Lipoma, 158, 158f
duodenal, linear array endoluminal ultrasonography of, 74, 74f
gastric, fine-needle aspiration biopsy of, with endoscopic ultrasonography, 171f
Liver, caudate lobe of, difficulties with imaging, 126, 127f
linear array echoendoscopy of, 51, 51f
Lower esophageal sphincter (LES), radial endoluminal ultrasonography of, 85f, 86t
in achalasia, 87, 88f, 88t
Lymph nodes, endosonography of, 113–114, 114f
linear array endoluminal ultrasonography of, 75–76, 76f
metastatic disease in
in gastric cancer, 187–188, 189f, 190
recognition of, 143, 197–198
TNM staging of, 117–118
radial endoluminal ultrasonography of, 92
Lymphoma, gastric, 175–176
differential diagnosis of, 180
endoscopic ultrasonography of, 177f–181f, 177–182
growth of, 177, 178f
infiltrative, 180f
resection of, level of, 181
staging of, 178f, 179, 179f–180f
non-Hodgkin's
fine-needle aspiration biopsy of, with Pentax/Hitachi FG-32UA linear array echoendoscope, 36f
imaging of, with Pentax/Hitachi FG-32UA linear array echoendoscope, 33f

**M**

Magnetic resonance imaging (MRI), in portal hypertension, 221–222
for staging of rectal cancer, 285
Mechanical transducers, 9f, 9–10
Mediastinum, linear array echoendoscopy of, 48f–50f, 48–50
Menetrier's disease, 176–177, 181f
Mesenteric arteries, superior. *See* Superior mesenteric artery (SMA)
Mesenteric vein, in portal hypertension, 206, 207f
Metastatic disease, in lymph nodes, in gastric cancer, 187–188, 189f, 190
recognition of, 143, 197–198
staging of, 117–118
Mirror-image artifacts, 17, 17f
M-mode imaging, linear array endoluminal, 72, 72f

**N**

Needle knife catheter, for drainage of pancreatic pseudocysts, 258, 259f
Neuroendocrine tumors
of duodenum, 266f
endoscopic ultrasonography of, 264f–266f, 265–266, 267t
invasive tests of, 264
noninvasive localization of, 263–264
of pancreas, 265f
of stomach, 266f
Neurolysis, celiac plexus, endosonography-guided, with Pentax/Hitachi FG-32UA linear array echoendoscope, 39–41, 41f–42f
Non-Hodgkin's lymphoma, fine-needle aspiration biopsy of, with Pentax/Hitachi FG-32UA linear array echoendoscope, 36f
imaging of, with Pentax/Hitachi FG-32UA linear array echoendoscope, 33f

**O**

Oblique scanning, pitfalls of, 125, 126f
Off-axis artifacts, 16, 16f
Olympus CF-UM3 echocolonoscope, 272f
Olympus EU-M20 radial scanning ultrasound console, 19–27. *See also* EU-M20 radial scanning ultrasound console
Olympus GF-UM20 echoendoscope, for imaging of rectal cancer, 280

**P**

Pancreas, aberrant, 160, 162f
adenocarcinoma of, 241f
fine-needle aspiration biopsy of, 35f, 256f
with Pentax/Hitachi FG-32UA linear array echoendoscope, 35f
computed tomography of, 236, 236f
Doppler ultrasonography of, interventional, 252, 253f–254f
endocrine tumors of, 240
endoscopic ultrasonography of, 230–232, 231f–232f
as adjunct to conventional imaging, 240–242
advantages of, 235
benign *vs.* malignant disease in, 239–240

Pancreas, endoscopic ultrasonography of (*cont.*)
difficulties with, 235
normal anatomy in, 230–232, 231f–232f
pathology in, 232–233
endosonography of, 113, 113f
fine-needle aspiration biopsy of, 239
imaging of, with Pentax/Hitachi FG-32UA linear array echoendoscope, 31, 32f
intraductal ultrasonography of, 242
linear array echoendoscopy of, interventional, 251–252, 253t
neuroendocrine tumors of, endoscopic ultrasonography of, 264f–266f, 265–266, 267t
pseudocysts of, 238–239
drainage of, 258f–260f, 258–261, 261t
transabdominal ultrasonography of, 235–236
Pancreatic cancer
endoscopic ultrasonography of, 246f–247f, 246–248
clinical usefulness of, 248–249
and treatment planning, 249
radial endoluminal ultrasonography of, 99, 99f
staging of, systems for, 245–246, 246t
Pancreatic duct, radial endoluminal ultrasonography of, 97–98
Pancreatic rests, 160, 162f
Pancreatitis, acute, 237
cholangiopancreatography of, with Pentax/Hitachi FG-32UA linear array echoendoscope, 37, 38f
chronic, 237–239, 238f
endosonography-guided celiac plexus neurolysis for, 39–41, 41f–42f
Paraduodenum, normal anatomy of, 230–231, 231f–232f
Pentax/Hitachi FG-32UA linear array echoendoscope, 29–42. *See also* Linear array echoendoscopes, Pentax/Hitachi FG-32UA
Peristalsis, during swallowing, radial endoluminal ultrasonography of, 93
Piezoelectric crystals, function of, 7–8, 8f
Polyps, linear array endoluminal ultrasonography of, 76f
Portal hypertension, angiography in, 221
ascites in, 219–220, 223f
assessment of severity in, 220
azygous vein in, 204, 205f, 207–208, 214, 215f
collateral circulation in, 209
complications of, 220
computed tomography in, 221
dilated gastric veins in, 205, 206f–207f
Doppler ultrasonography in, 222–223
endoscopic ultrasonography in
organs visualized during, 214, 214f–215f
technique of, 203
*vs.* other imaging modalities, 203–204
*vs.* traditional endoscopy, 224
esophageal varices in, 204, 204f, 207
gastric varices in, 205, 205f, 218–219, 221f–222f, 222t
gastroepiploic vein in, 205, 207f
gastropathy in, 219, 223f, 224
magnetic resonance imaging in, 221–222
mesenteric vein in, 206, 207f
periesophageal collateral veins in, 204, 205f
portal vein in, 214, 217f
real-time transabdominal ultrasonography in, 222
splenic vein in, 205, 207f, 214, 217f
studies of, 214f–217f, 214–216, 218t
findings of, 220–224, 221t–222t
subepithelial hemorrhage in, 223f
Portal vein, color flow endosonography of, 61f
imaging of, with Pentax/Hitachi FG-32UA linear array echoendoscope, 31, 32f
in portal hypertension, 214, 217f
Power settings, on ultrasound units, 10
Probes, for imaging of rectal cancer, 280–281, 281t
for linear array endoluminal ultrasonography
application of, 70–72, 71f–72f
development of, 68–70, 69f–70f
for radial endoluminal ultrasonography, 95–96, 96f, 96t
for staging of esophageal carcinoma, 117
Prostate, anatomy of, 273f
Pseudocysts, pancreatic, 238–239
drainage of, 258f–260f, 258–261, 261t
Pseudotumor, esophageal, 125f

**R**

Radial echoendoscopes, *vs.* linear array echoendoscopes, 47t, 47–48
Radial endoluminal ultrasonography, 81–94
of achalasia, 86–88, 88f, 88t
components of, 82f, 82–83
of diaphragm, 86f
of esophagus, 96–97, 97f
human, 84, 85f
normal anatomy in, 84–86, 85f–86f, 86t
in sheep, 83f, 83–84
examination technique in, 96
history of, 81–82
during laparoscopy, 93–94
limitations of, 100
of normal swallowing, 87f
of pancreatic cancer, 99, 99f
of pancreaticobiliary tract, 97–99, 98f–99f
probes for, 95–96, 96f, 96t
of scleroderma, 91f, 91–92
for swallowing studies, 92–94
Radiation, staging of esophageal carcinoma after, 133–135, 134f–135f
Radiation therapy, and esophageal fibrous wall thickening, 149
for rectal cancer, endoscopic ultrasonography after, 285–286
Real-time imaging, 9, 9f
Real-time transabdominal ultrasonography, in portal hypertension, 222
Rectal cancer, endoscopic ultrasonography in, after radiation therapy, 285–286
appearance of malignancy in, 282
for follow-up, 286
future advances in, 287
instrumentation for, 280–281, 281t
technique of, 281
incidence of, 279

Rectal cancer (*cont.*)
prognosis in, 279–280
staging of
Dukes, 282t
endoscopic ultrasonography in
accuracy of, 282, 284t
interobserver agreement in, 284–285
limitations of, 282, 284t
and treatment planning, 286, 287t
*vs.* other imaging modalities, 285, 285t
TNM, 119–120, 120f, 120t, 248f, 283
surgical resection of, 279
Rectum, adenoma of, endoscopic ultrasonography of, 286
endoscopic ultrasonography of
indications for, 273–276, 274f–276f
normal anatomy in, 272, 273f, 281
technique of, 271–272, 272f
linear array endosonography of, 73f
subepithelial lesions of, 163
wall of, endosonography of, 107
Reflection, of sound waves, 4f–5f, 4–5
Reflection coefficient, in endosonography, of gut wall, 104
Refraction artifacts, 16, 17f
Resolution, of endoluminal transducers, 68, 68f
Resonant frequency, 7
Retrograde cholangiography, linear array endoluminal, 78f
Retroperitoneum, endoscopic ultrasonography of, 229–233
normal anatomy in, 230–231, 231f–232f
in pancreatic disease, 232–233
technique of, 229–230
Reverberation artifacts, 13–14, 14f
Ring-down artifacts, 14, 15f
Rugal folds, enlarged, 176–177, 182

## S

Scattering, in endosonography, of gut wall, 104
of ultrasound beam, 5–6, 6f
Scleroderma, radial endoluminal ultrasonography of, 91f, 91–92
Sclerotherapy, monitoring of, 208–209
Section-thickness artifacts, 16
Sector scanning endosonography, instruments for, 19
Seminal vesicles, anatomy of, 273f
Shadowing artifacts, 7f, 14–15, 15f
Sheep esophagus, radial endosonography of, 83f, 83–84
Sigmoid colon, leiomyoma in, linear array endosonography of, 74f
SMA. *See* Superior mesenteric artery (SMA)
Small-aperture transducer(s), physical principles of, 67–68, 68f
Smooth muscle tumors, malignant, 160, 162, 163f
Sonoprobe, Fujinon, 77
Sound waves, 3–6, 4f–6f
absorption of, by tissue, 6–7
as energy, 6–7, 7f
frequency of, 3
length of, 4, 4f
reflection of, 4f–5f, 4–5
velocity of, 3–4
Spatial resolution, 12, 12f–13f
Spindle cell tumors, 164f
Spleen, linear array endosonography of, 56, 57f
Splenic artery, endosonography of, 112–113, 113f
enlarged, 162f
Splenic vein, endosonography of, 112–113, 113f
in portal hypertension, 205, 207f, 214, 217f
thrombosis of, Doppler imaging of, with Pentax/Hitachi FG-32UA linear array echoendoscope, 31f
Squamous cell carcinoma, esophageal, linear array endoluminal ultrasonography of, 76f
Stomach. *See also* entries under Gastric
anatomic divisions of, 112, 112f
cysts of, 160, 161f
endosonography of, 112f–114f, 112t, 112–114
leiomyoma of, 154f, 156t, 156–157, 157t, 168f
linear array endoluminal ultrasonography of, 73f
lipoma of, 158, 158f
fine-needle aspiration biopsy of, with endoscopic ultrasonography, 171f
lymphoma of, 175–176. *See also* Lymphoma, gastric
neuroendocrine tumors of, 266f
subepithelial lesions of, 155t, 160f
varices of, 159, 159f, 163f
Stomach wall, endosonography of, 106–107
Strictures, esophageal, high-grade, with carcinoma, 133
linear array endoluminal ultrasonography of, 71f, 74f
Subcarinal region, linear array echoendoscopy of, 49f
Subclavian artery, linear array echoendoscopy of, 49f
Subepithelial hemorrhage, in portal hypertension, 223f
Subepithelial lesions, 153–164
diagnosis of
comparison of imaging modalities in, 156
contrast studies in, 153, 154f
endoscopic ultrasonography in, 154–155, 155t–156t
and prediction of histologic layer, 156t
fine-needle aspiration biopsy of, 168–169
gastric, 155t, 160f
guillotine needle biopsy of, 170f–172f, 170–171
histologic typing of, 163–164, 164f
malignant *vs.* benign, 160, 162–163, 164f
rectal, 163
Superior mesenteric artery (SMA), linear array echoendoscopy of, 50f, 55f
Swallowing studies, radial endoluminal ultrasonography for, 87f, 92–94

## T

TNM staging system, 115–120
for carcinoma in ampulla of Vater, 119, 119t
for colorectal cancer, 119–120, 120f, 120t
for esophageal carcinoma, 116t–117t, 116–117, 139, 140f–141f
pretreatment, 131–132
for gastric carcinoma, 118, 118t
for lymph node metastasis, 117–118
for pancreatic cancer, 245–246, 246t
for rectal cancer, 282, 283t
Transabdominal linear array echoendoscopy, 50–59, 51f–57f

Transabdominal ultrasonography, of pancreas, 235–236
  real-time, in portal hypertension, 222
Transcutaneous ultrasonography (TUS), with Pentax/Hitachi FG-32UA linear array echoendoscope, 38–39, 39f–40f
Transducers, 9f, 9–10
  components of, 7–8, 8f
  for endosonography, of gut wall, 106
  physical principles of, 4
  for radial endoluminal ultrasonography, 82f, 82–83
  small-aperture, physical principles of, 67–68, 68f
Treatment planning, in esophageal carcinoma, 139–141
  in gastric cancer, 198
  in pancreatic cancer, 249
  in rectal cancer, 286, 287t
Trolley-based EU-M20 radial scanning ultrasound console, 20f
Tumor staging, history of, 115–116
  with Pentax/Hitachi FG-32UA linear array echoendoscope, 33f–34f, 33–34
  TNM system for, 115–120. *See also* TNM staging system
TUS. *See* Transcutaneous ultrasonography (TUS)

**U**

Ulcerative esophagitis, radial endosonography of, 92, 92f
Ulcers, gastric, differential diagnosis of, 196–197
Ultrasonography, Doppler. *See* Doppler ultrasonography
  gel for, 5
  image production in, 7–11, 8f–12f
  physical principles of, 3–7, 4f–7f
  real-time imaging in, 9, 9f
  waves in, 3–6, 4f–6f
Ultrasound beam, scattering of, 5–6, 6f
Ultrasound units, controls on, 10f–12f, 10–11

**V**

Varices, endoscopic ultrasonography of, 158–159, 163f
  esophageal
    grading of, 217, 219f–220f, 220t
    in portal hypertension, 204, 204f, 207, 216–218, 218t, 219f
    treatment of, monitoring of, 208–209
  gastric, 159, 159f, 163f
    in portal hypertension, 205, 205f, 214, 215f, 218–219, 221f–222f, 222t
  radial endosonography of, 88–91, 89f–90f
Velocity, of sound waves, 3–4
Vena cava, inferior, color flow endosonography of, 62f
Vilmann needle, 60, 63f–64f

**W**

Wall thickness, measurement of, 125–126, 126f
Water, for endosonography, of gut wall, 105
  for linear array endosonography, 71–73, 73f
Water-filled balloon, examination of esophagus with, 109
  for recurrence of cancer, 148–149
Water instillation method, for use with the GF-UM2O radial scanning echoendoscope, 25
Water pump, for use with the GF-UM20 radial scanning echoendoscope, 24–25

ISBN 0-7216-7989-7